Anatomy
and Physiology
for Midwives

SECOND EDITION

For Elsevier:
Commissioning Editor: Mary Seager
Development Editor: Rebecca Nelemans
Project Manager: Morven Dean
Designer: Sarah Russell

Anatomy and Physiology for Midwives

By

Jane Coad BSc PhD PGCEA

Senior Lecturer in Human Nutrition, Massey University, New Zealand

with

Melvyn Dunstall BSc MSc PGCEA RM RGN

Lecturer/Practitioner in Midwifery, Frimley Park Hospital; Midwifery Visitor for NMC

Foreword by

Rona McCandlish RGN RMN RM Ba (Hons) MSc (Epid)

Wellcome Trust Training Fellow in Clinical Epidemiology National Perinatal Epidemiology Unit, University of Oxford, Oxford, UK

Second Edition

ELSEVIER
CHURCHILL
LIVINGSTONE

Edinburgh London New York Oxford Philadelphia St Louis Sydney Toronto 2005

CHURCHILL LIVINGSTONE

ELSEVIER

An imprint of Elsevier Limited

First published 2001
 Reprinted 2002
Second edition 2005
 Reprinted 2006, 2007, 2008

ISBN: 978-0-443-10130-4

British Library Cataloguing in Publication Data
A catalogue record for this book is available from the British Library

Library of Congress Cataloging in Publication Data
A catalog record for this book is available from the Library of Congress

Notice
Knowledge and best practice in this field are constantly changing. As new research and experience broaden our knowledge, changes in practice, treatment and drug therapy may become necessary or appropriate. Readers are advised to check the most current information provided (i) on procedures featured or (ii) by the manufacturer of each product to be administered, to verify the recommended dose or formula, the method and duration of administration, and contraindications. It is the responsibility of the practitioner, relying on their own experience and knowledge of the patient, to make diagnoses, to determine dosages and the best treatment for each individual patient, and to take all appropriate safety precautions. To the fullest extent of the law, neither the Publisher nor the Editors/Authors assumes any liability for any injury and/or damage to persons or property arising out or related to any use of the material contained in this book. It is the responsibility of the treating practitioner, relying on independent expertise and knowledge of the patient, to determine the best treatment and method of application for the patient.

The Publisher

ELSEVIER your source for books, journals and multimedia in the health sciences
www.elsevierhealth.com

Working together to grow
libraries in developing countries

www.elsevier.com | www.bookaid.org | www.sabre.org

ELSEVIER   BOOK AID International   Sabre Foundation

Printed in *Great Britain*

08 09 10 10 9 8 7 6 5 4

The Publisher's policy is to use **paper manufactured from sustainable forests**

Contents

Foreword

In the early 1980s I began my career as a student midwife. At that time there was a comfortable and pervasive notion in midwifery (and nursing) that there were essential 'facts' that you could learn once, and never, ever have to reconsider. Human anatomy and physiology were fertile areas for one-off rote learning of 'facts'. As student midwives we were expected to achieve a basic level of knowledge of these topics by the time we qualified. We spent the minimum time possible to ensure that, for example, we could list the structures of the female pelvic floor, reproduce a diagram of the heart indicating blood circulation to the lungs, and describe the components of a cell. Dynamic learning this was not! The idea that we might apply our understanding to enable us to discuss the physical changes that a woman would experience during pregnancy, birth and in the post-natal period did not feature in our learning objectives. Using our basic knowledge in the real world of work was not something that impinged on us much and, therefore, anatomy and physiology were given a bizarrely abstract place as we honed our skills as midwives.

Since then, substantial developments have occurred in national maternity care policy, education and practice in the UK. In the policy arena Changing Childbirth (DoH 1993) and the National Service Framework for Children, Young People and Maternity Care (DH 2004) have placed choices and needs of women and their families at the centre of care and as the factors that should determine the content of services. Learning and practising midwifery has also undergone enormous changes including movement of pre- and post-registration education into the university sector, implementation of Post Registration Education and Practice (PREP) (NMC 2004) and the modernisation of registration systems at the Nursing and Midwifery Council (NMC). Contemporary midwifery students now enter midwifery knowing that their knowledge and competence will develop and change over the whole of their lives as midwife practitioners. Although registration is an important landmark for every midwife, it signals only that at that point she has achieved the learning and competence

required – to maintain registration will mean a life-long journey of learning.

In the environment of evolving and challenging midwifery practice, Jane Coad and Melvyn Dunstall have again taken what is useful and meaningful to practice as the basis of their approach to learning and teaching anatomy and physiology. The case study examples given at the beginning of chapters provide authentic keys to open up thinking about how best to integrate and apply knowledge and understanding in practice. There is no doubt that the anatomy and physiology explored in this book is based on best current evidence and understanding. The authors also acknowledge that understanding and knowledge change and develop. There are areas where this can be more clearly anticipated, for example, in genetic screening and artificial reproductive technologies, but the possibility that new evidence will emerge in future, even about issues that appear immutable should remain.

Delivery of the highest quality and relevant midwifery care will continue to require practitioners who can communicate effectively and share information with women, their families and with their colleagues, acknowledge the limits of their understanding and competence, respect the decisions and choices that women make, and seek to find the best evidence and information to inform their practice. Midwives, whether students or registered practitioners, will use the immense depth of knowledge here to fuel their journey of life-long learning and curiosity about anatomy and physiology to meet the exhilarating demands of being 'with woman'.

DOH (1993) Changing Childbirth: The report of the expert maternity group Vol 1 HMSO London, England.

DH (2004), National Service Framework for Children, Young People and Maternity Services. *www.doh.gov.uk/nsf* <http://www.doh.gov.uk/nsf>

NMC (2005) The PREP Handbook *http://www.nmc-uk.org/nmc/main/publications/thePREPhandbook2.pdf*

Rona McCandlish, 2005

Preface

Many of the most magical aspects of physiology are associated with reproduction, from before conception, through fetal development and maternal responses to the growing fetus, to the signalling and progression of labour, continued development of the neonate and the mother's subsequent return to fertility. Reproductive physiology is also a fast-moving field as recent advances in fertility treatment, postnatal care of premature infants and the implications of HIV make evident.

Midwives are expected to understand in depth the science underpinning midwifery practice but have often had little background in this exciting field. Midwives also often find themselves to be bombarded with questions from interested and fascinated parents. This book aims to support students and practising midwives wanting more detailed scientific knowledge that can be applied within the practice setting.

The book provides a thorough review of anatomy and physiology applicable to midwifery from first principles through to current research. It acknowledges the importance of the research basis and aims to integrate theory and practice.

The chapters are organized so learning objectives lead into the body of the chapter. Case studies provide the reader with the opportunity to reflect on the implications for practice. Wherever possible, information is provided as illustrations. At the end of each chapter, key points are provided and the applications of the scientific content to practice are summarized. Each chapter is comprehensively referenced and has a list of annotated recommendations for further reading.

Chapter 1 begins by introducing the reader to the basic unit of structure, the cell, and describes the relationship between cellular structure and function. It provides an introduction to the major tissue types and physiological systems found within the body and reviews the principles of regulation and maintenance of homeostatic systems.

Chapter 2 focuses on the reproductive and urinary systems of the human. The basic anatomy and physiology of the urinary system are explored in the first part of this chapter. The female reproductive tract and the organs associated with it are then described, relating both their structure and function specifically to childbirth. The last part of this chapter focuses on the male reproductive organs and the process of spermatogenesis.

Chapter 3 introduces the principles of endocrinology, laying the foundation for the understanding of changes that occur in pregnancy. It describes the different types of hormones, how and where they are produced, and their modes of action.

Chapter 4 covers the endocrine control and regulation of reproductive cycles. Ovarian function and follicular development lead on to gamete formation within the female and consideration is given as to why this is so dramatically different to spermatogenesis within the male. One of the essential roles of reproductive cycles is that the coordination of oogenesis and the cyclical changes within the endometrium occur to optimize fertilization and implantation. Thus the menstrual cycle is described in depth in this chapter. Some of the hormonal causes of infertility are discussed as is the endocrine manipulation to achieve contraception. The chapter concludes with a brief description of the physiological changes at puberty and menopause.

Chapter 5 integrates the concepts introduced in the first four chapters by focusing on how sexual differentiation is achieved and the biological basis for the differences in reproductive physiology and behaviour in women and men. This chapter leads on to the next two chapters. Chapter 6 describes how sexual bimorphism facilitates fertilization, very early development and implantation of the zygote and the maternal physiological responses that allow successful fertilization and implantation. The principles and techniques used in artifical fertilization are briefly described. Chapter 7 introduces the science of genetics, highlighting an essential component of the human reproductive strategy: that of how genetic mixing and thus variation within the species is achieved. An introduction to the aetiology and types of genetic disease and how these may be detected within the clinical situation are discussed. The basic concepts of genetic testing and screening are also included.

Chapter 8 presents the development and function of the placenta and its interaction with maternal physiology. It also discusses some of the causes and effects of placental pathology. Following this, Chapter 9 provides a comprehensive overview of the development of the embryo and its physiological systems. The factors that promote and influence fetal growth are also discussed in this chapter.

Chapter 10 brings the reader back to maternal physiology by introducing and giving an overview of immunological issues and principles related to pregnancy. The maternal acceptance of the fetus and its implications are discussed, as are the effects of pregnancy upon the maternal immune system. A section is included on the interaction of the maternal and fetal immune systems, using some clinical conditions as examples of these interactions. The neonate's vulnerability to infection is described in relation to midwifery care together with the principles of immunization. Finally, the specific effects of the human immunodeficiency virus (HIV) in pregnancy are considered.

One of the most striking aspects of reproductive physiology is the physiological changes that occur in the pregnant female. Chapter 11 explores why these changes occur and how they are orchestrated in order to facilitate an optimal outcome of pregnancy. These changes are related to how the woman experiences pregnancy and the signs, symptoms and discomforts she might encounter. Following on from this, Chapter 12 provides a brief overview of nutrition and nutritional requirements in pregnancy. This lays the basis for exploring how maternal nutrition and health can influence pregnancy outcomes not only for the mother but also for the fetus, both in utero and potentially throughout life.

Chapter 13 specifically explores the physiology of parturition and how the maternal physiology changes to facilitate this. Current theories and evidence relating to the timing and initiation of labour in humans are discussed. An overview is provided of pain physiology related to labour and how this is affected by pain-relieving interventions. This chapter includes a section that explores the effects of labour upon the fetal physiology.

Following birth, the physiological changes that occur during pregnancy are dramatically and efficiently reversed and so the puerperium is the subject of Chapter 14. Alongside the maternal postnatal changes, the neonate has to quickly adapt to extrauterine life and so Chapter 15 focuses on the transition to neonatal life, including how these changes are assessed.

The final chapter, Chapter 16, highlights the physiology of lactation and how this meets the unique requirements of the neonate not only from a nutritional perspective but from an immunological basis and a developmental basis as well. It is essential that midwives understand the physiological aspects of lactation in order to promote breastfeeding, as the evidence is overwhelming that successful breastfeeding can positively influence the health and well-being of the infant for the rest of its life.

The demand for this book came primarily from our students, including pre-registration students, midwives returning to practice and those following post-registration study. Enthusiastic questions, demands for explanation and an evident relish for understanding the theory related to practice stimulated the birth and development of the book. We hope that readers will continue to enquire about and enjoy this exciting field.

Jane Coad
Melvyn Dunstall
Palmerston North and Frimley 2004

Acknowledgements

Above all, we would like to thank our patient families and friends who again provided us with the encouragement and support to complete the second edition of this book. Also all our colleagues at Massey University in New Zealand, Frimley Park Hospital NHS Trust and the European Institute of Health and Medical Sciences at the University of Surrey for their continued help, support and guidance in the development of the second edition. Our midwifery and physiology students and other readers of the book have continued to ask questions and demand answers and their views and opinions have shaped the development of the second edition and so we continue to be indebted to them all. Within the clinical situation there is a now an even greater need for evidence-based practice and students and practitioners demand a knowledge base that will support this. Finally, we continue to owe much to the production team at Elsevier, especially Mary Seager, Rebecca Nelemans and Catharine Steers. We would like to thank them all for their help, guidance and continuing patience in supporting us complete the second edition.

List of abbreviations

ABP	androgen-binding protein
ACTH	adrenocorticotrophic hormone (corticotrophin)
ADH	antidiuretic hormone
AFP	alpha-fetoprotein
AIDS	acquired immune deficiency (immunodeficiency) syndrome
ANP	atrial natriuretic peptide
APC	antigen-presenting cell
ATP	adenosine triphosphate
AV	arteriovenous
AVN	atrioventricular node
BAT	brown adipose tissue
BMI	body mass index
BPD	biparietal diameter
CAH	congenital adrenal hyperplasia
CAM	calcium-binding protein (calmodulin)
cAMP	cyclic adenosine monophosphate
CAP	contraction-associated protein
CBP	corticosteroid-binding protein
CCK	cholecystokinin
CCT	controlled cord traction
CD	cluster of differentiation
CDH	congenital dislocation of the hips
cGMP	cyclic guanosine monophosphate
CMV	cytomegalovirus
CNS	central nervous system
CoA	coenzyme A
COC	combined oral contraceptive
COX	cyclo-oxygenase
CRH	corticotrophin-releasing hormone
CRH-BP	corticotrophin-releasing hormone-binding protein
CRL	crown–rump length
CSF	cytostatic factor
CVS	chorionic villus sampling
D&C	dilatation and curettage
DHA	docosahexaenoic acid
DHEAS	dehydroepiandrosterone sulphate
5α-DHT	5α-dihydrotestosterone
DIC	disseminated intravascular coagulation
DNA	deoxyribonucleic acid
DVT	deep vein thrombosis
E$_1$	oestrone
E$_2$	oestradiol-17β
E$_3$	oestriol

ECG	electrocardiogram
ED	erectile dysfunction
ED-PAF	embryo-derived platelet-activating factor
EDRF	endothelium-derived relaxing factor
EGF	epidermal growth factor
ER	endoplasmic reticulum
ERPC	evacuation of retained products of conception
FBM	fetal breathing movement
FHR	fetal heart rate
FHV	fetal heart variability
FIL	feedback inhibitor of lactation
FISH	fluorescent in situ hybridization
FPU	fetal–placental unit
FSH	follicle-stimulating hormone
GALT	gut-associated lymphoid tissue
GFR	glomerular filtration rate
GH	growth hormone
GI	glycaemic index
GIFT	gamete intrafallopian transfer
GIP	gastric inhibitory peptide
GL	greatest length
GLUT	glucose-transport protein
GM-CSF	granulocyte–macrophage colony-stimulating factor
GnRH	gonadotrophin-releasing hormone
GP	general practitioner
Hb	haemoglobin
hCG	human chorionic gonadotrophin
HDL	high-density lipoprotein
HDNB	haemorrhagic disease of the newborn
HELLP	haemolysis, elevated liver enzymes and low platelet counts
HFEA	Human Fertilisation & Embryology Authority
HIV	human immunodeficiency virus
HLA	human leukocyte antigen
hMG	human menopausal gonadotrophin
HPA	hypothalamic–pituitary–adrenal
hPL	human placental lactogen
HPV	human papillomavirus
HRT	hormone replacement therapy
ICSI	intracytoplasmic sperm injection
IDDM	insulin-dependent diabetes mellitus
Ig	immunoglobulin

IGF	insulin-like growth factor
IGF-BP	insulin-like growth factor binding protein
IL	interleukin
IU/i.u.	international units
IUGR	intrauterine growth retardation
IVF	in vitro fertilization
kDa	kilodalton
LBW	low birth weight
LC-PUFA	long-chain polyunsaturated fatty acid
LDL	low-density lipoprotein
LH	luteinizing hormone
LHRH	luteinizing hormone releasing hormone
LIF	leukaemia-inhibitory factor
LSCS	lower-segment caesarean section
LUS	lower uterine segment
MCV	mean blood cell volume
MESA	microepidermal sperm aspiration
MHC	major histocompatibility complex
MIS	Müllerian-inhibiting substance (also known as Müllerian-inhibiting hormone, MIH)
MLCK	myosin light-chain kinase
mRNA	messenger ribonucleic acid
MRSA	methicillin-resistant *Staphylococcus aureus*
MSH	melanocyte-stimulating hormone
MSU	midstream specimen of urine
mtDNA	mitochondrial DNA
NIDDM	non-insulin-dependent diabetes mellitus
NK	natural killer
NO	nitric oxide
NPN	non-protein nitrogen
NPU	net protein utilization
NPY	neuropeptide Y
NSAID	non-steroidal anti-inflammatory drug
NSP	non-starch polysaccharide
NST	non-shivering thermogenesis
NT	nuchal translucency
NTD	neural tube defect
NVP	nausea and vomiting in pregnancy
PE	pulmonary embolism
PCOS	polycystic ovary syndrome
PDE	phosphodiesterase
PDZ	partial zona dissection
PESA	percutaneous epididymal sperm aspiration
PGD	preimplantation genetic diagnosis
PGH	placental growth hormone
PGDH	prostaglandin dehydrogenase

Pi	inorganic phosphate
PID	pelvic inflammatory disease
PKU	phenylketonuria
PLA$_2$	phospholipase A$_2$
PLC	phospholipase C
PMDD	premenstrual dysphoric disorder
PMS	premenstrual syndrome
PPH	postpartum haemorrhage
PRL	prolactin
PROM	premature rupture of the membranes
PUFA	polyunsaturated fatty acid
RAS	renin–angiotensin system
RDI	recommended daily intake
RDS	respiratory distress syndrome
REM	rapid eye movement
RER	rough endoplasmic reticulum
RNA	ribonucleic acid
rRNA	ribosomal ribonucleic acid
RSA	recurrent spontaneous abortion
SAN	sinoatrial node
SER	smooth endoplasmic reticulum
SGA	small for gestational age
sIg	surface immunoglobulin
SLE	systemic lupus erythematosus
SNP	single nucleotide polymorphism
SRY	sex determining region on the Y chromosome
STD	sexual transmitted disease
SUZI	subzonal sperm injection
T$_3$	tri-iodothyronine
T$_4$	thyroxine
TB	tuberculosis
TBG	thyroid-binding globulin
TENS	transcutaneous electrical nerve stimulation
Th cells	helper T cells
TBP	thyroid-binding protein
TGF	transforming growth factor
TNF	tumour necrosis factor
tRNA	transfer ribonucleic acid
TSH	thyroid-stimulating hormone
TxA$_2$	thromboxane A$_2$
U-LGL	uterine large granular leukocytes
UVR	ultraviolet radiation
UTI	urinary tract infection
VIP	vasoactive intestinal peptide
VLDL	very-low-density lipoprotein
WHI	Women's Health Initiative (studies on HRT)
ZIFT	zygote intrafallopian transfer
ZP	zona pellucida

Introduction to physiology

Introduction

Physiology explores how living organisms are able to function in order to survive and reproduce. This book explores reproductive function and how it is achieved within human beings. This chapter aims to provide an illustrated introduction to, and an overview of, some of the basic physiological concepts referred to and developed in subsequent chapters with specific references to reproduction. (If more detail is required, readers are recommended to look at the list of further reading at the end of the chapter.)

Chapter case study

Zara is a 29-year-old primapara who presents herself at the midwife's clinic, which is held at her GP's surgery, giving a history of a positive pregnancy test. Zara has regularly attended the Well-Woman's Clinic and appears to be well. What information would be available to the midwife in Zara's medical records that would be useful to the midwife in her ongoing assessment of Zara's pregnancy? How could this information be used by the midwife to inform Zara of the physiological changes that have started to occur in her body?

to perform specific functions and processes that contribute to the well-being of the organism as a whole. Differentiated cells form tissues, which combine with other tissues to form organs, which are linked together in physiological systems (Fig. 1.1). However, although cells can be highly specialized, they all share common features of the single cellular organisms from which we evolved. A typical human cell is about 10 μm in diameter. The largest human cell is the oocyte (see Ch. 6); it can just be seen with the naked eye. The follicular cells surrounding the oocyte have a more typical human cell size. The sperm cell is one of the smallest human cells. Smaller cells and organelles can be visualized by light and electron microscopy.

The cell

The cell is the fundamental unit of structure and function within all living organisms. The evolution of multicellular organisms has led to the differentiation of cells, which means that different cells have evolved

Cell structure

Most cells contain cytoplasm and are bound by a plasma membrane. Within them are various structures, called organelles (see Table 1.1), and a specialized part

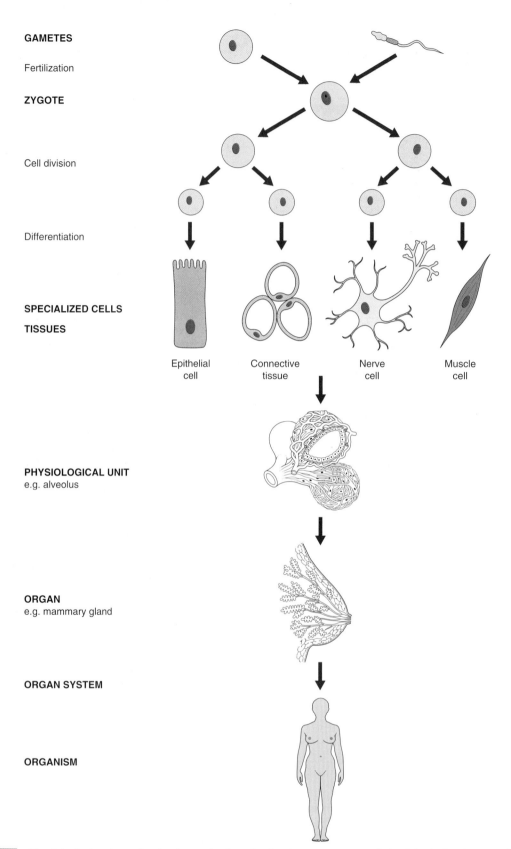

GAMETES

Fertilization

ZYGOTE

Cell division

Differentiation

SPECIALIZED CELLS

TISSUES

Epithelial cell

Connective tissue

Nerve cell

Muscle cell

PHYSIOLOGICAL UNIT
e.g. alveolus

ORGAN
e.g. mammary gland

ORGAN SYSTEM

ORGANISM

Fig. 1.1 *Physiological systems: levels of organization of cells, tissues, organs and physiological systems, using breast tissue as an example.*

Table 1.1   *Cell components*

Cell component	Structure	Function
Cell membrane	The cell membrane is composed of a phospholipid bilayer embedded with various protein structures such as hormone receptors, ion channels and antigen markers	The membrane acts as a differential permeable membrane between the cell and its immediate environment
The nucleus	The nucleus is bound by a membrane, similar to the plasma membrane of the cell; this contains openings referred to as nuclear pores, which allow the movement of substances in and out of the nucleus	The nucleus contains deoxyribonucleic acid (DNA), the genetic instruction for the organism. Most of the time, the DNA is organized as chromatin threads; these condense into chromosomes prior to cell division. The nucleus stores and replicates DNA, which is expressed to synthesize proteins via a second type of nucleic acid, ribonucleic acid (RNA). These proteins determine the structure and function of the cell
Endoplasmic reticulum	This is a system of membranes, enclosing a space, which is continuous with the nuclear membrane Endoplasmic reticulum (ER) exists as rough (granular) endoplasmic reticulum (RER) and smooth (agranular) endoplasmic reticulum (SER)	RER appears rough because of the attached ribosomes. RER is involved in protein packaging. SER is involved in lipid and steroid synthesis and the regulation of intracellular calcium levels
Mitochondria	Spherical or elongated rod-like structures surrounded by a folded inner membrane and a smooth outer membrane. There are more mitochondria in cells that are metabolically active and have a high energy requirement	Chemical processes involved in the formation of adenosine triphosphate (ATP). The cristae (inner membrane folds) are the site of oxidative phosphorylation and the electron transfer chain of aerobic respiration. Krebs (tricarboxylic acid or TCA) cycle and the oxidation of fatty acids take place within the matrix. Mitochondria contain mitochondrial DNA, which is maternally inherited and contains the genes for mitochondrial proteins
Golgi apparatus (complex)	A series of flattened curved membranous sacs	Modifies proteins from the RER and sorts them into secretory vesicles
Lysosomes	Spherical or oval organelles enclosed by a single membrane	Enclose acidic fluid containing digestive enzymes which act as a 'cellular stomach' breaking down cellular debris
Peroxisomes	Similar structure to lysosomes	Destroy reactive oxygen species and protect cell
Cytoskeleton	Filamentous network	Involved in maintaining cell shape and motility

of the cell, called the nucleus (Fig. 1.2). The fluid surrounding the organelles is called cytosol.

Cells and tissues

Although about 200 types of cells with different structures can be identified within the body, cells can be grouped together in functional categories (Table 1.2).

The study of the physical characteristics of cells is called histology (see Box 1.1). There are four types of tissue: epithelial tissue, muscle, connective tissue and neural tissue.

Epithelial tissue

Epithelial cells line the internal and external surfaces of the body organs (Fig. 1.3), forming the outer layer

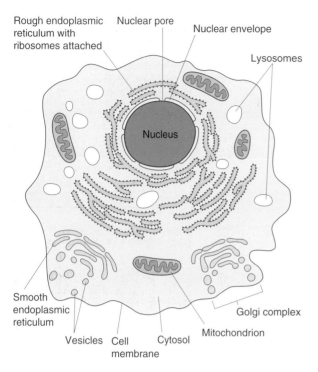

Rough endoplasmic reticulum with ribosomes attached
Nuclear pore
Nuclear envelope
Lysosomes
Nucleus
Smooth endoplasmic reticulum
Vesicles
Cell membrane
Cytosol
Mitochondrion
Golgi complex

Fig. 1.2   *A typical cell.*

of skin, the mucous membranes, the lining of the lungs, gut, reproductive and urinary tracts, and also the endocrine and exocrine glands. Epithelial cells are relatively undifferentiated and tend to undergo frequent mitotic divisions (see Ch. 7). This is because they are often exposed to wear and tear and so replacement epithelial cells are generated from a basal layer where cell division takes place. Epithelial cells form a barrier, which allows secretion and absorption of substances from one compartment to another. The skin is a specialized epithelial layer. The basal layer produces cells that are enriched with the protein keratin. The outer layers of skin cells are dead and so lack cytoplasm; it is these keratinized dead cells that provide the barrier function of the skin. Epithelial cells are classified by shape (cuboidal or columnar) and number of layers. If there is a single layer of cells, the epithelium is described as simple; if there is more than one layer of cells (such as skin), it is stratified. Pseudostratified cells are a single layer of cells that appear to consist of more than one layer.

Muscle tissue

Muscle cells contain contractile elements so the cells can generate the mechanical force required for movement of the body or substances within the body (Fig. 1.4). Skeletal muscle may be attached to bones and controls movement of the skeleton. Skeletal muscle can also be attached to the skin, for instance the muscles of the face involved with expression. Contraction of skeletal

Table 1.2   *Functional classification of cells*

Cell group	Epithelial cells	Support cells	Contractile cells	Nerve cells	Germ cells	Blood cells	Immune cells	Hormone-secreting cells
Example	Lining gut and blood vessels Covering skin	Fibrous support tissue, cartilage, bone	Muscle	Brain	Spermatozoa Ova	Circulating 1. red cells 2. white cells 3. platelets	Lymphoid tissues, nodes and spleen	Islets, thyroid adrenal
Function	Barrier; absorption; secretion	Organize and maintain body structure	Movement	Direct cell communication	Reproduction	1. Oxygen transport 2. Defence	Defence	Indirect cell communication
Special features	Tightly bound together by cell junctions	Produce and interact with extracellular matrix material	Contractile proteins	Release chemical messengers directly on to other cells	Haploid (i.e. half-normal chromosome number)	1. Proteins bind oxygen 2. Proteins destroy bacteria 3. Blood clotting	Recognize and destroy foreign material	Secrete chemical messengers into blood

Box 1.1

Histology

The study of tissue structure is described as histology. The functions of tissues are reflected in the microscopic structure of the cells of which the tissue is composed. For example, cells that are metabolically active contain many mitochondria, whereas cells that produce hormones or enzymes, for instance, will contain a large proportion of ER. Specific tissues and cellular structures are often identified by the application of various chemicals that stain particular tissues. Histology is important in diagnosing cancer, as the cancerous tissue often has histological characteristics different from those of the tissue in which the cancer has developed. Malignant cancerous tumours have highly differentiated cells, which means they often appear different to the normal tissue cells from which they arose; they often have a simpler structure and are usually prolific in their division rate. These cells are less likely to adhere to neighbouring cells as normal cells do, so they are shed into the circulatory system and carried to other parts of the body where they seed more tumours (secondary tumours or metastases). Benign tumours usually have undifferentiated cells, which may closely resemble the cells of the tissue from which they arose and tend only to grow in the one position. Although cancers in pregnancy are rare, many cancerous cells may respond to oestrogen (sometimes referred to as oestrogen-dependent); thus cancer growth during pregnancy can be quite rapid.

50 µm

Fig. 1.4 *Muscle: A skeletal muscle; B smooth muscle; C cardiac muscle. (Adapted with permission from Brooker 1998.)*

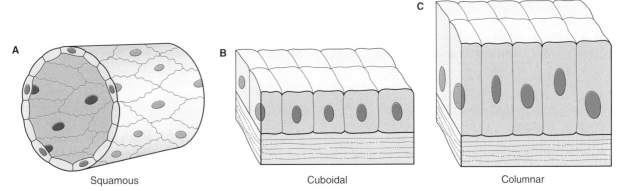

Squamous   Cuboidal   Columnar

Fig. 1.3 *Types of epithelial cell: A squamous epithelium provides a smooth lining of blood vessels (endothelium, alveoli of lung and glomeruli of kidney); B cuboidal epithelium is often found on absorptive surfaces such as in kidney tubules; C columnar epithelium is often associated with secretory and absorptive tissues and may have microvilli, as in the gut; it may also be ciliated, as in the upper airways. (Reproduced with permission from Brooker 1998.)*

muscle is usually under voluntary or conscious control. Skeletal muscle is often described as 'striated' because of the striped appearance of the sarcomeres of the muscle observed under the light microscope.

Smooth muscle is usually under involuntary control (meaning there is no conscious awareness of the control) and surrounds many of the 'tubes' in the body, maintaining the function of several body systems. Smooth muscle cells are linked by gap junctions, and muscle contraction is relatively slow. Blood pressure is maintained by the contraction of a smooth muscle layer in the walls of the blood vessels. If the smooth muscle constricts, described as 'vasoconstriction', the internal lumen of the vessel will decrease and blood pressure will increase. 'Vasodilatation' is the opposite condition: the smooth muscle relaxes and the lumen diameter increases so blood pressure falls. Organized synchronized waves of smooth muscle contraction, for instance in the gut, renal system and uterine tubes, generate peristaltic waves; these produce unidirectional movement of the contents within the lumen of the tube (Fig. 1.5).

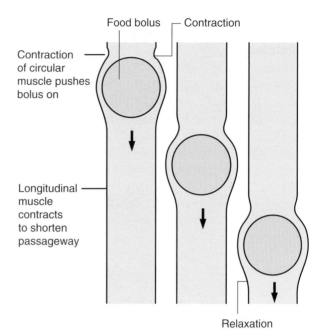

Fig. 1.5 *Peristaltic waves: peristalsis is achieved through the interaction of both longitudinal and circular smooth muscle fibres found in vessels with patent lumen. The peristaltic waves are responsible for (usually) unidirectional movement of the contents within the lumen. (Reproduced with permission from Brooker 1998.)*

Connective tissue

Connective tissue functions to connect, anchor and support body structures (Fig. 1.6). Connective tissue cells often produce an extracellular matrix composed of proteins in a ground substance of sugars, proteins and minerals. Bone is a type of connective tissue, whereas collagen is an example of an extracellular matrix. Adipose tissue is composed of specialized cells that store fat for future energy requirements and have an endocrine role. Adipose tissue also acts as an insulating layer to conserve body heat loss and so contributes to the maintenance of the homeothermic status of the organism. Fibrous tissue is an example of dense connective tissue. It is a tough tissue that forms ligaments, tendons and protective membranes.

Neural tissue

Neurons are cells that are specialized to initiate and conduct electrical signals (Fig. 1.7). Neurons require the presence of glial cells for nourishment and support. As neurons are so highly specialized, they do not usually undergo further mitotic divisions once developed. Therefore, in the fetal and early neonatal period, the number of neurons produced far exceeds the level required for normal neurological function. Neurons need regular stimulation if they are to survive and function. Throughout life millions of neurons become dysfunctional and die.

The structural organization of the body

The body's organization can be understood by considering each component organ system separately (see below). However, these systems all work together, as a whole. Together the systems provide nutrients and oxygen for the cells and the excretion of waste products (Fig. 1.8). Movement is controlled and the temperature is maintained. Survival until reproductive function is completed has allowed the species to multiply. Cells are bathed in extracellular fluid, which can be divided into the interstitial fluid surrounding the tissue cells and the plasma within the blood vessels.

Fig. 1.7 Types of neuron: A bipolar; B unipolar; C multipolar.

Fig. 1.6 Connective tissue: A adipose tissue; B fibrous tissue; C compact bone. (Reproduced with permission from Brooker 1998.)

Homeostasis

Homeostasis is the term used to describe the processes of the various physiological systems that maintain the constancy of the internal environment. Multicellular animals are able to maintain an internal stability that is essential for the optimal functioning of all body systems, whereas simple unicellular organisms tend to inhabit stable environments or have adapted to overcome fluctuations in the environment, for instance by forming spores during dry periods. Unicellular organisms rely on basic nutrients being present in the environment to allow cell growth and reproduction.

The evolution of multicellular organisms and the development of motility meant these animals were able to move within the environment to seek out the conditions that suited them best and so optimize their ability to reproduce. Mammals have developed homeostasis to a high degree. Motility, together with the homeostatic challenge of counteracting fluctuations in the external environment, places a huge energy burden upon these individuals. This increased energy requirement is above the basal metabolic rate, which is the

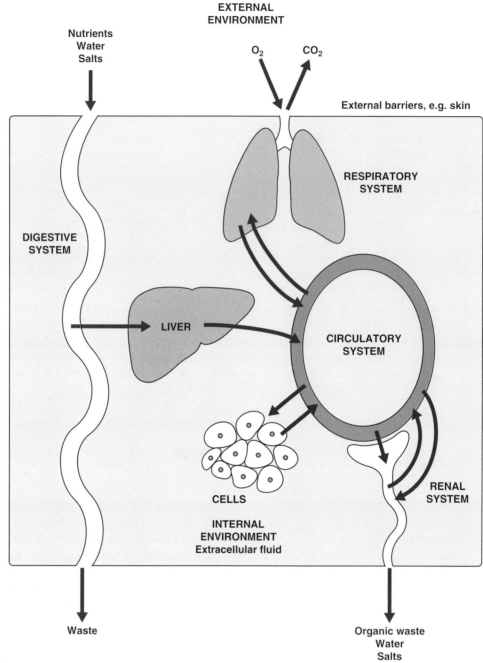

Fig. 1.8 *Organization of the body.*

rate of energy required to maintain essential functioning only.

Homeostasis can be considered to have three main components:

- chemostasis: the maintenance of electrolytes and pH balance

- haemostasis: the maintenance of an adequate circulatory system facilitating the passage of nutrients and oxygen in and waste products out of the organism

- thermostasis: the maintenance of a constant internal temperature.

Homeostasis is regulated by the nervous system, the endocrine system and behavioural factors that are dependent on conscious or subconscious action by the organism. A homeostatic control system requires monitoring a variable, detecting changes and generating responses which will restore the composition of the internal environment (Fig. 1.9). (This type of system, involving a process called negative feedback, is dealt with in more detail under Hormonal regulation in Ch. 3, p. ●●.)

Thermoregulation

Temperature regulation is one example of homeostasis (Fig. 1.10). Enzymes regulating biochemical changes, and physiological and metabolic functions, have optimal activity within a narrow temperature range. Outside this physiological temperature range, the protein structure of the enzyme begins to denature so the configuration (shape) of the enzyme distorts, which affects its functional activity. A warm-blooded (homeothermic) animal is well prepared to react quickly and efficiently to changes within the environment, unlike a cold-blooded (poikilothermic) animal, which depends upon the ambient temperature of the environment.

The nervous system

The nervous system coordinates body functions. It monitors physiological processes by processing input from the senses, integrating them and initiating responses or motor output. The nervous system is an organization of millions of neurons, or nerve cells, and glial cells, which support and regulate the composition of the nervous system. It is composed of the brain, the spinal cord (in the centre of the vertebral column) and the neurons throughout the body. The skull and the vertebral column protect the brain and the spinal cord. The brain and spinal cord form the central nervous system (CNS) and the remainder is the peripheral nervous system (Fig. 1.11). Neurons usually consist of a cell body and dendrites (extensions) and an axon or nerve fibre, which carries information from the cell body to or from the CNS. They are a variety of different sizes; some neurons have axon projections over 1 metre in length. A nerve is a collection of axons running alongside each other over the same distance. A ganglion is a collection of cell bodies of neurons within the peripheral nervous system. Ganglions are located in dorsal (back) or ventral (front) branches of the spinal cord. The spinal cord and spinal nerves are organized on a segmental basis; this corresponds to the embryonic origin of the dermatomes (see Ch. 9). Cranial nerves carry information between the brain and regions of the head. Neurons that carry information towards the brain, entering the dorsal roots of the spinal cord, are sensory or afferent neurons. Neurons carrying information from the CNS to the skeletal muscles, and leaving the spinal cord at the ventral roots, are motor or efferent neurons (Fig. 1.12). Neurons that carry information between a sensory neuron and the CNS (or between the CNS and a motor neuron) are known as interneurons.

The action potential

Neurons carry information or nerve impulses by changing the electrical charge along their axon length so the transmembrane polarity changes rapidly from negative to positive and back. This change in electrical charge is termed an 'action potential'. When the impulse reaches the axon, specific channels known as 'sodium gates' open, allowing the movement of extracellular sodium ions across the concentration gradient

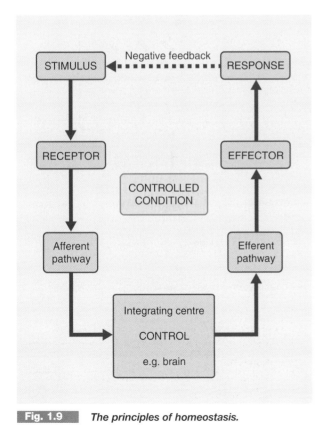

Fig. 1.9   *The principles of homeostasis.*

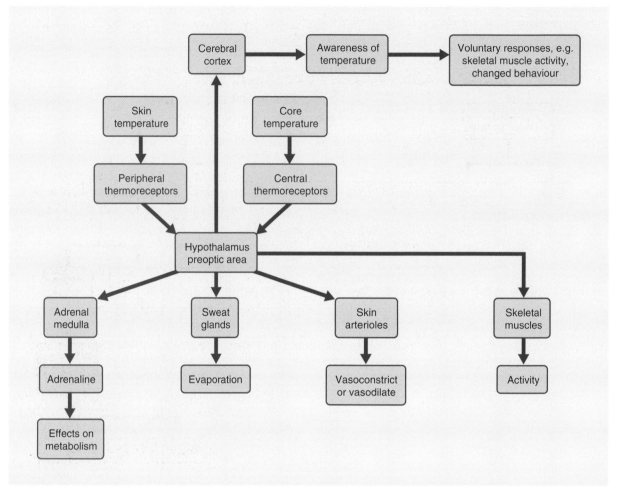

Fig. 1.10   *Temperature regulation: a homeostatic system in operation.*

into the axon. As the sodium ions carry a positive charge, the immediate local area around the sodium gate inside of the axon becomes electrically positive compared with the immediate area outside and so the membrane becomes temporarily depolarized. At the height of the action potential (about 1 ms) the sodium channels close and the membrane becomes leaky to potassium ions; these move out of the axon down the electrochemical gradient. The result is restoration of the membrane potential, described as 'repolarization'. That segment of the axon then enters a refractory period when no further action potential can be produced. However, depolarization in one small segment of the neuron leads to depolarization in the next segment; the rapid movement of the altered electrical activity is therefore propagated along the length of the neuron.

The action potential moves along the axon. The information detected at the periphery triggers activity at the neuron receptor and the action potential travels along the axon to the synapse, a junction with another neuron. There is a gap between two neurons at the synapse. Information transmission across this gap is by chemicals called neurotransmitters. These are released from the first neuron, travel across the synapse and trigger an action potential in the second neuron. The connection between a stimulating neuron and a muscle is called a neuromuscular junction. Action potentials move faster in axons of greater diameter and if the axon is insulated by a myelin sheath. Myelin sheaths surround the nerve for short lengths punctuated by the nodes of Ranvier. Action potentials in myelinated nerves are not propagated as waves but move by saltatory conduction whereby they 'hop' along the nerve in a fast and efficient manner. Multiple sclerosis is due to breakdown of the myelin sheath, limiting the normal conduction of action potentials along nerves.

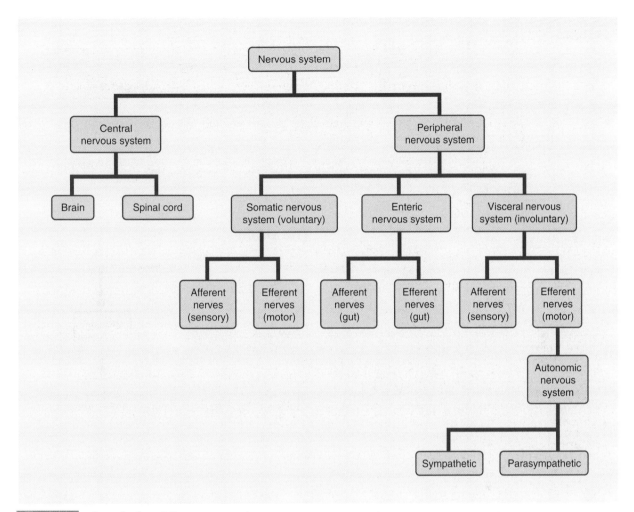

Fig. 1.11   *Organization of the nervous system.*

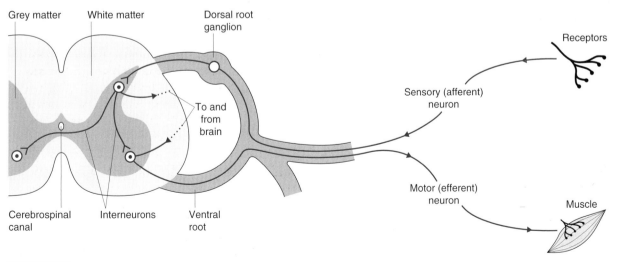

Fig. 1.12   *Afferent and efferent neurons.*

The somatic and autonomic nervous systems

The somatic nervous system controls muscles that change position. These muscles are called skeletal or voluntary muscles as they are controlled voluntarily, whereas smooth muscle and cardiac muscle are controlled involuntarily by the autonomic nervous system (ANS). The ANS controls the internal functions of the body such as circulation, respiration, digestion and metabolism.

Traditionally the ANS has been divided into the sympathetic and parasympathetic systems (Table 1.3); these two branches of the ANS are described as working in tandem, either synergistically or antagonistically. The sympathetic nervous system controls the responses and provision of energy required for stressful situations; it is often known as the fear–fight–flight system. Effects of the sympathetic system include increased heart rate and blood pressure, pupillary and bronchial dilation, increased skeletal muscle blood flow (at the expense of blood flow to other tissues), increased glycogenolysis and lipolysis to increase energy provision and other responses that facilitate fight or escape and heightened awareness to threatening situations. The sympathetic system operates in conjunction with the endocrine system facilitating the release of adrenaline, which augments the manifesting fear–fight–flight reflexes. Conversely, the parasympathetic branch of the ANS is more influential in periods of rest and inactivity and favours rest, increased digestive activity and restoration. Effects of parasympathetic nervous activity include increased blood flow to the gut and skin, stimulated salivary gland secretion and peristalsis, and slowing of the heart rate. In the ANS, two neurons carry information from the CNS to the target organ; these are described as autonomic ganglia. There is a further division of the ANS called the enteric nervous system, which affects smooth muscle and secretion in the gut.

The brain

The brain is the centre of the nervous system; it is a most complex organ and is not fully understood. The vertebrate brain develops from three anterior bulges of the neural tube (see Ch. 9), which are the brain stem, the cerebellum and the cerebrum. The brain stem is formed of the medulla oblongata (which controls autonomic functions), the pons (which relays information to and from the higher centres of the brain) and the midbrain (which integrates sensory information). The brain stem is an evolutionary older structure which regulates essential automatic and integrative functions; it is often called the 'lower brain' and is particularly important in maintaining

Table 1.3	The autonomic nervous system	
	Sympathetic division	**Parasympathetic division**
Characteristics	Preganglionic outflow originates in thoracolumbar portion of spinal cord	Preganglionic outflow originates in midbrain, hindbrain and sacral portions of spinal cord
	Chain of ganglia	Terminal ganglia near or in effector organs
	Postganglionic fibres distributed throughout body	Postganglionic fibres mainly associated with head and viscera
	Divergence of pathways so system as a whole is usually stimulated.	Little divergence so limited parts of the system are stimulated
	'Fear, fight and flight'	'Resting and digesting'
Examples of effect	Eye: dilation of pupil	Eye: constriction of pupil
	Cardiovascular system: increased heart rate and increased strength of myocardial contraction, vasoconstriction of peripheral vessels and increased blood pressure	Cardiovascular system: decreased heart rate and vasodilation of peripheral vessels and decreased blood pressure
	Lungs: dilation of bronchioles	Lungs: constriction of bronchioles
	Bladder: increased muscle tone	Bladder: increased contraction
	Uterus: contraction in pregnant woman; relaxation in non-pregnant woman	
	Penis: ejaculation	Penis: vasodilation and erection

homeostasis, coordinating movement. The cerebellum coordinates and error-checks motor activities and perceptual and cognitive factors.

The most highly evolved structure of the brain is the cerebrum. The outer layer of the brain is the grey matter of the cerebral cortex, which is divided into a left and a right hemisphere (Fig. 1.13). The fibres that connect these hemispheres are the corpus callosum, the largest white matter structure. Different regions of the cortex are associated with different functions; they can be illustrated in a figure known as the 'sensory homunculus' (Fig. 1.14). The reticular formation acts as a sensory filter and is concerned with states of waking and alertness. The hypothalamus is involved in motivation and regulation and integration of many metabolic and autonomic processes. The hypothalamus controls body temperature, hunger and thirst, and circadian cycles and links the nervous and endocrine systems. The cerebellum is mainly concerned with coordination of movement and repetitive performance of previously learned tasks.

Fig. 1.13 *The brain: an overview of some of the functional areas.*

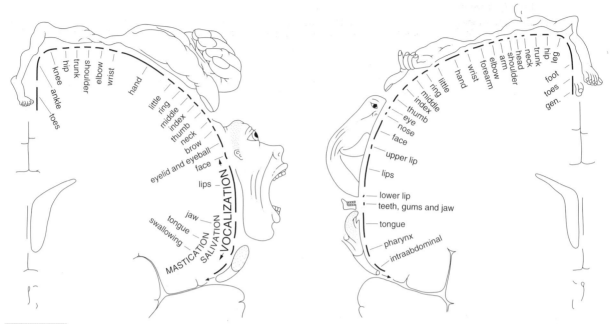

The 'homunculus': a representation of the (A) motor and (B) sensory areas of the brain illustrating the proportion of brain tissue dedicated to these areas. (Reproduced with permission from Brooker 1998.)

The digestive system

As animals grew larger they could not rely upon obtaining nutrients through diffusion and random contact with the environment; they became hunters and grazers. As they evolved they became able to feed intermittently. They could do this because they had developed the ability to digest (break down) large organic macromolecules into smaller molecules through the action of digestive enzymes. They were able to store and digest food slowly. Mechanisms for food storage, such as the deposition of fat within adipose tissue, enabled periods of food shortage to be overcome. The ability to synthesize new tissue with energy expenditure is termed anabolism. When tissue is broken down there is a reverse process termed catabolism; this usually results in the production of energy and waste products, which require excretion.

The gastrointestinal tract, or gut, is a long tube that runs from mouth to anus (Table 1.4) in which food is digested and absorbed, to extract the energy and nutrients; the remaining waste is expelled. Food enters the mouth; here it is masticated (mechanically broken down, thus increasing its surface area) and lubricated and enzymes are added before it is passed through the oesophagus to the stomach. The stomach is a bag-like swollen structure where the first major digestive processes occur. Hydrochloric acid secreted into the stomach maintains a pH of about 2; this has an important role in destroying microorganisms. There is some protein breakdown in the stomach and the food is mixed well. The mixed food, or chyme, then moves into the duodenum where most of the digestion occurs. Digestive enzymes and bicarbonate ions (which neutralize the acidic pH) are produced from the pancreatic exocrine tissue and secreted into the duodenum. Bile salt secretion is important for the digestion of fats. The small intestine is a major site of absorption and has a very large surface area provided by finger-like projections called villi (Fig. 1.15). Tiny projections or microvilli on the surface of the individual epithelial cells further increase the surface area. The net result is a surface area of about 300 square metres. The epithelial cells lining the absorptive surfaces of the gastrointestinal system have membrane-bound enzymes, for further digestion of the food molecules, and specific transport mechanisms for absorbing different molecules into the bloodstream.

Cells of the mucosa that lines the gut have a very rapid turnover; the entire cell lining is renewed every 4 or 5 days. Therefore agents that inhibit cell division such as radiation and chemotherapy drugs compromise the epithelium and total surface area. The absorbed nutrients pass from the capillaries of the

Table 1.4 *The digestive system*

Region of gastrointestinal system	Main digestive events
Mouth	■ Taste ■ Mechanical digestion (chewing, mastication) ■ Food moistened and lubricated, to facilitate passage down oesophagus ■ Starch digestion (amylase)
Oesophagus	■ Peristalsis enables transfer of food bolus to stomach ■ Buccal amylase activity continues
Stomach	■ Stores, mixes, dissolves, releases food ■ Hydrochloric acid (HCl) 　—lowers pH to 2 　—kills microbes 　—denatures proteins 　—converts pepsinogen to pepsin ■ Mucus: protects gastric lining ■ Pepsin: protein digestion
Pancreas	■ Enzyme production: digestion ■ Bicarbonate: neutralizes pH
Liver	■ Bile production
Gall bladder	■ Bile concentration and coordinated release facilitating emulsification of fats
Small intestine	■ Digestion and absorption of most nutrients
Large intestine	■ Passage of undigested matter ■ Absorption of water and vitamins ■ Provides environment for commensal symbiotic bacteria
Rectum	■ Storage of undigested matter ■ Defecation

small intestine into the hepatic portal vein to the liver. The wall of the gut is lined with smooth muscle, which undergoes synchronous contraction, generating waves of peristaltic movement propelling the food along the gut. The control of the smooth muscle is via the enteric nervous system.

The large intestine is important in the maintenance of fluid and iron balance and the absorption of vitamins. It is colonized and inhabited by bacteria, many of which synthesize vitamins, including vitamin B_{12}, vitamin K, thiamin and riboflavin, which can be absorbed across the gut wall. Motility of food through the gut is increased if there are more undigested non-starch polysaccharides (fibre) present. Some breakdown of these polysaccharides occurs by bacterial action, which can produce gas (flatus), nitrogen, carbon dioxide, hydrogen, methane and hydrogen sulphide.

Secretion and motility of the gut are controlled by nervous stimulation (Fig. 1.16). There are three phases or stages of nervous control. The cephalic phase is stimulated by the smell, taste and sight of food, which increase motility and hydrochloric acid secretion. When food reaches the stomach it causes distension, increased acidity and increased peptide formation, which stimulate the gastric phase of control. The hormone gastrin is released, which stimulates secretion of acid and affects the lower regions of the gut. The third phase of control is the intestinal phase, which is stimulated by food within the intestine. The intestinal phase causes the reflex inhibition of gastric secretion.

A transverse section through the intestinal wall:

- Two layers of smooth muscle
- Connective tissue
- Muscle layer
- Connective tissue
- Lumen
- Villus

B a villus:

- Artery
- Vein
- Lymphatic vessel

C detail of the epithelium:

- Brush border

Fig. 1.15 *Structure of the small intestinal villi: A transverse section through the intestinal wall; B a villus; C detail of the epithelium. (Reproduced with permission from Saffrey & Stewart 1997.)*

The respiratory system

Respiration is the exchange of gases between the environment and the body. Respiration is essential for the functioning of all living organisms. There are two types: aerobic and anaerobic. In aerobic respiration, organic molecules from the food are oxidized to produce energy (Fig. 1.17). Anaerobic respiration is when energy is produced in the absence of oxygen. This form of respiration is relatively inefficient compared with aerobic respiration.

Anaerobic respiration is common among single-celled organisms. Large animals, such as humans, can produce some energy anaerobically, for instance in times of acute stress and rapid muscle activity when oxygen demand exceeds oxygen provision. However, anaerobic respiration results in the rapid accumula-

tion of toxic metabolites. In simple organisms, these may simply diffuse out of the cell into the environment, but for large animals this rapid excretion cannot be achieved so anaerobic processes are self-limiting. Asphyxia is the term that describes irreversible damage of cells due to the build-up of these toxins.

Aerobic respiration is an extension of anaerobic respiration. The metabolites, produced under anaerobic processes such as glycolysis, are further broken down producing carbon dioxide, water and significantly more energy. Aerobic respiration requires the presence of oxygen and mitochondria, the sites of the enzymes involved in these biochemical pathways. Cells require a continuous source of oxygen for metabolism.

The respiratory system consists of the lungs, the branching airways, the gaseous exchange membranes,

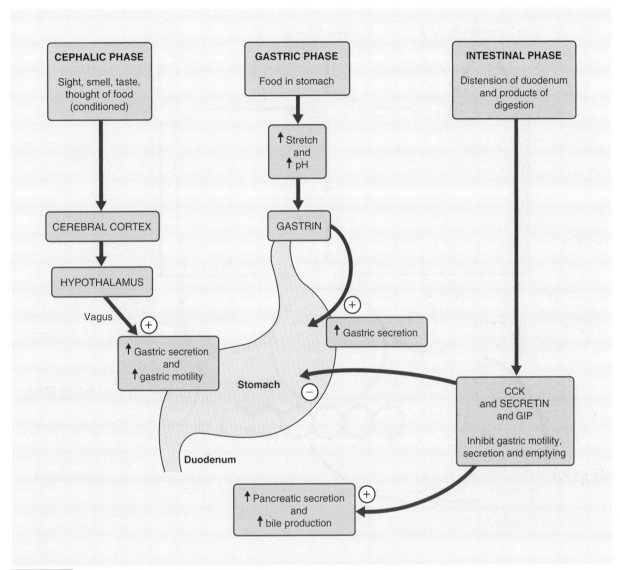

Fig. 1.16 *Phases of hormonal control of the stomach and associated organs.*

the rib cage and respiratory muscles. Ventilation is the mechanical activity that moves gases in and out of the lungs; the movements of the intercostal muscles and diaphragm allow filling and emptying of the lungs (Fig. 1.18). An adult at rest will inspire about 250 ml of oxygen and expire about 200 ml of carbon dioxide every minute. The respiratory tract provides a very large surface area that, whilst optimizing gas exchange, is vulnerable as it is constantly exposed to microorganisms. An important function of the respiratory system is to defend itself and prevent pathogens gaining access to the body.

Gas exchange occurs across the capillary membranes of the alveoli, which are very thin so have a very low diffusion distance. Oxygen from the inspired air diffuses into the capillaries where it binds temporarily to haemoglobin in the red blood cells. The binding of oxygen and haemoglobin can be described by the oxygen–haemoglobin dissociation curve (Fig. 1.19). Haemoglobin has a high affinity for oxygen at higher concentrations and its binding sites are saturated with oxygen in the alveoli. At low concentrations of oxygen, haemoglobin has a low affinity for oxygen so it releases oxygen at the tissues. Binding of

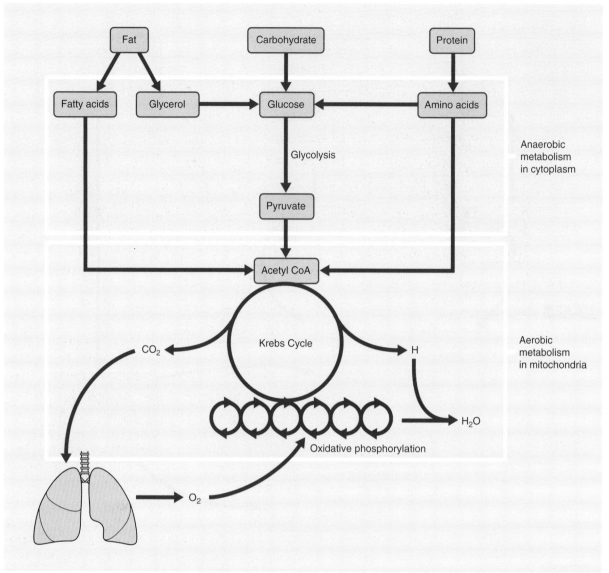

Fig. 1.17 *A summary of metabolism: substrate molecules (such as glucose from food) are oxidized (using respiratory oxygen), producing carbon dioxide (expired) and energy in the form of ATP.*

oxygen to haemoglobin is altered by carbon dioxide, pH, temperature and the glycolytic intermediate 2,3-bisphosphoglycerate (also known as 2,3-diphosphoglycerate). These alter the shape of the haemoglobin molecule, which affects its oxygen-binding sites. Substances that reduce haemoglobin–oxygen affinity increase the release of oxygen (so the curve is shifted towards the right).

Carbon dioxide diffuses from the tissues into the capillaries. It is taken up by the red blood cells where it reacts with water to form carbonic acid. This reac-

tion is catalysed by the enzyme carbonic anhydrase in the red blood cell. Carbonic acid is unstable and dissociates to bicarbonate and hydrogen ions (Fig. 1.20); the bicarbonate diffuses out of the red blood cell into the plasma.

The respiratory control centre, in the medulla oblongata of the brain stem, affects the activity of the inspiratory and expiratory neurons that control the respiratory muscles, which contract to allow inspiration and expiration. The respiratory centre receives information from stretch receptors in the lungs and from the

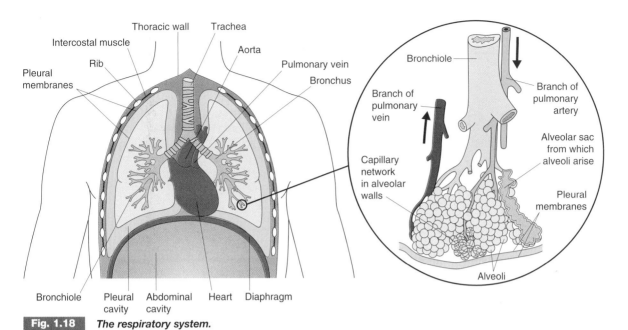

Fig. 1.18 *The respiratory system.*

Labels (left diagram): Intercostal muscle, Thoracic wall, Trachea, Aorta, Rib, Pulmonary vein, Bronchus, Pleural membranes, Bronchiole, Pleural cavity, Abdominal cavity, Heart, Diaphragm

Labels (right diagram): Bronchiole, Branch of pulmonary vein, Branch of pulmonary artery, Alveolar sac from which alveoli arise, Capillary network in alveolar walls, Pleural membranes, Alveoli

peripheral and central chemoreceptors that monitor the pH and oxygen content of the blood (Fig. 1.21).

There is homeostatic regulation of acid–base balance to maintain pH within narrow parameters at around 7.3 (Fig. 1.22). This regulation involves both the respiratory and the renal systems (see Ch. 2).

The cardiovascular system

The cardiovascular system includes the heart, the blood vessels and the blood. The blood is pumped around a network of blood vessels (Fig. 1.23). Arteries transport blood away from the heart and have thick muscular walls. Veins carry blood towards the heart; they function as a capacitance system. Capillaries link the arterial and venous systems and allow exchange of substances between the blood and the tissues.

The heart functions as a double pump, pumping blood to the tissues of the body and the lungs (Fig. 1.24). Blood from the right side of the heart enters the pulmonary circulation to the capillaries surrounding the alveoli of the lungs where the blood is oxygenated. Oxygenated blood returns to the left side of the heart in the pulmonary veins. The oxygenated blood is then pumped from the left side of the heart around the body. The pulmonary circulation takes blood from the right side of the heart, to the lungs, and back to the left side of the heart. The systemic circulation is the circulation of blood around the body

Oxygen saturation of haemoglobin (%) Oxygen content of blood (ml/100 ml)

100 mmHg

40 mmHg

5.3 13.3

PO_2 (kPa)

A=Venous blood (at the tissues)
B=Arterial blood (at the lungs)

Fig. 1.19 *The oxygen–haemoglobin dissociation curve. (Reproduced with permission from Brooker 1998.)*

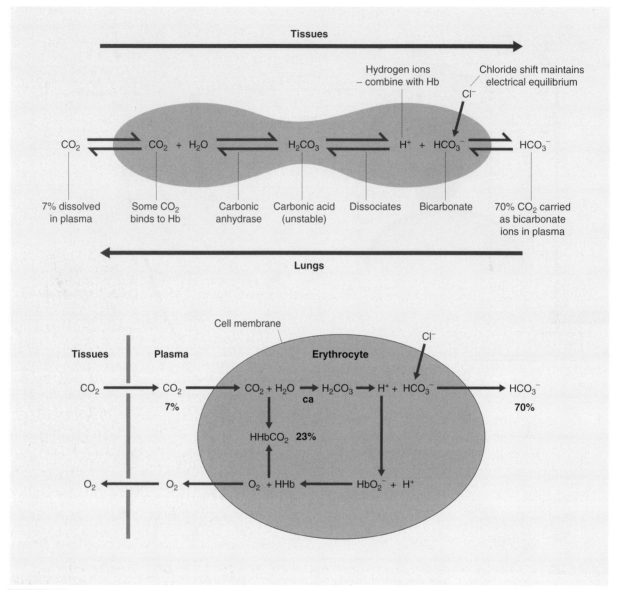

Fig. 1.20 *Carbon dioxide transport. (Reproduced with permission from Brooker 1998.)*

from the left side of the heart to the tissues and back to the right side of the heart. There are two circulatory routes which do not fit the general pattern of double circulation. The portal blood blow from the hypothalamus to the anterior pituitary gland (see Ch. 3) is one of these. The other is associated with the gut. The deoxygenated blood from the digestive system drains into the portal vein which goes to the liver, allowing the liver to take up absorbed nutrients (and neutralize any absorbed toxins). From the liver, blood drains to the hepatic portal veins into the inferior vena cava and thence to the heart.

The coronary circulation is the circulation of blood within the vessels of the heart. Blood flow to the brain is via a circular arrangement of vessels (the circle of Willis); this ensures that there will always be sufficient oxygen and nutrients, albeit at the expense of other parts of the body when the circulatory system is under stress. The blood–brain barrier protects the brain against the entry of some harmful substances, such as toxins.

The heart beats about 70 times a minute at rest, forcing blood from the ventricles into the pulmonary artery and the aorta. The increased volume of blood

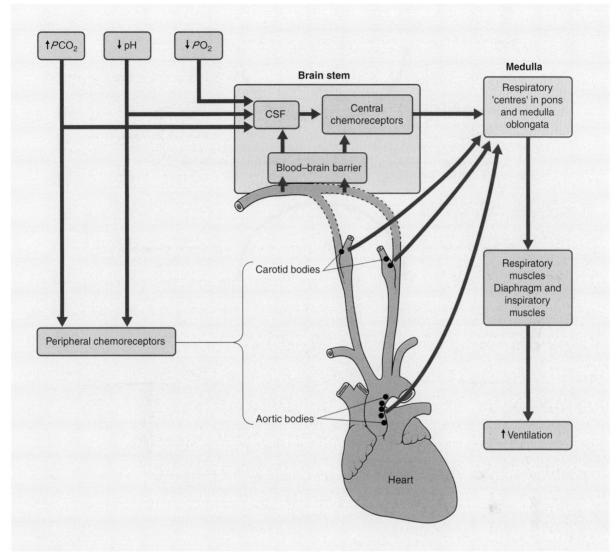

Fig. 1.21 *Chemoreceptor control of respiration: the regulation of ventilation is achieved via peripheral and central chemoreceptors, which sample the blood, and then via a neuronal pathway influencing the rate and depth of breathing. CSF, cerebrospinal fluid.*

entering the blood system causes a fluctuating increase in blood pressure. Blood pressure can be measured using a sphygmomanometer to record pressure within an artery and a stethoscope to hear the turbulence of blood within the blood vessels (Fig. 1.25). The amount of blood that leaves the heart per minute is described as the cardiac output. This is the volume of blood ejected from the ventricles each time the heart beats multiplied by the number of beats per minute (Fig. 1.26). The amount of oxygen that reaches the cells of the tissue depends on the proportion of the cardiac output the tissue receives.

The heart's internal pacemaker, the sinoatrial node (SAN), sets the heart rate. The SAN spontaneously depolarizes and triggers a wave of electrical activity, which stimulates the heart muscle to contract (Fig. 1.27). The SAN is innervated by both parasympathetic and sympathetic nerves. Receptors throughout the body respond to changes in blood pressure and respiratory gas level. These baroreceptors and chemoreceptors transmit information to afferent nerves in the medulla of the brain (the brain stem) that control efferent nerves to the heart, lungs and blood vessels (Fig. 1.28).

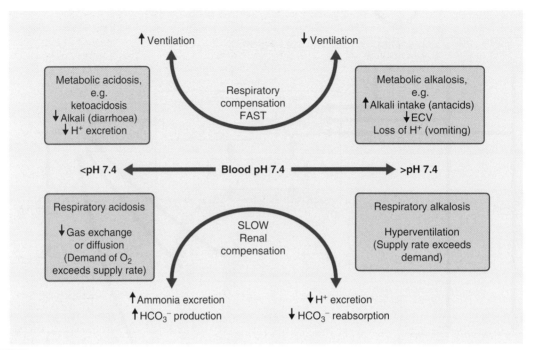

Fig. 1.22 *Acid–base balance.*

The total capacity of blood vessels in the body exceeds the volume of the blood. To maintain homeostasis and tissue requirements, the cardiovascular system is carefully regulated to ensure optimal oxygenation of the tissues. The control of blood flow is regulated by alteration of the diameter of the blood vessels, which changes peripheral resistance. The diameter of the blood vessels is altered by the activity of sympathetic nerves that innervate the smooth muscle in the vessel walls. Increased sympathetic activity, or increased adrenergic stimulation, increases vasoconstriction, reducing blood flow and increasing peripheral resistance. Decreased sympathetic activity causes vasodilation, which increases blood flow and reduces peripheral resistance. Blood vessel diameter is also controlled locally by tissue metabolites. This autoregulation increases blood flow to metabolically active tissues.

Blood

Blood is a suspension of cells in plasma (see Table 1.2). Blood cells are all derived from stem cells in the bone marrow. The majority (>99%) of cells are red blood cells (or erythrocytes). Red blood cells contain haemoglobin, which binds to oxygen. Iron, folic acid and vitamin B_{12} are required for the production of erythrocytes. The kidneys produce a hormone, erythro-

poietin, in response to low oxygen levels, which stimulates an increase in the production of red blood cells from the bone marrow. Leukocytes, or white blood cells, include polymorphonuclear granulocytes (neutrophils, eosinophils and basophils) and the agranular monocytes and lymphocytes. The role of white blood cells is the defence of the body (see Ch. 10). Platelets are cellular fragments of megakaryocytes, which are an essential component of the blood-clotting mechanism (Fig. 1.29). Plasma contains proteins (albumin, globulins and some clotting factors, such as fibrinogen), nutrients, hormones, waste products and ions.

The lymphatic system

The lymphatic system is part of the circulatory system and consists of a network of thin branching vessels, lymph nodes and lymphatic fluid (Fig. 1.30). It collects the interstitial fluid from cells and returns it to the blood. Lymph vessels have one-way values like veins and depend on the movement of skeletal muscle to propel the fluid which moves slowly under low pressure. The lymphatic system transports lymphocytes and is important in defending the body against microorganisms (see Ch. 10). Lymph nodes in the lymphatic system are lymphocyte-filled and act as collecting filters for viruses and bacteria which are then destroyed. Lymphatic vessels are present in

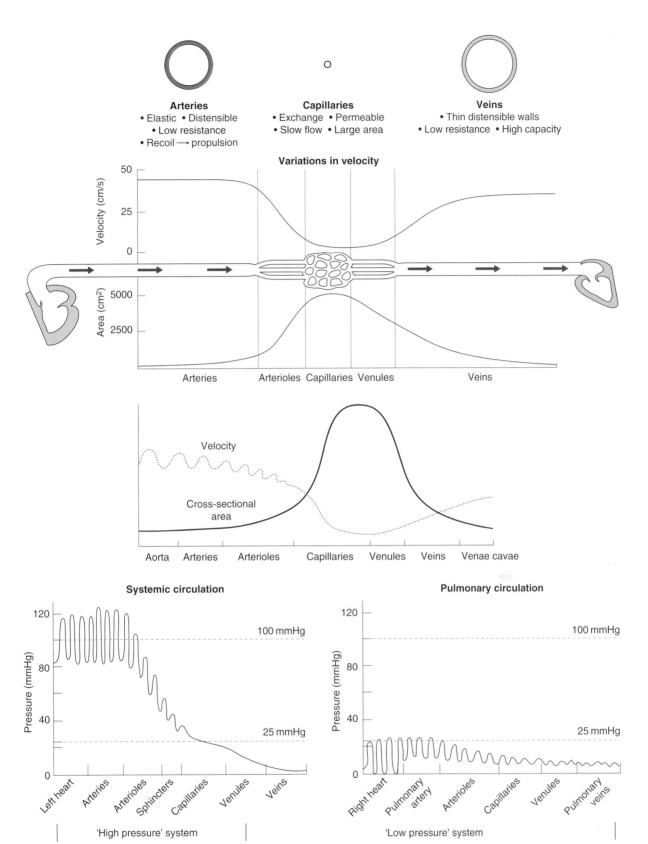

Arteries
- Elastic • Distensible
- Low resistance
- Recoil ⟶ propulsion

Capillaries
- Exchange • Permeable
- Slow flow • Large area

Veins
- Thin distensible walls
- Low resistance • High capacity

Variations in velocity

Velocity (cm/s)

50

25

0

Area (cm²)

5000

2500

Arteries   Arterioles Capillaries Venules   Veins

Velocity

Cross-sectional area

Aorta   Arteries   Arterioles   Capillaries   Venules   Veins   Venae cavae

Systemic circulation

Pressure (mmHg)

120

80

40

0

100 mmHg

25 mmHg

Left heart   Arteries   Arterioles   Sphincters   Capillaries   Venules   Veins

'High pressure' system

Pulmonary circulation

Pressure (mmHg)

120

80

40

0

100 mmHg

25 mmHg

Right heart   Pulmonary artery   Arterioles   Capillaries   Venules   Pulmonary veins

'Low pressure' system

Fig. 1.23 *Blood vessels: the major role of arteries is in the generation of elastic recoil, which propels the blood around the body. The capillaries are involved in gas exchange and the veins act as capacitance vessels returning blood to the heart.*

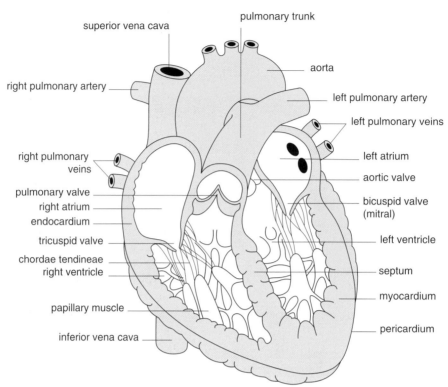

superior vena cava

pulmonary trunk

right pulmonary artery

aorta

left pulmonary artery

left pulmonary veins

right pulmonary veins

left atrium

aortic valve

pulmonary valve

bicuspid valve (mitral)

right atrium

endocardium

tricuspid valve

left ventricle

chordae tendineae

right ventricle

septum

myocardium

papillary muscle

inferior vena cava

pericardium

Fig. 1.24 *Interior of the heart to show layers, chambers and valves. (Reproduced with permission from Brooker 1998.)*

the lining of the digestive tract and transport digested lipids to the thoracic duct into the venous circulation.

Metabolism

Energy production and storage

Cells have a continuous requirement for energy and adenosine triphosphate (ATP). The energy from ATP drives virtually all the body processes but there is very little ATP present at any one time, just enough to provide energy requirements for only a few minutes. Every organ requires energy but some, such as muscles, have a very variable energy requirement. Meals provide fuel from food components, which are oxidized to provide ATP and heat. However, the intake of food is irregular and does not coordinate with the requirement for energy. The energy substrates from a meal are usually absorbed within 3 hours; as the next meal can be hours away, animals have evolved successful methods of storing energy substrates.

The main storage forms of energy are glycogen in liver and skeletal muscle and triacylglycerides in adipose tissue. Carbohydrates are the major fuels for the brain and nervous tissue. Oxidation of glucose occurs in several stages (Fig. 1.31). Glycolysis takes place in the cell cytosol and produces a little ATP anaerobically. If oxygen is present, there is further oxidation through the Krebs cycle and oxidative phosphorylation (the electron transfer chain). This increased efficiency of ATP production takes place in cells that have mitochondria and adequate provision of oxygen. In tissues lacking mitochondria, such as red blood cells, or those with insufficient oxygen, such as active muscle, there is a build-up of the key intermediate pyruvate. Pyruvate can be converted into lactate and oxidized by the heart and kidneys or converted to glucose by the liver and kidneys.

About 500 g of the glucose polymer, glycogen, is stored: 100 g in the liver, which can release the glucose when required (by glycogenolysis), and 400 g in the skeletal muscles, which is available for use by the muscle. Triacylglycerides are stored in virtually unlimited amounts, as observed in obesity. As they do not mix with water, the storage form is very calorie dense and

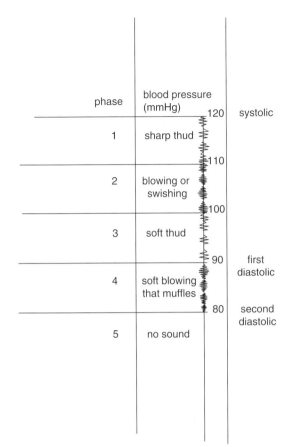

phase	blood pressure (mmHg)		
		120	systolic
1	sharp thud		
		110	
2	blowing or swishing		
		100	
3	soft thud		
		90	first diastolic
4	soft blowing that muffles		
		80	second diastolic
5	no sound		

Fig. 1.25 *Blood pressure measurement. (Reproduced with permission from Brooker 1998.)*

efficient. Triacylglycerides are composed of three fatty acids bound to a glycerol backbone. The glycerol can be converted into glucose, thereby providing a substrate for the brain to oxidize for energy. Fatty acids are released with free glycerol from the adipose tissue and can be oxidized by the liver, muscles and kidneys. Fatty acids cannot cross the blood–brain barrier and cannot be converted to glucose so they provide little substrate for the brain. Ketone bodies are water-soluble derivatives of fatty acids formed by the liver during starvation or prolonged severe exercise. When sufficient concentrations of ketone bodies accumulate, the brain and kidney use them to generate ATP. Certain amino acids are also ketogenic, and can be converted into ketone bodies. Overproduction of ketone bodies, as in uncontrolled diabetes, overwhelms the buffering capacity of the body and can cause life-threatening acidosis.

There is not a reserve storage form of protein independent of function. Protein can be metabolized to provide energy but at the expense of the breakdown of structural and functional components of the body. The use of protein as a fuel potentially damages the body, so it is used only as a 'last resort' when the protein is broken down and the amino acids are converted into components of the glycolytic pathway to produce energy. However, proteins constitute a large proportion of body structure and therefore can provide a substantial source of energy when other supplies have been exhausted. Protein in excess of requirements can be irreversibly converted into glucose or triacylglycerides.

The brain consumes about a quarter of the body's daily energy production when the body is at rest. The brain's requirement for fuel drives energy metabolism. The main fuel storage form of the body is triacylglycerides, but the brain cannot use fatty acids directly. Although the brain can oxidize ketone bodies, derived from fatty acids, for 80% of its energy requirements, 20% *must* come from glucose. Glucose comes from the diet or from glycogenolysis or gluconeogenesis in the liver. Other cells therefore utilize other substrates preferentially to glucose. The hierarchy of fuel use means that the brain utilizes ketone bodies when they are available, or glucose. Muscle has a major reserve of protein and glycogen. Muscle spares brain fuel by preferentially oxidizing fatty acids, thus sparing ketone bodies and glucose for the brain. The glycogen stored in the muscle is specifically available for muscle use.

The external environment is continually fluctuating and energy requirements are constantly changing. However, the body maintains homeostasis or internal stability by ensuring a constant level of amino acids and glucose in the blood, despite intermittent high loads following a meal. The level of ATP within cells is kept relatively constant although the rate of usage is variable; for instance, activity increases energy requirement of a muscle by up to 20 times. Cellular energy requirement is regulated very sensitively; different metabolic pathways predominate after a meal (called the absorptive state) to those between meals (the postabsorptive state) (Fig. 1.32). Dominance of the pathways is via changed enzyme activity and altered uptake of substrates, controlled by hormones. Interconversion from one metabolic step to the next is regulated by substrate activation, where the substance stimulates its own use, and product inhibition, where the product prevents the reaction from continuing. Enzymes catalysing the same reaction may exist as isoenzymes in different types of tissue, having different affinities for their substrates. This means that different concentrations of substrate are required for the biochemical pathway to progress.

Fig. 1.26   *Cardiac output.*

Conduction system

Fig. 1.27   *Sinoatrial node (SAN) depolarization: the conduction pathway of the heart enables the organ's coordinated and rhythmic beating.*

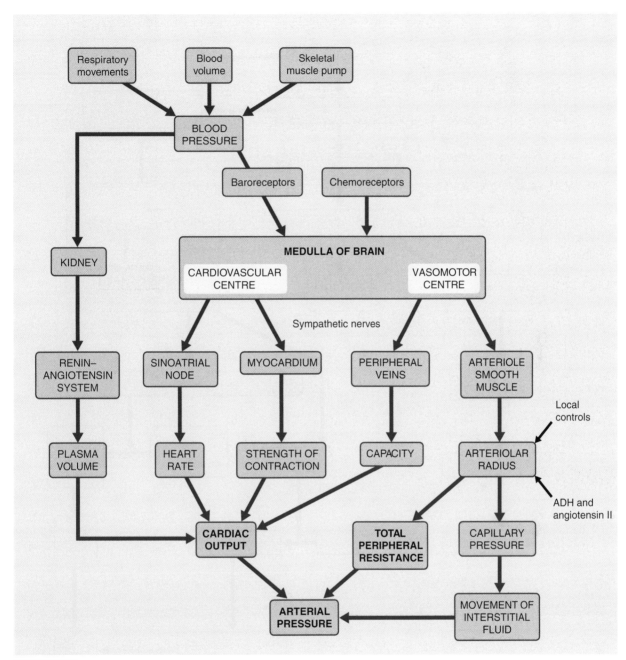

Fig. 1.28 *Regulation of blood pressure.*

Blood sugar regulation

When plasma glucose concentration rises after a meal, secretion of insulin from pancreatic β-cells is stimulated and plasma levels of insulin increase. Insulin triggers the translocation of vesicles containing the insulin-sensitive glucose transporter, GLUT4, from intracellular sites to the cell membrane of the insulin-sensitive tissues, skeletal and cardiac muscle and adipocytes. This increases the uptake of glucose and other substrates into the cell and promotes the anabolic (storage) biochemical pathways (Fig. 1.33). Tissues that have a constant requirement for glucose, such as brain cells, do not

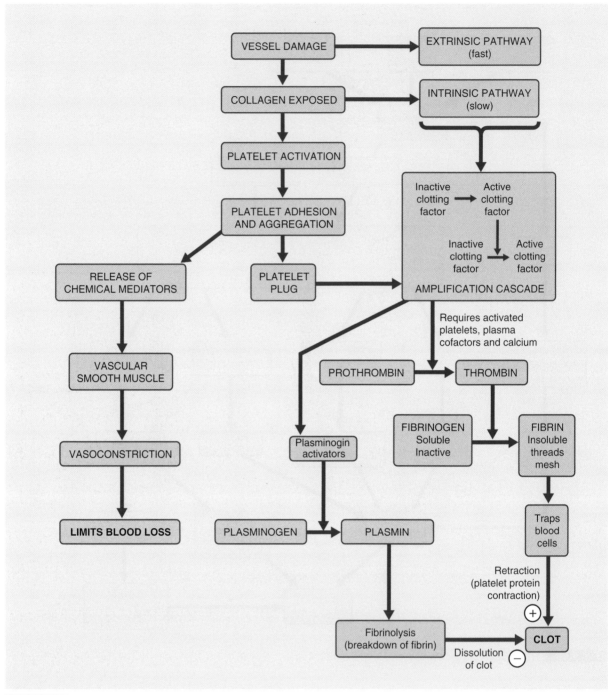

Fig. 1.29 *Haemostasis: the blood coagulation cascade.*

have insulin-sensitive glucose transport but do express the high-affinity transporter, GLUT3, as well as GLUT1. Under conditions of low glucose, pancreatic production of glucagon is increased, which acts to mobilize tissue reserves of metabolic fuels. Adrenaline, secreted from the adrenal medulla in response to sympathetic innervation, causes a rapid mobilization of fuels for 'fight or flight' (see p. 12). Adrenaline stimulates glucose production from muscle glycogen and increases lipolysis in adipose tissue so that levels of fatty acids increase to provide additional metabolic fuel.

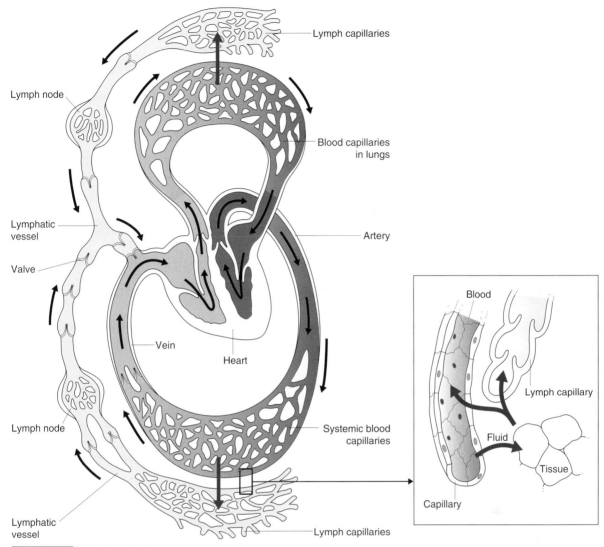

Fig. 1.30　*The lymphatic system.*

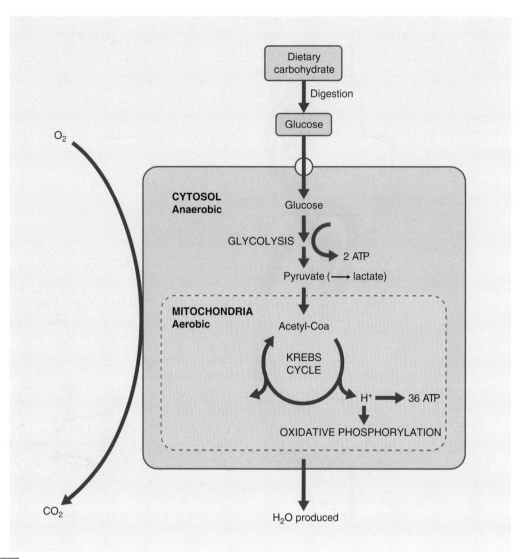

Fig. 1.31 *Oxidation of glucose.*

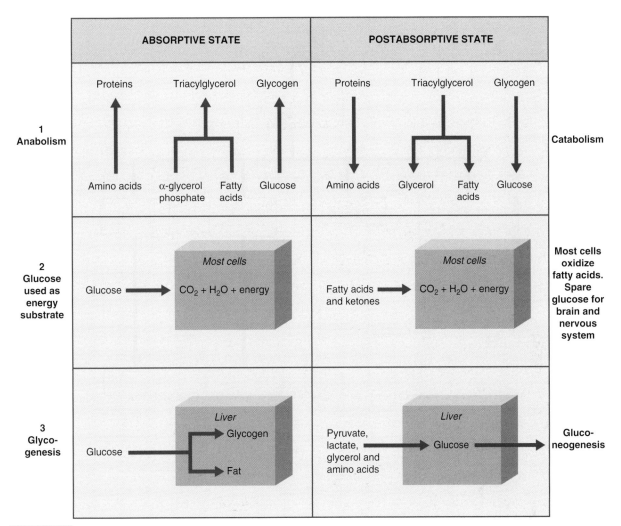

Fig. 1.32   *Absorptive and postabsorptive states.*

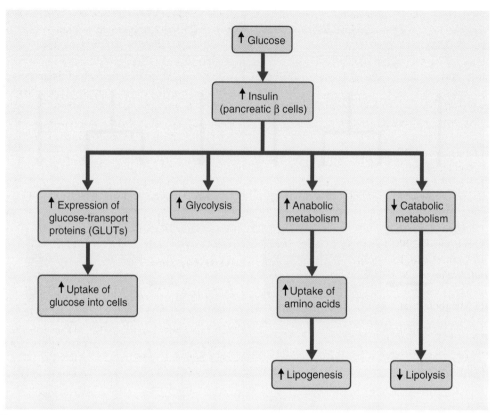

Fig. 1.33 *The effects of insulin.*

- Cells have different anatomical structures, which are related to their physiological functions.

- Cells are organized together to form tissues, which are organized into organs and the physiological systems of the body.

- The role of the physiological systems is to provide internal stability or homeostasis, which will ensure that the cells' variable but essential requirements for energy are met by an adequate supply of oxygen and nutrients.

- As the enzymes that regulate cellular activity have a protein structure, they are affected by fluctuations in pH and temperature, so homeostasis has to maintain optimum temperature and acid–base balance as well.

Application to practice

The basic physiology described in this chapter relates to the non-pregnant state. During pregnancy there are many physiological changes, which are explored through the rest of the book. A basic knowledge of physiology is essential so that the complexities of the physiological changes in pregnancy can be understood and explained as required. This knowledge is also essential for the midwife to be able to monitor the development of pregnancy effetively.

Annotated further reading

Alberts B, Bray D, Lewis J, Raff M, Roberts K, Watson JD 2002 Molecular biology of the cell. 4th edn. Garland, New York

A beautifully written and well-illustrated text on molecular and cellular biology which is accessible, easy to read and up to date; the cell biologist's 'bible'.

Berne RM, Levy NM 2003 Physiology, 5th edn. Mosby, St Louis
A comprehensive illustrated textbook, which emphasizes physiological concepts and basic principles.

Greenstein B, Greenstein A 1996 Medical biochemistry at a glance. Blackwell, Oxford
A useful overview of human biochemistry which provides a synopsis using detailed flow-charts and explanatory diagrams.

Koeppen BM, Stanton B 2000 Renal physiology, 3rd edn. University of Connecticut, Farmington
Provides a useful reference to the area of renal physiology.

Salway J 2003 Metabolism at a glance, 3rd edn. Blackwell, Oxford
A large-format book which provides a comprehensive review of basic human metabolism, including inborn errors of metabolism and clinical aspects of metabolism.

Metabolic pathways are summarized as segments with a clear diagrammatic pathway map on one page and an outline of the metabolism on the facing page.

Tortora GJ, Grabowski SR 2003 Principles of anatomy and physiology, 10th edn. Harper Collins, New York
A clear, illustrated textbook (with CD-ROM) providing an in-depth overview of physiology and anatomy. It is targeted at students in health professions and includes clinical applications and study outlines.

Vander AJ, Sherman JH, Luciano DS 2003 Human physiology, 9th edn. McGraw-Hill, New York
Provides a useful guide to the principles of human physiology using clear diagrams and flow-charts.

References

Brooker CG 1998 Human structure and function, 2nd edn. Mosby, St Louis, pp 15, 30, 32, 33, 88, 207, 211, 228, 277, 279, 296, 372, 383

Saffrey J, Stewart M (eds) 1997 Maintaining the whole. SK220 Human biology and health, Book 3. Open University Press, Milton Keynes, p 65

2 The reproductive and urinary systems

Learning objectives

- To describe the structure and function of the urinary system.
- To compare the structure of the female and male reproductive systems.
- To identify differences between the male and female reproductive tracts in relation to reproduction and adaptations to facilitate childbirth.

Introduction

This chapter reviews the basic anatomy of the reproductive and urinary systems of the human. The human urinary system differs only slightly between the male and female, mostly in relation to the structure of the external genitalia. The function of the urinary system is also essentially the same within the male and female. However, the renal system can be severely stressed by pregnancy, mostly because of its close proximity to the reproductive organs and the major changes in fluid balance resulting in fluid retention during pregnancy. The midwife needs to know the basics of normal renal physiology in order to understand the changes that take place in the renal system during pregnancy and how these may affect the general condition of the woman. For example, not only are the regulation and retention of fluid altered in pregnancy but also the excretion of glucose and other substances is affected by these changes. Drug excretion via the kidneys may also be affected, so long-term medication may need to be changed as pregnancy progresses. The effectiveness of medication may be reduced and altered drug dosage may also be required. (Specific changes in the renal system in pregnancy are covered in Ch. 11.)

Chapter case study

Zara, during the booking appointment, informs the midwife that she had previously suffered an ectopic pregnancy with her last pregnancy, which was treated conservatively with methotrexate. What does the midwife need to do to ensure that Zara's pregnancy is progressing normally? What are the signs and symptoms of an ectopic pregnancy; and when are they most likely to become apparent?

The urinary system

The urinary system is composed of two kidneys, which produce urine, two ureters running from the kidneys to the bladder, which collects and stores the urine, and a urethra from which urine is discharged to the exterior (Fig. 2.1).

The kidneys

The kidneys have a broad range of other functions (see Box 2.1) as well as producing urine. The kidneys are situated upon the posterior wall of the abdominal cavity, one on either side of the vertebral column at the level of the thoracic and lumbar vertebrae (just below the rib cage). The right kidney is slightly lower than the left owing to its relationship to the liver. Each kidney is about 10 cm long, 6.5 cm wide and about 3 cm thick (about the size of a clenched fist). The kidneys each weigh about 100 grams (a small proportion of

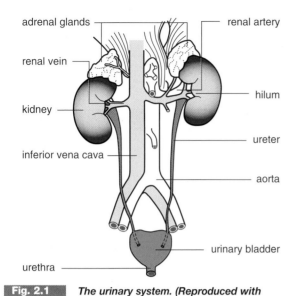

the total body mass), but they receive about 25% of the cardiac output. The renal blood supply arises from the aorta via the renal arteries and returns to the inferior vena cava via the renal veins. Each kidney is enclosed by a thick fibrous capsule and has two distinct layers: the reddish-brown cortex, which has a rich blood supply, and the inner medulla, within which the structural and functional units of the kidney, the nephrons, are found (Fig. 2.2).

The nephron

Each kidney has approximately a million nephrons, each of which is about 3 cm long. The nephron is a tubule that is closed at one end and opens into the collecting duct at the other. The nephron has six distinct regions, each of which is adapted to a specific function (Fig. 2.3). There are two types of nephron. Most nephrons (90%) are cortical nephrons; these have short loops of Henle and are mainly concerned with the control of plasma volume during normal conditions. The juxtamedullary nephrons, which have longer loops of Henle, facilitate increased water retention when the availability of water is restricted.

The renal corpuscle comprises the Bowman's capsule, a blind-ended tube, and the glomerulus, a coiled arrangement of capillaries around which the Bowman's capsule is invaginated. The glomerulus provides a large area of capillary vessels from which substances can leave, crossing the specialized flattened epithelial cells to enter the capsule of the nephron. There is a double capillary arrangement (see Fig. 2.3) whereby afferent arterioles supply the glomerular

---

Box 2.1

Functions of the kidney

- Regulation of water balance
- Regulation of pH and inorganic ion balance (sodium, potassium, calcium)
- Excretion of metabolic waste products (urea from protein, uric acid from nucleic acids, creatinine from muscle creatine and haemoglobin breakdown products)
- Hormone secretion (of erythropoietin, renin, 1,25-dihydroxyvitamin D_3 (1,25-dihydroxycholecalciferol, also called calcitriol) and prostaglandins)
- Removal of toxic chemicals (drugs, pesticides, food additives)
- Regulation of blood pressure (renin–angiotensin system)
- Control of formation of red blood cells (via erythropoietin)
- Vitamin D activation and calcium balance
- Gluconeogenesis (formation of glucose from amino acids and other precursors)

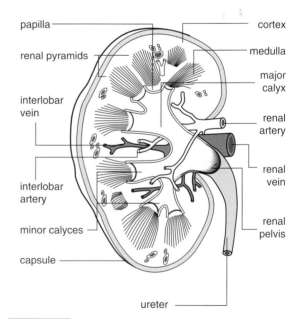

Fig. 2.2   *The structure of the kidney (longitudinal section). (Reproduced with permission from Brooker 1998.)*

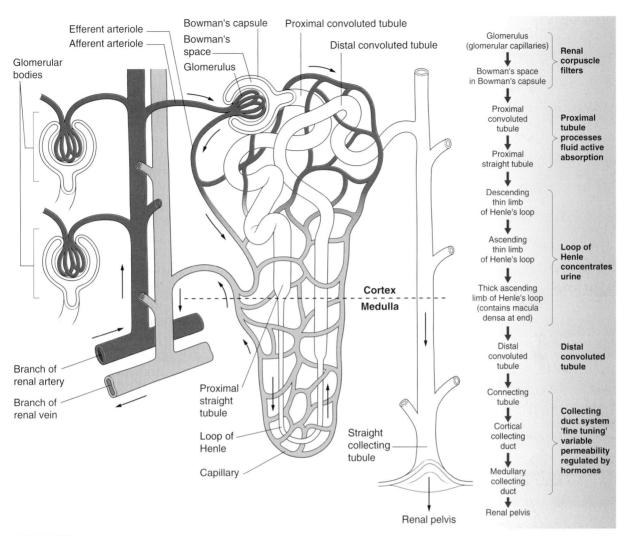

Fig. 2.3 *The nephron and double capillary arrangement. The panel on the right shows the functions of the regions of the nephron.*

capillaries and efferent arterioles lead from the glomerulus to a second capillary bed supplying the rest of the nephron. Differential vasoconstriction of the afferent and efferent arterioles maintains a constant blood pressure within the glomerulus, which results in a constant rate of filtration. Urine production relies on three steps: simple filtration, selective reabsorption and secretion (Fig. 2.4).

Filtration

Filtration is a passive process that occurs through the semipermeable walls of the glomerulus and glomerular capsule. All substances with a molecular mass of less than 68 kilodaltons (kDa) are forced out of the glomerular capillaries into the Bowman's capsule. So water and small molecules enter the nephron whereas blood cells, plasma proteins and other large molecules are usually retained in the blood. The content of the Bowman's capsule is referred to as the 'glomerular filtrate' and the rate at which this is formed is referred to as the 'glomerular filtration rate' (GFR). The kidneys form about 180 litres of dilute filtrate each day (a GFR of about 125 ml/min). Most of it is selectively reabsorbed so the final volume of urine produced is about 1–1.5 litres per day.

Box 2.2 describes an example of disrupted renal function in pregnancy that is detected by abnormal urine content.

FILTRATION

Glomerulus

Glomerular capsule

Hydrostatic
pressure
70 mmHg

Osmotic
pressure
30 mmHg

Hydrostatic
pressure
5 mmHg

**NET FILTRATION
PRESSURE
35 mmHg**

FILTRATE IN TUBE

Selective
reabsorption
from tubule
to blood

BLOOD IN CAPILLARY

SELECTIVE REABSORPTION

Secretion
from blood
to tubule

SECRETION

Fig. 2.4 *Urine production.*

Hypertension in pregnancy

Hypertensive disorders in pregnancy can disrupt renal
function. The detectable presence of protein within
the urine (proteinuria) may indicate that larger
molecules than normal are being forced into the
Bowman's capsule. This is caused by the increased
blood pressure resulting in abnormal ultrafiltration.
Women who have a degree of renal damage prior to
pregnancy are less likely to be able to adapt to the
pregnancy-induced physiological changes as
effectively as women with normal renal function.
These women tend to develop high blood pressure
during early pregnancy and so do not normally
demonstrate such a marked physiological reduction in
blood pressure parameters, putting both the mother
and fetus at risk.

Selective reabsorption

The glomerular filtrate is reabsorbed from the rest of
the nephron into the surrounding capillaries. The proximal convoluted tubule (PCT in Fig. 2.6) is the widest
and longest part of the whole nephron (approximately
1.4 cm long). The cells lining it contain a large number
of mitochondria to provide energy for facilitating
active transport as most of the reabsorption of the
glomerular filtrate takes place here. Some substances,
such as glucose and amino acids, are completely
reabsorbed and are not normally present in urine.
Reabsorption of waste products is largely incomplete
so, for instance, a large proportion of urea is excreted.
The reabsorption of other substances is under the
regulation of several hormones. Antidiuretic hormone
(ADH) controls the insertion of aquaporins, pore-
forming membrane proteins, into the walls of the distal convoluted tubule (DCT in Fig. 2.6) and collecting

ducts (CD in Fig. 2.6), which allows water to leave the filtrate, thus producing less urine (Fig. 2.5). The formation of concentrated urine is facilitated by the physical arrangement of the loop of Henle and its surrounding capillaries, which create and maintain the conditions for the reabsorption of water by osmosis (Fig. 2.6, Box 2.3). Calcitonin increases calcium excretion and parathyroid hormone enhances reabsorption of calcium from renal tubules. Aldosterone affects the reabsorption of sodium (Fig. 2.7). Atrial natriuretic peptide (ANP) inhibits NaCl reabsorption in the distal convoluted tubule and cortical collecting duct of the nephron. ANP also increases the glomerular filtration rate by dilating the afferent glomerular arterioles and constricting the efferent glomerular arteriole, thus increasing NaCl excretion.

Secretion

Some waste products may be actively transported directly into the tubules from the surrounding blood capillaries. These include hydrogen and potassium ions, creatinine, toxins and drugs. The cells of the renal tubules synthesize some substances, such as ammonia ions and peptides, which can be secreted into the filtrate.

The ureters

The ureters, which are tubes about 25–30 cm long and 3 mm in diameter, transport the urine from the kidneys to the bladder. From each kidney the collecting ducts open into the renal pelvis, which leads to the ureter. The walls of the renal pelvis have smooth muscle, which has intrinsic activity (i.e. not controlled by nerves), generating peristaltic waves of contraction every 10 seconds. These waves of contraction propel urine along the ureters to the bladder. Each ureter is also lined with smooth muscle and transitional epithelium; the lumen has a star-shaped cross-section.

The ureters lie upon the posterior abdominal wall outside the peritoneal cavity, entering the bladder at an oblique angle, one at each side of the base of the specialized muscle area called the trigone which has its apex at the urethral opening. As urine accumulates in the bladder, the ureters are compressed, effectively forming a valve (the vesicoureteral valve), which prevents urinary reflux.

The bladder

The bladder is a distensible hollow organ, also composed of smooth muscle, which acts as a reservoir for urine. It is intermittently emptied under conscious control. Stretch receptors within the muscle and trigone provide the signals that indicate that the bladder is full. The normal capacity of the bladder is approximately 700–800 ml; however, the natural desire to void urine becomes conscious when the level of urine in the bladder reaches approximately 300 ml.

As the bladder lies below the uterus, its capacity is compromised by the growing uterus in early pregnancy. Later on, once the pregnant uterus has become an abdominal organ, the pressure on the bladder is relieved. Finally, at the end of pregnancy, bladder capacity is again compromised as the presenting part of the fetus engages, occupying space within the true pelvic cavity and thus restricting the space available to the bladder.

Fig. 2.5   *The action of ADH.*

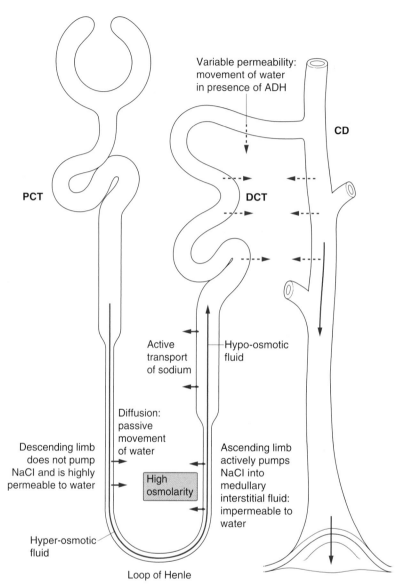

Fig. 2.6   *Formation of concentrated urine.*

Box 2.3

Hypertonic urine

The evolution of the mammalian kidney has enabled mammals to become highly adapted to terrestrial living. The kidney aids water conservation by producing urine that is able to be concentrated far more than the internal body fluid environment. The scarcer water is within the environment, the longer the nephron to conserve water.

The urethra

Urine is voided via the urethra. The female urethra is considerably shorter and straighter than the male urethra: only 4 cm in length compared with about 20 cm. This anatomical difference predisposes women towards an increased incidence of ascending urinary tract infections. Thus a colony count of more than 100 000 bacterial cells per millilitre of urine is considered to be pathologically significant. There are small mucus-secreting glands in the urethra that help

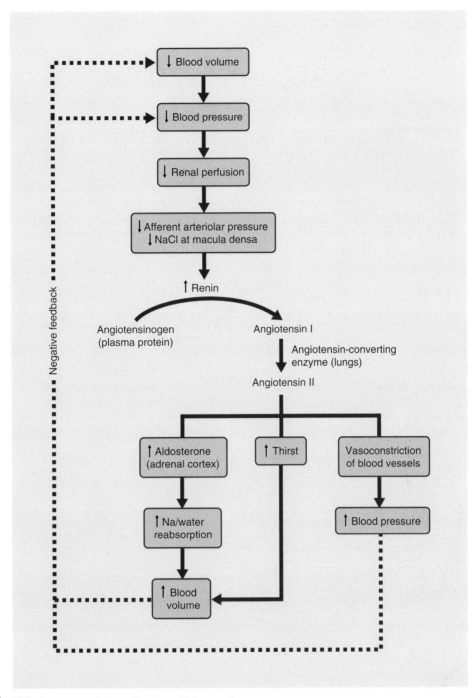

Fig. 2.7 *Aldosterone regulation of sodium (Na) excretion.*

to protect the epithelium from the corrosive urine. The upper internal sphincter, at the exit from the bladder, is composed of smooth muscle and is under autonomic control. The external sphincter is composed of skeletal muscle and is under voluntary control. The urethra within the male has a dual role as the route for urine and the delivery of spermatozoa, via coitus. Structural differences related to the development of the external genitalia are covered in Chapter 5.

Urine

Urine has a specific gravity of 1010–1030 and is usually acidic. The volume and final concentration of urea and solutes depend on fluid intake. Sleep and muscular activity also inhibit urine production. The amber colour is due to urobilin, the bile pigment. Urine has a characteristic smell, which is not unpleasant when fresh. Odour or cloudiness generally indicates a bacterial infection.

Control of micturition

Micturition (urination) is a coordinated response that is due to the contraction of the muscular wall of the bladder, reflex relaxation of the internal sphincter of the urethra and voluntary relaxation of the external sphincter (Fig. 2.8). It is assisted by increased pressure in the pelvic cavity as the diaphragm is lowered and the abdominal muscles contract. Overdistension of the bladder is painful and can cause involuntary relaxation of the external sphincter resulting in incontinence and overflow. The tone of this sphincter is also affected by psychological stimuli (such as waking or getting ready to leave the house) and external stimuli (such as the sound of water or the feel of the lavatory seat). Any factor that raises the intraabdominal and intravesicular pressures (such as laughter or coughing) in excess of the urethral closing pressure can result in stress incontinence.

Accumulation of urine increases bladder wall tension, stimulating the stretch receptors of the bladder, which relay parasympathetic sensory impulses to the

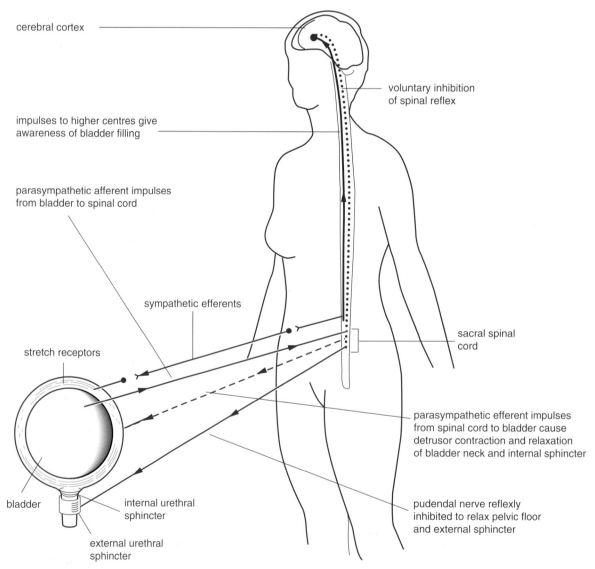

cerebral cortex

voluntary inhibition
of spinal reflex

impulses to higher centres give
awareness of bladder filling

parasympathetic afferent impulses
from bladder to spinal cord

sympathetic efferents

sacral spinal
cord

stretch receptors

parasympathetic efferent impulses
from spinal cord to bladder cause
detrusor contraction and relaxation
of bladder neck and internal sphincter

bladder

internal urethral
sphincter

pudendal nerve reflexly
inhibited to relax pelvic floor
and external sphincter

external urethral
sphincter

Fig. 2.8   *Control of micturition. (Reproduced with permission from Brooker 1998.)*

brain, generating awareness. However, there is conscious descending inhibition of the reflex bladder contraction and relaxation of the external sphincter. Entry of urine into the urethra irritates and stimulates stretch receptors, augmenting the sensory pathways as the bladder fills. Micturition is postponed until a socially acceptable time and place. This inhibition of the spinal reflex and contraction of the external sphincter is learned. Infants tend to develop bladder control when they are about 2 years old. Irritation of the bladder or urethra, for instance as a result of infection, can also initiate the desire to urinate regardless of the bladder capacity.

Normal physiological control of micturition requires an intact nerve supply to the urinary tract, normal muscle tone (of bladder, urethral sphincters and pelvic floor muscles), absence of any obstruction to flow, normal bladder capacity and, finally, the absence of psychological factors that may inhibit the micturition cycle (such as embarrassment and discomfort).

The female reproductive tract

The main features of the female reproductive tract distinguishing it from the male are that the female reproductive organs are internal and in the non-pregnant state are situated within the true pelvic cavity. The female reproductive tract consists of two ovaries, two uterine (fallopian) tubes, the uterus and cervix, the vagina and external genitalia. The female reproductive system undergoes considerable changes throughout life from childhood through reproductive life (see Box 2.4) to the menopause. Superimposed on these changes are the effects of the menstrual cycle.

The ovaries

The ovaries are dull-white almond-shaped bodies, approximately 4 cm long. They lie posteriorly and laterally relative to the body of the uterus and below the uterine tubes. They are anchored by the ovarian ligaments and attached to the posterior layer of the broad ligament, a fold within the peritoneum that extends from the uterus (Fig. 2.9). The blood supply to the ovary is via the ovarian artery, which runs alongside the ovarian ligament, and the ovarian branch of the uterine artery (see Fig. 2.12, p. 46). This dual blood

---

Box 2.4

Changes to the genital tract at puberty

- Hair appears on mons veneris and subcutaneous fat accumulates
- Secretory glands mature and become active
- Labia majora and minora become pigmented with melanin
- Enlargement of the clitoris occurs
- Vaginal epithelium thickens and becomes responsive to oestrogen
- Vaginal pH decreases as lactobacilli metabolize glycogen from cell secretions
- Uterus grows and cervix doubles in length

---

supply is important in maintaining reproductive function; if the ovary becomes twisted, for instance because it is displaced by a tumour or cystic growth, the ovarian ligament may occlude the blood supply from the ovarian artery. This torsion of the ovary can cause ischaemia of the tissues and intense pain.

The ovaries are composed of two distinct layers: the outer layer is the cortex and the inner section is referred to as the medulla. The ovary is contained within a sheath of connective tissue, the tunica albuginea. The cortex contains the developing follicles that contain the primary oocytes and is also responsible for the production of the female steroid hormones oestrogen and progesterone (see Chs 4 and 5). The medulla is composed primarily of connective tissue and blood vessels and provides precursors to facilitate steroid production within the cortex.

The uterine (fallopian) tubes

The uterine tubes (also known as the fallopian tubes or oviducts) are approximately 12 cm long and have walls of smooth muscle lined with ciliated epithelial and secretory cells. The distal end of the uterine tube has specialized structures called fimbriae, which surround the opening into the tube. The fimbriae lie in close proximity to the ovary and, at ovulation, assist the entry of the ovum into the uterine tube by a wafting action, which facilitates movement of the interperitoneal fluid. The lining of the uterine tubes lies in many folds (called plicae) and is composed of ciliated columnar epithelial cells interspersed with goblet cells that secret pyruvate to nourish the ovum. The cilia facilitate the movement of the ovum down the uterine

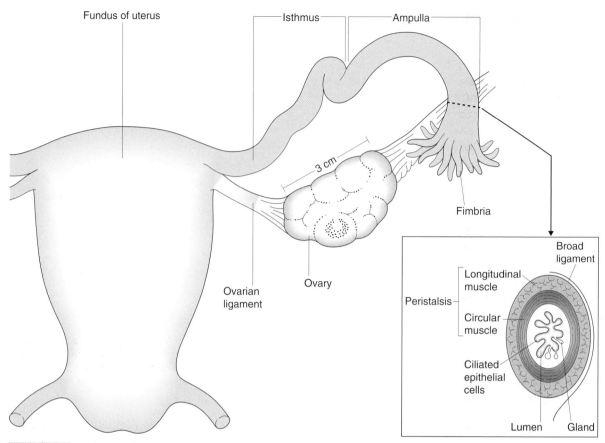

Fig. 2.9 *Position of the ovary, and ovarian and broad ligaments. (Reproduced with permission from Sweet 1996.)*

tube; this is augmented by coordinated peristaltic contractions of the smooth muscle. The distal end of the uterine tube has a slightly wider area, called the ampulla, where fertilization of the ovum by the sperm usually occurs.

If both uterine tubes are completely blocked, fertilization is prevented as the sperm are unable to access the ovum. If one uterine tube is patent or only partially blocked then sperm may encounter and fertilize an ovum within the peritoneal cavity. However, if a fertilized ovum enters a partially or totally blocked uterine tube its passage to the uterus will be impeded and so the pregnancy may develop within the uterine tube or peritoneal cavity (see Box 2.5). The uterine tubes are mobile and not fixed to the ovaries.

The uterus

The functions of the uterus are to prepare to receive the fertilized ovum, to provide a suitable environment for growth and development of the fetus and to assist in the expulsion of the fetus, placenta and membranes at delivery. In the non-pregnant state the pear-shaped uterus is situated within the true pelvic cavity. It is described as being anteverted (tilted forwards) and anteflexed (curved forward), situated in a superior position to the urinary bladder (Fig. 2.10). A uterus in an abnormal position, such as a retroverted uterus, is not in an optimal position to expand in pregnancy and surgical intervention may be required to adjust its position to allow the pregnancy to proceed. The anatomical position of the uterus is maintained by the uterine ligaments, which are important in supporting the weight of the uterus, particularly during contractions (Fig. 2.11). Its blood supply is shown in Figure 2.12.

The non-pregnant uterus weighs approximately 50 g with a cavity of approximately 10 ml and is composed of three layers (Fig. 2.13). The inner layer of the uterus is the endometrium. This layer is markedly different in the body of the uterus compared with the cervix. The cells of the endometrium are ciliated and the entire cell layer undergoes considerable growth

Box 2.5

Ectopic pregnancy

An ectopic pregnancy is one that implants in the uterine tubes or, more rarely, the cervix, ovaries or abdomen. It is usually confirmed by a positive pregnancy test in conjunction with an ultrasound scan revealing an empty uterine cavity. Levels of human chorionic gonadotrophin (hCG) are also markedly lower in ectopic pregnancy. The warning sign of an ectopic pregnancy is abdominal pain at around 8 weeks' gestation. If the uterine tube ruptures then the woman may become clinically shocked owing to excessive bleeding into the peritoneal cavity. The growing fetus can be surgically removed together with the damaged uterine tube if necessary (this is referred to as a salpingectomy). Occasionally an abdominal pregnancy may ensue if implantation occurs on the peritoneum. The pregnancies rarely go to term; however, delivery of live infants via abdominal surgery has been documented. This phenomenon underpins scientific interest enabling men to have babies through a process of peritoneal implantation. The main causes of tubal blockage are infection (usually due to pelvic inflammatory disease), the formation of scar tissue from surgery or trauma and congenital malformation. High levels of steroid hormones can also affect cilia movement. If a tubal pregnancy is diagnosed early before trauma occurs, it can be treated by the administration of the drug methotrexate. Methotrexate inhibits folic acid metabolism thus inhibiting DNA synthesis and cell division so the embryo does not develop further and is eventually reabsorbed. Although the uterine tube is saved, the risk of another ectopic pregnancy is high.

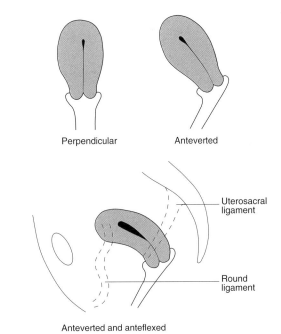

Fig. 2.10 *The anteverted and anteflexed position of the non-pregnant uterus. (Reproduced with permission from Sweet 1996.)*

changes during the menstrual cycle; the superficial decidual layers are shed in menstruation at the end of the cycle (see Ch. 4). The vascular connective tissue, or stroma, contains many glands that secrete alkaline mucus into the uterine cavity.

The middle layer is composed of smooth muscle, called the myometrium, which is arranged in three muscle layers (see Box 2.6). In the non-pregnant state these layers are not very distinctive.

The uterus has an outer layer of peritoneum that drapes over the uterus anteriorly to form a fold

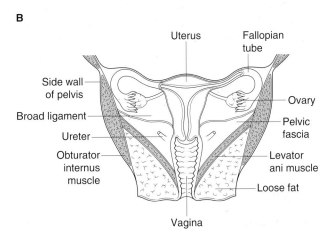

Fig. 2.11 *The uterine ligaments (transverse and coronal sections). (Reproduced with permission from Sweet 1996.)*

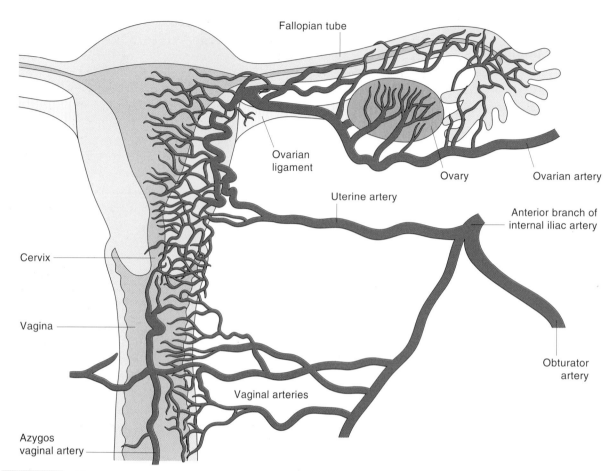

Fallopian tube

Ovarian
ligament

Ovary   Ovarian artery

Uterine artery

Anterior branch of
internal iliac artery

Cervix

Vagina

Obturator
artery

Vaginal arteries

Azygos
vaginal artery

Fig. 2.12 *The uterine and ovarian blood supply.*

between the uterus and bladder, and over the uterine tubes to cover the myometrium. This is referred to as the perimetrium; it forms the broad ligament, thus maintaining the anatomical position of the uterus. The body of the uterus is about 5 cm in both length and width (excluding the dimensions of the cervix).

The uterus is innervated by both parasympathetic nerves (arising from the second, third and fourth sacral segments) and sympathetic nerves via the pre-sacral nerve (branching from the aortic plexus) and branches from the lumbar sympathetic chain. Both types of innervation to the uterus are via the Lee–Frankenhäuser plexus, which is situated in the lower region of the pouch of Douglas.

The cervix

The cervix is the neck of the uterus at the top of the vagina. It has an important role in protecting the uterus from infection and undergoes important changes preceding labour (see Ch. 13). The isthmus, an indistinct layer of tissue that forms the lower uterine segment in pregnancy (see Ch. 13), separates the body of the uterus and the cervix. The cervix is about 2.5 cm in length and is composed of dense collagenous circular fibres. The cervix is spindle-shaped with an os (smooth muscle arrangement forming a constriction) at the top and bottom. The internal os forms the inner opening of the cervix at the junction with the body of the uterus. The external os is located at the bottom of the cervical canal where it projects into the vagina. Two different types of cell meet at this junction: the columnar cells of the cervical canal and the squamous epithelial cells of the outer cervix. Abnormal precancerous cells are most likely to arise at this junction. Cervical cancer is one of the more common cancers affecting women of reproductive age. One of the risk factors for cervical cancer is the presence of antibodies to certain strains of human papillomavirus (HPV). HPV itself is benign but it is thought to trigger changes in the cells of the cervix. The pap smear (named after

Georgios Papanikolaou) is a cervical swab which samples cells and allows checking for precancerous changes. The shape of the spatula used to take cell samples during a cervical smear accommodates the curve of the external part of the cervix. About 5–7% of cervical smears identify abnormal results such as dysplasia indicating the need for increased vigilance. The lining of the cervix does not undergo cyclical changes in growth rate although glandular activity changes. The inner tissue lies in folds that appear branched, giving it the name arbor vitae. These folds allow dilatation during delivery.

The vagina

The vagina is a distensible muscular tube, about 8–10 cm long, situated within the true pelvic cavity, extending through the pelvic floor from the cervix to the vulva. The vagina is described as a potential tube because its walls are in contact but easily separated.

The cervix protrudes into the vagina, normally pointing to the posterior wall of the vagina because of the anteverted and anteflexed position of the uterus. The spaces between the cervix and the upper portion of the vaginal wall are referred to as the anterior, lateral and posterior fornices (singular: fornix). The vagina has three main functions: the facilitation of coitus, as a passage for the release of the menses and as the route for the baby to be born, commonly referred to as the birth canal. It also helps to support the uterus and prevent ascending infection through the release of antibacterial secretions favouring the growth of commensal bacteria.

The vagina is lined by a layer of moist epithelial cells folded into ridges (called rugae) that distend during intercourse and childbirth, thus facilitating the stretching of the vagina. There is also a lining of smooth muscle, which maintains the tone of the vagina. The opening of the vagina, which is a skeletal muscle sphincter, is protected by the external genitalia. It lies below the urethral opening, which is situated

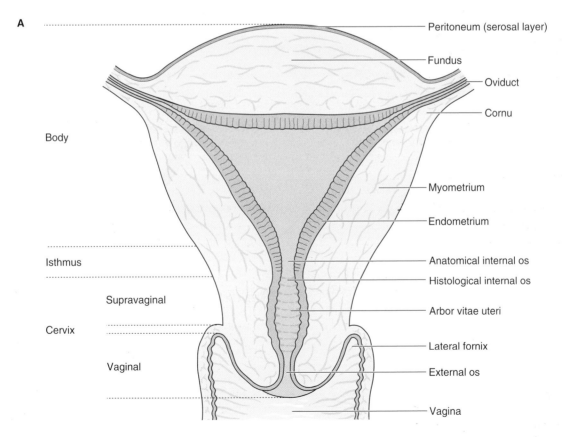

Fig. 2.13 *Structure of A the non-pregnant uterus and B endometrium. (A reproduced with permission from Bogin 1999; B reproduced with permission from Brooker 1998.)*

Continued

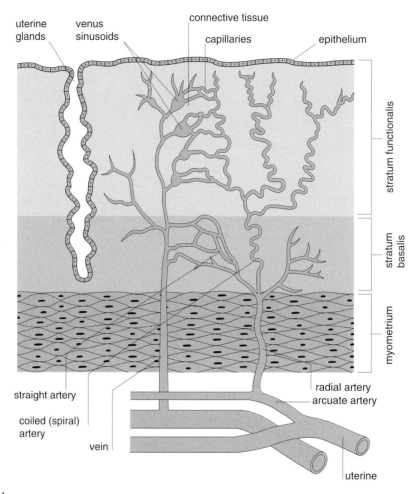

Fig. 2.13   Cont'd

The uterine muscle layers

1 *Inner layer*: fibres in the longitudinal plane that run from the anterior cervix, up over the fundus and back to the posterior edge of the cervix

2 *Middle layer*: interlaced spiral fibres concentrated in, and originating from, the fundal region of the uterus and getting less dense approaching the cervical region; the circular arrangement of the fibres is accentuated at the junctions with the uterine tubes and the cervix (internal os) thus providing closures to the expanding pregnant uterus

3 *Outer layer*: combination of longitudinal and circular fibres

below the clitoris (see Fig. 2.14). The vagina does not have glands but is maintained in a moist state by secretions from the cervical glands and transudate of fluid from the blood vessels that lie below the vaginal lining.

The external genitalia

The external genitalia are those structures that can be seen (Fig. 2.14). Most of the structures are well innervated; therefore they are very sensitive and are a source of sexual arousal responses. The external genitalia are well vascularized, which means they bleed easily if subjected to trauma but also heal rapidly.

The mons veneris is a pad of subcutaneous fat covered by skin lying over the pubic bone; it functions as

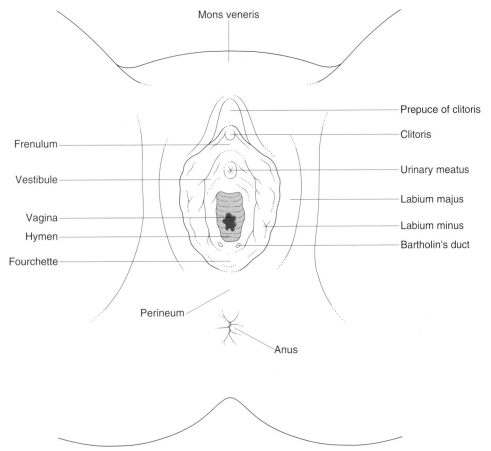

Mons veneris

Prepuce of clitoris

Clitoris

Urinary meatus

Labium majus

Labium minus

Bartholin's duct

Frenulum

Vestibule

Vagina

Hymen

Fourchette

Perineum

Anus

Fig. 2.14 *The female external genitalia.*

a cushion during intercourse. At puberty it becomes covered with pubic hair, which is coarse and curly because of the unusually oblique hair follicles. The labia majora (singular: labium majus) are two fatty folds of tissue extending from the mons veneris in which the round ligaments terminate. The labia majora narrow where they come together between the vagina and anus. The outer surface is covered in pubic hair; the inner surface is rich in sebaceous and sweat glands. The labia majora enclose and protect the urogenital cleft. The labia minora are two smaller longitudinal fleshy folds of tissue; they are erectile and very vascular. They are pigmented, hairless and have some sweat and sebaceous glands. The labia minora enclose the clitoris anteriorly and unite posteriorly at the fourchette, which is commonly torn at the first delivery. The functions of the labia minora are probably to increase the depth of the vaginal canal during intercourse and to increase retention of the ejaculate following intercourse.

The clitoris is a highly sensitive erectile body that is about 2.5 cm long exteriorly but projects internally for up to 9 cm (O'Connell et al 1998) before diving into two arms, the crura, which extend around to the interior of the labia majora. The external part of the clitoris, the clitoral glans, is covered and protected by a fold of skin called the clitoral hood, or prepuce which is homologous with the foreskin in males. The erectile bodies, analogous to the spongy tissue structures of the penis, become erect and engorged on stimulation. The clitoris is an important source of sexual arousal, generating reflex lubrication responses from the surrounding tissue. When the labia are held open, the vestibule (area from clitoris to fourchette) can be seen. It contains the external orifice of the urethra. This urinary meatus lies about 2.5 cm below the clitoris and is a characteristic vertical slit with prominent margins. It is important to identify this in women requiring catheterization of the bladder. To each side, slightly behind the urinary meatus, are the dimple-like exits of the Skene's ducts, which produce mucus. The vaginal orifice is partly occluded by the protective hymen, which is probably most important in preventing ascending infection before puberty when the pH of the vagina is less acidic. The Bartholin's glands lie posteriorly, each side of the vagina. These mucus-producing glands are the size and shape of haricot beans and, unless inflamed, cannot normally be seen. Their rate of secretion increases with the erection of the clitoris. The vestibular bulb posterior to the vagina is also formed of erectile spongy tissue.

Box 2.7 describes an example of problems caused by mutilation of the external genitalia.

The pelvic floor

The pelvic floor is composed primarily of the muscle fibres of the levator ani and soft tissues suspended within the outlet of the pelvis, forming a sling-like sheet of tissue that encloses and supports the pelvic

---

Box 2.8

Functions and characteristics of the pelvic floor

- Its muscles are arranged in two layers: superficial and deep (see Fig. 2.15)
- It supports and maintains the anatomical position of the internal female reproductive organs
- It provides voluntary muscle control for micturition and defecation
- It facilitates birth by resisting descent of the descending presenting part, so forcing the fetus to rotate forward in the presence of strong regular uterine contractions. The human pelvic floor plays an essential role in delivery as the fetus would not otherwise be able to rotate to negotiate its passage through the pelvic girdle due to the morphology of the pelvis influenced by the evolution of our upright stance.

---

contents (Box 2.8). In women, the main characteristic distinguishing it from that of the pelvic floor of the male is that there are three openings instead of two. As well as the anal canal and urethra, the female also has a vaginal opening. This is why women are much more likely to suffer from pelvic inflammatory disease (PID) as there is a direct route from the external environment via the genital tract, uterine cavity and uterine tubes to the internal pelvic cavity lined by the peritoneum.

Pelvic shape and adaptation

The pelvis is a girdle composed of a number of bones held together by ligaments and cartilaginous and fused joints (Fig. 2.16). The dimensions of the inlet, cavity and outlet affect the passage of the fetus. This means that the fetus has to negotiate the pelvic cavity by undergoing a rotational manoeuvre. The sling-like arrangement of the gutter-shaped pelvic floor muscles means that the fetus is forced to rotate in a forward position. This arrangement has evolved due to humans adopting an upright stance.

The female pelvis is wider and shallower than the male pelvis. Each half of the pelvis is known as the innominate bone, which is composed of ilium, ischium and pubic. Traditionally pelvic morphology has distinguished four major categories (Fig. 2.17). In prac-

---

Box 2.7

Female genital mutilation ('female circumcision')

Many ethnic groups, particularly those of Muslim origin in North Africa, Indonesia and other countries, regard female genital mutilation as essential to moderate sexual desire or to increase hygiene. The surgery, performed in infancy, early childhood or puberty, may involve removal of the prepuce of the clitoris, removal of the labia minora and clitoris or removal of most of the labia and clitoris. The procedures may be carried out without anaesthetics and under unclean conditions such as using thorns to form stitches of the vaginal walls which increase the risks of infection, scarring and infertility. Genital mutilation may be accompanied by infibulation, the surgical closure of the labia majora (apart from a small opening for urine and menses) to ensure chastity. Although the practices are unacceptable and illegal in Western Europe, they may be undertaken illicitly or girls may be mutilated in other countries. At delivery, the urogenital tissue is extremely vulnerable to trauma, which can be minimized by anterior and mediolateral episiotomy incision. Failure to deliver vaginally may result in rejection of the woman from her family.

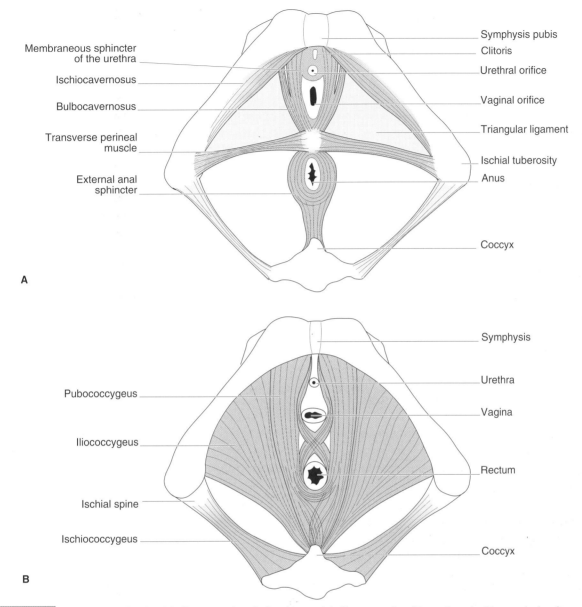

Membraneous sphincter of the urethra

Ischiocavernosus

Bulbocavernosus

Transverse perineal muscle

External anal sphincter

Symphysis pubis
Clitoris
Urethral orifice
Vaginal orifice
Triangular ligament
Ischial tuberosity
Anus
Coccyx

A

Pubococcygeus

Iliococcygeus

Ischial spine

Ischiococcygeus

Symphysis
Urethra
Vagina
Rectum
Coccyx

B

Fig. 2.15 *A the superficial pelvic floor muscles; B the deep pelvic floor muscles. (Reproduced with permission from Bennett & Brown 1999.)*

tice, there is a wide variation in pelvic form combining features from all four of the categories. There are also recognized abnormalities of the pelvis including justominor pelvis (normal shape but overall dimensions smaller than normal), Nägele's pelvis (asymmetrical due to abnormal bone formation on one side), and Robert's pelvis (similar to Nägele's pelvis but the abnormal bone formation is bilateral). Pelvic shape can also be affected by disease, for example rachitic pelvis due to rickets, which is an extreme form of the platypelloid pelvis. The shape of the pelvis affects the

mechanism of labour (see Ch. 13); abnormal pelvic shape is associated with problems at delivery as the rotation of the presenting part may be suboptimal.

The male reproductive tract

The male reproductive tract comprises a number of structures that permit gamete formation to occur below body temperature and provide conditions that allow sperm maturation and ejection (Fig. 2.18).

A

Cavity shallow
Outlet wide

Sacral promontory
is not prominent

Curved sacrum

Smooth ischial spines

Rounded brim

Sub-pubic angle 90°

B

Crest of ilium

Posterior superior iliac spine

Anterior superior iliac spine

Posterior inferior iliac spine

Greater sciatic notch

Ischial spine

Lesser sciatic notch

Symphysis pubis
Obturator foramen
Inferior ramus of pubic bone

Ischial tuberosity

Inferior ramus of ischium

C

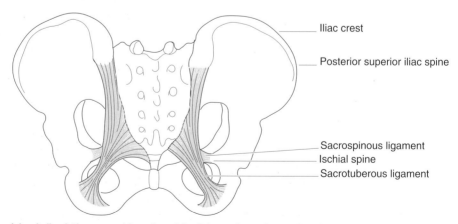

Iliac crest

Posterior superior iliac spine

Sacrospinous ligament
Ischial spine
Sacrotuberous ligament

Fig. 2.16 *The pelvic girdle: A the normal female pelvis; B innominate bone showing important landmarks; C posterior view of the pelvis to show ligaments. (Reproduced with permission from Bennett & Brown 1999.)*

Gynaecoid

Android

Anthropoid

Platypelloid (flat)

Fig. 2.17 *Characteristics of the four categories of pelvic shape.*

The testes

The testes are suspended within the scrotal sac or scrotum. Optimal spermatogenesis in the human is achieved 2–3°C below the body's core temperature. There are a number of mechanisms to regulate the temperature of the testes. The testes are suspended outside the abdominal cavity but can be retracted upwards towards the warmth of the body by contrac-

tion of the cremaster muscle which covers the testes. This muscle will also reflexly raise the testes towards the body if the inner thigh is stroked or scratched; this cremaster reflex is used as a neurological test. The pigmented skin of the scrotum lies in rugae (folds), which increase the surface area. The scrotum is well vascularized but has no insulating hair or subcutaneous fat. It is lined by dartos muscle, which contracts in response to cold. Blood flow to the testes allows heat to be transferred from the descending testicular arteries to the ascending pampiniform venous plexus forming a countercurrent heat-exchange mechanism, which helps to maintain the lower temperature of the testes relative to the body.

The testes are a pair of glandular organs, analogous to the ovaries, that produce gametes (spermatozoa) and male sex hormones. Within the scrotum, the testes are surrounded by a thick fibrous capsule called the tunica albuginea, which penetrates internally dividing the testes into lobules. Each testis has about 200 lobules, each containing about three seminiferous tubules, about 0.2 mm in diameter and up to 70 cm long (Fig. 2.19). The seminiferous tubules are the site of spermatogenesis (sperm production). Within the tubules are spermatogenic cells and their supporting Sertoli cells. Between the tubules are the interstitial cells of Leydig, which produce testosterone.

The sperm produced from the seminiferous tubules are stored in the epididymis where they are concentrated, becoming mature and motile. The epididymis is a comma-shaped convoluted tube, about 6 cm long, leading into the vas deferens. The vas deferens provides the conduit for sperm delivery during emission and ejaculation. It is a thick-walled tube leading from the tail of the epididymis to the ejaculatory duct. The vas deferens dilates into a storage reservoir, or ampulla, just before it joins with the exit of the seminal vesicle to form the ejaculatory duct. Just as infection or trauma can cause blockage of the uterine tubes, the male reproductive capacity can be also affected by blockage, of the epididymis or vas deferens for instance, impeding the passage of spermatozoa. The vas deferens, blood vessels and cremaster muscle lie closely together forming the spermatic cord.

The seminal vesicles are two pyramid-shaped membranous sacs, about 4 cm long, lying between the base of the bladder and the rectum. They produce semen, a fructose-rich viscous fluid, which facilitates sperm transport and nourishment. Secretory activity of the seminal vesicles depends on the level of testosterone. The ejaculatory ducts begin at the base of the prostate

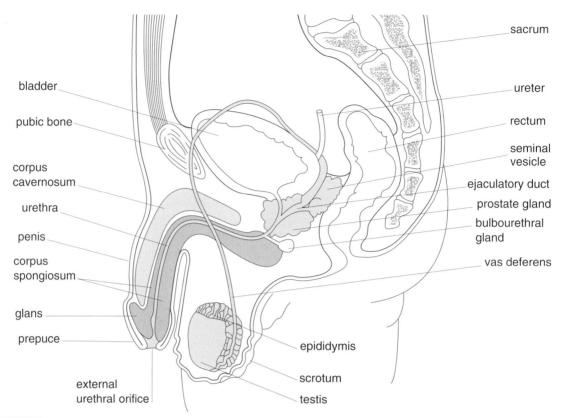

bladder

pubic bone

corpus cavernosum

urethra

penis

corpus spongiosum

glans

prepuce

external urethral orifice

sacrum

ureter

rectum

seminal vesicle

ejaculatory duct

prostate gland

bulbourethral gland

vas deferens

epididymis

scrotum

testis

Fig. 2.18 *The male reproductive system. (Reproduced with permission from Brooker 1998.)*

gland and terminate in the single prostatic urethra. These muscular ducts carry sperm and seminal fluid through the prostate gland. The prostate gland is a walnut-sized exocrine gland lying just below the neck of the bladder, between the rectum and pubic bone. It is a compound gland, formed of about 20–40 smaller glandular units each with its own exit into the ejaculatory duct. Prostatic fluid is a thin lubricating secretion that mixes with the sperm and seminal fluid. The prostatic gland can be palpated through the rectal wall. In elderly men, the prostate gland may undergo hypertrophy causing benign prostatic hyperplasia which can compress the urethra and impede micturition. Prostatitis or inflammation of the prostate gland can affect men of all ages. Prostatic carcinoma is one of the most common cancers affecting elderly men in developed countries; it is a major cause of death if it is not detected early. Prior to ejaculation, the bulbo-urethral glands (or Cowper's glands) secrete clear lubricating fluid into the urethra just below the prostate gland.

The penis carries the urethra, which provides a shared passage for sperm and urine, and allows intro-

mission: the delivery of sperm into the vagina. Unlike other mammalian species, the human penis does not have an erectile bone and relies entirely on engorgement to achieve erection; it also cannot be withdrawn into the groin. Humans have one of the largest penis:body size ratios. The penis has three columns of erectile tissue: two lateral corpora cavernosa and a ventromedial corpus spongiosum (Fig. 2.20). The corpus spongiosum contains the urethra and does not engorge as much as the corpora cavernosa. This prevents trauma to the urethra and generates an appropriate angle for intromission. The expanded cone-shaped end of the corpus spongiosum forms the glans penis where the urethra opens. The penis is covered with a fold of skin or prepuce (foreskin), which can be retracted in an adult and older child to expose the glans. The foreskin attaches to the underside of the penis at a small fold of tissue called the frenum. The prepuce and shaft skin are not attached to underlying tissue so they are free to glide along the shaft of the penis, which reduces friction, abrasion and loss of lubricating fluid during intercourse. On the underside of the penis, there is a small ridge called the raphe

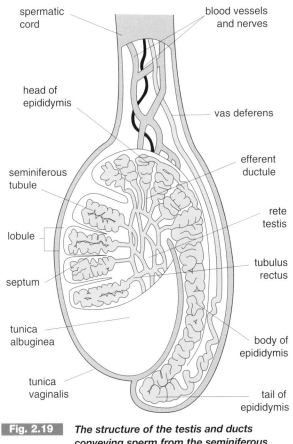

Labels (left figure):
- spermatic cord
- blood vessels and nerves
- head of epididymis
- vas deferens
- seminiferous tubule
- efferent ductule
- rete testis
- lobule
- tubulus rectus
- septum
- tunica albuginea
- body of epididymis
- tunica vaginalis
- tail of epididymis

Fig. 2.19 *The structure of the testis and ducts conveying sperm from the seminiferous tubules to the urethra. (Reproduced with permission from Brooker 1998.)*

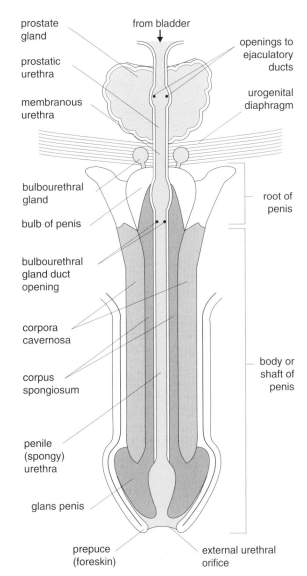

Labels (right figure):
- prostate gland
- from bladder
- openings to ejaculatory ducts
- prostatic urethra
- urogenital diaphragm
- membranous urethra
- bulbourethral gland
- root of penis
- bulb of penis
- bulbourethral gland duct opening
- corpora cavernosa
- body or shaft of penis
- corpus spongiosum
- penile (spongy) urethra
- glans penis
- prepuce (foreskin)
- external urethral orifice

which runs from the opening of the urethra across the scrotum to the perineum (between the scrotum and anus). The spongy bodies of the penis become distended with blood during an erection (see Ch. 6).

Fig. 2.20 *Internal structure of the penis.*

Gametogenesis

The process of gametogenesis is achieved through a specialized form of cellular division called meiosis (Fig. 2.21). The stages of meiosis are reviewed in Chapter 7. Gametogenesis is remarkably different in the male and female reproductive systems, both representing adaptation of the process of meiosis to facilitate reproduction. Gametes are specialized sex cells that contain half the genetic material of the normal cell content. Their fusion, referred to as fertilization, is described in detail in Chapter 6.

The production of spermatozoa begins at puberty in the male and results in the continual production of millions of sperm. Spermatozoa have completed all the meiotic divisions prior to ejaculation and fusion with the oocyte. In this sense, they are true gametes containing the haploid number of chromosomes. (These terms are explained in Ch. 4.)

The differences between gamete formation have evolved with the development of sexual reproduction and internal fertilization. Oocytes are relatively protected within the abdominal cavity and so it is not necessary for a large number to be produced. Movement of oocytes is passive, influenced by the structure of the uterine tube. Sperm, in contrast, must become highly motile in order to travel along the female reproductive tract. Many are lost and, of the millions contained

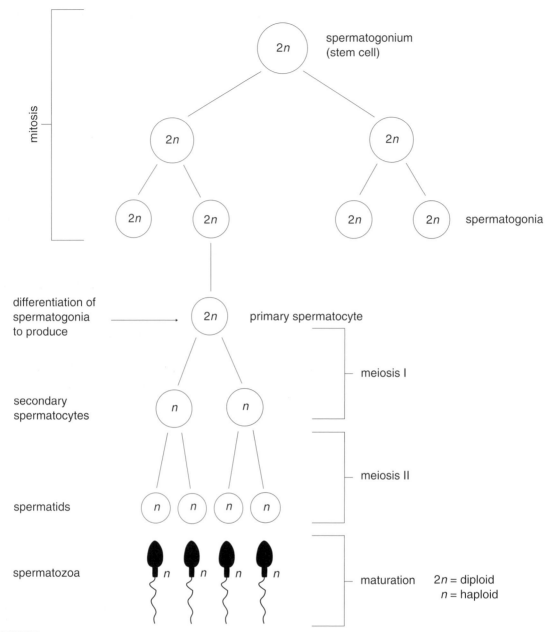

spermatogonium
(stem cell)

mitosis

spermatogonia

differentiation of
spermatogonia
to produce

primary spermatocyte

meiosis I

secondary
spermatocytes

meiosis II

spermatids

spermatozoa

maturation $2n$ = diploid
n = haploid

Fig. 2.21   *Gametogenesis. (Reproduced with permission from Brooker 1998.)*

within the ejaculate, only a few hundred will make it to the vicinity of the oocyte.

Spermatogenesis

Spermatogenesis begins at puberty and continues into senescence, albeit less efficiently. The primitive germ cells, around the inner circumference of the seminifer-

ous tubule, divide and replicate by a process called mitosis (see Ch. 4), forming many spermatogonia (Fig. 2.22). Each spermatogonium first divides into two diploid primary spermatocytes. The primary spermatocytes then undergo meiosis producing two haploid and genetically diverse secondary spermatocytes and then, after the second meiotic division, four haploid spermatids. For each cell undergoing meiosis, therefore, four gametes are produced. The spermatids undergo spermiogenesis (nuclear and cytoplasmic changes) producing the characteristic morphology (shape) of a spermatozoon. As meiosis progresses, the immature sperm are supported within nurse-like Sertoli cells (see Box 2.9), which move them into the lumen of the seminiferous tubule.

The spermatozoa are stored in the epididymis where they mature for 2 weeks and may stay for up to 6 months. The shortest time between the initial meiosis and ejaculation is about 10 weeks, which is therefore the critical preconception period in men. Spermatogenesis is affected by temperature, malnutrition, alcohol, cottonseed oil (a potential source of contraception), some drugs and heavy metals.

Steroidogenesis

The interstitial cells of Leydig interspersed between the seminiferous tubules produce 90% of the circulating testosterone (the remainder has an adrenal origin). Testosterone is responsible for male secondary sex characteristics (see Ch. 3) and, together with FSH, controls production of sperm. Testosterone production is stimulated by luteinizing hormone (LH) from the pituitary gland (Fig. 2.23). Testosterone binds to androgen binding protein (ABP) in the seminiferous

Box 2.9

The role of Sertoli cells

- Support spermatogenic cells and move them inwards
- Provide nutrients to spermatocytes and spermatids (hence their former name of 'nurse cells')
- Secrete fluid to aid release of sperm into lumen
- Act as a barrier between sperm-producing areas and lumen
- Engulf and digest cellular debris left from spermiogenesis
- Produce inhibin, which inhibits follicle-stimulating hormone (FSH) secretion
- Produce androgen-binding protein (ABP), which increases seminiferous tubule testosterone concentration
- Produce Müllerian-inhibiting hormone (MIH), which affects sexual differentiation (see Ch. 5)

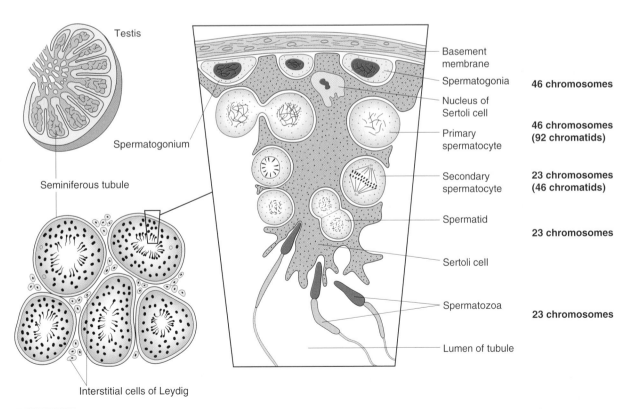

Fig. 2.22   *Spermatogenesis, showing cell stages and chromosome numbers.*

tubules, which means that testosterone levels within the tubule can be very high while maintaining a concentration gradient that drives diffusion from outside to inside. Testosterone exerts a negative feedback mechanism on the hypothalamic–pituitary axis in a manner analogous to the feedback control by oestrogen in the female cycle (see Ch. 4). FSH stimulates the production of ABP by the Sertoli cells. Inhibin produced from the Sertoli cells inhibits FSH production. Illness and stress affect male reproductive capacity probably via the hypothalamic–pituitary axis.

Control of gametogenesis

The control of gametogenesis and steroidogenesis in the male and female have some similarities. The hypothalamus regulates reproduction by secreting gonadotrophin-releasing hormone (GnRH) (see Fig. 2.23). This stimulates both FSH and LH produc-

tion from the anterior pituitary gland. FSH stimulates gametogenesis: spermatogenesis in males and follicular development in females. Luteinizing hormone plays a pivotal role in steroidogenesis: increasing testosterone production from the Leydig cells in males and stimulating the increases in progesterone and oestrogen secretion in the second half of the menstrual cycle in females (see Ch. 4).

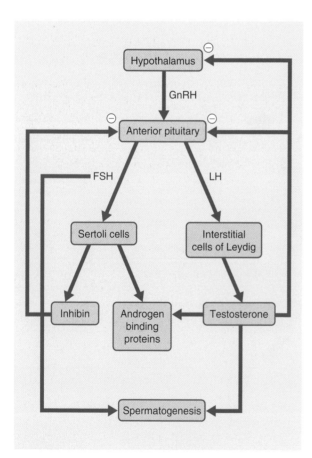

Fig. 2.23 *Production of testosterone.*

■ The hypothalamus regulates reproduction by secreting gonadotrophin-releasing hormone (GnRH), which stimulates production of FSH and LH from the anterior pituitary, which in turn have effects on the gonads. The sex steroids produced by the gonads exert negative feedback inhibition at the hypothalamic-pituitary axis.

Application to practice

Why is an in-depth knowledge of the female genitalia required by the midwife and how will this knowledge affect the decisions made by the midwife within practice?

You might consider what the midwife needs to know in order to suture the peritoneum, to catheterize a woman during labour or to recognize the sex of a baby at birth (see Ch. 5). There are many signs and 'symptoms' in pregnancy that are indicative of changes occurring within the renal system; knowledge of this will help the midwife to explain these fully to the woman.

During routine antenatal check-ups the midwife routinely performs urinalysis. Are you able to explain the significance of the findings as a whole or do you think it is appropriate that midwives just observe for evidence of proteinuria?

The hormones of pregnancy affect muscle tone and relax ligaments so bladder control is often less effective in pregnancy and these effects may continue after pregnancy. In such cases muscle tone can be improved by encouraging pelvic floor exercises to promote optimal continence following childbirth. Displacement of the pelvic organs resulting in anterior and posterior prolapses become increasingly common the higher the parity due to the loss of effective muscle tone and ligament support, and so pelvic floor exercises should be encouraged to minimize these problems.

Annotated further reading

Datta S 2003 Crash course: renal and urinary systems. Mosby, St Louis
This well-illustrated book provides a useful reference text for students requiring more details of the renal and urinary systems.

Johnson MH, Everitt BJ 2000 Essential reproduction, 5th edn. Blackwell Science, Oxford
An integrated and well-organized research-based textbook that explores comparative reproductive physiology of mammals, including anatomy, physiology, endocrinology, genetics and behavioural studies.

Raynor MD, Morgan M 2000 Female genital mutilation: unveiled and deconstructed. In: Fraser D (ed) 2000 Professional studies for midwifery practice. Churchill Livingstone, Edinburgh
This chapter gives an excellent overview of female genital mutilation, the different classifications and prevalence and explores racial, ethnic and cultural aspects of this phenomenon. Guidance is provided for the midwifery care of women who have undergone mutilation and the health problems related to these practices.

Royal College of Obstetrics and Gynaecology (RCOG) 1999 The management of tubal pregnancies (clinical guideline 21). RCOG, London
This guideline provides a detailed account of methotrexate in the non-surgical management of ectopic pregnancy.

Readers also are recommended to read chapters on the renal and reproductive systems in a physiology textbook, such as those listed at the end of the previous chapter.

References

Bennett VR, Brown LK 1999 Myles' textbook for midwives, 13th edn. Churchill Livingstone, Edinburgh, pp 940, 941, 942, 949
Bogin B 1999 Patterns of human growth, 2nd edition. Cambridge University Press, Cambridge
Brooker CG 1998 Human structure and function, 2nd edn. Mosby, St Louis, pp 344, 345, 363, 470, 471, 473, 476, 483
O'Connell HE, Hutson JM, Anderson CR, Plenter RJ 1998 Anatomical relationship between urethra and clitoris. Journal of Urology 159:1892–1897
Sweet B 1996 Mayes' midwifery, 12th edn. Baillière Tindall, London, p 29

3 Endocrinology

Learning objectives

- To introduce the terminology used within endocrinology.
- To define the different types of hormones, their functions, main sites of production and mechanism of effects.
- To describe the role of the sex steroids.
- To relate endocrinology to the physiological process of reproduction.

Introduction

This chapter presents an overview of endocrinology and summarizes the role of hormones in the regulation of human physiology. Throughout the chapter, links to reproductive physiology will be highlighted and referenced to other chapters in the book where the relevant interactions will be described more specifically.

The endocrine system, in conjunction with the nervous system, coordinates, regulates and adjusts the internal physiology in response to changes in the external environment. The nervous system tends to react in situations where an immediate response is required, whereas the endocrine system is involved in sustaining body functions over a longer period (Table 3.1). For example, shivering is induced by neuromuscular activity to counteract a drop in the environmental temperature, whereas many body cycles, such as the menstrual cycle, are almost entirely orchestrated through hormonal systems. However, the two systems interact with one another and so some rapid responses have a hormonal component. For instance, the release of adrenaline and the fear–fight–flight reflex and hormonal release are often regulated by a neuronal pathway via the hypothalamus. The advantage of the endocrine system over the nervous system is that it can instigate a much more diffuse response in all body tissues at about the same time and coordinate integrated responses.

Chapter case study

Zara is now just 6 weeks pregnant. She feels concerned about feeling increasingly nauseated, especially late in the evening; she actually vomited last night. Zara rings you, as her midwife, the next day expressing her concern, especially since her sister has told her that this is not the typical morning sickness of pregnancy. What explanations could you give Zara to the likely cause of her nausea and what advice should you give her to help her cope with her nausea? How is nausea and vomiting of pregnancy differentiated from hyperemesis gravidarum? What are the possible complications of hyperemesis and what specific treatment is required to minimize complications?

What is endocrinology?

The endocrine system originally appeared to be a relatively simple system of discrete glands (Fig. 3.1) that secreted chemical messengers, or hormones, into the blood where they would be carried to specific target cells at a distant site, inducing a reaction. However, it is now clear that the endocrine system is more complex. Some organs that have other functions also produce hormones. For instance, the atrium of the heart produces atrial natriuretic peptide (ANP), which inhibits reabsorption of sodium chloride in the kidneys and hence affects blood pressure. Some hormones are produced by several different glands, for instance somatostatin, which is produced by the

Table 3.1 *Comparison of the nervous and endocrine systems*

	Nervous system	Endocrine system
Source of signal	Brain	Endocrine gland
Signal	Neurotransmitter and action potential	Hormone
Usual route	Efferent nerve	Blood
Response rate	Fast	Slow
Specificity	Specific	Diffuse
Target	Single	Multiple
Type of effect	Immediate effect	Long-term control and integration

hypothalamus, pancreas, stomach and intestine. Although the trophoblast is the prime site of human chorionic gonadotrophin (hCG) production, it can also be produced by other tissues, albeit in very low concentrations (Iles & Chard 1991). The placenta appears to be capable of synthesizing a very broad range of hormones and releasing factors that interact with both maternal and fetal physiology. Some substances such as noradrenaline can act as both hormone and neurotransmitter depending on their mode of delivery and whether they are released from a gland or from a nerve. The hypothalamus produces neurohormones that are important in the interaction between the endocrine and nervous systems.

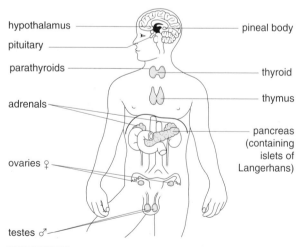

hypothalamus — pineal body
pituitary
parathyroids — thyroid
— thymus
adrenals
— pancreas (containing islets of Langerhans)
ovaries ♀
testes ♂

Fig. 3.1 *The endocrine glands. (Reproduced with permission from Brooker 1998.)*

Overall, the endocrine system (in partnership with the neural system):

- coordinates the homeostatic balance
- regulates various physiological systems such as the digestive system and reproductive system
- facilitates differentiation of the sexes in the embryonic stage and the manifestation of the secondary sexual characteristics at puberty
- modifies and induces behavioural changes within the individual.

The evolution of endocrinology

The evolution of the endocrine system has its rudiments within the activity of single-cell (unicellular) organisms. The unicellular organisms developed the ability to be attracted to chemicals, described as a chemotactic response, or to chemicals that were vital for the functioning of the organism, described as a chemotrophic response. Equally, these organisms developed the ability to recognize noxious chemicals (toxins) and were thus able to avoid them. The cell reacting to chemical signals interacting with receptor sites upon the cell membrane and within the cytoplasm led to the development of active mobility.

As multicellular organisms developed, the group of unicellular organisms that were the prototypes of multicellular organisms evolved chemical communication as an extension of the chemotrophic response. As multicellular evolution progressed further, the cells became more differentiated and specialized. Regulation therefore became the function of more specialized types of cells. This is reflected in the developmental sequence of a fetus, beginning with the division of a single cell (see Ch. 7). With each successive division, the resulting cells are slightly different from the original zygote cell (although differentiation during the initial divisions may be induced by the presence of maternally derived factors within the cytoplasm of the zygote). Although this differentiation is primarily under genetic control, it is achieved through a process of induction from chemical signals produced by one cell type that influence the division of other neighbouring cells. The altered gene expression of the dividing cells results in a changed morphology and developmental pathway.

As organisms became larger and more complex, cell-to-cell communication became more complicated.

It evolved in two ways: the endocrine system (of chemical transmission via the circulating blood system) and the neural system (via transmission of an action potential; see Ch. 1). Under the traditional approach to biological science, the endocrine and neural systems were always considered in isolation; however, they are now considered to be extensions of the same system that are highly interactive. Many endocrine responses are initiated by a neuronal influence. Many neurotransmitters and neuromodulators have also been found to be endocrine hormones.

Classification of hormones

Hormones regulate metabolism, activate or inhibit the immune system, stimulate or inhibit growth, induce or suppress apoptosis (see below), and prepare the body to respond (such as fleeing or fighting) or undergo transition to a new stage of life such as puberty, pregnancy or the menopause. Hormones are produced by almost every organ and type of tissue; they function as cellular messengers. The action of hormones depends on the responses of the target cells and the pattern of hormonal secretion. Endocrine means 'secreted inwards' and is applied to hormones that fit the classical description of being secreted into the bloodstream and having an effect at a distant target. There are also exocrine hormones, which are 'secreted outwards' into ducts. These include hormones that are secreted into the vas deferens and uterine tubes.

A number of hormones have a local or paracrine effect, diffusing short distances to act on neighbouring cells or cells separated only by an intracellular space. Examples of a paracrine response are the effects of testosterone and Müllerian-inhibiting hormone (also known as Müllerian-inhibiting substance, MIS) on sexual differentiation (see Ch. 5). If the hormone produced acts upon the same cell that produced it, it is described as autocrine. For example, an autocrine hormone may induce cellular division or signal the programmed death of the cell (apoptosis). If it affects adjacent cells, it is described as a juxtacrine hormone.

Neuroendocrine hormones are synthesized in specialized neurons, and their effects can also be paracrine in nature (these are usually described as neurotransmitters and neuromodulators). Oxytocin is an example of a neuroendocrine hormone. It is released from the posterior lobe of the pituitary gland and influences the contractility of the myometrium (see Ch. 13) and myoepithelial cells in the breast (see

Ch. 16). In these respects, oxytocin has an endocrine effect, but in many mammals it also modifies female behaviour by inducing parental behaviour in the presence of the sex steroids (Insel 1992).

A pheromone is a hormone produced by one organism that induces a response within another. Releaser pheromones stimulate rapid behavioural responses. Primer pheromones act via the neuroendocrine system to produce delayed responses. Receptors for pheromones are found on the vomeronasal organ close to the nasal cavity of mammals, which use pheromones to indicate identity of kin or family territory. It is controversial as to whether the human vomeronasal organ retains a function; some scientists think it is involved in social behaviour such as pair bonding, parental attachment, sexual attraction and synchrony of menstrual cycles (Halpern & Martinez-Marcos 2003).

Secretion of hormones is influenced by a number of factors, including the nervous system, hormone-binding proteins, plasma concentrations of nutrients and ions, environmental changes and other hormones, such as stimulating and releasing hormones.

Hormone structure

Hormones can be classified according to their structure (see Table 3.2). Steroid hormones and eicosanoids (the prostaglandin family of hormones) are lipids. The other classes are protein and peptide hormones and monoamines.

Steroid hormones

The steroid group of hormones consists of the sex steroids, the glucocorticoids, mineralocorticoids, thyroid hormones and 1,25-dihydroxyvitamin D_3. Steroid hormones are derived from cholesterol and acetate (Fig. 3.2). As well as being the precursor for the steroid hormones, cholesterol is also an important structural component of cell membranes.

The first and common step in the biosynthesis of sex steroids is the formation of pregnenolone, which is rate-limiting, and therefore important in controlling production of sex steroids. Pregnenolone is produced on the inner mitochondrial membrane whereas the next stages take place in the smooth endoplasmic reticulum (SER).

The three classes of sex steroids are structurally related, which offers the opportunity for interconversion. This means that a genetic defect in one of the

Table 3.2 *Classification of hormones and examples*

Lipid hormones	Steroid hormones	Sex steroids e.g. androgens, oestrogens and progestogens
		Glucocorticoids e.g. cortisol
		Mineralocorticoids e.g. aldosterone
		Thyroid hormones
		1,25-Dihydrovitamin D$_3$
	Eicosanoids	Prostaglandins
		Leukotrienes
Protein hormones	Gonadotrophic glycoproteins	Follicle-stimulating hormone (FSH)
		Luteinizing hormone (LH)
		Human chorionic gonadotrophin (hCG)
		Thyroid-stimulating hormone (TSH)
	Somatotrophic polypeptides	Prolactin (PRL)
		Human placental lactogen (hPL)
		Growth hormone (GH)
	Cytokines	Insulin
		Activins and inhibins
		Müllerian-inhibiting hormone (MIH)
		Interferons
		Growth factors
Small peptides		Gonadotrophin-releasing hormone (GnRH)
		Oxytocin (OXY)
		Antidiuretic hormone (ADH or vasopressin)
		β-Endorphin
		Vasoactive intestinal peptide (VIP)
Monoamines	Catecholamines	Adrenaline, noradrenaline and dopamine
		Melatonin
		Dopamine

Adapted from Johnson & Everitt 1995.

steps can result not only in a deficiency of the normal amount of the product but also in an excess of another sex steroid. For instance, a genetic deficiency of the enzyme that converts 17α-hydroxyprogesterone to the precursor of cortisol results in increased levels of 17α-hydroxyprogesterone, which is converted into androstenedione and then into androgens. The unusu-

ally high level of androgens can cause masculinization of the female fetus. These structural similarities mean that the steroid hormones can affect the activity of other steroid hormones by exerting agonistic and antagonistic properties (see below). However, the effects of the hormones vary depending on their structure (see Table 3.3).

The main role of androgens is in the development and maintenance of masculine characteristics and fertility. Similarly, the dominant role of oestrogens is in development and maintenance of feminine characteristics and fertility. The key role for progesterone is the preparation for pregnancy and its maintenance.

As steroid hormones are lipid-soluble, they are able to diffuse freely across the cell membrane. In the cytoplasm, the steroid hormones may be altered. The receptor sites for thyroid hormone and the sex steroids are within the nucleus. Specific receptors for the other steroid hormones are within the cytoplasm; binding usually results in cleavage of smaller 'heat-shock' proteins from the receptors. Steroid hormones exert their effect by altering ribonucleic acid (RNA) synthesis and subsequent protein synthesis (Box 3.1). The steroid-receptor ligand binds to specific segments of DNA in promoter regions of the gene in that section of DNA, affecting the rate of transcription and gene expression. Protein synthesis can be increased (or decreased) within 30 minutes, so the effects of steroid hormones are therefore relatively slow in action compared with those of protein hormones. The term 'anabolic steroids' describes the effect of steroid hormones in influencing new tissue growth.

The other class of lipid hormones is the eicosanoids, which have an important role in reproduction. They are formed from an arachidonic acid precursor, generated by the activity of either phospholipase C or phospholipase A$_2$ (Fig. 3.3). Arachidonic acid production appears to be the rate-limiting step. Phospholipase A$_2$ is present in an inactive form in lysosomes in cells that are released if the cell membranes become unstable. Most tissues of the body including the myometrium, cervix, ovary, placenta and fetal membranes synthesize prostaglandins. They have a short half-life and are metabolized quickly. They have an important role in amplifying signals at the onset of labour (see Ch. 13). Leukotrienes are also synthesized from arachidonic acid by the enzyme 5-lipoxygenase in leukocytes and macrophages. They are involved in inflammatory reactions particularly in asthma and allergy and also seem to be important in pregnancy.

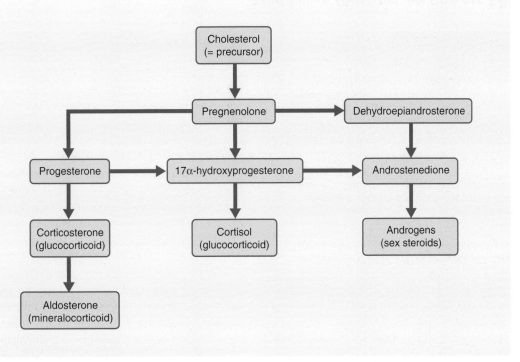

Fig. 3.2 *Steroid hormone production.*

Table 3.3 *Biological activity and effects of the sex steroids*

Sex steroid	Family members (and approximate biological activity)	Main effects
Androgens	5α-dihydrotestosterone (100%) Testosterone (50%) Androstenedione (8%) Dehydroepiandrosterone (4%)	Differentiation of male embryo Secondary sex characteristics Spermatogenesis Sexual and aggressive behaviour Growth promoting, protein anabolism, ossification and erythropoiesis
Oestrogens	Oestradiol-17β (E$_2$) (100%) Oestriol (E$_3$) (10%) Oestrone (E$_1$) (1%)	Female secondary sex characteristics Prepares uterus for ovulation and fertilization Vascular effects—increased blood flow, neovascularization Growth-promoting effects on endometrium and breasts Primes endometrium for progesterone action Mildly anabolic Increases calcification of bones May be associated with sexual behaviour
Progestogens	Progesterone (100%) 17α-hydroxyprogesterone (17α-OHP) (40–70%) 20α-hydroxyprogesterone (5%)	Prepares uterus for pregnancy Maintains pregnancy Stimulates glandular growth of breasts Affects sodium and water excretion Mildly catabolic Relaxes smooth muscle tone Affects appetite and thirst, metabolic rate, sensitivity to carbon dioxide

Adapted from Johnson & Everitt 1995.

Action of steroid hormones

- Transported in plasma bound to binding protein
- Hormone released and diffuses into target cell
- Hormone diffuses into nucleus
- Binds to specific receptor
- Affects DNA transcription
- Affects mRNA synthesis
- Affects protein synthesis
- Altered functional response of cell

Action of peptide hormones

- Binds to receptor on cell membrane
- Hormone-receptor complex
- Altered internal state
  - e.g. by opening ion channel in membrane
  - e.g. by affecting an enzyme such as tyrosine kinase which may phosphorylate (and activate) a protein
  - e.g. by activating a G-protein and causing calcium release
- Altered cell response

Protein, peptide and monoamine hormones

Protein and peptide hormones bind to receptors located on or within the cell membrane. They initiate plasma membrane depolarization and a cascade of second-messenger systems and chemical changes within the cytoplasm, generating a faster response than steroid hormones. They primarily affect the functioning of the cell by stimulation or inhibition. Their action is initiated through the activation of G-proteins located within the cell cytoplasm, which initiate various chemical reactions (Box 3.2). G-proteins may open ion channels or stimulate phosphorylation of internal proteins, thus generating the signalling cascade. Many peptide hormones function as neurotransmitters in the brain. The monoamine hormones are derivatives of the amino acids tryptophan and tyrosine.

Gonadotrophic glycoproteins

This group includes FSH, LH and hCG, all of which are structurally similar to thyroid-stimulating hormone (TSH). Their structure is a globular protein composed of two common chains and two unique chains with unique carbohydrate side-chains that bestow stability and biological activity. hCG is produced by the placental tissue, whereas the other gonadotrophic glycoproteins are produced by the anterior pituitary gland.

Somatomammotrophic polypeptides

This group of hormones includes prolactin (PRL), human placental lactogen (hPL) and growth hormone (GH), which have marked effects on tissue growth including the breasts. Their structure is a single polypeptide chain. PRL and hPL are involved with lactation. GH has a role in puberty including breast development. Although PRL and GH are pituitary hormones, the placenta also produces them in addition to hPL. However, the activity of the placental hormones is often not exactly the same as the pituitary hormones. For instance, placental GH has a higher affinity for the PRL receptor than does pituitary GH.

Cytokines

Cytokines are small polypeptide chains. There is a large number of cytokines including inhibin, activin, epidermal growth factors and MIS (see Chs 5 and 13). Cytokines have a broad range of activity. They are

Fig. 3.3 *Formation of eicosanoids.*

usually made in a variety of cell types rather than in a specific gland. Cytokines act on many different cell types, often interacting with and modulating each other's responses. Several cytokines have similar and overlapping functions. They usually have paracrine activity and often modulate or mediate the actions of other types of hormone. Cytokines act by binding to their specific receptors on the cell membrane; typically, these receptors are also tyrosine kinase (enzymes that transfer a phosphate group to a tyrosine residue of protein which then regulates the activity of other enzymes).

Small peptide hormones

This group of hormones includes gonadotrophin (GnRH), a decapeptide (i.e. a chain of 10 amino acids) from the hypothalamus, and other releasing hormones, oxytocin, antidiuretic hormone (ADH), β-endorphin (described in Ch. 13) and vasoactive intestinal peptide (VIP). Most of these small peptide hormones are initially produced in the form of pre-prohormones (large inactive polypeptide precursors). The prohormone is then processed in the endoplasmic reticulum to form prohormones. The processing may involve glycosylation (addition of polysaccharides) or removal of the N-terminal signal sequence. Prohormones often contain redundant amino acid residues that were required to direct the folding of the molecule into its active configuration but then have no further function. Endopeptidases cleave the prohormone thus producing the mature functional form of the hormone just before it is released from the cell. Some of the 'pro'-fragments of the prohormones also exert a biological effect.

Monoamine hormones

This group includes catecholamines (dopamine, adrenaline and noradrenaline) and melatonin, all of which are derived from tyrosine (an amino acid) and may have a role in neuroendocrine control mechanisms. The medulla of the adrenal gland is a modified sympathetic ganglion; its cell bodies release adrenaline and noradrenaline (in the ratio 4:1) into the blood. Its effects, therefore, augment sympathetic nervous system activity. Dopamine released from the hypothalamus affects prolactin secretion (see Ch. 16). Melatonin, from the pineal gland, may have a role in seasonal and environmental influences on reproductive capability, which are particularly important in species other than humans.

Hormone transport

Peptide and protein hormones are water-soluble and are carried dissolved in the blood, whereas steroid hormones circulate bound to plasma proteins. When hormones are secreted into the blood supply, a large proportion become protein-bound, leaving only a small proportion free (unbound and able to access the target cell) and physiologically active. There are many types of hormone-binding proteins, all of which are colloidal in nature. Some hormones bind with great affinity to specific proteins. Other proteins may bind to numerous different hormones with different affinity rates that may be affected by the concentration of the hormone. Therefore, the amount of hormone present may affect its activity. For instance, oxytocin at high concentrations binds to ADH (or vasopressin) receptors within the renal tubule. During labour, levels of oxytocin do not normally rise until the end of the first stage. However, exogenous oxytocin can be administered to augment uterine contractions. If the administration of oxytocin is high and prolonged, however, water retention can occur because oxytocin also stimulates the ADH receptors. This overlap in the biological activity of hormones is described as promiscuity.

Hormonal regulation

One of the most important functions of the endocrine system is maintenance of the internal environment. This 'steady' state is described as homeostasis (see Ch. 1). Homeostatic mechanisms buffer changes within the external environmental conditions. For example, mammals have evolved to be homeothermic (warm-blooded) so that the chemical processes essential for physiological function proceed under optimal conditions of temperature. Fluctuations in temperature are monitored and the homeostatic mechanisms ensure that body temperature is held within narrowly defined limits. Homeostasis is achieved through the integration of the neural system with the endocrine system, commonly referred to as feedback systems.

As mentioned above, hormonal release is often instigated by neurological stimulation. Hormone release may also be stimulated by another hormone. Factors that facilitate the release of hormones are referred to as positive influences and factors that inhibit the release of hormones are termed negative influences. The negative feedback tends to slow down a process and maintain stability whereas positive feedback tends to speed up a process and generate rapid change.

Positive feedback

Positive feedback describes a specialized chain of events involving one or more hormones in which there is a cycle of positive effects, amplifying the original signal (Fig. 3.4). An example of positive feedback is the maintained production of PRL secretion from the anterior pituitary gland during lactation. Suckling of the infant stimulates PRL secretion, which maintains lactation. If suckling decreases or stops then the amount of stimulation decreases and PRL production is reduced. Other examples of positive feedback include coagulation of blood and the hormonal control of parturition.

Negative feedback

Negative feedback describes a similar specialized chain of events involving one or more hormones, except here there is a cycle of negative influence (Fig. 3.4). An example of negative feedback is that the anterior lobe of the pituitary gland produces TSH, which stimulates the thyroid gland to produce thyroid hormone. TSH production is, however, inhibited by the presence of thyroid hormone.

Fig. 3.4 *Negative and positive feedback.*

Activation and deactivation

Hormones may be released by the presence of a certain stimulus. For example, insulin release depends on plasma glucose levels. Many specific metabolic pathways are activated by the build-up of specific metabolites within the internal environment. Similarly, some hormones may be inhibited by the presence of a signal. This may be another hormone, such as adrenaline, neurological, such as light stimulation inhibiting melatonin release from the pineal gland, or chemical, such as insulin inhibiting the release of glucagon.

Agonist and antagonist effects

An agonist is a ligand or substance that binds to a receptor on the cell membrane or within the cytoplasm and activates a response. An antagonist also binds to the receptor but does not activate it, thus blocking or inhibiting the normal physiological response of the receptor. By occupying the receptor site, a competitive antagonist blocks the action of the specific hormone (agonist) that normally binds to the site; antagonists can also be non-competitive. A partial agonist activates a receptor to a lesser degree and elicits a smaller physiological response. The physiological overlap of oxytocin and ADH is an example of an agonist effect. Oxytocin can elicit the same biological response as ADH because it can bind to the same receptor sites. Therefore, oxytocin is agonistic to the ADH receptor and may be described as an ADH agonist. Progesterone acts as a glucocorticoid agonist and affects metabolism (see Ch. 11).

A number of environmental chemicals can mimic the effects of hormones. These are detailed in Box 3.3.

Hormone action

The effects of hormones depend on a number of factors including affinity of the hormone for the receptor, agonist–antagonist effects, receptor number and hormone levels. Receptor number is important in the selection of the dominant follicle (see Ch. 4) and the increased sensitivity of the uterus to oxytocin in early labour (see Ch. 13). A lack of receptor expression can cause abnormal development, such as testicular feminization in the absence of androgen receptors (see

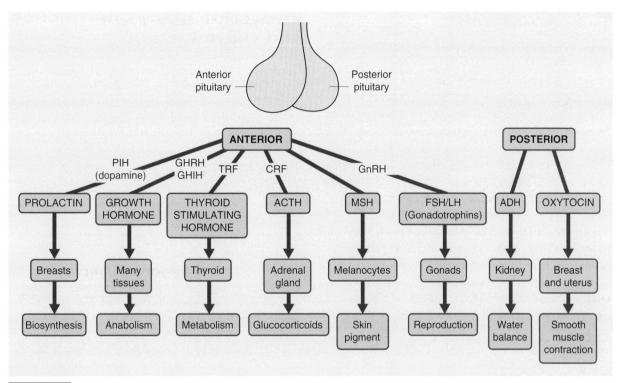

Fig. 3.5 *The pituitary gland and its secretions.*

Ch. 5). Hormone levels are affected by local circulation, stability, metabolism and excretion. Many hormones are inactivated within the blood, liver and their specific target cells. The breakdown of hormones is achieved by the action of various enzymes.

Hormone secretion may fluctuate with time. For instance, secretion of testosterone and prolactin exhibit circadian rhythms (characteristic pattern of changes during a 24-hour period), whereas GnRH, FSH, LH and PRL are released in a pulsatile fashion. A continuous infusion of these hormones would diminish their response as the constant occupancy of the receptors uncouples them from the second-messenger system, effectively exhausting the cell. A high blood flow increases dissipation of hormones and is likely to increase a systemic endocrine response but to decrease a paracrine response.

Levels and metabolism of binding proteins will also affect the activity of hormones. The protein-bound hormone complex renders the bound hormone inactive but also protects the hormone from enzymatic degradation. Hormone turnover may be affected by multiple sites of production. Different tissues may

have different feedback mechanisms controlling hormone production. Replicating hormone production occurs physiologically from the placental cells, but also pathologically from tumours. Hormones and their metabolites may be excreted via the kidney during the formation of urine. As the rate of excretion of many hormones is proportional to the rate of secretion, excretion rate indicates secretion rate. Generally, peptide hormones are readily metabolized by blood enzymes and are easily excreted so their half-life in the blood is short compared with that of protein-bound steroid hormones.

Levels of hormones may change within the tissues themselves as hormones can be converted to a form with a higher biological activity. For instance, the enzyme 5α-reductase in many of the target tissues for testosterone converts testosterone to 5α-dihydro-testosterone, which has twice the biological activity. A deficiency of this enzyme can cause poor development of the male external genitalia (see Box 3.4). The target cell may metabolize a hormone. Peptide hormones are endocytosed and catabolized and the receptors are recycled.

Environmental influences on hormonal expression

A number of environmental chemicals, such as phthalates (plasticizers) and PCBs (polychlorinated biphenyls), exert hormone-like effects. The chemicals may mimic or antagonize endogenous hormones, disrupt synthesis and metabolism of endogenous hormones and/or affect receptor expression. These oestrogenic contaminants were initially linked to abnormal sexual development in wild animals and fish but effects on humans are also under investigation. The pesticide DDT has been associated with reduced sperm counts and decreased libido. Chemicals used in plastics have been demonstrated to have oestrogenic properties. Degradation of alkylphenols used in detergents releases oestrogenic compounds. These environmental chemicals have been implicated in the increased incidence of testicular cancer, hypospadias (incomplete fusion of the urogenital folds of the penis), cryptorchidism (undescended testicles), breast cancer and endometriosis. It has also been suggested that fetal development, particularly of reproductive organs, may be affected by exposure to these compounds. The protective effect of phytoestrogens (see Ch. 4) may be related to interaction with environmental contaminants.

5α-Reductase deficiency

In the Dominican Republic, there is an increased incidence of an autosomal recessive condition resulting in 5α-reductase deficiency (Imperato-McGinley et al 1986). 5α-Reductase is the enzyme that converts testosterone to the more biologically active 5α-dihydrotestosterone within the target cell. The lack of enzyme means that there is a diminished response to testosterone during fetal sexual development (see Ch. 5) so an affected baby may have small and ambiguous genitalia, appearing female at birth (testicular feminization). However, at puberty the surge in testosterone production is adequate to stimulate the cells, therefore the child then develops male external genitalia. This condition is known as 'Guevodoces' (penis-at-twelve).

Endocrine glands, hormones and reproduction

Hormones can influence the ability of the target cell to respond by regulating the number of hormone receptors. Prolonged exposure to a low concentration of hormone may increase the number of receptors expressed by the cell (described as 'up-regulation'). Conversely, prolonged exposure to a high concentration of hormone might decrease the number of receptors for that hormone (described as 'down-regulation'). For instance, the expression of oxytocin receptors is down-regulated on prolonged exposure to oxytocin; this may explain the lack of response to exogenous oxytocin in induction of labour (see Ch. 13). Hormones can also affect receptors for other hormones, increasing or decreasing their effectiveness. When one hormone has to be present for another to have its full effect, it is described as permissive.

The endocrine glands and their main functions are summarized in Table 3.4.

The pituitary gland

The pituitary gland is a pea-sized gland at the base of the brain which is connected to the hypothalamus via the tuberoinfundibular pathway. It secretes hormones which regulate a broad range of body activities including trophic hormones which regulate other endocrine glands. The pituitary gland has two main lobes, the anterior lobe (or adenohypophysis) and the posterior lobe (or neurohypophysis) (Fig. 3.5). The anterior lobe originates from the primitive oral cavity, whereas the posterior lobe is a projection of the hypothalamus. The anterior lobe produces hormones such as LH and FSH that regulate gametogenesis and steroidogenesis by the gonads (see Ch. 4). The maintenance of lactation is achieved through the production of PRL (see Ch. 16). The anterior lobe also produces PRL, TSH, GH, adrenocorticotrophic hormone (ACTH) and endorphins. The posterior lobe of the pituitary gland does not produce hormones but stores and secretes oxytocin and ADH, which is also known as vasopressin. The tiny intermediate lobe of the human pituitary gland, which is almost indistinguishable from the anterior pituitary, produces melanocyte-stimulating hormone (MSH).

Table 3.4	*The endocrine system*
Endocrine gland	**Main function(s)**
Hypothalamus	■ Regulates homeostasis ■ Controls pituitary function ■ Integrates nervous and endocrine systems
Pituitary	'Master gland' ■ Stimulates other endocrine glands
Pineal body	■ Produces melatonin during nocturnal period ■ Involved in biological rhythms and body 'clock'
Thyroid	■ Affects metabolism and growth
Parathyroid glands	■ Maintenance of calcium homeostasis
Thymus	■ Development of immune system
Adrenal glands	Medulla: ■ Secretion of catecholamines (adrenaline and noradrenaline) Cortex: ■ Secretion of corticosteroids —glucocorticoids affect metabolism and responses to stress —mineralocorticoids affect electrolyte and fluid homeostasis ■ Sex steroids
Pancreas	■ Insulin and glucagon control cellular uptake of glucose and regulate cellular metabolism affecting blood glucose ■ Somatostatin = growth hormone-inhibiting hormone
Gonads (testes or ovaries)	■ Produce sex steroids that affect reproductive cycles and gamete formation
Kidney	■ Erythrocyte production stimulated by erythropoietin
Heart	■ Atrial natriuretic peptide lowers blood pressure
Adipose tissue	■ Appetite suppressed by leptin ■ Affects steroid hormone metabolism

The thyroid gland

The thyroid gland lies in front of the trachea, posterior to the larynx, and produces thyroid hormones. Thyroxine (T_4) is circulated and converted to an active form tri-iodothyronine (T_3) within the target tissues. Thyroid hormones affect all tissues in the body and regulate metabolic rate, growth, brain development and function. During pregnancy, the fetus initially utilizes maternally derived thyroxine so the maternal thyroid gland hypertrophies (increases in size) to compensate for this. This is achieved by the thyrotrophic effect of hCG and a placentally derived hormone called human chorionic thyrotrophin. Thyroid activity is stimulated by oestrogens and hCG; the changes contribute to glucose provision for the fetus. The increase in thyroid activity increases the basal metabolic rate of the pregnant woman, resulting in an increase of maternal and fetal oxygen consumption. The parafollicular cells of the thyroid gland produce calcitonin which is involved in the metabolism of calcium and phosphorus. Calcitonin levels increase in pregnancy and it is suggested that this may protect the maternal skeleton from excessive bone resorption.

The parathyroid glands

There are about four parathyroid glands within the thyroid that produce parathyroid hormone. Parathyroid hormone levels increase in response to a fall in serum calcium; it causes a decrease in urinary calcium excretion, increased mobilization of calcium from bone and, indirectly, causes an increase in calcium absorption (via an increase in vitamin D). Although parathyroid hormone is the primary regulator of 1,25-dihydroxyvitamin D synthesis in the non-pregnant state, it may not be important in pregnancy as levels do not change much in pregnancy, and women without functioning parathyroid glands still have a raised level of circulating 1,25-dihydroxy-vitamin D during pregnancy.

The adrenal glands

The adrenal glands are triangle-shaped glands situated on top of the kidneys that regulate the response to stress by synthesizing corticosteroids and catecholamines. Glucocorticoids, such as corticosterone

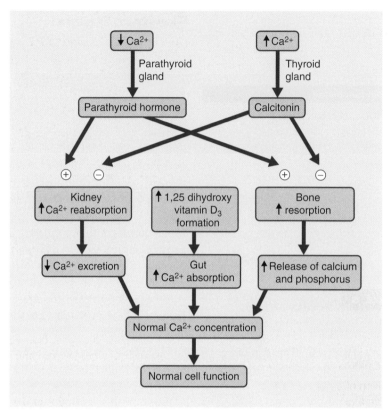

Fig. 3.6   *The parathyroid glands.*

and cortisol, are involved in the regulation of carbohydrate metabolism, the body's responses to stress and the regulation of the immune system. Carbohydrate metabolism is altered during pregnancy but it would appear that the fetal–maternal interaction concerning carbohydrate metabolism is mediated through the action of other hormones (see Ch. 11). Corticotrophin-releasing hormone (CRH) from the hypothalamus controls the release of ACTH from the anterior pituitary which regulates the production of hormones from the adrenal cortex; this is described as the hypothalamic–pituitary–adrenal axis. In pregnancy, maternal CRH levels increase dramatically, predominantly as a result of placental production. Placental CRH also enters the fetal circulation and may play a role in fetal organ maturation and also parturition. During pregnancy, ACTH levels double and cortisol levels increase. The adrenal glands also produce mineralocorticoids such as aldosterone, which are principally involved in the regulation of the electrolyte balance of the body (see Ch. 2). Aldosterone levels increase in

pregnancy as a response to increased renin and angiotensin II levels.

The gonads

The gonads are responsible for the production of the sex steroids. In the male, the testes predominantly produce testosterone. In the females, the ovary produces oestrogens and progesterone. The endocrine cells of the gonads lack the enzymes to produce mineralocorticoids and glucocorticoids. The gonadal function of the regulation of reproduction is discussed in Chapter 4.

Fetal endocrinology

Many of the endocrine and metabolic changes of pregnancy are results of hormonal signals originating from fetal–placental unit (FPU), which is a major site of protein and steroid hormone production and secretion. The interactions of neuronal and hormonal factors mediated by the FPU is critical in directing the initiation and maintenance of pregnancy, maternal adaptations to pregnancy, fetal growth and development, coordination of the timing of parturition and preparation for lactation. Production of oestradiol involves cooperation between the maternal and feto-placental systems (see Ch. 11). The fetal endocrine system is also involved in the differentiation and development of the sexes (see Ch. 5).

Key points

- The endocrine system and the nervous system interact and are involved in communication and maintenance of the internal environment.

- The classic description of a hormone as a substance released from a gland and transported in the blood to its target organ(s) cannot be applied to all hormones.

- Hormones can be classified structurally as monoamine, protein, peptide or lipid (steroid) hormones.

- Steroid hormones are produced from cholesterol precursors and include mineralocorticoids (such as aldosterone), glucocorticoids (such as cortisol) and sex steroids (oestrogen, progesterone and testosterone).

- Steroid hormones circulate bound to plasma proteins and exert their effect by altering protein synthesis in their target cells.

- Peptide hormones and catecholamines circulate in the plasma and affect signal transduction in their target cells.

- Hormonal effects are modulated by binding proteins, receptor expression, hormone metabolism and agonist–antagonist effects.

- Testosterone and oestrogen are responsible for the development and maintenance of sexual characteristics and fertility. Progesterone is involved in preparation for and maintenance of pregnancy.

Annotated further reading

Abbe Research Division 2004 Birth defects of humans induced by chemicals: index and medical analysis of new research information. Abbe Publishing Association, Washington DC.
Many of the chemicals that cause birth defects and which interact with the endocrine system are explored in this text.

Brook CGD, Marshall NJ 2001 Essential endocrinology. Blackwell Science, Oxford
Excellent textbook which is supported by introductory chapter summaries, integrated case studies and clear diagrams.

Carlson NR 2004 Physiology of behaviour, 8th edn. Longman Higher Education, Harlow
An interesting and comprehensive exploration of how physiological processes regulate and influence the behaviour and psychology of an organism; this textbook describes sexual behaviour in depth, relating it to endocrine and neurological interactions.

Greenstein B 1994 Endocrinology at a glance, Blackwell Science, Oxford
Introduces the study of endocrinology in a clear, precise and easy-to-understand way.

Johnson MH, Everitt BJ 2000 Essential reproduction, 5th edn. Blackwell, Oxford
An integrated, up-to-date and well-organized research-based textbook that explores comparative reproductive physiology of mammals, including anatomy, physiology, endocrinology, genetics and behavioural studies.

Sanders S Endocrine and reproductive systems, 2nd edn. Mosby, St Louis
A crash-course textbook for students written by students.

References

Brooker CG 1998 Human structure and function, 2nd edn. Mosby, St Louis

Halpern M, Martinez-Marcos A 2003 Structure and function of the vomeronasal system: an update. Progress in Neurobiology 70:245–318

Iles RK, Chard T 1991 Human chorionic gonadotrophin expression by bladder cancers: biology and clinical potential. Journal of Urology 145:453

Imperato-McGinley J, Gautier T, Peterson RE, Shackleton C 1986 The prevalence of 5-alpha-reductase deficiency in children with ambiguous genitalia in the Dominican Republic. Journal of Urology 136:867–873

Insel TR 1992 Oxytocin—a neuropeptide for affiliation: evidence from behavioral, receptor autoradiographic and comparative studies. Psychoneuroendocrinology 17:3–35

Johnson MH, Everitt BJ 1995 Essential reproduction, 4th edn. Blackwell, Oxford, p 29

McClintock MK 1971 Menstrual synchrony and suppression. Nature 229:244–245

4 Reproductive cycles

Learning objectives

- To describe follicular development, ovulation and subsequent events in the ovary.
- To describe the hormonal changes in the non-fertilized menstrual cycle.
- To outline the principles of hormonal regulation of reproduction and to identify factors that affect this regulation.
- To describe the effects of the hormonal changes on the female reproductive system.
- To relate the cyclical fluctuation in hormone levels to other changes in female physiology.

Introduction

The function of the ovaries is to release oocytes and to produce the steroid hormones oestrogen and progesterone. Relatively few oocytes are produced during a woman's reproductive life compared with the number of male gametes. The ovarian follicles produce all the oocytes, steroid hormones and inhibin. The cyclical pattern of hormone release has cyclical effects on the whole body, and behaviour, of the woman. The effects are particularly pronounced on the genital tract, facilitating its functions in gamete transport and the implantation and development of the conceptus. The first part of the cycle, the follicular phase, is dominated by the release of oestrogen produced by the developing follicles (Fig. 4.1). This oestrogen-dominant phase prepares the woman for ovulation, receipt of the sperm and fertilization of the oocyte. In the second half of the cycle, the luteal phase, the effects of progesterone are dominant. The physiological changes in this phase of the cycle prepare the woman's body for pregnancy and promote implantation and nurture of the conceptus should fertilization be successful. Progesterone is secreted from the corpus luteum; thus, this phase of the cycle is known as the luteal phase.

Ovulatory cycles usually have a duration of 24–32 days; the follicular phase is 10–14 days and the luteal phase between 12 and 15 days. Longer cycles usually have a prolonged follicular phase and delayed ovulation.

Chapter case study

Zara is now 12 weeks pregnant and has just attended the midwives' clinic to arrange her 12-week nuchal fold scan at her local maternity unit. Zara is quite excited because not only is her twin sister pregnant but her husband's sister and two of her best friends as well and all the babies are due within the same 2 weeks. They, and their partners, had all been working abroad together doing voluntary work over a period of 1 year and had lived together in shared accommodation.

They had helped build and set up an orphanage for children whose parents had died from AIDS-related illnesses in an African country, and had only returned home a week before Zara's pregnancy was confirmed.

What possible explanation could account for all five of the women conceiving together? What environmental factors could have influenced the menstrual cycles of the women and what possible physiological mechanisms may have resulted in the group apparently ovulating simultaneously?

Fig. 4.1 *Phases of the menstrual cycle.*

The follicular phase

Developmental stages

The stages of cell division leading to the production of the female gamete begin early in fetal life. The process is halted until puberty when ovulation begins, then halted again until fertilization. The developing egg is called an oocyte; it differentiates into a mature haploid ovum (or egg). Although dramatic progress in the development of an oocyte takes place during the follicular phase, the development of the follicle begins about 3 months prior to the menstrual cycle in which it is released at ovulation (Fig. 4.2). At the beginning of the cycle, a number of follicles are recruited to undergo initial development, stimulated by luteinizing hormone (LH). One follicle is selected to continue development as the dominant follicle. It is this follicle that releases the ovum at ovulation. The remnants of the follicle then become the corpus luteum.

In the female fetus, the primordial germ cells migrate to the ovary at 21 days postfertilization and become oogonia. They proliferate by mitotic division and then differentiate into primary oocytes; by 20 weeks of gestation, in each ovary, there are about 10 million primary oocytes ready to enter meiotic division (see Ch. 5). The oocytes degenerate throughout fetal life so the female neonate is born with a finite number of 250 000–500 000 oocytes; this is all the

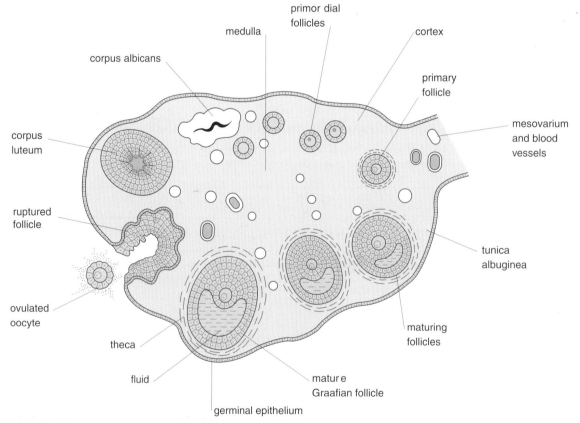

Fig. 4.2 *Ovarian follicles. (Reproduced with permission from Brooker 1998.)*

oocytes she will ever have. Degeneration of the oocytes continues throughout postnatal life; there are fewer than 200 000 oocytes left at puberty and numbers continue to fall. However, if one assumes a reproductive life of about 35–40 years, the maximum number of ova released from the ovaries will be no more than a few hundred.

Arrested meiosis

Meiosis is a specialized cell division involved in the production of gametes (see Ch. 7, p. 155, for a detailed description). In it, the number of chromosomes is reduced from 46 (known as the diploid number) to 23 (the haploid number). In the first part of meiosis the DNA replicates so each chromosome is composed of two chromatids. The homologous chromosomes pair up along their long axes and crossing over occurs so the chromosomes exchange genetic material. In humans, two or three exchanges of DNA occur per chromosome pair ensuring that the combination of genes will be unique (Box 4.1). This is achieved by areas of fusion (called chiasmata) forming between adjacent chromosomes (see Ch. 7). The oocyte remains arrested in the prophase stage of division I of meiosis for a number of years until sexual maturity (Fig 4.3). During this time, the primary oocytes synthesize the extracellular matrix and the secretory vesicles. Arrested meiosis provides a specialized mechanism to allow the oocyte to grow while it contains duplicate copies of chromosomes and, therefore, twice as much DNA available to direct synthesis of RNA than a somatic cell. The hormones of puberty release the oocyte from the first meiotic block; this process is called oocyte maturation. The oocyte resumes division I of meiosis. The chromosomes recondense, the nuclear envelope breaks down and the meiotic spindle forms. The chromosomes then segregate into the two daughter nuclei. The cytoplasm divides asymmetrically to form a large secondary oocyte and a small polar body, each of which contains 23 chromosomes as pairs of

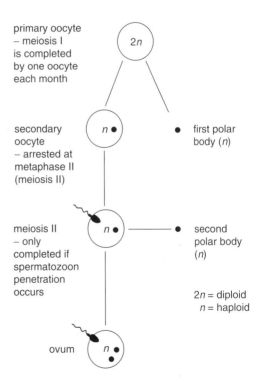

NB Polar bodies eventually degenerate within the ovum

Fig. 4.3 *Arrest of oocyte meiosis. (Reproduced with permission from Brooker 1998.)*

Box 4.1

Gamete formation

- Cell proliferation (mitosis)
- Genetic reshuffling and reduction (meiosis)
- Packaging of chromosomes
- Gamete maturation

chromatids. Meiotic division then arrests for a second time so the oocyte released at ovulation has still not completed meiosis. Activation of the oocyte and release from the second meiotic block occurs at fertilization. In the second meiotic division, the sister chromatids finally segregate into two nuclei and the cytoplasm again divides asymmetrically, this forming the mature ovum and a second polar body, each with 23 chromosomes. Because both divisions of the cytoplasm are asymmetrical, the ovum is large. Effectively, the polar bodies are small packages of cytoplasm which contain discarded chromosomes.

In the female, mitosis of the gametes stops in the fetal period, whereas, in the male, mitotic division of gametogenesis begins at puberty and continues until senescence (see Box 4.2). The termination of mitosis in the female, and entry into meiosis, is under the control of protein complexes, maturation-promoting factor (MPF) and cytostatic factor (CSF), which regulate the oocytes progression through meiosis (Dale, Marino & Wilding 1999). MPF phosphorylates multiple proteins involved in chromosome condensation and the breakdown of the nuclear envelope. The hormones of puberty increase MPF activity at the exit of the first meiotic block. It is hypothesized that the second meiotic block occurs because the maturing oocyte accumulates CSF which inhibits cell division. Oocyte activation and the release from the second meiotic block are thought to be triggered by a component of sperm that enters the oocyte at fertilization and causes CSF degradation.

Both premature arrest at the end of oocyte maturation and parthenogenic release from meiotic arrest are thought to cause infertility. As women age, the extended duration of arrested meiosis, which may last for over 50 years, probably results in the meiotic

spindles (see Fig. 7.11, p. 155) becoming increasingly fragile; this leads to an increased rate of abnormalities such as Down's syndrome and failed implantation.

Primordial follicles

Development of a mature female gamete depends on complex interactions between the developing gamete and the surrounding cells forming the outer layers of the follicle. Mitosis is completed during fetal development. During first meiotic prophase, the primordial germ cells stimulate organization of the surrounding cells to form the granulosa cells (flattened cuboidal epithelial cells) which condense and encircle around them forming the primordial follicles. The follicular cells secrete a basement membrane around the outside forming a cellular unit (Fig. 4.4). These granulosa cells are connected to the oocyte by gap junctions through which nutrients can be transported. The primitive oocyte is about 18 µm in diameter. A few follicles may resume development spontaneously and incompletely throughout fetal and neonatal life. However, regular recruitment of the primordial follicles into the pool of growing follicles begins at puberty when levels of follicle-stimulating hormone (FSH) increase, so the primordial follicles containing oocytes may stay arrested in meiosis for decades.

Preantral (primary) follicles

From puberty, a few primordial follicles restart their development each day forming a continuous stream of growing preantral or primary follicles. Most of these early follicles fail to develop fully and undergo atresia; less than 0.1% of follicles will ovulate and develop into a corpus luteum. The granulosa cells of follicles undergoing atresia accumulate lipid droplets and reduce protein synthesis. Both the granulosa cells and the oocyte become apoptotic (undergo 'programmed cell death'). White blood cells invade the dying follicular cell mass and scar tissue forms.

As the majority of the follicles regress rather than progress through development, the ovary has a dense population of atretic follicles resulting in an irregular corrugated outer surface of the ovary. The development of primordial follicles into preantral follicles takes about 85 days; the preantral phase is the longest phase of development of the oocyte. Initiation and progress through this early follicular development is

---

Box 4.2

Oogenesis compared with spermatogenesis

- Mitosis: fetal in female, after puberty in male
- Meiosis: halted in female, can last many years
- Relatively few oocytes released
- Release is episodic at ovulation not a continuous stream
- Organization is comparable to testis (stromal tissue containing primordial follicles, tubules) and glandular tissue (interstitial glands, Leydig cells)
- Mitotic proliferation is less
- Time-course of gamete production is much longer

independent of pituitary hormones but there may be paracrine regulation by cytokines, such as epidermal growth factor (EGF) (Box 4.3). These developing follicles do not secrete significant amounts of steroid hormones. Further follicular development requires pituitary support (secretion of FSH and LH).

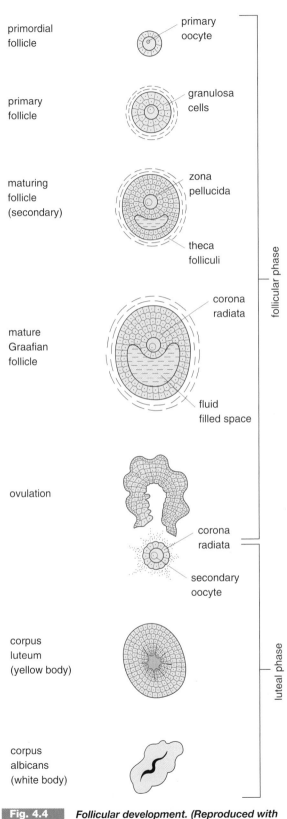

primordial follicle — primary oocyte

primary follicle — granulosa cells

maturing follicle (secondary) — zona pellucida, theca folliculi

mature Graafian follicle — corona radiata, fluid filled space

ovulation — corona radiata, secondary oocyte

corpus luteum (yellow body)

corpus albicans (white body)

follicular phase

luteal phase

Fig. 4.4 *Follicular development. (Reproduced with permission from Brooker 1998.)*

Box 4.3

Cytokines and growth factors

Inhibin and activin

The gonadotrophins (FSH and LH) stimulate the production of the cytokines activin and inhibin. The cytokines modulate actions of steroid hormones and gonadotrophins. Inhibin appears to affect only reproduction (see Fig. 4.7, p. 79), whereas the closely related activin affects cell growth and differentiation in other tissues. Inhibin is produced by the granulosa cells of small antral follicles in response to FSH (Roberts et al 1993) and suppresses FSH secretion. It is also produced by the Sertoli cells of the testis. Levels peak mid-cycle but remain high in the luteal phase, because the corpus luteum produces inhibin in response to LH. Inhibin production in the pituitary has a local inhibitory effect on FSH release (Hillier 1991). Inhibin stimulates androgen output by the thecal cells and moderates aromatizing activity of the granulosa cells (Hillier 1991). Activin is produced by granulosa cells, which also secrete follistatin, which may modulate the effects of activin. The thecal cells of the dominant follicle also produce activin (Roberts et al 1993). The anterior pituitary gland also produces activin, which is co-secreted with the gonadotrophins and enhances FSH production. It inhibits pituitary production of growth hormone (GH), ACTH and PRL. It may also have a role in embryogenesis (Hamilton-Fairley & Johnson 1998). Activin is present in follicular fluid but is inhibited by follistatin. Activin suppresses the androgen output by thecal cells but stimulates aromatizing capacity of granulosa cells. It therefore inhibits progesterone production. Activin is present early in the cycle, and inhibin later in the cycle, thus producing a balance between androgen output and conversion.

Follistatin

Follistatin was identified in 1987 as an inhibitor of FSH secretion (Roberts et al 1993). It is synthesized in the ovary and inhibits activin activity by acting as an activin-binding protein.

Continued

Box 4.3—Cont'd

Interleukins

Interleukins are a group of cytokines, small protein molecules that communicate between the immune system cells and between immune and other cells. They are usually secreted by immune cells and usually have a local action. Interleukins include histamine, prostaglandin, tumour necrosis factor (TNF), IL-1 and IL-6. IL-1 is a polypeptide cytokine, usually produced by activated macrophages, which induces an acute phase reaction in the liver in response to inflammation. However, it is also produced by granulosa cells in a hormone-dependent manner with a peak production mid-cycle. IL-1 affects follicular maturation and a number of aspects of ovulation, including increasing production of prostaglandins, collagenase, nitric acid and hyaluronic acid (Hurwitz et al 1992) and steroidogenesis. It is not known whether other members of the interleukin family are involved in follicular development.

Epidermal growth factor (EGF)

EGF is produced by many tissues including granulosa cells. It appears to inhibit FSH-stimulated oestrogen and inhibin production and proliferation and differentiation of granulosa cells. EGF may be involved in the selection of the dominant follicle (Hamilton-Fairley & Johnson 1998).

Transforming growth factors (TGF)

Transforming growth factors, TGF-α and TGF-β, have been identified in thecal cells (Adashi et al 1989). TGF-α has similar properties to EGF and suppresses granulosa cell differentiation. It also regulates differentiation of other cell types including fetal ovaries and ovarian carcinoma cells. Members of the TGF-β family are structurally similar to inhibin and increase FSH receptor expression, positively modulating granulosa cell proliferation and differentiation.

Insulin-like growth factors (IGFs)

Insulin-like growth factors stimulate mitotic division and cell differentiation. Their effects are mediated by insulin-like growth factor binding proteins (IGF-BP). In follicular development, they appear to coordinate the production of steroid hormones from the granulosa and thecal layers of the follicle (Giudice 1994). IGF-I enhances follicular development and hormone production. IGF-II enhances the response to insulin. IGF-BP bind to the IGFs decreasing the concentration of free growth factor. Decreased levels of binding

proteins are associated with follicular growth and increased concentrations of binding proteins are found in atretic follicles (Mason et al 1993). The large follicles from women with polycystic ovaries have lower concentrations of growth factors and higher concentrations of binding proteins (Mason et al 1994). IGFs seem therefore to have an important role in follicular growth, maturation and ovulation. In pregnancy, IGFs and their binding proteins play essential roles in modulating fetal growth and development (see Ch. 9).

Tumour necrosis factor (TNF)

TNF was initially identified as having a role in inflammation and in inhibiting tumour growth. It is produced by follicular cells and stimulates steroidogenesis, and may have a role in ovulation.

Early in the cycle, the concentration of FSH is sufficient to support the further development of some preantral follicles. The preantral follicles that are optimal for further development are of the appropriate size and maturity to respond and have adequate FSH receptors. Recruitment of the follicles is related to the interaction between the FSH concentration and the number of FSH receptors on the developing follicles. Therefore, the number of follicles surviving is related to the amount of FSH present. The antral development phase, ovulation and luteal phase comprise one cycle in the human. In other mammalian species, antral expansion occurs in the luteal phase of the previous cycle thus shortening non-fertile cycles.

Antral follicles

Usually about 15–20 preantral follicles are rescued from atresia each month and undergo initial stages of development and marked enlargement in response to the increasing FSH concentration at the beginning of each cycle. Several components contribute to the growth of the follicle: the oocyte enlarges, the follicular cells divide and further stromal cells are recruited to form the expanded outer layers of the follicle. The oocyte itself increases in diameter to 60–120 μm. It synthesizes large amounts of ribosomal RNA (rRNA) and messenger RNA (mRNA) to increase its protein stores ready for the maturation of the oocyte and fertilization, but does not resume meiosis. The follicular cells divide into several layers of granulosa cells, which secrete an amorphous and acellular translucent jelly, the zona pellucida. The zona pellucida is formed from condensation of glycoprotein and accumulates between the granulosa cells and the oocyte, acting as an extracellular coat of the oocyte. It has an important role in sperm binding and penetration during fertilization (see Ch. 6). Although the zona pellucida acts to separate the oocyte from the avascular granulosa cells, cytoplasmic processes penetrate the zona pellucida forming gap junctions at the oocyte surface. These allow delivery of low molecular weight substrates, such as nucleotides and amino acids, and cellular signalling molecules into the oocyte. Gap junctions also exist between granulosa cells.

The third component of follicular growth is condensation of ovarian stromal cells on the basement membrane (membrana propria) of the follicle. These recruited cells form a loose matrix of spindle-shaped cells around the follicle, known as the thecal layer. The cells differentiate into two layers: the theca interna, an inner layer of highly vascular glandular cells, and the theca externa, a poorly vascularized fibrous capsule.

The granulosa cells acquire receptors for FSH and oestrogen and the theca interna cells acquire receptors for LH. Synthesis of steroid hormones by the follicle requires cell cooperation (Fig. 4.5) (Hillier, Whitelaw & Smyth 1994). Interstitial glands lie within the stroma and between the developing follicles. They are formed of steroidogenic cells and produce androgens for secretion and aromatization to oestrogen in follicles. LH stimulates the theca interna cells to synthesize androgens (testosterone and androstenedione) from acetate and cholesterol but these cells initially have limited capacity to synthesize oestrogens. Androgens from the theca interna cells diffuse to the avascular granulosa cells. The granulosa cells are unable to synthesize androgens but can aromatize androgens to oestrogens (oestradiol-17β and oestrone). The enzyme aromatase is involved in the steroid biosynthesis pathway leading to increased oestrogen production. FSH stimulates production of insulin-like growth factor I (IGF-I), which stimulates aromatase activity and hence oestrogen production. Small amounts of LH are required to amplify follicular oestrogen production. The steroids are secreted into the bloodstream, where they have a systemic effect, and into the follicular fluid, where they may have a paracrine role. Androgens also stimulate aromatase. Oestrogens stimulate granulosa cells to proliferate and express further oestrogen receptors. Therefore, oestrogen fur-

ther stimulates oestrogen output, an example of positive feedback. This increases the amount of circulating oestrogen from the most advanced or 'dominant' follicle (therefore monitoring oestrogen output is a guide to the maturity of the most mature follicles). The dominant follicle, which undergoes the most growth, will enlarge from 20 to 200–400 μm diameter. The dominant follicle produces oestradiol, which inhibits FSH secretion. However, the dominant follicle develops exquisite sensitivity to FSH and can continue to respond to the decreasing concentration of FSH. The smaller follicles, destined to become atretic, lose their responsiveness to FSH and do not develop LH receptors (Scheele & Schoemaker 1996).

Early in the antral phase, the granulosa cells produce activin which suppresses androgen output and increases the aromatizing capability of the granulosa cells, thus promoting oestrogen synthesis. Later in the antral phase, the granulosa cells switch to producing inhibin which stimulates androgen output and attenuates the aromatizing activity. Thus androgen output is regulated by activin and inhibin.

The dominant antral follicle

The single follicle emerging as dominant undergoes preovulatory growth. This dominant follicle produces more oestrogen, which inhibits production of FSH from the pituitary gland. This is an example of negative feedback where a product limits its own production. The effect of oestrogen inhibiting production of FSH is that further development of the other follicles is limited. These follicles with fewer FSH receptors exposed to a diminishing supply of FSH are least able to respond to FSH and therefore undergo a downward spiral and become atretic. The dominant follicle continues to produce inhibin which stimulates androgen production by the thecal cells and aromatization by the granulosa cells thus leading to the surge of oestrogen. The dominant follicle also has a high ratio of insulin-like growth factor 2 (IGF-2) to IGF-BP which mediates LH-stimulated androgen output and FSH-dependent aromatization.

Angiotensin II (A-II), the product of the renin–angiotensin system (RAS, see Ch. 2), may be involved in oocyte maturation and ovulation. There is a RAS that is specific to the ovary and A-II occurs in high concentrations in preovulatory follicles. This ovarian RAS is implicated in the pathogenesis of ovarian tumours, ovarian hyperstimulation syndrome, ectopic pregnancy and hypertension (Hassan et al 2000). Symptoms of ovarian hyperstimulation

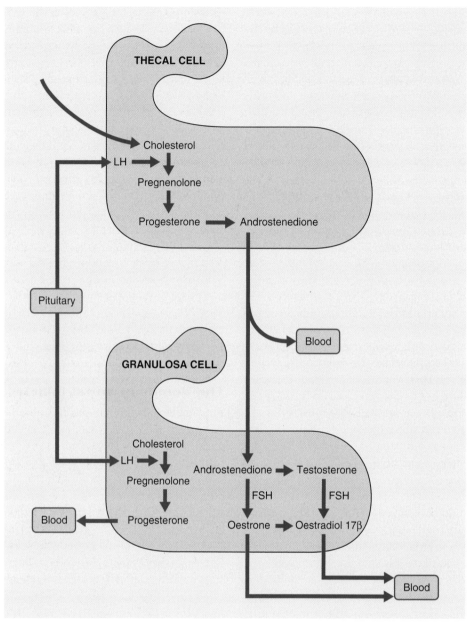

Fig. 4.5 *'Two-cell model' of steroid synthesis.*

syndrome include serious metabolic and fluid disturbances which are associated with abnormal control of
the RAS. It has also been suggested that A-II may have
a role in the formation and maintenance of the corpus
luteum, regulation of progesterone production and
angiogenesis (Hamilton-Fairley & Johnson 1998).
The biggest or dominant follicle, which is best able to
respond to FSH, further develops on the pathway to
expansion and ovulation. Oestrogen and FSH stimulate the mid-cycle expression of LH receptors on the
outer layers of granulosa cells of the dominant follicle,

which means that it will be able to respond to the mid-
cycle surge of LH secretion. Entry into the preovulatory phase depends on both the expression of these
receptors and a surge of LH from the anterior pituitary gland.

The granulosa cells continue to divide and increase
in size. However, most of the increase in follicular size
is due to accumulation of follicular fluid formed from
mucopolysaccharides, secreted from granulosa cells,
and serum transudate. The fluid coalesces forming an
antrum (or cleft) filled with follicular fluid. The

antrum separates the granulosa cells into two regions: the corona radiata (a rim of granulosa cells) around the oocyte and the outer membrana granulosa. The oocyte becomes isolated and suspended in the fluid connected to the rest of the granulosa cells by a thin strand of cells, the cumulus oophorus (egg stalk). The oocyte does not increase in size but continues to synthesize RNA and protein.

Follicular development is dependent on pituitary support. Removal of the pituitary gland (hypophysectomy) results in the cessation of follicular growth and the death of the oocyte. This can be halted by adding back LH and FSH, which stimulate further growth. It takes 8–12 days for the primary follicle to grow into the antral follicle. Failure of follicular growth for any reason results in a restarting of the cycle of follicular development, and hence both a longer first phase of the cycle and a longer cycle. It seems likely that women who regularly have a longer than normal menstrual cycle have either a slow rate of follicular development and increasing oestrogen secretion or the dominant follicle starts developing but fails so the next most appropriate follicle takes over the role as the dominant follicle.

Although the increasing concentration of oestrogen (predominantly oestradiol, E_2) initially has a negative feedback on the hypothalamus and pituitary, there is a critical concentration of oestrogen that is stimulatory provided it lasts for a critical duration. When the diameter of the follicle is 18–22 µm and the oestradiol concentration reaches 600–1200 pmol/l, there is positive feedback on the anterior pituitary gland leading to a sudden increase or 'surge' of LH release (Hamilton-Fairley & Johnson 1998) (Fig. 4.6).

The LH surge

The effect of the LH surge is two-fold. First, it stimulates the terminal growth phase of the follicle and the meiotic and cytoplasmic maturation of the oocyte, culminating in expulsion of the oocyte from the ovary. Second, it causes endocrine changes within the follicular cells that result in a different hormone secretory profile in the second half of the cycle.

Within a few hours of the LH surge, there are dramatic changes in the oocyte, which resumes meiotic division. There may also be a positive signal from the granulosa cells or a reduction of gap junction communication, which decreases the flow of meiosis-arresting substances to the oocyte. Progression through the remainder of the first meiotic division results in half

the chromosomes (as paired chromatids) and almost all the cytoplasm being enclosed in the secondary oocyte, which is destined to become the ovum. The remaining chromosomes and very little cytoplasm are enclosed in a membrane forming a very small cell, known as the first polar body (see Fig. 4.3, p. 77). Thus the secondary oocyte keeps the bulk of the materials that were synthesized earlier in follicular development; these are conserved for the zygote. The chromosomes of the secondary oocyte enter the second meiotic division and go on to the next stage of division, called metaphase (see Fig. 7.11, p. 155), where they align on the spindle. However, meiosis is then immediately arrested for a second time; this is regulated by cytostatic factors. Meiosis resulting in the production of a mature female pronucleus will not resume until successful fertilization following ovulation. By this time, the oocyte will already contain the sperm nucleus. Thus, there is actually no time when the oocyte is a true gamete in the sense of being a cell with only 23 chromosomes, as is the case of a spermatozoon.

Concurrently, the LH surge promotes maturation of the cytoplasmic compartment of the oocyte. The cytoplasmic processes between the oocyte and the granulosa cells withdraw and contact is lost. The Golgi apparatus (see Table 1.1, p. 3) synthesizes lysosome-like cortical granules, which align under the surface of the oocyte. Protein synthesis continues but the profile of the proteins synthesized changes as the oocyte prepares for fertilization. The gonadotrophin surge stimulates the cumulus cells surrounding the oocyte (see Fig. 4.4, p. 79) to secrete hyaluronic acid, which disperses the cumulus cells embedding them in a mucus-like matrix.

Ovulation

Ovulation is triggered by the mid-cycle surge of LH, which occurs in response to sustained high levels of oestrogen released from the developing dominant follicle. The single mature preovulatory follicle has a diameter of 2–2.5 cm in an ovary that is approximately 3 cm long. It was this structure that de Graaf identified and named in 1672. The increased size and changed position of the follicle means that it protrudes from the surface of the ovary (see Fig. 4.2, p. 76). This results in the thinning of the layer of epithelial cells between the wall of the follicle and the peritoneal cavity. As expansion continues, the wall becomes thinner and avascular and the cells appear to dissociate.

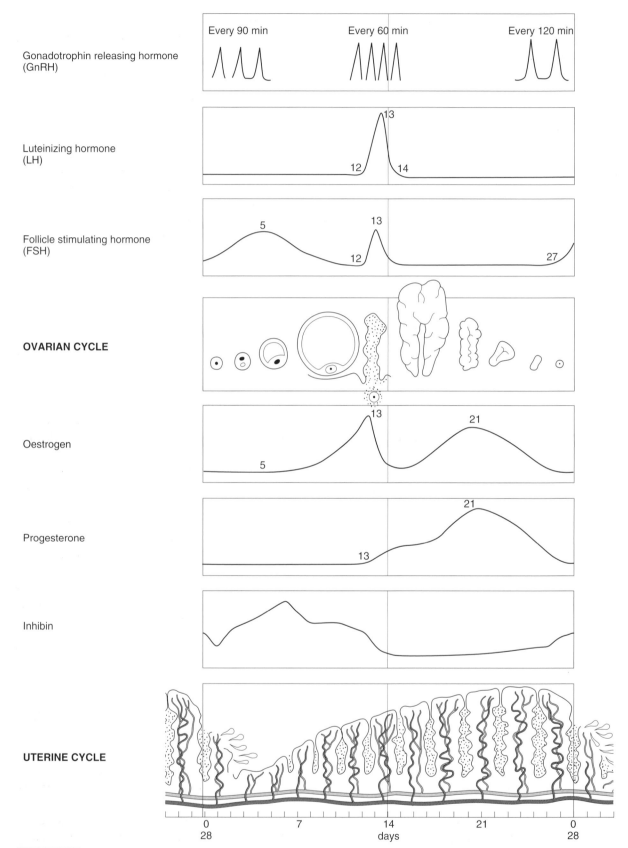

Fig. 4.6   *The reproductive cycle and hormone levels.*

About 36 hours after the LH surge ovulation occurs and the oocyte is expelled from the ovary (see Fig. 4.2, p. 76). The LH surge stimulates the production of a cascade of proteolytic enzymes, including renin and other trypsin-like enzymes from thecal cells, which digest the follicle wall. The biochemical changes, including generation of oxygen free radicals, that precede ovulation are similar to those seen in inflammation. Plasminogen activator, which converts procollagenase to collagenase, is produced by granulosa cells resulting in the breakdown of the connective tissue. Progesterone production rises immediately after the LH surge and the preovulatory increase in progesterone may be important in follicular rupture as it decreases formation of collagen. Prostaglandins increase vascular permeability, which maintains the intrafollicular pressure as fluid begins to leak through the eroded follicular wall. Small contractile waves also ripple across the ovary increasing the intrafollicular pressure. The force is cushioned by the follicular fluid so the pressure generated is targeted at the weakened ovarian surface, causing it to rupture. As the follicle ruptures and the ovarian surface is breached, the fluid washes the oocyte, which is surrounded by the granulosa (cumulus) cells, from the ovary to the exterior. The oocyte is swept into the uterine tube by the fimbria. It is then propelled towards the uterus by peristaltic muscular activity and cilia movements of the epithelial cells lining the tube. After taking years to complete maturation, the oocyte is then viable and fertilizable for only about a day.

The luteal phase

Within 2 hours of the LH surge, there is a transient rise in oestrogen and androgens secreted by the follicle as the thecal layers become stimulated and hyperaemic. The outer granulosa cells with their newly expressed receptors for LH no longer convert androgens to oestrogen but synthesize progesterone instead. The cells no longer bind oestrogen or FSH. The result is a marked increase in progesterone secretion, which begins several hours before ovulation.

The corpus luteum

After ovulation, the residual parts of the follicle remaining in the ovary collapse into the space and form the corpus luteum ('yellow body'; see Fig. 4.4,

p. 84). There is some bleeding and fibrotic activity in the cavity, which allows formation of a fibrin core around which the remaining granulosa cells congregate. The structure is enclosed by a capsule of fibrous thecal cells. The basement membrane between the granulosa cells and thecal cells breaks down allowing vascularization of the interior. This allows increased transport of cholesterol precursor to the luteinizing granulosa cells to maintain a high rate of progesterone secretion. A few of the thecal cells disperse to the stroma tissue. The granulosa cells first luteinize, then stop dividing and hypertrophy into large luteal cells. The luteal cells are rich in mitochondria, endoplasmic reticulum and Golgi bodies and have numerous lipid droplets and lutein, a yellow carotenoid pigment.

Hormonal changes

Luteinization is associated with a progressive increment in progesterone secretion from the corpus luteum. The outer thecal cells form a stem cell population of smaller luteal cells which have numerous LH receptors and produce progesterone and androgens. Levels of progesterone rise until the middle of the luteal phase (see Fig. 4.6, p. 84). The corpus luteum produces oestrogen and inhibin as well as progesterone. All three hormones inhibit secretion of FSH from the anterior pituitary gland and therefore prevent further development of follicles.

It has been suggested that a cause of fertility problems may be inadequate production of progesterone at the time of ovulation and during the subsequent luteal phase. However, exogenous administration of progesterone or human gonadotrophin (hCG) has had limited success in clinical practice. It appears that most women have a proportion of their cycles with a low progesterone output without it affecting their fertility (Hamilton-Fairley & Johnson 1998). A shortened luteal phase can lead to intermenstrual bleeding, premenstrual 'spotting' and short cycles.

The corpus luteum also synthesizes relaxin, secretion of which peaks in the middle of the luteal cycle (Johnson et al 1993), probably regulated by LH. Relaxin may be involved in promoting the growth of the myometrium and cervix and growth and secretory activity of the endometrium (Huang, Stromer & Anderson 1991).

Effectively, the corpus luteum is an endocrine gland producing oestrogen and progesterone. The LH surge stimulates its growth and activity. Unless fertilization occurs the life of the corpus luteum is very short, and it undergoes spontaneous luteolysis (degeneration and regression) after about 6 days. The corpus luteum appears to have an age-related decrease in responsiveness to LH (Zeleznik & Hillier 1997) and so requires progressively more LH for survival. Following the LH surge, LH concentration in the luteal phase is low so luteolysis will occur. Blood flow to the corpus luteum falls and the follicular tissue becomes ischaemic. The concentrations of oestrogen and progesterone begin to fall as the degenerating corpus luteum stops hormone production. Thus luteolysis terminates a non-fertile cycle. As the level of oestrogen falls, the inhibition on the hypothalamus will be abrogated and FSH secretion will resume ready for the next cycle. The atrophying corpus luteum loses its yellow pigment, so it becomes known as a corpus albicans. It gradually contracts over a period of months, leaving white scar tissue which is absorbed into stromal tissue of the ovary.

Changes on fertilization

If fertilization occurs then hCG, which has structural similarities to LH, rescues the corpus luteum from luteolysis, stimulating its further growth and production of steroid hormone up to the 10th week when placental endocrine function becomes established. Human chorionic gonadotrophin has a longer half-life than LH so it provides a sustained and more intense stimulus. If fertilization occurs then the concentration of relaxin also continues to rise until the end of the first trimester.

Regulation of gonadotrophin secretion

The brain controls and regulates the ovarian cycle. The gonadotrophs in the anterior pituitary secrete the glycoprotein hormones LH and FSH (which together are known as gonadotrophins). There appear to be two distinct populations of cells in the anterior pituitary, each producing one particular type of hormone; however, fluorescent labelling shows that some cells contain both hormones. Synthesis and secretion of LH and FSH are dependent on gonadotrophin-releasing hormone (GnRH) from the hypothalamus, which acts as the common mediator of influences via the CNS. (GnRH is also known as luteinizing hormone releasing hormone, or LHRH.) The hypothalamus releases

GnRH into the hypophysial portal circulation that runs to the pituitary gland.

This pathway means that control of the reproduction can be modulated and affected by other inputs from the higher brain centres. The GnRH neurons convert neural signals into endocrine signals. Stress, nutritional status and environmental influences, for instance, affect the timing and success of the reproduction. Ovulation appears to be seasonally regulated in populations experiencing seasonal variation in food availability; suspending reproductive function when nutrition is poor favours maternal health and outcome of pregnancy.

There are two levels of regulation. First, the GnRH neurons of the hypothalamus have an inherent pulsatile activity. The steroid hormones, the gonadotrophins (LH and FSH) and GnRH feedback on the hypothalamic–pituitary axis exert a second level of endocrine control. Prolactin (PRL) also has an effect on the control of reproduction.

GnRH and gonadotrophins are released in a pulsatile manner (see Box 4.4). The cells releasing GnRH appear to be widely and diffusely distributed (Rance et al 1991) but are remarkably synchronized to produce pulses of GnRH. During the follicular phase, the pulses are of low amplitude and high frequency, occurring every 60 minutes (Clarke 1996). In the luteal phase, they are more irregular and have high amplitude and occur with a low frequency of about every 2 hours. The output of the gonadotrophins, LH and FSH, is changed by increasing or decreasing the amplitude or frequency of the pulses or by modulating the response of the gonadotrophs to the pulses. Prior to the LH surge, gonadotroph GnRH receptor density increases and the cells become more sensitive to GnRH. Inhibin and activin affect secretion of FSH without affecting secretion of GnRH. Two phenomena are observed: first, a depressant effect on output of gonadotrophins by increased oestrogen, progesterone and inhibin; second, an increased surge of LH and FSH secretion induced primarily by oestradiol (Fig. 4.7). The pattern of pulsatile secretion of GnRH is regulated by a complex mechanism that allows multiple signals, such as neurotransmitters and sex steroids, to determine ovulation.

In the early part of the follicular phase, rising levels of FSH stimulate oestrogen production from the developing follicles. Rising concentrations of oestradiol have a negative feedback effect on gonadotrophin production from the anterior pituitary so FSH secretion falls.

Box 4.4

Biological rhythms

The study of biological rhythms is termed 'chronobiology'. All living cells, organs, organisms and groups of individuals demonstrate rhythmical changes within their internal (endogenous) physiology that can also result in external changes in behaviour. The rhythms can be categorized according to the length of the cycle or period of oscillation.

- ultradian: the rhythm is less than 1 day, e.g. rapid eye movement in sleep
- circahordal: the period of oscillation is around 1 hour
- circadian: the period of oscillation is about 1 day; levels of many hormones such as cortisol fluctuate on a daily basis
- infradian: the rhythm is repeated in a cycle greater than 1 day, e.g. menstrual and oestrus cycles
- circaseptram: the period of oscillation is about 1 week
- circatidal: the rhythm relates to tidal movement of water
- circalunar (synodic): the rhythm relates to the cycle of the moon
- circannual: the rhythm has a cycle of about 1 year

These fluctuations are often affected by the external environment and appear to enable the individual to respond to forthcoming changes within the environment. Factors that influence or reset the cycle are described as entraining the cycle. In the human brain, the suprachiasmatic nuclei of the hypothalamus may influence daily fluctuations. The pineal gland, which produces the hormone melatonin at night, appears to affect the suprachiasmatic nuclei, acting as an entrainer. The circadian pattern of melatonin secretion is achieved through inhibition via a neural pathway (outside the optic nerve) that is activated by light stimulation upon the retina. Therefore, within temperate zones, light not only acts as an entrainer on a daily basis but, due to the fluctuation of the photoperiod (length of daylight exposure), entrainment of annual cycles can also be achieved.

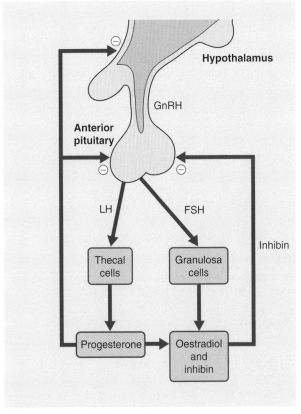

Fig. 4.7 *Hormonal regulation of the menstrual cycle. (Reproduced with permission from Johnson & Everitt 1995.)*

by two- to four-fold. These concentrations are maintained for 48 hours, which produces a positive feedback effect resulting in the dramatic surge of LH and FSH release seen in mid-cycle prior to ovulation. The effect of oestradiol is very sensitive: a low concentration has a marked and rapid effect that is evident within 1 hour and maximal within 4–6 hours. During the luteal phase, increased progesterone concentrations reinforce the negative feedback effects of oestradiol. The production of both LH and FSH secretion is very low, therefore the positive effect of oestradiol is blocked.

Cyclical effects of oestrogens and progesterone

Effects on the uterus

Organs that respond to hormonal changes have receptors for the hormones. Responses can change because hormone levels fluctuate or because receptor density on the target organs alters. The principal actions of

Activin and inhibin also affect FSH secretion. Inhibin is involved in the negative feedback of FSH secretion. However, the dominant follicle is exquisitely sensitive to even a diminishing concentration of FSH and continues to produce oestrogen, which markedly increases oestrogen and progesterone during the monthly cycle are on the endometrium. The endometrium undergoes cyclical changes: the growth of the uterine wall in expectation of an embryo, and its degeneration if fertilization does not take place. In the first half of the cycle, the uterus goes through a proliferative phase. Oestrogen stimulates the epithelial cells of the basal layer of the endometrium to divide and proliferate, forming a thick mucosal wall with numerous endometrial glands (Fig. 4.8). Oestrogen also stimulates angiogenesis (growth of new blood vessels): extensive vascular tissue, spiral arteries and veins develop within the endometrium. Within the space of a few days, the effect of oestrogen is to increase the height of the wall from 0.5 to 5 mm, a remarkable 10-fold increase. The thickness of endometrium is monitored by ultrasound in assisted conception (see Ch. 6) to assess whether it is optimal for implantation; the insertion of embryos into a uterine cavity with an endometrium less than 5 mm thick is unlikely to be successful The myometrium does not grow so extensively during the menstrual cycle. During the proliferative phase, oestrogen primes the endometrial cells by inducing the synthesis of progesterone receptors.

After ovulation, the cells of the enlarging corpus luteum begin to secrete progesterone, which has a dramatic effect on the secretory activity of the endometrial glands. In this secretory phase, the effects of progesterone are dominant, although oestrogen is still secreted from the corpus luteum. The spiral arteries continue growing and thus become more prominent and coiled as the height of the endometrium remains unchanged. The endometrial glands become dilated and convoluted with secretions rich in proteins, glycogen, sugars, amino acids, mucus and enzymes. The secretory products are important for the survival and nutrition of the zygote and blastocyst prior to implantation. Failure of conception results in diminishment of the corpus luteum and decreased steroid hormone production. By the 7th postovulatory day, the secretory process ceases and the glands become exhausted and regress.

Cyclical effects are particularly evident within the female reproductive tract. Activity of the myometrium is inversely related to progesterone secretion. During menstruation, when progesterone levels are low, the uterine contractions, mediated by prostaglandins, have a higher frequency and strength than in labour (Lyons et al 1991). These uterine contractions are responsible for dysmenorrhoea (period pains). Nonsteroidal anti-inflammatory drugs (NSAIDs) such as aspirin inhibit prostaglandin synthesis, and are therefore effective in reducing pain. After menstruation there is a slow decline in myometrial activity during the follicular phase; it reaches negligible activity midcycle. Thus the uterus is at its most quiescent at the time of implantation. Uterine quiescence is maintained until the late luteal phase when levels of progesterone fall. If pregnancy intervenes, levels of progesterone remain high and the myometrium remains inactive. Uterine blood flow, on the other hand, correlates positively with the pattern of oestrogen secretion. Due to low levels of oestrogen, blood supply to the endometrium during menses and early follicular phase is reduced. A marked increase occurs just prior to ovulation followed by a slight nadir. A secondary peak occurs in the luteal phase which mirrors the rise in oestrogen production. This means that endometrial blood flow is relatively high at the time of implantation but lower at menstruation, which helps to limit the blood loss at the latter time.

Uterine contractile activity varies with stage of the menstrual cycle (Kunz & Leyendecker 2001). In the preovulatory period, uterine peristaltic activity directs sperm transport preferentially to the uterine tube lateral to the ovary containing the dominant follicle. The uterine activity is relatively quiescent in the late luteal phase which favours implantation. However, there are still some gentle peristaltic waves which may promote high fundal implantation. Uterine peristalsis causes some retrograde menstruation. It is thought that this may be of evolutionary benefit and help preserve body iron (Kunz & Leyendecker 2001). Dysfunction of uterine activity may be involved in the development of endometriosis, uterine adenomyosis and infertility.

Effects on the uterine tubes, cervix and vagina

Uterine tubes

Oestrogen stimulates the epithelial cell activity, increasing cilia movement and secretion. This facilitates the movement of the ovum along the uterine tubes following ovulation. These effects are reversed by progesterone, which inhibits the peristaltic activity of the uterine tube smooth muscle.

Cervix

Oestrogen relaxes the myometrial fibres supplying the cervix and increases stromal vascularization and oedema. Collagenase is activated, which causes some dispersal of the tightly bound collagen bundles into a looser matrix. The result is that the cervix becomes

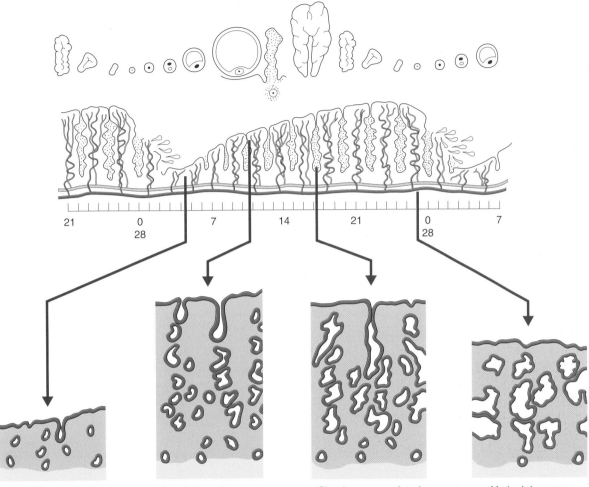

Straight tubular glands

Glands have become longer and increasingly convoluted

Glands are convoluted and dilated with secretions

Marked decrease in tissue height

Glands exhausted of secretions

Columnar cells

Cells have centrally placed nuclei showing mitotic activity

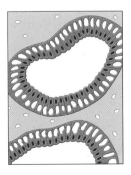

Cells have apical nuclei and basal vacuoles

Cells show basal nuclei

Vacuoles have discharged their contents into the lumen

Breakdown of spiral arteries in the stroma

Fig. 4.8   *Cyclical effects on the endometrium.*

softer to touch. The external os everts prior to ovulation. Progesterone causes the cervical muscle to retract and the stroma to become more compact as the collagen matrix reforms. The external os becomes tighter. The change in texture of the cervix is used as part of natural family planning (see Box 4.5). The cervix is softer at ovulation and a few days before, coinciding with the fertile period. At this stage it has the consistency of lips compared with the harder 'nose-like' cartilaginous consistency of the cervix later in the cycle when the effects of progesterone are dominant.

The cyclical changes in blood flow are reflected by the composition of cervical mucus, which is copious and receptive to sperm penetration in mid-cycle (Table 4.1). When progesterone levels are high, small volumes of thick cervical mucus are secreted that are hostile and impenetrable to sperm. The increased viscosity of the mucus in the latter half of the menstrual cycle reduces the risk of ascending infection at the time of implantation.

Both oestrogen and progesterone are secreted from the corpus luteum in the second half of the cycle. The concentrations of oestrogen and progesterone will continue to rise if successful fertilization results in secretion of hCG and consequent survival of the corpus luteum. Therefore, the effects of the hormones in the second half of the cycle on the female body portend the changes that would take place in pregnancy.

Vagina

Oestrogen increases mitotic activity and secretion in the vaginal epithelial cells. Stimulation by progesterone results in an increased size of nucleus of vaginal epithelial cells. It is important when examining cervical cells, obtained from a smear, to relate the morpho-

Table 4.1   *Changes in cervical mucus*

Proliferative phase (follicular)	Secretory phase (luteal)
'E' mucus	'G' mucus
Oestrogen	Progesterone
Network of long parallel polypeptide chains	Meshwork of polypeptide strands
Carbohydrate side chains	Increased carbohydrate side chains
Forms channels 5 μm wide	Smaller space between molecules
High water content (98%)	Lower water content
Copious volume	Scanty volume
Clear	Cloudy
Acellular	Cells present
Spinnbarkeit = 10–20 cm (stretching between glass plates)	Spinnbarkeit ~ 3 cm
Dehydration: ferning	No ferning
Assists transport of sperm	Forms mucus plug to protect against infection

logical differences to the stage of a woman's menstrual cycle. Earlier in the cycle, cells appear flatter, whereas under the influence of progesterone they tend to become clumped and folded. There are also cyclical changes in the pH of the vagina as oestrogen stimulates the growth of commensal lactobacilli (Döderlein's bacilli). These lactobacilli metabolize glycogen from the cervical secretions producing lactic acid as a metabolic by-product, which decreases pH to a level that protects the reproductive tract from opportunistic pathogenic microorganisms.

The resident flora of the vagina also produces volatile aliphatic acids, which have distinctive odours. The profile of acids changes throughout the cycle under the influence of the changing hormones, and may result in changed sexual behaviour. It is suggested that male responses to their partners are affected by the cyclical fluctuations in olfactory stimuli stimulating sexual responsiveness and interaction. These olfactory signals do not seem to be consciously perceived in humans.

Box 4.5

Concepts of natural family planning

- Based on periodic abstinence
- Also known as 'rhythm method' or 'safe period'
- Assumes interval between ovulation and menstruation is constant
- Based on recognition of signs of ovulation and fertile phases of menstrual cycle
  - temperature rise after ovulation
  - increased cervical mucus and watery vaginal secretions
  - softer consistency of cervix
- Probably most effective for birth spacing

Another example is women who live together are often observed to demonstrate menstrual synchrony: they ovulate and menstruate at the same time. Recently, it has been demonstrated that humans have the potential to communicate by pheromones. Odourless body secretions from women in different phases of the menstrual cycle can advance or delay the phases of other women (Stem & McClintock 1998). Sexual desire, sexual activities and sexual satisfaction are all reported to increase around ovulation (see Ch. 5).

Other effects

There are additional effects and benefits of oestrogen on women's health. Oestrogens appear to protect the cardiovascular system; thus women of reproductive age and normal endocrine function have a lower incidence of hypertension and a reduced risk of cardiovascular disease owing to higher levels of high-density lipoproteins (HDL), which lower circulating levels of cholesterol. Oestrogens stimulate osteoblasts, the cells involved in bone formation, thus maintaining bone mass. Oestrogens may depress appetite and are mildly anabolic. There is a preovulatory drop in food intake; this decrease in female 'foraging' behaviour is hypothesized to allow the female more time for activity, including 'shopping' for alternative mates (Fessler 2003). Increased consumption of food is observed in the late luteal phase.

Postovulatory levels of progesterone are high, causing a slight increase in the basal metabolic rate. The basal body temperature rises owing to the influence of progesterone on the thermoregulatory centre of the hypothalamus. A temperature rise of $0.2–0.6°C$ confirms ovulation has taken place but does not predict it. In the second half of the cycle the skin may appear more pigmented and acne may worsen as progesterone increases constriction of sebaceous glands. Progesterone also increases appetite during the luteal phase (Buffenstein et al 1995). Women with premenstrual syndrome (PMS) may report cravings for carbohydrate, which are often associated with feelings of depression (Dye & Blundell 1997) (see Box 4.6). These patterns of fluctuations in energy intake, appetite and depression may be associated with low serotonin activity. Metabolism of drugs and alcohol may cyclically alter during the menstrual cycle.

Oestrogen and progesterone affect connective tissue oedema and hyperaemia and can cause increased breast size and tenderness. Progesterone binds to renal

---

Box 4.6

Premenstrual syndrome (PMS)

PMS is very common, with physical and psychological symptoms occurring in about 50% of women of reproductive age during their lifetime. Premenstrual dysphoric disorder (PMDD) is a more severe form of PMS that is associated with the luteal phase of the menstrual cycle. PMDD is classified as a depressive disorder by the American Psychiatric Association and affects about 3–5% of women. It is characterized by anxiety, anger and severe irritability. It is more severe than PMS and usually requires treatment to allow an affected woman to function in her environment. Both PMS and PMDD are characterized by mood swings including depression, but clinical depression occurs in PMDD. Some women have been acquitted of crimes conducted when they were affected by PMS and PMDD.

The cause of PMS is not clear. It may be due to a hormonal imbalance and low progesterone secretion in the luteal phase, abnormal neurotransmitters response, disorganized aldosterone function leading to water retention, deficient adrenal hormone secretion due to abnormal hypothalamic–pituitary–adrenal function, carbohydrate intolerance, a nutrient deficiency, stress or a combination of these factors (Girman et al 2003). Women may be prescribed antidepressants such as serotonin reuptake inhibitors. Many women select lifestyle modification and complementary or alternative medicine approaches rather than conventional medicine. Women with PMS tend to consume more dairy products, refined sugar and high-sodium foods so many clinicians recommend reducing intake of these. As fat contributes to oestrogen levels and fibre helps to reduce the effects of oestrogen on gut flora, high-fibre low-fat diets may be recommended. Reducing caffeine intake, from coffee, tea and caffeinated soft-drinks, can also be helpful. Vitamin B_6 can affect neurotransmitter release but the evidence that it improves PMS symptoms is inconclusive. As excess vitamin B_6 can cause nerve damage before symptoms of toxicity are evidenced, the daily dose should be limited. There is some evidence that calcium supplements can be beneficial. Of the herbal preparation more commonly used to relieve symptoms, the evidence is stronger for chasteberry (vitex) and ginkgo than for black cohosh,

Continued

aldosterone receptors, causing natriuresis (sodium excretion) and blocking aldosterone occupation. Aldosterone increases to restore sodium retention, so there is a net effect of sodium retention. Oestrogen stimulates angiotensinogen production, which also tends to enhance sodium retention. Thus, in the luteal phase of the cycle, salt and water retention may be increased causing generalized weight gain and premenstrual feelings of bloatedness.

Menstruation

Menstruation is the loss of most of the decidual (superficial) layers of the endometrium accompanied by some blood loss that occurs after withdrawal of steroid hormones at the end of each menstrual cycle. In the human, menstrual loss usually lasts about 5–7 days. Humans and other primates, together with elephant-shrews and some types of bats, are the only animals that menstruate. In these species there is marked progesterone-related proliferation of the endometrium and implantation is invasive. It was suggested that menstruation evolved as a protective mechanism against sperm-borne pathogens. However, an alternative hypothesis is that cyclical regression and proliferation of the endometrium is energetically more economical in term of reproductive costs than constantly maintaining a receptive endometrium (Strassmann 1996).

The mechanism of menstruation is thought to be either tissue destruction following necrosis and/or an inflammatory response (Salamonsen 2003). In the destructive model, anoxia causes necrosis of the endometrium. The degeneration of the corpus luteum results in a fall in oestrogen and progesterone levels which causes a modest but significant decrease in endometrial tissue height so the spiral arteries are coiled tighter and compressed. This results in a reduced blood flow, ischaemia and denudement of the endometrial tissue and interstitial haemorrhage. Prostaglandins released by the spiral arteries stimulate vasoconstriction and vasodilatation resulting in rhythmic waves of contraction and relaxation in the latter. (The effect is like breaking a wire by rhythmically bending it backwards and forwards.) The waves become longer and more profound causing the decidual endometrium to break away along the natural plane of cleavage. The straight arteries in the basal layer maintain the blood supply. It is from these that new spiral arteries will regenerate. Alternatively menstruation can be regarded as an inflammatory response. There is a marked increase in the number of leukocytes, particularly mast cells, immediately before menstruation as progesterone levels fall. These are probably attracted by chemokines produced by the endometrial cells. Mast cell degranulation may trigger the extracellular activation of matrix metalloproteinases, proteases that have the capacity to degrade components of the tissue.

Within 12 hours, the height of the endometrium falls from 4 mm to 1 mm. At the end of the secretory phase, there is an ischaemic phase followed by the menstrual phase leading to the next proliferative phase. Endometrial repair is very rapid and occurs without scarring.

Menstrual flow is usually between 35 and 95 ml and consists of endometrial debris and blood. Blood loss is limited by vasoconstriction of the spiral arteries and formation of thrombin–platelet plugs in the terminal portions of the straight arteries. When oestrogen secretion resumes at the beginning of the next cycle, it stimulates healing and new tissue growth. Menstrual blood does not coagulate in the pattern seen normally. The damaged endometrial cells secrete proteolytic and fibrinolytic enzymes, which inhibit the formation of fibrin and therefore clot formation. The average volume of blood lost is 50 ml, which accounts for 0.7 mg of iron, a loss that is just matched by dietary iron absorption.

Case study 4.1 looks at the problem of calculating the length of gestation from the date of the last menstrual period.

Hormonal causes of infertility

Hormonal causes of infertility account for about a third of the known causes (Box 4.7).

Case study 4.1

Njuka is in England with her husband who is a diplomatic representative of a central African country. When they first meet, the midwife asks Njuka when her baby is due and is informed that four full moons are left to pass before the baby will come. The midwife, intrigued by this answer, asks Njuka how she knows this. Njuka explains that six full moons have passed since her last period and that is how she knows.

- How accurate is Njuka's calculation of her gestation?
- Why is it important for a midwife to be able to estimate the length of gestation?
- What other information can help in this estimation?

Hypogonadotrophic hypogonadism

Hypogonadotrophic hypogonadism is due to malfunction of the hypothalamic–pituitary axis and is characterized by low levels of oestrogen. Women with normal pituitary functions can be successfully treated with pulsatile exogenous GnRH from a small infusion pump. The hypothalamus is frequently entrained by the pump so normal rhythms of pulsatile secretion continue after the pump is removed. Alternatively, women can be treated with exogenous gonadotrophins. Human menopausal gonadotrophin (hMG) extracted from the urine of postmenopausal women (the effects of ovariectomy or the menopause are to decrease oestradiol concentration, which results in raised circulating levels of FSH and LH) is used because it contains both FSH and enough LH to stimulate synthesis of androgenic precursors for oestrogen production. Ultrasound monitoring of follicular devel-

Box 4.7

Hormonal causes of infertility
- Hypogonadotrophic hypogonadism
- Anorexic states
- Weight fluctuations
- Obesity
- Hyperprolactinaemia
- Polycystic ovary syndrome (PCOS)

opment is important to assess development of excess follicles and the risk of multiple pregnancy. Ovarian stimulation can cause ovarian hyperstimulation syndrome which has serious implications because vascular permeability can suddenly increase, resulting in a movement of fluid out of the vascular system (McClure et al 1994).

Anorexic states and weight fluctuations

Weight loss can also disrupt the hypothalamic–pituitary axis. Anorexic patients often have disrupted menstrual cycles, but acute weight loss or disruptions in energy intake (such as those associated with 'crash' dieting) even within a normal body weight range may disrupt hormone secretion. A body mass index (BMI) index greater than 19 kg/m² and at least 22% fat as a proportion of body weight seem to be necessary for the maintenance of normal ovulatory cycles. It has been suggested that the critical fat mass for fertility is equivalent to the energy requirements of pregnancy (Frisch 1990). Low body fat delays puberty and the menarche. Weight loss particularly affects LH secretion and can result in an abbreviated luteal phase.

Appetite is stimulated by the orexigenic neuropeptide Y (NPY) from the hypothalamus. NPY is involved in the regulation of food intake and energy balance. It has both stimulatory and inhibitory effects at the pituitary gland. In the well-nourished state, NPY release is acute and intermittent, a mode of secretion that potentiates GnRH-induced LH release. However, fasting decreases plasma glucose concentrations and extremes of exercise result in chronic secretion of NPY and continuous NPY receptor activation, which is inhibitory to LH release and thus fertility.

Eating causes storage of triacylglycerides in adipose cells, which stimulates the cells to release leptin. Leptin seems to be the satiety signal, which modulates the release of NPY. In starvation, leptin levels are low and NPY levels are high, which inhibits GnRH. The nutritional control of reproduction probably had an important evolutionary role in suppressing fertility at times of poor food supply. Suspending reproductive function at times of food shortage is protective.

Case study 4.2 looks at the problem of underweight in the calculation of gestation.

Case study 4.2

Lisa, a 17-year-old primipara, presents herself at the midwives' clinic, giving a vague history and saying that she thinks she might be pregnant. On palpation and abdominal examination, Lisa seems to be 26 weeks' pregnant and this is supported by a fundal height of 26 cm. The presence of fetal heart sounds confirms that Lisa is indeed pregnant. On questioning Lisa, the midwife discovers that Lisa has had only two scanty periods in the last 2 years and does not know the date of her last menstrual period. Lisa smokes 60 cigarettes a day, and has the appearance of being very underweight.

■ Can you identify any possible reasons why Lisa might have irregular periods?

■ Why must the midwife not assume that Lisa is 26 weeks' pregnant?

■ Are there any clues that the midwife may investigate in order to estimate more precisely the actual gestation of Lisa's pregnancy?

Obesity

Paradoxically, obesity also affects fertility; obese women are over-represented in fertility clinics and have increased incidence of menstrual abnormality and a higher risk of miscarriage. The effects of obesity may persist even after weight loss has occurred. One of the reasons is that the adipose tissue is metabolically active, producing altered ratios of oestrogens and androgens. Obesity also affects insulin secretion (obese people are more likely to demonstrate insulin resistance) and affects production of leptin.

Hyperprolactinaemia

Hyperprolactinaemia can result from PRL-secreting tumours, which are usually benign. However, other factors including stress, breast stimulation or examination, hypothyroidism, polycystic ovary syndrome (PCOS) and dopaminergic antagonists can also raise circulating PRL levels. Hyperprolactinaemia can cause oestrogen deficiency, amenorrhoea and galactorrhoea (milk production). The management of hyperprolactinaemia is usually by administration of bromocriptine,

a dopamine agonist, although tumours may be surgically removed.

Polycystic ovary syndrome

Polycystic ovary syndrome (PCOS) affects 5–10% of women; it is the most common endocrine disorder in women of reproductive age and is one of the leading causes of infertility. It is suspected from clinical signs and symptoms, and confirmed by ultrasound examination that shows enlarged ovaries containing more than 10 large cysts. Some women exhibit symptoms of disrupted cycles, central obesity and hyperandrogenism, which can cause acne, alopecia and hirsutism. The endocrine causes are hypersecretion of LH, glucose intolerance and increased levels of testosterone, insulin and PRL. Oestrogen levels are high but not cyclical and ovulation frequently does not occur. The follicles retain the oocyte, forming ovarian cysts which may take on a string-of-pearls appearance. Weight loss often improves the hormonal profile and alleviates the symptoms. Women with PCOS are at greater risk of developing impaired glucose tolerance and type II diabetes (Legro et al 1999). Pregnant women with PCOS are at greater risk of developing gestational diabetes and therefore should be screened (Radon et al 1999, Vollenhoven et al 2000).

Clomifene citrate (Clomid) is an anti-oestrogenic drug that can be used to re-establish a normal pattern of ovulation in women with PCOS; however, its use is associated with an increased risk of multiple pregnancies. In cases where women fail to respond to clomifene citrate, especially if the BMI is above 25 kg/m^2, combined treatment with metformin and clomifene citrate improves ovulation and pregnancy rates (National Collaborating Centre for Women's and Children's Health 2004).

Artificial control of fertility

Oral contraceptives

The first oral contraceptives were extracts from yam. Although yams are rich in progesterone-like compounds, the active ingredient was actually mestranol, an oestrogenic agent. The combination of progestogen and mestranol was essential for good cycle control. Natural progesterone and most other steroid hormones are digested in the gastrointestinal tract and are usually effective only if injected. Chemically modified hormones are resistant to proteolytic digestion in the gut but retain their biological activity. Many synthetic steroid hormones have been developed that have similar biological activity to the naturally occurring hormones and are metabolized very slowly by the liver, increasing their half-life. The term progestogens is used to describe the family of natural and synthetic progesterone-like compounds.

The first contraceptive pills, used in Britain since 1961, were combined oral contraceptive pills (COC), combinations of an oestrogen and a progesterone. Currently the most common progestogen and oestrogen combinations used are norethisterone and ethinyloestradiol respectively (Fig. 4.9). A course of COC pills is taken for 21 days followed by 7 pill-free (or placebo) days when hormone levels fall, mimicking natural hormonal cycles and allowing a withdrawal bleed. Monophasic pills have a constant concentration of the active agents whereas biphasic and triphasic preparations attempt to mimic the characteristic fluctuations in oestrogen and progesterone throughout the cycle. Alternatively, progesterone-only preparations, known as 'minipills', containing small doses of progesterone only are taken on a continuous basis. Progesterone can also be administered as a depot injection or as a slow-releasing preparation from a subcutaneous or uterine source.

It takes at least one complete menstrual cycle for the pill to become effective. Some drugs reduce the effect of the pill and can cause breakthrough bleeding, or even permit pregnancy. These include barbiturates, antibiotics and some anti-epileptic drugs.

Emergency contraception ('the morning-after pill') usually consists a two or four high-dose pills which can be combinations of oestrogen and progesterone or progesterone only. The morning-after pill has strong side-effects and relatively low reliability so it is not recommended as a main method of birth control; it also does not protect against sexually transmitted diseases (STDs). Use of the morning-after pill is controversial. For those who believe that pregnancy begins at implantation, the morning-after pill prevents pregnancy, but for those who believe that pregnancy begins at conception, prevention of implantation is classified as abortion because fertilization has already occurred. The morning-after pill should not be confused with mifepristone, which is a synthetic steroid used as an abortifacient for the chemical termination of early pregnancy.

Effects on reproductive cycle

Synthetic oestrogens feed back on the hypothalamus during the antral phase of the menstrual cycle, reducing levels and the rate of pulsatile secretion of GnRH. Therefore the release of FSH is inhibited so follicular maturation and expression of LH receptors do not occur. The oestrogens also prevent the LH surge and subsequent ovulation. Production of endogenous oestrogen is reduced.

Synthetic progestogens interfere with the pulsatile secretion of GnRH and decrease the production of LH. Small doses of progesterone may not suppress ovulation but large doses do inhibit maturation of follicles and ovulation. Norethisterone also slows down the breakdown of natural progesterone by the liver. It can be used in low doses because it specifically binds to the progesterone receptors, rather than to androgen receptors as well. Progestogens also reduce secretory activity of the endometrium so it is not favourable to implantation. Under the influence of progestogens, the cervical mucus is thick and tenacious so is unreceptive to sperm. The peristaltic muscle activity and cilia movement of the uterine tube become uncoordinated so transport of the ovum and sperm are affected; this may directly affect successful fertilization. This effect on tubal motility is the reason why there is a slight increase in risk of ectopic pregnancy (implantation in the uterine tube) associated with progesterone preparations.

Side-effects

Reported side-effects of oral contraceptives include weight gain, headaches and nausea, depression, vaginal infection or discharge, urinary tract infection, breast changes, skin problems and gum inflammation. Oestrogens affect coagulation factors and promote intravascular coagulation. They also tend to increase plasma lipid levels. Therefore, they can be used safely in young, healthy, motivated women who have no history of circulatory disease. However, smoking and obesity significantly increase the risk of side-effects, particularly thromboembolic complications. Although chemical contraceptive agents have been linked to an increased risk of breast cancer, the doses of synthetic

Cholesterol

Progesterone

Norethisterone

Oestradiol-17β

Gestodene

Testosterone

Ethinyloestradiol

Fig. 4.9   *Chemical structures of synthetic contraceptive hormones.*

hormone used in current contraceptive preparations are now extremely low so it is difficult to assess their risk. Although hormonal treatment has known thromboembolic health concerns, the morbidity complications from pregnancy and labour far outweigh the risks of using oral contraceptives.

Puberty

Puberty describes the morphological, physiological and behavioural changes that occur as the gonads change from infantile to adult condition. The most obvious sign of sexual maturation in females is menarche (the first menstrual cycle), which indicates that the levels of oestrogen and progesterone are adequate to induce development of the uterus. The equivalent step in males is the first ejaculation, which is often nocturnal. However, menarche or the first ejaculation does not necessarily mean that the adolescent body is able to reproduce; early menstrual cycles are frequently anovulatory and the ejaculate of pubertal boys may be mostly seminal plasma, lacking sperm. The underlying hormonal changes are initiated 2–4 years before menarche and the first ejaculation. The sequence of pubertal changes is fairly constant but the starting age and the time for the changes to take place vary. The hormonal changes at puberty lead to a growth spurt and attainment of adult height. In girls, the pubertal growth spurt occurs early in puberty, whereas in boys the growth spurt occurs late in puberty (Fig. 4.10). There is thought to be an evolutionary advantage to

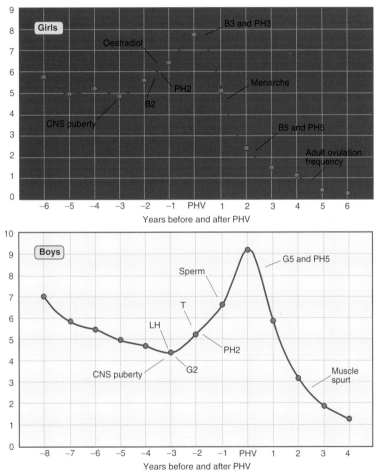

Fig. 4.10 *Order of sexual maturation events for girls and boys during the adolescent growth spurt. CNS puberty represents the changed activity of the hypothalamus and nervous system controlling the pubertal changes; stages prefixed B, G and PH represent the development of the breasts, male genitalia and pubic hair, respectively on a 5-point scale. Note that sexual maturation in girls (marked by menarche) follows the peak height velocity (PHV), but in boys (marked by sperm production) occurs before the peak height velocity. (Reproduced with permission from Bogin 1999.)*

the differential timing of adult appearance (attainment of adult height) and sexual development (fertility). Bigger girls may be treated as equals by other females in society and taught 'female life-skills', whereas smaller males will not be construed as competitive by other males in society while they undergo development; indeed, becoming fertile while not appearing to be an adult may allow an adolescent male to sneakily mate (Bogin 1998).

Physical changes

Physical changes include the development of secondary sex characteristics, the adolescent growth spurt and marked changes in height, psychological states and fertility. All muscle and skeletal dimensions change and the body composition also alters. The earliest changes are measurable in young girls from the age of 6 years. Secondary sex characteristics become evident as secretion of oestrogen (from ovaries) and androgens (from ovaries and adrenal glands) increases. Changes are seen in the breasts, genitalia, pubic hair and voice.

Hormonal changes

The hypothalamic–pituitary–gonadal axis, which has been developing since fetal life, is activated in early infancy but inhibited in childhood before being reactivated ('re-awoken') at puberty. Immediately after birth, levels of hCG and placental steroid hormones fall. LH and FSH levels increase; they are released in a pulsatile pattern, with nocturnal dominance, throughout infancy and childhood. FSH levels are higher in females and LH levels are higher in males. In the prepubertal period, FSH levels are relatively high compared with LH levels.

At puberty, the pulse amplitude of GnRH increases, resulting in dramatically increased magnitude and frequency of LH secretion, particularly during sleep. In late puberty, day-time secretion of LH also increases until the adult pattern of higher basal LH levels is reached. The 'on' switch for puberty is unknown but may be related to body mass, energy metabolism, leptin secretion or other nutritional factors. There is a progressive change in pituitary responsiveness to GnRH which may be related to maturation of the central nervous system and hypothalamus. Adrenal function matures independently before gonadal function. Adrenal secretion of sex steroids increases. Adrenal androgens stimulate pubic and axillary hair growth and have a small effect on growth and bone development. The timing of gonadal maturity and the onset of puberty correlate more closely with bone development than with chronological age. The central nervous system can restrain the onset by affecting the hypothalamic GnRH pattern. The age at menarche is affected by body mass, exercise, stress, nutrition and altitude (Frisch 1990).

Age of menarche

Over half of early menstrual cycles are anovulatory and do not result in the release of an ovum. Ovulation usually occurs about 10 months after menarche. After a period of 5 years, the incidence of anovulatory cycles has decreased to about 20%. There are secular trends in the age of menarche which got progressively earlier, particularly in the early to mid 20th century. The average age of menarche in Europe is currently 12–13 years compared with a century ago when it was 14–15 years. However, with the marked increase in childhood obesity over the last 20 years, one might expect the age of menarche to have fallen in parallel with increased body size; this has not happened.

Various influences on the age of menarche have been investigated, such as photoperiod and body mass. One suggestion was that the earlier age of menarche has coincided with the introduction of electricity, increasing the photoperiod and the individual's exposure to light (Bullough 1981). However, a more plausible theory is that it is related to better nutrition. Women seem to have a critical body mass for successful reproduction; if their body mass falls much below, the menstrual cycle becomes erratic and stops. Body fat levels seem to play a role. Anorexic women have lower levels of FSH and LH (see p. 93). Moderate obesity is associated with earlier menarche but severe obesity delays it. The combination of heavy exercise and undernutrition is synergistic, as can be observed in ballet dancers and athletes (see Ch. 12). Chronic illness can also delay menarche; the exact mechanisms are unknown. An alternative view is that there are genetic factors influencing the rate of development and that body fatness and age at menarche are both driven by the 'blue-print' or genetic plan rather than age at menarche being a consequence of fat deposition. Children who are taller tend to have earlier pubertal development and the age at menarche correlates better with height than with weight (Cole 2003).

Sequence of changes at puberty

The normal sequence in females is breast budding (at 8–13 years), growth of pubic hair, peak growth velocity (9.5–14.5 years) and then menarche (10–16.5 years). The pattern in boys is testicular growth, pubic hair growth, penile growth and growth spurt. These characteristic changes in pubic hair distribution and breast development in girls and external genitalia in males have been classified as Tanner stages which are used to assess pubertal development (Table 4.2).

From about 6 months of age, childhood growth depends on adequate growth hormone (GH) secretion. Growth declines progressively and reaches its slowest velocity just before the onset of the pubertal growth spurt. In boys, the growth spurt starts slightly later, and is faster (9.4 cm/year compared with 8.3 cm/year in girls) with delayed fusion of the epiphyseal plates so men attain a higher adult height. The pubertal growth spurt depends on sex hormones secreted from the gonads. Optimal growth depends on both sex steroids and GH; GH levels are highest in the pubertal period.

Menopause

The term 'menopause' is literally the cessation of menstrual cycles. It is defined as permanent cessation of menstruation due to the loss of ovarian follicular activity after 12 consecutive months of amenorrhoea without another cause and, hence, can only be determined retrospectively. However, the term 'menopause' is frequently applied to the climacteric (perimenopausal phase), which is the transitional decline of reproductive activity over a period of 2–3 years leading up to the final menstrual period, usually occurring between the ages of 45 and 55 years (median 51 years). The climacteric begins when fertility is already rapidly declining and continues until the ovaries cease secreting oestrogen. Premature menopause is defined as menopause before 40 years of age; it is usually due to autoimmune disorders, genetics, problems with ovarian development or chromosomal abnormalities. Menopause can also be induced, for instance by surgery (removal of ovaries usually with a hysterectomy) or by treatment for cancer. The average woman may spend about 35–40% of her lifespan in the post-menopausal period. Menopause is a complex and natural process of ageing. It is unique to humans (and the short-finned pilot whale) and is thought to have an evolutionary advantage. There are advantages to the species in preventing late childbearing and ensuring that the dependent human offspring are more likely to have the care and protection of their mother (and she to have the support of her mother) (Shanley & Kirkwood 2001).

A number of factors affect the age of menopause. These include leanness and nutritional status, ethnicity and genetics. Smokers, women who have not had children and women of lower socio-economic status tend to have an earlier menopause as do women who have shorter menstrual cycle length. There is no relationship between age at menarche and age at menopause.

Effects on the reproductive system

Morphologically, the ovaries at menopause appear smaller and relatively devoid of follicles (Santoro & Chervenak 2004). There is a finite number of ova; however, hormonal changes precede the depletion of follicles. There are about 25 000 follicles remaining at the time of menopause. One of the earliest changes is a decrease in inhibin production by the granulosa

Table 4.2 *Tanner stages of pubertal development*

Stage	Pubic hair	Breast development in females	External genitalia in males
1	None	Prepubertal; no breast tissue and papilla elevated	Pre-adolescent stage
2	Sparse growth of long downy hair along labia	Areolar enlargement with breast bud	Scrotum and testes enlarged (>4 ml); changes texture/colour of scrotal skin
3	Coarser and curly pigmented hairs	Enlargement of breast and areolar as a single mound	Further growth of testes (6–10 ml) and scrotum; increase in penis size
4	Small adult configuration	Projection of areolar above breast as a double mound	Further enlargement of testes (10–15 ml), scrotum and penis; glans penis devolvement
5	Adult pubic hair distribution	Mature adult breast as a single contour	Adult stage

cells. This results in decreased negative feedback at the hypothalamic–pituitary axis and an increase in GnRH level which promotes secretion of FSH and follicular development. This is the reason for the paradoxical increase in twinning rate that is observed in women conceiving late in reproductive life. After this brief increase in follicular development, the menstrual cycles tend to become shorter particularly in the follicular phase. This results in oestrogen secretion diminishing, so the production of androgens increases. Menstrual cycles become increasingly erratic with variable cycle lengths and an increase in anovulatory cycles. Anovulation is associated with progesterone deficiency which is associated with prolonged or irregular vaginal bleeding. As the cycles become less frequent, there is increased time for endometrial proliferation which can lead to excessive menstrual blood loss. Ultimately, oestrogen and progesterone levels decrease and cycling ceases.

From menopause onwards, levels of FSH and LH are high and levels of oestrogen and inhibin are decreased. FSH increases because of the lack of a negative feedback from oestrogen influencing the anterior pituitary gland. The postmenopausal ovary continues to produce considerable amounts of androgens and some progesterone, thus natural menopause is not equivalent to the effects of a surgically induced menopause following oophorectomy (removal of ovaries). There is some oestrogen production by the adipose tissue; this (and the protective cushioning provided by fat) is the reason why fatter women are protected, at least partially, from osteoporosis.

Effects on other physiological systems

In addition to the reproduction tract itself, there are many other target organs bearing oestrogen receptors, which respond to the fall in circulating oestrogen levels. The resulting vasomotor instability produces symptoms of hot flushes (or 'hot flashes'), sweats and palpitations. The thermoregulatory centre in the hypothalamus falsely signals that body temperature is too high. It is thought that the decreased oestrogen level abrogates the catechol–oestrogen inhibition of tyrosine hydroxylase so noradrenaline levels are increased. This results in physiological processes such as increased peripheral vasodilation that attempt to reduce core body temperature. Hot flushes are not always visible but may be extreme; skin temperature

may increase by as much as 7–8°C for a few minutes accompanied by a rapid increase in heart rate. Emotional and psychological problems such as anxiety, depression, loss of libido and mood swings may occur. Insomnia is also a frequently cited problem.

All the tissues of the female reproductive tract have a high density of oestrogen receptors and are profoundly affected by oestrogen withdrawal. The uterus shrinks. The vaginal epithelium diminishes and becomes less elastic. The vaginal cells decrease production of glycogen, affecting lactobacillus colonization, so the pH increases, resulting in increased susceptibility to vaginal infections. Vaginal atrophy causes vaginal secretions to diminish, which may result in painful intercourse. Menopausal women have an increased frequency of urinary problems, which is probably related to oestrogen withdrawal as there are many oestrogen receptors in the urinary tract (which shares the same embryonic origin as the lower reproductive tract). The walls of the lower bladder and urethra becomes thinner and the urethral muscles weaken which increases the risk of stress incontinence.

Oestrogen protects the cardiovascular system; the risk of cardiovascular disease doubles in postmenopausal women. The incidence of coronary heart disease in premenopausal women and postmenopausal women treated with hormone replacement therapy is much lower than in men. Oestrogen inhibits the uptake and degradation of low-density lipoprotein (LDL) by the coronary blood vessel endothelium. It may also inhibit coronary vasospasm. Oestrogen has been shown to decrease vascular resistance (and therefore blood pressure), increase cardiac output and increase synthesis of nitric oxide (NO, a potent locally acting vasodilator). Postmenopausal women have significantly higher levels of serum cholesterol and triacylglycerides. Oestrogen inhibits endothelial hyperplasia, smooth muscle cells growth and platelet activation. Oestrogen withdrawal is associated with raised levels of certain blood-clotting factors and an increased tendency for thrombosis, and thus with increased risk of myocardial infarction and cerebrovascular accident (stroke). Insulin resistance is more common in postmenopausal women.

Skeletal changes occur as the decrease in oestrogen results in increased bone resorption increasing the tendency to stoop and the likelihood of fractures. Osteoblasts (bone-producing cells) have oestrogen receptors. Osteoclast activity increases postmenopause and osteoblast activity decreases. Oestrogen deficiency uncouples bone formation and bone resorption. This effect is increased by changes in hormones controlling calcium balance. Levels of calcitonin fall in parallel with oestrogen levels. Calcitonin inhibits the activity of osteoclasts (bone-absorbing cells). The progressive loss of calcium from the bones and the long postmenopausal lifetime means that a woman can lose about half of her trabecular bone density and about a third of her cortical bone and is therefore predisposed to osteoporosis. Collagen is lost from the skin, tendons and bones.

There are also changes in metabolism and body composition during the postmenopause. Women tend to gain fat, especially visceral fat, and to lose muscle mass.

Hormone replacement therapy

Hormone replacement therapy (HRT) aims to reduce the diverse symptoms and adverse effects of menopause (Box 4.8). HRT provides low doses of various combinations of hormones. It is effective during its use but not in the long-term. Oestrogen on its own is mitogenic and promotes endometrial hyperplasia (which is associated with increased risk of cancer). Oestrogen with progesterone is safer as progesterone abrogates cell division and increases endometrial secretory activity. The Women's Health Initiative (WHI) studies in the United States looked at long-term health outcomes of women taking HRT using randomized controlled primary-prevention trials. The WHI studies found that HRT increased the risk of heart disease, stroke, deep vein thrombosis, pulmonary embolism

and some types of cancer. This was at odds with previous studies which tended to select healthy women as subjects and omitted women who smoked or might be at increased risk of vascular disease. However, the figures need to be considered in context; although the risk of disease was increased significantly, the actual numbers of women affected were very low. Rather than being a panacea for all menopausal problems, there are benefits and risks to HRT which need to be assessed, as for all medications. Some women have extreme symptoms of menopause which have a very negative influence on their quality of life.

Box 4.8

Hormone replacement therapy (HRT)

- Exogenous oestrogen replaces ovarian oestrogen
- Prevents long-term consequences
- Oral route or directly to genital tract or systemically (transdermal patch or subcutaneous implant)
- Abrogates flushing and sweating
- Stimulates replication of, and secretion from, vaginal epithelial cells
- Progesterone given to induce menstruation (and prevent endometrial hyperplasia)
- Progesterone-withdrawal bleeding is major reason for non-compliance
- Protects against coronary heart disease and osteoporosis

K e y   p o i n t s

- The ovary produces the female gametes (ova) and steroid hormones, oestrogen and progesterone.

- Relatively few female gametes are produced during a woman's reproductive life, between puberty and the menopause.

- The meiotic division of the ovum begins in the female fetus and is suspended until ovulation, halts again, and is completed at fertilization.

- Follicular development begins about 3 months prior to ovulation but key stages in development of the follicles are stimulated by FSH in the first half of the menstrual cycle in which the ovum is released. The developing follicles produce oestrogen; usually a single dominant follicle matures and ovulates.

- The first half of the menstrual cycle (follicular phase) is dominated by oestrogen and prepares the reproductive system for ovulation, for instance by stimulating growth of the endometrial lining.

- Ovulation is triggered by the surge of LH. The ovum surrounded by a rim of cumulus cells is released and swept into the uterine tube.

- Follicular cells remaining in the ovary become the corpus luteum, which produces progesterone and oestrogen.

- The second half of the cycle (luteal phase) is dominated by the effects of progesterone, which prepare the body for pregnancy.

- LH promotes secretion from the corpus luteum. However, the effect is short-lived so the corpus luteum regresses, unless rescued by hCG from the dividing cells of the embryo, and menstruation ensues.

Continued

Key points—Cont'd

- Pituitary secretion of FSH and LH is under the control of pulsatile GnRH release from the hypothalamus. Oestrogen and progesterone exert negative feedback effects on the hypothalamic–pituitary axis except at mid-cycle, when oestrogen exerts positive feedback leading to the LH surge and ovulation.

- The hypothalamus integrates other signals regulating reproductive function. Fertility can be disrupted by abnormal endocrine activity such as abnormal production of GnRH and hyperprolactinaemia, abnormal follicular development and extremes of weight loss or gain.

- Understanding the hormonal regulation of reproduction has allowed manipulation of fertility using chemical analogues of the steroid hormones in contraceptives.

Application to practice

There are many environmental influences, both internal and external, that may affect the regulation of reproductive cycles. There is increasing evidence that many pollutants and chemicals in the environment can have negative effects upon human reproduction; knowledge of this is important in understanding some possible causes of subfertility and congenital abnormalities of the genitalia.

It is important to realize that the menstrual cycle prepares women for pregnancy. The physiological changes, in preparation for and support of pregnancy, are initiated prior to ovulation and conception.

An understanding of the variance in the menstrual cycle is important when considering the estimated due date. Knowledge of the reproductive cycles is essential in understanding the various methods of birth control.

Annotated further reading

Balen A 2005 Polycystic ovary syndrome: a guide to clinical management. Taylor & Francis, London
A well-illustrated overview of current knowledge about the polycystic ovary syndrome (PCOS), and its aetiology, development, implications and possible treatments.

Balen AH, Jacobs HS 2003 Infertility in practice, 2nd edn. Churchill Livingstone, New York
A practical guide, based on the authors' clinical practice, which provides an overview of human infertility problems, aetiology and evidence-based possible interventions.

Eppig JJ 2001 Oocyte control of ovarian follicular development and function in mammals. Reproduction 122(6): 829–838
A recent review covering the bi-directional interaction between the oocyte and granulosa cells throughout follicular development.

Glasier A 2000 Handbook of family planning and reproductive health care, 4th edn. Churchill Livingstone, New York
A practical handbook covering all forms of contraception, pill prescribing, possible complications, advantages and disadvantages of each method and the clinical management of women with psychosexual disorders, sexually transmitted infections, menopausal symptoms and gynaecological problems.

Johnson MH, Everitt BJ 2000 Essential reproduction, 5th edn. Blackwell, Oxford
An integrated, up-to-date and well-organized research-based textbook that explores comparative reproductive physiology of mammals including anatomy, physiology, endocrinology, genetics and behavioural studies.

Kreitzman L, Russell FG 2004 Rhythms of life: the biological clocks that control the daily lives of every living thing. Profile Books
A very readable text covering fascinating details about the rhythms of the natural world and how time influences life.

Leung PCK, Adashi EY 2004 The ovary, 2nd edn. Academic Press, London
A detailed description of ovarian structure and function at the cellular and molecular level, including normal development and pathophysiology.

Mistlberger RE, Skene DJ 2004 Social influences on mammalian circadian rhythms: animal and human studies. Biological Reviews of the Cambridge Philosophical Society 79(3):533–556
A readable review, which describes how light and social stimuli ('zeitgebers' or time-cues) entrain mammalian circadian rhythms.

Ridley M 1993 The red queen: sex and the evolution of human nature. Penguin, London
A new and exciting approach to understanding reproductive behaviour and physiology from an evolutionary perspective.

Shuttle P, Redgrove P 1999 The wise wound: menstruation and every woman, 3rd edn. Victor Gollancz, London
This text provides an exploration of the sociological and anthropological perspectives of human reproduction including the facts, fantasies, taboos and cultural aspects surrounding menstruation.

....

References

Adashi EY, Resnick CE, Hernandez ER, May JV, Purchio AF, Twardzik DR 1989 Ovarian transforming growth factor-beta (TGF beta): cellular site(s), and mechanism(s) of action. Molecular and Cellular Endocrinology 61(2):247–256

Bogin B 1999 Evolutionary perspective on human growth. Annual Review of Anthropology 28:109–153

Bogin B 1999 Patterns of Human Growth, 2nd edn. Cambridge University Press, Cambridge

Brooker CG 1998 Human structure and function, 2nd edn. Mosby, St Louis, pp 480, 488, 489

Buffenstein R, Poppitt SD, McDevitt RM, Prentice AM 1995 Food intake and the menstrual cycle: a retrospective analysis with implications for appetite research. Physiology and Behaviour 58:1067–1077

Bullough VL 1981 Age at menarche: a misunderstanding. Science 213:365–366

Clarke IJ 1996 The hypothalamic–pituitary axis. In: Hillier SG Kitchener HC, Neilson JP (eds) Scientific essentials of reproductive medicine. WB Saunders, Philadelphia, pp 120–132

Cole TJ 2003 The secular trend in human physical growth: a biological view. Economics & Human Biology 1(2):161–168

Dale B, Marino M, Wilding M 1999 The ins and outs of meiosis. Journal of Experimental Zoology 285(3):226–236

Dye L, Blundell JE 1997 Menstrual cycle and appetite control: implications for weight regulation. Human Reproduction 12:1142–1151

Eppig JJ 1996 The ovary: oogenesis. In: Hillier SG, Kitchener HC, Neilson JP (eds) Scientific essentials of reproductive medicine. WB Saunders, Philadelphia, pp 147–159

Fessler DMT 2003 No time to eat: an adaptionist account of periovulatory behavioural changes. Quarterly Review of Biology 78:3–21

Frisch RE 1990 The right weight, body fat, menarche and ovulation. Baillière's Clinics in Obstetrics and Gynaecology 4:419–439

Girman A, Lee R, Kligler B 2003 An integrative medicine approach to premenstrual syndrome. American Journal of Obstetrics and Gynecology 188:S56–65

Giudice LC 1994 Growth factors and growth modulators in human uterine endometrium: their potential relevance to reproductive medicine. Fertility and Sterility 61:1–17

Hamilton-Fairley D, Johnson MR 1998 The ovary. In: Chamberlain G, Broughton Pipkin F (eds) Clinical physiology in obstetrics, 3rd edn. Blackwell, Oxford, pp 396–417

Hassan E, Creatsas G, Mastorakos G, Michalas S 2000 Clinical implications of the ovarian/endometrial renin–angiotensin–aldosterone system. Annals of the New York Academy of Sciences 900:107–118

Hillier SG 1991 Regulatory functions for inhibin and activin in human ovaries. Journal of Endocrinology 131:171–175

Hillier SG, Whitelaw PF, Smyth CD 1994 Follicular oestrogen synthesis: the 'two-cell, two-gonadotrophin' model revisited. Molecular and Cellular Endocrinology 100:51–54

Huang CJ, Stromer MH, Anderson LL 1991 Abrupt shifts in relaxin and progesterone secretion by aging luteal cells: luteotrophic response in hysterectomized and pregnant rats. Endocrinology 128:165–173

Hurwitz A, Loukides J, Ricciarelli E et al 1992 Human intraovarian interleukin-1 (IL-1) system: highly compartmentalized and hormonally dependent regulation of the genes encoding IL-1, its receptor, and its receptor antagonist. Journal of Clinical Investigation 89(6):1746–1754

Johnson MH, Everitt BJ 1995 Essential reproduction, 4th edn. Blackwell Science, Oxford, pp 64, 65, 108, 109

Johnson MR, Carter G, Grint C, Lightman SL 1993 Relationship between ovarian steroids, gonadotrophins and relaxin during the menstrual cycle. Acta Endocrinologica 129:121–125

Kunz G, Leyendecker G 2001 Uterine peristaltic activity during the menstrual cycle: characterization, regulation, function and dysfunction. Reproductive BioMedicine Online 4:5–9

Legro RS, Kunselman AR, Dodson WC, Dunaif A 1999 Prevalence and predictors of risk for type 2 diabetes mellitus and impaired glucose tolerance in polycystic ovary syndrome: a prospective, controlled study in 254 affected women. Journal of Clinical Endocrinology and Metabolism 84: 165–169

Lyons EA, Taylor PJ, Zheng XH, Ballard G, Levi CS, Kredentser JV 1991 Characterization of subendometrial contractions throughout the menstrual cycle in normal fertile women. Fertility and Sterility 55:771–774

Mason HD, Margara R, Winston RML, Seppala M, Koistinen R, Franks S 1993 Insulin-like growth factor-I (IGF-I) inhibits production of IGF-binding protein-I while stimulating estradiol secretion in granulosa cells from normal and polycystic human ovaries. Journal of Clinical Endocrinology and Metabolism 76:1275–1279

Mason HD, Willis DS, Holly JMP, Franks S 1994 Insulin preincubation enhances insulin-like growth factor-II (IGF-II) action on steroidogenesis in human granulosa cells. Journal of Clinical Endocrinology and Metabolism 78:1265–1267

McClure N, Healy DL, Rogers PAW et al 1994 Vascular endothelial growth factor as capillary permeability agent in ovarian hyperstimulation syndrome. Lancet 34:235–236

National Collaborating Centre for Women's and Children's Health 2004 Clinical guideline 11. Fertility: assessment and treatment for people with fertility problems. National Institute for Clinical Excellence

Radon PA, McMahon MJ, Meyer WR 1999 Impaired glucose tolerance in pregnant women with polycystic ovary syndrome. Obstetrics and Gynecology 94:194–197

Rance NE, Young WS, McMullen NT 1991 Topography of neurons expressing luteinizing hormone releasing hormone gene transcripts in the human hypothalamus and basal forebrain. Journal of Comparative Neurology 339:573–586

Roberts VJ, Barth S, El-Roeiy A, Yen SS 1993 Expression of inhibin/activin subunits and follistatin messenger ribonucleic acids and proteins in ovarian follicles and the corpus luteum during the human menstrual cycle. Journal of Clinical Endocrinology and Metabolism 77(5):1402–1410

Salamonsen LA 2003 Tissue injury and repair in the female human reproductive tract. Reproduction 125:301–311

Santoro N, Chervenak JL 2004 The menopause transition. Endocrinology and Metabolism Clinics of North America 33(4):627–636

Scheele F, Schoemaker J 1996 The role of follicle stimulating hormones in the selection of follicles in human ovaries: a survey of the literature and a proposed model. Gynecological Endocrinology 10:55–66

Shanley DP, Kirkwood TB 2001 Evolution of the human menopause. Bioessays 23(3):282–287

Stem K, McClintock MK 1998 Regulation of ovulation by human pheromones. Nature 392:177–179

Strassmann BI 1996 The evolution of endometrial cycles and menstruation. Quarterly Review of Biology 71:181–220

Vollenhoven B, Clark S, Kovacs G, Burger H, Healy D 2000 Prevalence of gestational diabetes mellitus in polycystic ovarian syndrome (PCOS) patients pregnant after ovulation induction with gonadotrophins. Australia and New Zealand Journal of Obstetrics and Gynaecology 40:54–58

Zeleznik AJ, Hillier SG 1996 The ovary: endocrine function. In: Hillier SG, Kitchener HC, Neilson JP (eds) Scientific essentials of reproductive medicine. WB Saunders, Philadelphia, pp 133–146

5 Sexual differentiation and behaviour

Learning objectives

- To discuss the advantages of sexual dimorphism.
- To describe how sexual differentiation is achieved during embryological development.
- To describe possible causes of indeterminate sex.
- To outline the phases of gonadal development.
- To identify the main differences in gonadal function between the male and female.
- To discuss factors affecting sexual behaviour.

Introduction

Evolutionary biologists have long questioned why evolution has led to sexual dimorphism: the differentiation of the sexes into male and female forms. Hermaphroditism remains limited to lower life-forms, such as the annelids (worms) and molluscs (slugs and snails), although it is widespread throughout the plant kingdom. It is widely accepted that the development of sexual reproduction increased the speed of evolution resulting in the wide diversity of life-forms upon the planet. The essential characteristic of sexual reproduction is that the new individual is generated from two distinct packages of genes: half from the male gamete and half from the female gamete. The meiotic division that produces the gametes not only halves the normal (diploid) number of chromosomes but also increases genetic variability within each chromosome (see Ch. 7).

Sexual reproduction results in a wide diversity of genetic material within a species, enabling the species to adapt to long-term environmental changes. The advantage of this diversity is that the population is likely to be more resilient to environmental challenges. Asexual reproduction, on the other hand, allows genetic adaptation only by mutation. The question as to why higher life-forms evolved a reproductive strategy involving dimorphism remains unanswered. However, mammalian gametes are morphologically different, which lessens the potential for same-sex fertilization, which is not far removed from self-sex fertilization, thus ensuring optimal mixing of genes.

Sexual dimorphism is genetically controlled in many animals. However, in some species, such as crocodiles and tortoises, sexual dimorphism is principally determined by environment. The temperature of incubation of the egg promotes the development of either male or female offspring. Intermediate temperatures of egg incubation result in the ratios of the sexes altering in relation to the differing temperature gradients. In birds, the female carries the ZW chromosomes and the male the ZZ chromosomes, whereas some species of fish are able to change sex during a single lifetime. Differentiation of the sexes in mammals also involves sexual dimorphism of the urinary system because the two systems are closely linked in their development.

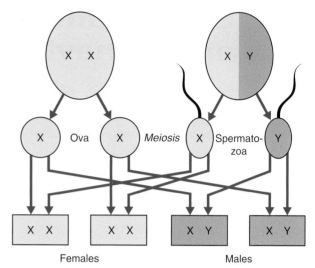

Fig. 5.1 *Paternal genetic determination of sex in humans. Sex determination is genetically influenced by the SRY gene normally located on the Y chromosome; therefore it is fertilization by either a gynosperm or an androsperm that influences sexual dimorphism.*

Differentiation into male and female

In humans, differentiation into either a male or female fetus is almost always under genetic control, depending on whether the ovum is fertilized by a sperm carrying an X chromosome (female) or a Y chromosome (male). However, events such as maternal pyrexia in the first trimester of pregnancy can result in abnormal cell division and development, in some cases contributing to indeterminate (ambiguous) sexual characteristics as well as other physical malformations. As in all mammals, the human female usually carries the XX chromosome arrangement whereas the male form carries the XY arrangement for reproductive function to be successful. Therefore, it is the sperm that determines the sex of the fetus (Fig. 5.1). Rarely, mosaic individuals (carrying a patchwork of XX and XY cells) or those individuals with mutations in genes important for sex determination may express a phenotype opposite to their karyotype leading to XX males or XY females.

The indifferent embryo

The development of the fetus, both male and female, is initially the same. Until approximately the 4th week of gestation, the fetus is in a sexually undifferentiated state. After this phase, the differentiation process is initiated by the activation of the *SRY* (sex-determining region of the Y) gene, usually found only upon the Y chromosome (Sinclair et al 1990). The *SRY* gene triggers a complex cascade of events leading to testicular development (Vilain 2000) either by activating genes leading to male development or inhibiting a repressor

of male development. *SRY* is also expressed in a number of brain structures and may be involved in sexual behaviour. If the *SRY* gene is not activated (even though the genotype is XY), the female morphological form will develop. Occasionally the *SRY* gene may be translocated on to an X gene, so if it is activated a male morphological state may develop from an XX genotype.

Abnormal numbers of sex chromosomes are often compatible with fetal development, and therefore occur with a relatively high birth frequency (Table 5.1). The major consequence of an aberrant number of X chromosomes is infertility. If there is an additional one or more X chromosome, as in Klinefelter's syndrome (47 chromosomes, XXY), the fetus will differentiate along the male pathway, as the Y chromosome is present. The absence of a Y chromosome, as in normal female development (XX) or Turner's syndrome (45 chromosomes, X0, where 0 indicates an absent sex chromosome), will result in the fetus developing as a female.

The factors that activate the *SRY* gene remain unknown; however, its effects are orchestrated through its influence on the production of androgens. The effects of these hormones upon tissue differentiation and development result in sexual dimorphism of the male during the embryonic phase. During the embryonic phase, female form develops in the absence of endocrine activity although oestrogen is required

Table 5.1 *Normal and abnormal sex chromosome complements*

State	Karyotype	Phenotype (expressed sex)	Incidence per live births	Notes and effects
Normal female	46, XX	Female		
Turner's syndrome	45, X0	Female	0.1 per 1000 females	Females are usually short in stature, possibly with a broad chest, webbed neck, cubitus valgus (extreme outward displacement of the extended forearm) and autism. They are infertile (primary amenorrhoea) and sexually immature. Associated with younger mothers
'Super female'	47, XXX	Female	1.0 per 1000 females	Normal in appearance and fertility, may be mentally retarded
Normal male	46, XY	Male		
Klinefelter's syndrome	47, XXY (up to four X chromosomes have been found)	Male	1.3 per 1000 males	Affected males are tall and thin with long limbs and small testes. May be infertile (azoospermia) and have gynaecomastia (breast development). May be mentally retarded. More common in sons of older mothers
'Super male'	47, XYY	Male	1.0 per 1000 males	Affected males tend to be tall, have reduced IQ and show 'antisocial' behaviour. Some studies show increased incidence (2–3%) in institutes for the criminally insane
Sex reversed	46, XX^{sxr}	Male	1.0 per 20 000	Small piece of Y chromosome containing *SRY* gene is translocated on to an X chromosome

for puberty and fertility. Therefore, a genetic male may develop female characteristics if the *SRY* gene is either absent or not activated (Fig. 5.2).

The undifferentiated gonad

The early human embryo is bipotential at all levels of sexual differentiation. The gonads are derived from three embryonic tissue sources: the coelomic epithelium, the underlying mesenchyme and the primordial germ cells (Fig. 5.3). The primitive germ cells, which are ultimately responsible for the production of the gametes (spermatozoa and ova), originate from the yolk sac. Here, they undergo rapid mitosis before migrating from the yolk sac wall towards the developing kidneys, about 4 weeks after fertilization. The coelomic epithelium develops into the genital ridge, which is found on the medial side of the mesonephros (which develops from the mesenchyme). The genital ridges appear to produce chemotactic substances that attract the primitive germ cells, stimulating them to develop pseudopodia and undergo amoeboid movement. Colonization of the primitive gonad by the germ cells is completed during the 6th week of embryonic development. The primary sex cords develop from the gonadal ridges into the underlying mesenchyme forming the medulla and cortex of the gonad. In the testes, the medulla develops and the cortex regresses; this is reversed in the development of the ovary. Two sets of primitive internal genitalia begin development. Further development will follow either the male or the female route depending on the hormonal influences.

The development of the male morphology

Embryological development

The *SRY* gene is essential to the production of the male morphology. It stimulates the medulla of the

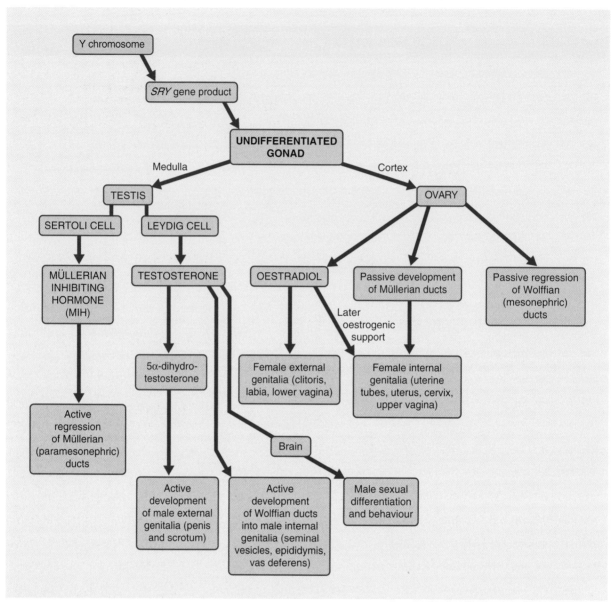

Fig. 5.2 *Sex determination factors: activation and influence of the SRY gene. Activation of this gene instigates a number of endocrine influences that determine the male morphology. In the absence of SRY gene activation, female morphology develops under a genetic influence.*

undifferentiated gonad to develop into the testes and produce two hormones, testosterone and Müllerian-inhibiting hormone (MIH; also known as Müllerian-inhibiting substance, MIS), which promote male genital duct development. MIH, from Sertoli cells, drives the regression of the Müllerian structures (paramesonephric ducts) and testosterone, from Leydig cells, stimulates development of the Wolffian ducts into the male internal genitalia, the epididymis, vas differens and seminiferous tubules. In the absence of testosterone, the Wolffian structures regress and

the Müllerian ducts continue to develop into the uterus, uterine tubes and the upper part of the vagina. Sexual differentiation along the male pathway requires active diversion, whereas differentiation into a female embryo follows an inherent pattern or 'default pathway'. However, some genes have been recognized as important in ovarian development (Goodfellow & Camerino 1999).

The Wolffian, or mesonephric, ducts initially develop as part of the embryological renal system. The adaptation of the mesonephric ducts to form the male

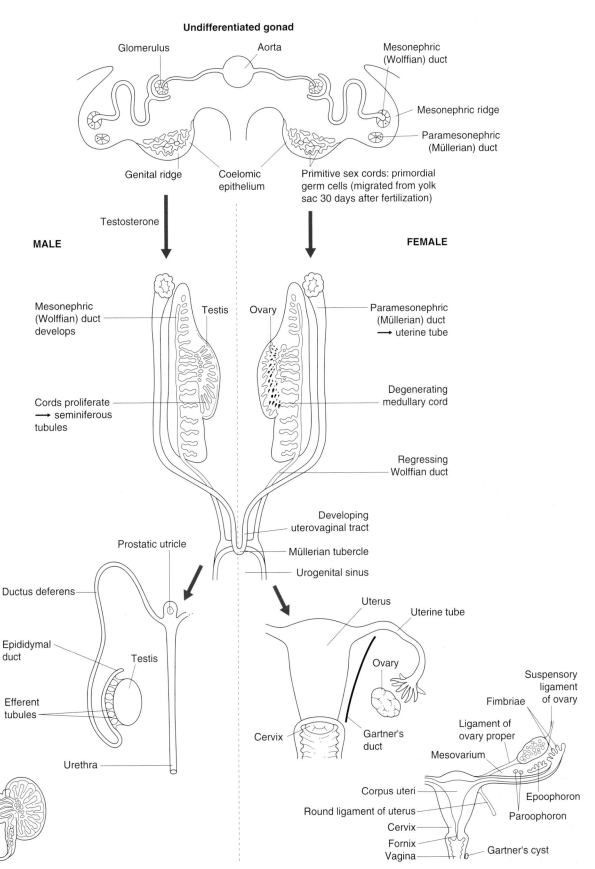

Undifferentiated gonad

Glomerulus

Aorta

Mesonephric (Wolffian) duct

Mesonephric ridge

Paramesonephric (Müllerian) duct

Genital ridge

Coelomic epithelium

Primitive sex cords: primordial germ cells (migrated from yolk sac 30 days after fertilization)

Testosterone

MALE

FEMALE

Mesonephric (Wolffian) duct develops

Testis

Ovary

Paramesonephric (Müllerian) duct → uterine tube

Cords proliferate → seminiferous tubules

Degenerating medullary cord

Regressing Wolffian duct

Developing uterovaginal tract

Prostatic utricle

Müllerian tubercle

Urogenital sinus

Ductus deferens

Uterus

Uterine tube

Epididymal duct

Testis

Ovary

Suspensory ligament of ovary

Fimbriae

Ligament of ovary proper

Efferent tubules

Cervix

Gartner's duct

Mesovarium

Urethra

Epoophoron

Corpus uteri

Paroophoron

Round ligament of uterus

Cervix

Fornix

Vagina

Gartner's cyst

Fig. 5.3 *Development of the internal genitalia. Once differentiation of the gonads has occurred, the resulting endocrine production coordinates the development of the internal genitalia. In the male, the reproductive tract is an evolutionary adaptation of a vestigial urological system.*

morphology is a significant development in sexual dimorphism, in evolutionary terms. Individuals very rarely have both testicular and ovarian tissues. These true hermaphrodites often have an internal testis on one side and an ovary on the other side (or a mixed structure known as ovatestis) which may be a result of chimerism (the fusion of a male and female embryo) (Strain et al 1998).

The phenotypic sex is determined by the sexual characteristics of the individual. The external genitalia are also bipotential (can become either male or female) and initially exist as a urogenital slit flanked by urethral folds, a genital swelling and a genital tubercle or bud. Steroid hormones directly influence the development of male external genitalia (unlike the female). Testosterone from the testes is converted into 5α-dihydrotestosterone (5α-DHT) within the target cells. Under the influence of this biologically more potent androgen, the tissues of the external genitalia form the penis and scrotum (Fig. 5.4). The urethral folds and

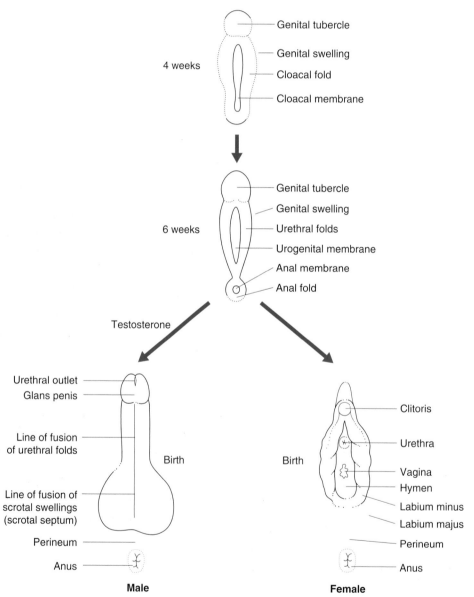

Fig. 5.4   *Development of the external genitalia: formation of the external genitalia is hormonally influenced; absence of testosterone or functioning testosterone receptors will result in the female morphology developing regardless of genotype. (Adapted with permission from Johnson & Everitt 1995.)*

genital swelling form the penis and scrotum. The genital tubercle expands to form the glans penis. The testes, like the ovaries, initially develop within the abdominal cavity but do not remain there. They descend to their normal position within the scrotal sac, suspended outside the abdominal cavity, just before or soon after birth. However, it is quite common (in approximately 1 in 50 liveborn males) for either one or both testes to fail to descend at this time (the condition is described as cryptorchidism). Spontaneous descent usually occurs within the first year of life. Testicular damage, potentially resulting in later failure of spermatogenesis and a higher incidence of malignant tumours, occurs if the testes remain within the abdominal cavity, so the testes are surgically lowered if spontaneous resolution has not occurred.

Testosterone is also converted into oestrogens within the brain. The presence of oestrogen is believed to be responsible for differentiation of certain brain structures along a male or female pathway. This resulting difference in morphology underpins the biological explanations for behavioural patterns differing between the sexes. Male sexual activity appears to depend on the presence of testosterone above a critical threshold. Female sexual activity in the human may be cyclical in response to changes in male behaviour. There are cyclical changes in the organic acid content of vaginal secretions (derived from normal bacterial flora), which may be a mechanism of olfactory communication to the woman's sexual partner (see Ch. 4).

Puberty

Following birth, the testes are endocrinologically inactive. As in the female, puberty commences when the secretory pattern of follicle-stimulating hormone (FSH) and luteinizing hormone (LH), under the influence of gonadotrophin-releasing hormone (GnRH), becomes mature. FSH and LH orchestrate spermatogenesis within the male (see Ch. 2). Unlike the ovarian cycle, this is a continuous process resulting in the production of many gametes. The testes produce testosterone from the Leydig cells, which influences the development of the male secondary sex characteristics (Box 5.1). Unlike the female, the male retains the capability of spermatogenesis indefinitely but failure to achieve copulation becomes more common with the progression of age.

Box 5.1

Male secondary sex characteristics

- Enlargement of the penis
- Pubic and axillary hair growth
- Deepening of voice (due to growth of larynx)
- Masculine pattern of fat distribution
- Development of the skeletal muscle (protein anabolism)
- Secretion of skin oil glands (predisposes to acne)
- Bone growth and adolescent growth spurt (via growth hormone secretion)
- Male sexual behaviour and aggression

The development of the female morphology

Embryological development

As the X chromosome does not contain the *SRY* gene, the Müllerian ducts differentiate into the female internal genitalia, the uterine tubes and fimbriae, the uterus, cervix and upper two-thirds of the vagina. The undifferentiated gonad develops into the ovary; the cortex develops and the medulla regresses. This is the route of differentiation in the absence of testosterone and MIH. Female external genitalia form independently of any hormonal influences; therefore the ovary has little endocrine activity until puberty. The genital tubercle becomes the clitoris and the urethral folds and genital swellings remain separate, forming the labia.

Common abnormalities

During development, the body of the uterus, cervix and upper vagina are formed by the fusion of the two Müllerian ducts. Abnormalities may range from a simple uterine septum to the complete duplication of the reproductive system (Fig. 5.5). The failure of one of the paramesonephric ducts to develop will result in a unilateral rudimentary horn.

Puberty: the initiation of fertility cycles

Puberty commences with the activation of the hypothalamus to produce GnRH in a mature pattern of

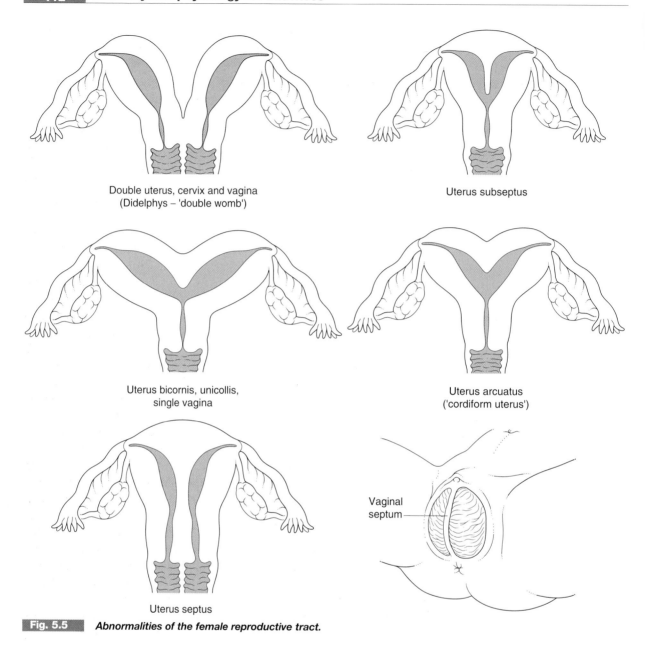

Double uterus, cervix and vagina
(Didelphys – 'double womb')

Uterus subseptus

Uterus bicornis, unicollis,
single vagina

Uterus arcuatus
('cordiform uterus')

Uterus septus

Vaginal
septum

Fig. 5.5 *Abnormalities of the female reproductive tract.*

secretion. It is suggested that the menarche is initiated when a critical mass of body fat, which may be genetically defined, is accumulated (Frisch 1990). GnRH stimulates the anterior pituitary to produce FSH and LH, which orchestrate the reproductive cycles in the female (see Ch. 4). The ovaries begin to produce oestrogens, which influence the development of the female secondary sex characteristics. The breasts develop, the deposition of adipose tissue is responsible for the distinct female body curvature, and the growth of hair in the axilla and genital region commences.

The menopause

The menopause (see Ch. 4) marks the end of the ability of the female to reproduce. The menstrual cycle ceases and the ovarian cycle is lost, resulting in atrophy of the ovaries. Therefore, there is a marked decrease in the amount of systemic oestrogen present in the postmenopausal woman. Modern fertility treatments can reverse the menopause to restore the menstrual cycle but not ovarian function. Hence, postmenopausal fertility treatment requires the donation of an ovum from a fertile, premenopausal woman.

Indeterminate sex

Indeterminate, or ambiguous, sexual features at birth are usually attributable to genetic abnormality, endocrine dysfunction (see Fig. 5.6) or developmental failure. In cases of ambiguous genitalia, the karyotype of the individual is assessed to determine the chromosomal sex (i.e. the presence of a Y chromosome for a male or the absence of a Y chromosome for a female regardless of the number of X chromosomes present within the karyotype).

Genetic abnormalities

The aetiology of genetic disease is discussed in Chapter 7. There are genetic conditions that result in a range of variable sexual development, such as Klinefelter's syndrome and Turner's syndrome. These disorders have been useful in understanding the control of normal sexual development. In Klinefelter's syndrome (47,XXY) the testes form normally but the germ cells die before completing meiosis. The Y chromosome initiates development of the male gonads but the presence of two XX chromosomes limits the completion of development. It is common in men with Klinefelter's syndrome to develop breast tissue (gynaecomastia) at the onset of puberty.

In Turner's syndrome, the single X chromosome initiates development of the ovary normally. However, the oocytes die before birth and the follicular cells become atretic, causing ovarian dysgenesis. The ovary becomes extremely regressed during fetal development, forming a streak ovary similar to a postmenopausal ovarian structure. Women with Turner's syndrome usually require hormone replacement, ovum donation and IVF to become pregnant (Abir et al 2001).

Endocrine dysfunction

Fetal endocrine dysfunction

It is thought that about 1% of livebirths exhibit some degree of sexual ambiguity (Fausto-Sterling 2002). The embryonic stage of male sexual differentiation is under endocrine influence. This may be disrupted by the failure, total or partial, of production of, or response to, the necessary hormones (Fig. 5.6). Therefore, the genetic male may fail to develop male genitalia, and appear female at birth. The gene that codes for the androgen receptor is situated on the Y chromosome. The activation of the *SRY* gene results in the formation of the testes, which produce testosterone. However, if the receptor is defective, the response to testosterone will be ineffectual so the Wolffian ducts will fail to develop into the male reproductive tract. The defective receptor may also be present on other tissues so the external genitalia will also be unable to respond to testosterone and the infant will appear female. MIH will continue to inhibit the growth of the female internal reproductive tract. Thus the child will be born with the external appearance of a female but lack both male and female internal structures. The testes remain within the abdominal cavity and as a result become dysfunctional.

Sufficient amounts of testosterone may be produced, but if the target cells lack the functional androgen receptors, or if the enzyme (5α-reductase) required to convert the testosterone into 5α-DHT is lacking, then virilization will not occur. This condition is described as testicular feminization or androgen-insensitivity syndrome. The lack of normal endocrine communication between the gonads and genitalia causes pseudohermaphroditism, a disparity between the gonadal sex (having testes or ovaries) and the phenotypic sex (appearing male and female).

Müllerian duct syndrome can occur if the MIS receptor is defective (persistent Müllerian duct syndrome) or if production of MIH is inadequate. Both the Wolffian and Müllerian ducts develop simultaneously, which results in the development of both of the male and female internal genitalia. The baby is genetically and gonadally male but retains the female internal structures, which developed from the Müllerian ducts. Men undergoing surgery for unrelated problems are sometimes found to have an unusual development of female internal genitalia without it causing any problem.

If a female embryo is exposed to androgens during development the internal and external genitalia may develop on the male pathway. Congenital adrenal hyperplasia (CAH) is an autosomal recessive disease usually caused by a defect in the enzyme 21-hydroxylase, resulting in underproduction of corticosteroid synthesis and overproduction of steroid hormones, including androgens. CAH can cause early masculinization of males and causes the majority of cases of female virilization (androgenital syndrome), accounting for most cases of ambiguous genitalia at birth. In the female fetus with CAH, androgens stimulate the development of the Wolffian ducts and stimulate the

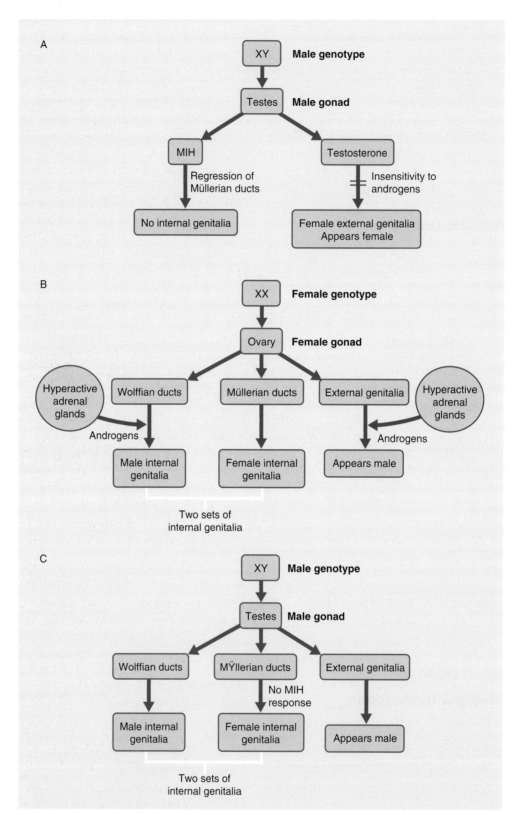

Fig. 5.6 *Aetiology of indeterminate sex at birth. A testicular feminization—insensitivity to androgens; B androgenital syndrome—excess androgens; C Müllerian duct syndrome—insensitivity to MIS (MIH).*

external genitalia to resemble the male form. The Müllerian system remains because there is no MIS. Although the baby is genetically and gonadally female (XX with ovaries), it has the internal genitalia of both sexes and male external genitalia. With high androgen concentrations, the sex of the baby may not initially be questioned and thus the problem may be evident only because there are no testes to descend. In the 1950s and 1960s, high levels of progestogenic drugs were given to mothers who had previously had a mid-term spontaneous abortion. It was thought that the pregnancies failed because of inadequate production of progesterone. However, progestogens are androgenic and can stimulate testosterone receptors causing pharmacological virilization of the fetus ('progestogen-induced hermaphrodites').

Case study 5.1 is an example of possible endocrine dysfunction.

Developmental failure

The physiological processes resulting in the development of the reproductive tracts are complex, arising from the induction and differentiation of embryonic tissue. If the tissues, such as the pronephros upon which the gonads develop, are missing then the gonads fail to develop because essential induction factors produced by the pronephros are lacking.

Induction, differentiation and growth of tissues are also affected by several other factors. Optimal development occurs at body core temperature. Maternal pyrexia at critical stages of embryonic development may severely disrupt the process. Many pathogens produce chemicals or toxins that can also severely affect embryological development (Box 5.2). There is growing concern among environmentalists over the increasing amounts of manmade chemical pollutants within the environment (see Box 3.3, p. 70). Many of these chemicals may disrupt endocrine function in a variety of ways, not only by inhibition but also by mimicking the effects of endogenous hormones. Case study 5.2 describes an example of ambiguous genitalia.

Sexual behaviour

Hormonal control of sexual dimorphism results not only in physical differences between the male and female, but also in behavioural differences. There are

---

Box 5.2

Teratogens and endocrine disrupters

■ Teratogens are chemical substances that are known to interfere with embryological development and so result in the manifestation of fetal abnormalities

■ Teratogens may be produced by pathogens, ingested by the mother either intentionally or unintentionally, or may be present within the external environment

■ Many drugs such as Thalidomide (used in the late 1950s as an antiemetic agent in early pregnancy) are now known to produce physical deformities

---

Case study 5.1

Milly, who is 43, has had an uncomplicated third pregnancy. Following a chorionic villus sample, she was informed that her baby appeared to have a normal female karyotype. As Milly's other children are boys, she was thrilled to be expecting a daughter because she had decided that this was to be her last pregnancy, regardless of the outcome. Milly spontaneously went into labour at 39 weeks' gestation and, following a rapid and uncomplicated delivery, a 4.2 kg male infant, of normal appearance, was presented to her.

■ What are the possible reasons to explain this?
■ Do you think there is a need for any further investigations and, if so, what should they be?

Case study 5.2

The midwife examines a newborn baby and is concerned over the appearance of the genitalia. Initially the parents had been congratulated upon the birth of a daughter but on closer examination the labia appear fused and the clitoris seems unusually large. A paediatrician who explains his concern to the parents examines the baby.

■ What are the possible causes for this ambiguity?
■ What investigations will be performed to establish the true sex of the baby?
■ Why is it important to confirm the sex of the baby before registering the birth?
■ What are the implications of assigning the wrong sex at birth?

many brain structures that are sexually dimorphic (different in males and females). Males have slightly larger brains and tend to perform better in spatial skills; they tend to show more physical aggression and display more sensation-seeking and risk-taking behaviour (Craig et al 2004). Females, on the other hand, perform better in verbal skills and memory tasks and seem to have greater communication between the two halves of the brain. The differentiation of certain brain structures, together with biochemical differences, is thought to explain the differences in sexual behaviour between the sexes. However, it is important to acknowledge that social construction also influences the development of sexual behaviour in humans (Carlson 1998). It is generally accepted that gonadal steroids induce brain sexual dimorphism but there may also be a direct genetic influence. Testosterone acts either directly or via local conversion into oestradiol and appears to stimulate formation of neural circuits involved in masculine behaviour.

The correct assignment of sex at birth is thought to be important in gender development, sexual orientation and attitudes later in life. Young children appear to demonstrate gender-related patterns of energy expenditure, parental rehearsal, explicit sexual behaviour and attentiveness to personal appearance. It is suggested that children recognize their own gender identity by the time they are about 2½ years old and ambiguity may have long-term developmental consequences. It is not clear whether there is any link between trans-sexualism and biological or social gender ambiguity.

Human sexuality is complex; sex appears to serve a social, as well as a reproductive, function. There is a wide diversity of sexual behaviour patterns within humans, ranging from complete homosexuality, to bisexuality, to complete heterosexual behaviour (see Case studies 5.3, 5.4). Traditionally, in Western cultures, heterosexual behaviour has always been regarded as normal and any other variation as being abnormal. This assumption was based upon many animal observations where copulation appeared to be involved only in reproduction. Justification of such behavioural patterns has been strongly argued from a sociological perspective. Recently, however, there has been an increasing amount of evidence arising from biological perspectives that attempts to explain the existence of diverse sexual behaviour (Crew 1994).

Anatomical studies have shown that there may be biological differences within certain brain structures associated with the expression of homosexual behav-

---

Case study 5.3

Lisa is a 20-year-old primigravida who has conceived by donor insemination. The biological father of the baby is Lisa's brother's partner and Lisa has agreed to act as a surrogate mother for the two men. Would Lisa's care by the midwife be any different than to a women who had conceived normally? How could the midwife include Lisa's brother and his partner in her care and facilitate the couple's preparation for parenthood?

Case study 5.4

Joan and Pippa are both pregnant and present themselves to the midwives' clinic where they inform the midwife that the babies have the same biological father who is an anonymous sperm donor. Joan and Pippa are in a stable relationship and are excited over the prospect of becoming parents. How should the midwife manage this situation and how would she plan the care of both these women?

---

iour in both males and females (LeVay & Hamer 1993). These studies can be criticized for many reasons; for instance, they are small, and the differences have been demonstrated only upon postmortem inspection. It has been questioned whether these changes might be caused by death and whether the samples studied were representative of the entire population. Many of the males studied died from AIDS-related conditions; the possibility of physical changes in the brain being affected by these conditions needs to be excluded. There does, however, seem to be a genetic predisposition to homosexuality (Hamer et al 1993), although sexual orientation is also affected by social, familial, environmental and endocrine factors. Finding genetic differences between homosexual and heterosexual brains may increase social acceptance of homosexuals; alternatively, it could provide a pseudoscientific rationale for discrimination and homophobia.

The emergence of genetic fingerprinting has enabled the identification of parents. Many biologists formerly accepted that many animals pair-bonded, reproduced and then cooperated to bring up their young, sometimes on a seasonal basis or for life. However, recent genetic studies have revealed that the offspring of many animals were conceived outside the pair-bonding arrangement. Promiscuity appears to be widespread throughout the animal kingdom. Society often portrays the human male as sexually promiscuous but studies have shown that females are six times more likely to commit adultery at the time of ovulation than during any other time of the menstrual cycle (Ridley 1993). This has a clinical significance in relation to family history-taking because as many as 1 in 6 children may be fathered outside of a relationship. Animal studies have also revealed that some animals use sex as a means of providing social stability. Studies of the Bonobo (pygmy chimpanzee) show that sex is used as a form of greeting, bonding and submission and that a full range of sexual behaviour from homosexuality to heterosexuality is present (De Waal 1995).

The programming of sexual behaviour may occur by endocrine organizational influences during the embryological period. However, reproductive behaviour may also be influenced by the endocrine system on a cyclical basis. Human females copulate throughout the menstrual cycle, but sexual motivation appears to increase during the ovulatory period and to decrease during the luteal phase.

Some animal studies have shown that the presence of sex steroids is required for positive sexual behaviour to be initiated. An example of this is the female rat who is receptive to the male only at certain times. During the fertile period, the female will adopt a specific position for mating called lordosis, which is induced by the presence of oestrogens and progesterone. The sex steroids also appear to make the female chemically attractive to the male by the production of pheromonal substances. Therefore sexual behaviour in the female rat can be described in three ways:

1. receptive: develops an ability to copulate
2. proceptive: increase in sexual motivation
3. attractive: physiological changes that arouse sexual interest in the male.

Some animals have a visual signal to the attractiveness component, such as the female baboon who advertises her sexual receptiveness by developing swollen genitalia. These components of female sexual behaviour are most clearly evident in animals that have an oestrus cycle, where ovulation is stimulated by copulation to maximize the chance of fertilization. In the human female, it appears that all three components are present throughout the cycle, which suggests that sexual activity in humans has evolved to have a social role. In many animals, it appears that various forms of stimuli produced by the female influence male reproductive behaviour that promotes successful reproduction. Human male sexual behaviour, however, may have developed to be more responsive to the social aspects of sex.

Key points

- Females have two X chromosomes, whereas the presence of the *SRY* region on the Y chromosome causes maleness. If there is an abnormal number of sex chromosomes, the presence of a Y chromosome leads to the phenotypic expression of maleness.

- If the embryo has a Y chromosome, the indifferent gonads differentiate into testes, which produce testosterone and Müllerian-inhibiting hormone. Testosterone promotes male differentiation of the internal and external genitalia. Müllerian-inhibiting hormone causes the structures that would have formed the female internal genitalia to regress.

- The endocrine changes at puberty cause development of secondary sex characteristics and the start of reproductive maturity.

- Indeterminate or ambiguous sex at birth can be due to genetic, endocrine or development problems.

- An abnormality of sex chromosome number is frequently associated with effects on fertility and mental ability.

- Sexual behaviour has been associated with endocrinology, brain development and cultural factors.

Application to practice

- Knowledge of sexual differentiation is essential in the examination of the newborn.

- Abnormalities of the sex organs and genitalia have their aetiology in the failure or dysfunctioning of the endocrine system. This may have a genetic origin or may be influenced by external factors such as pollutants.

Annotated further reading

De Waal F 2001 The ape and the sushi master. Allen Lane.
This book proposes an interesting theory that suggests primates learn behaviour from observing the behaviour of other older individuals. This theory may explain social and sexual behaviour that cannot be fully explained by innate or genetically influenced behaviour patterns.

Gooren LJ, Kruijver FP 2002 Androgens and male behaviour. Molecular and Cellular Endocrinology 198:31–40
This article reviews sexual dimorphism and the differentiation of the male brain in response to androgens, which affects gender identity and sexual orientation, sexual functioning and spatial ability and verbal fluency.

Imperato-McGinley J, Zhu YS 2002 Androgens and male physiology the syndrome of 5alpha-reductase-2 deficiency. Molecular and Cellular Endocrinology 198:51–59
This review examines the effects of mutations in the 5α-reductase isozymes which convert testosterone to the more potent androgen dihydrotestosterone (DHT). Affected individuals have ambiguous external genitalia at birth so they are believed to be girls and are often raised as such; however, virilization occurs at puberty, frequently with a gender role change.

Johnson MH, Everitt BJ 2000 Essential reproduction, 5th edn. Blackwell, Oxford
An integrated, up-to-date and well-organized research-based textbook that explores comparative reproductive physiology of mammals, including anatomy, physiology, endocrinology, genetics and behavioural studies.

Knower KC, Kelly S, Harley VR 2003 Turning on the male: SRY, SOX9 and sex determination in mammals. Cytogenetic and Genome Research 101:185–198
This is a review of the molecular genetics of differentiation of the bi-potential gonad into either a testis or an ovary depending on the presence or absence of the sex-determining region gene on the Y chromosome (SRY).

Migeon CJ, Wisniewski AB 2003 Human sex differentiation and its abnormalities. Best Practice & Research in Clinical Obstetrics & Gynaecology 17:1–18
This article reviews the presentation and management of patients affected by conditions of abnormal sex differentiation; it includes descriptions of the medical, surgical and psychological treatment options for people affected by various intersex conditions, practice points and information about relevant Internet websites and patient support groups.

Mobler M, Frazer L 2002 Donor insemination guide: written by and for lesbian women. Harrington Parker Press

This guide provides an insight into same-sex parents and the use of donor insemination.

Sykes B 2003 Adam's curse: a future without men. Bantam Press, London
Written by Brian Sykes, Professor of Human Genetics at the University of Oxford, this book explores the biological and behavioural mysteries of the male sex and discusses the cannibalization of the Y chromosome by the X chromosome drawing the conclusion that men are headed for extinction.

....

References

Abir R, Fisch B, Nahum R, Orvieto R, Nitke S, Ben Rafael Z 2001 Turner's syndrome and fertility: current status and possible putative prospects. Human Reproduction Update 7:603–610

Carlson NR 1998 The physiology of behaviour. Allyn & Bacon, Boston, pp 290–323

Craig IW, Harper E, Loat CS 2004 The genetic basis for sex differences in human behaviour: role of the sex chromosomes. Annals of Human Genetics 68:269–282

Crew D 1994 Animal sexuality. Scientific American 271(1): 96–102

De Waal FBM 1995 Bonobo sex and society. Scientific American 272(3):82–88

Fausto-Sterling A 2002 Gender identification and assignment in intersex children. Dialogues in Pediatric Urology 25(6):4–5

Frisch RE 1990 The right weight, body fat, menarche and ovulation. Baillière's Clinics in Obstetrics and Gynaecology 4:419–439

Goodfellow PN, Camerino G 1999 DAX-1, an 'antitestis' gene. Cellular and Molecular Life Sciences 55:857–863

Hamer DH, Hu S, Magnuson VL, Hu N, Pattatucci AM 1993 A linkage between DNA markers on the X chromosome and male sexual orientation. Science 261:321–327

Johnson MH, Everitt BJ 1995 Essential reproduction, 4th edn. Blackwell Science, Oxford, p 10

LeVay S, Hamer DH 1993 Evidence for a biological influence in male homosexuality. Scientific American 270(5):44–49

Ridley M 1993 The red queen: sex and the evolution of human nature. Penguin, London

Sinclair AH, Berta P, Palmer MS et al 1990 A gene from the human sex-determining region encodes a protein with homology to a conserved DNA-binding motif. Nature 346:240–244

Strain L, Dean JCS, Hamilton MPR, Bonthron DT 1998 A true hermaphrodite chimera resulting from embryo amalgamation after in vitro fertilization. New England Journal of Medicine 338:166–169

Vilain E 2000 Genetics of sexual development. Annual Review of Sex Research. 11:1–25

....

6 Fertilization

Learning objectives

- To describe the physiological processes involved in coitus.
- To describe the morphology and characteristics of the male and female gametes and how they are adapted to their specific function.
- To discuss factors thought to be involved in the conception of either a male or a female baby.
- To describe capacitance, the acrosome reaction and the cortical reaction in the stages of fertilization.
- To describe events in the first week after fertilization: the first mitotic divisions, cell cleavage, compaction, hatching, implantation and maternal recognition of pregnancy.
- To outline the relevance and implications of parental imprinting.
- To discuss the approaches used in assisted reproduction technologies.

Introduction

Fertilization is a series of processes that culminate with the union of the male gamete (the sperm) and the female gamete (the oocyte) to form a diploid zygote. Following fertilization, one cell progressively divides into 6 billion cells (6×10^{12}), forming a unique individual in about 38 weeks. Understanding fertilization is important for following events during pregnancy and understanding some of the causes of infertility and failed pregnancy. Knowledge about fertilization had led to development of sophisticated methods of in vitro fertilization (IVF) and, conversely, strategies for preventing fertilization (the basis for contraception).

Mammalian fertilization occurs within the female reproductive tract. Less than one in a million sperm, or spermatozoa, reach the oocyte. The sperm are deposited in the vagina during intercourse (coitus) and then make the long journey through the female reproductive tract (equal to about 100 000 times their own length). The hazards and challenges imposed on the successful fertilization are thought to help ensure that the individual sperm that actually fertilizes the oocyte is strong and healthy. Following fertilization, the zygote undergoes cleavage divisions while travelling through the uterine tube to the uterus where it implants in the uterine wall.

Chapter case study

Zara and James have attended the local hospital for the 12-week scan and have been informed that there is now only one baby present in the uterus. It would appear that one of the sacs, observed at Zara's earlier scans, had failed to develop further and the ultrasound scan could no longer detect any evidence of the sac's remnants. Zara and James are understandably upset over the loss of one of their babies but are reassured that the remaining baby has an extremely low risk of having Down's syndrome, is growing well and appears normal. How would you explain to Zara and James what were the possible reasons for one of the embryos failing to develop and is it more likely to occur in heterozygous or homozygous twins? How common is the loss of a twin in early pregnancy and what reasons could explain why this happens?

Coitus

Coitus in the human lasts on average 4 minutes, which is quite long compared to our closest animal cousin, the chimpanzee, who averages 8 seconds (De Waal 1995). Masters and Johnson (described in Levin 1998) described a four-phase model for sexual responses in human. This is known as the EPOR model:

- E: excitement phase, when stimuli increase sexual arousal or tension
- P: plateau phase, when arousal becomes intense; if the level of stimulation is inadequate, arousal subsides and there is no further progression to the next phase
- O: orgasmic phase, which is a few seconds of involuntary climax during which sexual tension is relieved, usually accompanied by a wave of profound pleasure
- R: resolution phase, when sexual arousal is dispersed; in males, it is believed that there is an absolute refractory period in which further sexual arousal and orgasm are impossible.

In the male

The principal event necessary for male sexual activity is acquisition and maintenance of penile erection. This is primarily a vascular phenomenon, initiated by neurological controls and facilitated by appropriate psychological and hormonal components. Initial stimulation of the penis can be both psychogenic (from erotic stimuli and sexual fantasy) and tactile (via touch receptors in the penis and perineum) and necessitates autonomic nervous system activity to coordinate increased blood flow into the vascular tissues. Centrally perceived sensual stimuli are relayed via the spinal thoracolumbar erection centre (T11 through L2), and reflex erections, initiated by tactile stimuli to the genital area, activate a reflex arc involving the sacral erection centre (S2 through S4) (Dey & Shepherd 2002). Involuntary non-sexual nocturnal erections occur during rapid eye movement sleep. There are three components of erection: increased arterial flow, relaxation of the sinusoidal spaces and venous constriction. In the excitement phase, increased inflow of blood converts the low-volume, low-pressure vasculature to a large-volume, high-pressure system (Andersson & Wagner 1995).

The arterioles and arteriovenous shunts dilate so there is an increase in blood flow which engorges the erectile vascular tissues (cavernous and spongiosum bodies, see Ch. 2). The corpus spongiosum does not increase in turgor as much as the two corpora cavernosa so the urethra is not compressed. Blood outflow is occluded by compression and constriction of the veins so the sinusoids (blood-filled spaces) enlarge further. This results in hardening and erection of the penis as the blood volume is increased by about 50%.

The control of an erection is by stimulation of parasympathetic nerves, and probably simultaneous inhibition of sympathetic outflow, which reduces arterial smooth muscle tone causing dilatation and increase in blood flow. Many central and peripheral neurotransmitters are involved in mediating the erectile response. Centrally, dopamine, nitric oxide (NO), oxytocin and adrenocorticotrophin (ACTH)/ melanocyte-stimulating hormone (α-MSH) seem to have a facilitatory role; serotonin may be either facilitatory or inhibitory, and enkephalins are inhibitory. Peripherally, the balance between vasoconstrictive factors (such as noradrenaline, endothelins and angiotensins) and vasodilatory factors (such as NO, vasoactive intestinal peptide, VIP, and prostanoids) controls the tone of the smooth muscle of the corpora cavernosa and determines the functional state of the penis. Other neurotransmitters implicated in the erectile response are acetylcholine, endothelins and ρ-kinases. NO is considered the most important factor facilitating vasodilatation thus maximizing blood flow and penile erection; it promotes the generation of cyclic guanosine monophosphate (cGMP) which increases smooth muscle relaxation and inflow of blood. Detumescence (loss of erection) occurs because NO-induced vasodilation abates as cGMP is broken down predominantly by the intracavernosal cGMP-phosphodiesterase (cGMP-PDE5). Sildenafil citrate (Viagra) and related oral therapies for erectile dysfunction (ED), such as vardenafil (Levitra) and tadalafil (Cialis), selectively inhibit the breakdown of cGMP-PDE5. Side-effects of these drugs may include headache, flushing, rhinitis, urinary tract infections, visual disturbances, diarrhoea and dyspepsia and they may be contraindicated for men with heart and various other medical conditions.

Descending pathways can be either excitatory (such as those initiated by the perceived attractiveness of the partner) or inhibitory (such as anxiety or guilt). Testosterone, mediated by oestradiol, is required to maintain intrapenile NO synthase levels, which mediate local vasodilatation by increasing NO production. In hypogonadal men, testosterone therapy can restore libido and erectile function. Other hormones, such as prolactin, adrenal steroids and thyroid hormone, contribute to male sexual functioning.

Erectile dysfunction (ED, 'impotence'), defined as inability to achieve and/or to maintain an erection for long enough to permit satisfactory sexual intercourse, can be caused by abnormalities of circulation or of neural inputs affecting the nervous control of erection. ED can results from psychogenic, organic (neurogenic, hormonal, vascular, cavernosal, or drug-induced) or mixed causes. Most cases of ED have an organic origin, mostly vascular disease. Atherosclerosis results in endothelial damage, cellular migration and smooth muscle proliferation influenced by cytokines, thrombosis, growth factors, antioxidants and metabolic changes. Ageing affects NO production by the endothelium. Smoking is a risk factor for ED because it affects the vascular endothelium and nicotine both increases sympathetic tone leading to smooth muscle contraction in the cavernosal body and decreases activity of the enzyme nitric oxide synthase. Failure of erection can be caused by damage to the spongy bodies, impaired flow in the vessels supplying the penis, drugs that interfere with neurotransmitter action or psychogenic factors. Local atherosclerosis can affect blood flow as can nicotine, which has vasoconstrictive properties. ED is usually treated with vacuum devices, intraurethral suppositories, intracavernosal injections of vasoactive drugs (such as prostaglandin E_1 (PGE_1, alprostadil) and papaverine, which increase cAMP levels) and, more recently, with oral antagonists of cGMP-PDE (see above). Neurogenic erectile dysfunction can also arise from lesions in the nervous system, such as peripheral nerve damage. At the cellular level, alterations in potassium efflux may lead to a state of hypercontraction and lack of erectile response. ED is a common age-related problem so the incidence of ED will increase as longevity increases; ageing is associated with a decline in testosterone which may compromise the oestrogen–androgen cross-talk involved in the control of erection. Diabetes is a risk factor for ED and is related to accelerated atherosclerosis, alterations in erectile tissue, and neuropathy. Diabetes-associated changes include smooth-muscle degeneration, endothelial cell dysfunction, abnormal collagen deposition and high levels of glycosylated end-products which reduce NO levels; these result in impaired relaxation of the corpus cavernosum smooth muscle (Sullivan et al 2002). Medications for hypertension can contribute to ED. ED can also be a manifestation of cardiovascular disease; hyperlipidaemia and hypercholesterolaemia affect the production of NO by the vascular endothelium. ED is a symptom not a disease; it may act as a barometer of cardiovascular health and be the first presenting sign of previously undiagnosed hypertension, atherosclerosis and diabetes. Although the incidence of ED is common and increasing, it is under-reported, underdiagnosed and undertreated as many men are reluctant to seek help. The condition can have considerable psychological and social impact on the affected man and his partner and their quality of life, causing depression, anxiety and loss of self-esteem.

As the penis becomes erect, the testes increase their blood volume and are drawn up towards the perineum. The dartos muscle contracts so the scrotal skin thickens and contracts. As stimulation proceeds, the plateau phase of emission occurs, where the muscles of the prostate, vas deferens and seminal vesicle undergo coordinated responses that propel spermatozoa and seminal fluid into the urethra. Ejaculation, the orgasmic phase, is the process of ejecting sperm from the urethra following contraction of the urethra smooth muscle. This is accompanied by contraction of the pelvic floor muscles and the accessory muscles including the vesicular urethral sphincter, which prevents retrograde ejaculation into the bladder. Orgasm, or contraction of the muscles, can occur without ejaculation. Oxytocin has a key role in the regulation of erection and, together with endothelin-1, in coordinated contraction of the epididymis and tubules at orgasm (Filippi et al 2003); oxytocin responsiveness seems to be mediated by oestrogen. The composition of ejaculate changes because the contractions are sequential and there is relatively little mixing of the components (Table 6.1).

Premature or rapid ejaculation is the most common ejaculatory dysfunction and is usually caused by anxiety or emotional stress (Master & Turek 2001); it

Table 6.1 *Composition of ejaculate during orgasm*

Fraction	Dominant gland	Particularly rich in
Initial	Prostate	Acid phosphatase
Mid	Vas deferens	Sperm
Late	Seminal vesicles	Fructose

is treated with behavioural therapy, pelvic floor muscle exercises, α-adrenoceptor antagonists ('sympathetic α-blockers'), topical anaesthetics, tricyclic antidepressants and selective serotonin reuptake inhibitors such as fluoxetine and sertraline. There have also been some clinical trials investigating the use of PDE5 inhibitors in the treatment of rapid ejaculation. Neurological lesions, such as spinal cord damage or damage following injury or surgery to the colon or abdomen, can also cause ejaculatory dysfunction; the sympathetic nerves associated with control of sexual functioning can easily be damaged. Other problems, such as diabetes and multiple sclerosis, can cause ejaculatory problems. Drugs, such as cold and hypertensive medications, may cause a lack of emission (deposition of the seminal fluid into the posterior or back part of the urethra) resulting in failure of ejaculation. Bladder neck damage in men who have undergone prostate surgery (particularly transurethral resection of the prostate) can result in retrograde ejaculation. Bloody ejaculation is usually due to haematospermia, a benign, self-limited condition resulting from inflammation of the seminal vesicles, colon, or prostate which is treatable by antibiotics.

In the female

Women have similar responses in coitus to those of men. Tactile stimulation of the perineal region and the glans clitoris as well as psychogenic stimuli elicit the response. The corpora of the clitoris and the labia undergo vascular engorgement. Increased blood flow to the vagina increases transudation and vaginal lubrication. The vagina increases in width and length and the uterus is elevated upwards, which lifts the cervical os to produce a 'tenting effect'. At orgasm, vaginal and uterine contractions increase in intensity. During orgasm, women may expel fluid from the urethra; the Skene's glands produce this fluid. Sexual responses in the female tend to be more prolonged. Detumescence of the female organs is similar to detumescence of the penis. Orgasm in women seems to be learned whereas in men it is a reflex action; female orgasm is not essential for pregnancy.

Systemic effects occur in both male and female: heart rate and blood pressure increase, accompanied by peripheral vasodilatation. This is followed by the resolution phase.

The gametes

Male gametes

The sperm (Fig. 6.1) develop in the seminiferous tubules of the testes (see Ch. 2). At about 17–20 µm long, the sperm cell is one of the smallest human cells. It retains fertilizing ability for about 2–5 days once deposited in the female reproductive tract. The genetic material of the male gamete is carried in the head of the sperm at the tip of which is located the acrosome, a vesicle containing digestive enzymes. The mid-piece

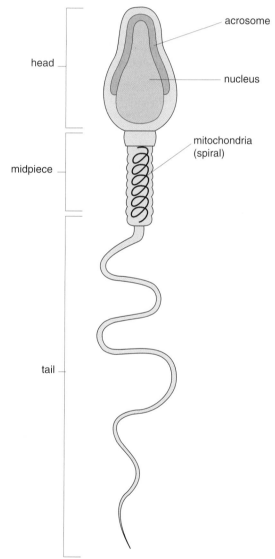

Fig. 6.1 *The male gamete: the spermatozoon or sperm. (Reproduced with permission from Brooker 1998.)*

is located between the head and the tail and is packed with mitochondria which generate the ATP required for movement. The tail of the mature sperm has a whip-like action which generates the propulsion for the sperm to swim about 30 cm/hour. Abnormalities in human sperm morphology (such as having no tail, two tails or a coiled tail, or no head, two heads or a small head) are very common. Table 6.2 summarizes these and their possible causes. Abnormal motility or morphology of sperm is associated with infertility, causing problems with both fertilization and implantation.

Sperm competition

It has been proposed that morphologically abnormal sperm, rather than being due to errors in production, have a role to play in fertilization (Baker & Bellis 1988). This highly controversial theory suggests that there are two types of sperm: 'egg-getters' and 'blockers'. The morphologically abnormal sperm may be adapted to non-fertilizing roles, particularly preventing passage and successful fertilization by a competitor's sperm. However, the theory has been contested because the metabolic cost of producing non-fertilizing sperm is high and sperm competition is probably better achieved by better swimming and fertilizing ability rather than by producing sperm to compete in other ways (Harcourt 1991). Comparative physiology predicts that mammalian species that have a large testis:body weight ratio are more likely to benefit from a promiscuous mating system in which sperm competition operates; by these criteria, men were not designed to be promiscuous (Short 1997).

Female gametes

The ovum (i.e. the oocyte surrounded by the corona radiata) is expelled from the mature follicle of the ovary (see Ch. 4) and picked up by the fimbria of the uterine tube. The oocyte is the largest human cell, approximately 120–150 μm in diameter, and is therefore just visible to the naked eye. In comparison, follicular cells are typical-sized human cells of about 10 μm diameter. A rim of these follicular cells known as cumulus cells or the corona radiata surrounds the released oocyte. During follicular growth, the oocyte accumulates RNA and protein and numerous large mitochondria, which provide for the needs of the dividing zygote. At birth, meiotic division has been suspended (see Ch. 7).

The fertile window

The lifespan of the human oocyte is thought to be about 6–24 hours. Sperm have a viability of up to about 5 days in oestrogenized cervical mucus, so sperm in the reproductive tract up to 5 days before ovulation have a chance of fertilizing an oocyte. This means that the 'fertile window', when conception is possible, is about 4–5 days before ovulation.

Table 6.2 *Abnormalities of sperm*

Type of abnormality	Description	Possible causes
Azoospermia (aspermia)	No sperm present within the ejaculate	Primary testicular failure; blockage to the vas deferens i.e. infection or trauma
Oligozoospermia (oligospermia)	Reduced numbers of sperm in the ejaculate (low sperm count)	Gonadotrophin insufficiency; drugs (social and medical, alcohol, toxins, etc.)
Idiopathic oligospermia	Low sperm count but physiological parameters normal	Unexplained
Teratozoospermia (teratospermia)	Abnormal morphology, e.g. giant heads, double tails	Genetic, toxins, viral infection
Asthenospermia	Reduced (or lack of) mobility	Toxins, infection
Sperm agglutination	Sperm clump together in groups	Infection Production of antigens against sperm (autoimmune response)

Conception on the day after ovulation has never been reported (Stanford et al 2002). Sperm concentrations fall with increasing frequency of intercourse but not to an extent that daily intercourse reduces benefit. Sperm counts are maximal after about 5 days of abstinence. Thus, daily intercourse during the fertile window optimizes conception because each day of intercourse increases the probability of pregnancy. The best outcome might by achieved by couples abstaining from intercourse for about 5 days prior to the fertile window and then aiming for daily intercourse.

Sex of the zygote

In meiotic division, the cells have their genetic complement reduced from 46 to 23 chromosomes. Each normal sperm will have 22 autosomes and either an X or a Y sex chromosome. If the oocyte is fertilized by a sperm bearing an X chromosome (a gynosperm) the zygote will be female, and if it has a Y chromosome (an androsperm) the offspring will be male (see Ch. 5). Theoretically, there will be equal numbers of gynosperm and androsperm. However, the sex ratio is not constant. The number of male babies born exceeds the number of female babies all over the world and, since the actual number of male conceptions is proportionately higher, male embryos have a higher failure rate (Bromwich 1991).

It was observed that the incidence of male babies was markedly higher in cultures where menstruating women were considered unclean and had a ritual cleansing period (niddah) before resuming sexual relations (Harlap 1979). It was therefore suggested that sperm bearing X and Y chromosomes swim at different rates. If there is a longer period between menstruation and the first intercourse, sperm deposition is less likely to occur much before ovulation, so a recently ejaculated sperm will achieve fertilization. It is hypothesized that androsperm, which are slightly smaller than gynosperm and have rounder heads, can swim faster.

There are a number of methods that are proposed to alter the sex chromosome ratio in sperm and allow sex selection. The difference in mass of gynosperm and androsperm in some species is much more marked than it is in humans. Bulls' sperm, for instance, can be differentially centrifuged. The bottom fraction in the tube will be enriched with the heavier gynosperm, which can be used to impregnate cows to increase the female dairy proportion of the herd. Separation of

human androsperm and gynosperm seems more difficult but is practised albeit with questionable success rates. Although a number of practices may have no scientific foundation, an increased number of female babies are born as the father ages, infants with blood group O are more likely to be male and environmental pollution seems to increase the number of female babies born. Sex selection is practised but usually not at the time of fertilization. In some parts of the world, selective abortion or infanticide is reported. In the West, sex selection is evident in that couples who have both a male and a female child are less likely to have further children.

Case study 6.1 looks at the question of sex determination.

In the days leading up to ovulation, the epithelial cells lining the uterine tubes become more ciliated and smooth muscle activity of the tubes increases. At ovulation the fimbriae of the uterine tube move closer to the ovary and rhythmically stroke its surface. These sweeping movements, together with the currents generated by the moving cilia, facilitate the capture of the ovum released at ovulation. Ovum capture is remarkably efficient. Some women have only one functional ovary and one functional uterine tube; even if the ovary and uterine tube are from opposite sides, pregnancy can still occur. The oocyte is transported towards the uterus by movements generated by peristaltic contractions of the uterine tube aided by the beating movement of the cilia. The oocyte has no inherent motility but is washed along by tubal fluid secreted by the epithelial cells and serum transudate. It takes about 3 or 4 days to reach the uterus. Initially the movement through the ampulla, where fertilization is most likely to occur, is slow, but the zygote

---

Case study 6.1

Molly, who has four healthy daughters, is expecting her fifth child. She jokes with the midwife that she knows that this will be a girl as well. The midwife asks her why and Molly informs her that her husband works on an oil rig and is always home for 10 days and then away for 10 days. She laughingly states that every time she has conceived she has always started her period on the day her husband returns home.

- What factors in Molly and her husband's life may influence the sex of their children?
- How unusual is it to have five children all of the same sex?

travels faster through the isthmus into the uterus. The junction between the uterine tube and the uterus relaxes under the influence of progesterone and allows the oocyte through. If the oocyte has not been fertilized, it degenerates and is phagocytosed.

Stages of fertilization

Gamete motility and sperm deposition

Spermiogenesis (see Ch. 2) occurs in the seminiferous tubules but, although the sperm are morphologically mature, they are not fully motile. The sperm develop swimming ability during a maturation phase of 4–12 days in the epididymis. At intercourse, about 200–300 million sperm are released in about 3 ml of seminal fluid (Box 6.1), which is deposited in the vagina. Repeated ejaculation normally results in a fall in sperm concentration, but the proportion of motile sperm decreases in men who are infertile, suggesting that impaired transport through the male genital tract affects motility (Matilsky et al 1993). The sperm coagulate in the vagina, which appears to facilitate their retention and to buffer them against the normally unfavourable acidic environment (pH≈4–5) of the vagina. The pH of the vagina is increased by the buffers in the seminal fluid favouring sperm motility and access to the cervix. The coagulum dissolves in about 20–60 minutes.

Between days 9 and 16 of the menstrual cycle, during the fertile period of the few days preceding and including ovulation, the watery composition of cervical mucus facilitates passage of sperm (see Table 4.1, p. 90). The cervical mucus interacts with the sperm and provides protection and nourishment. It also acts as a reservoir and may filter morphologically abnormal sperm. Most sperm (99%) do not enter the uterus.

Box 6.1

Composition of ejaculate

- 40–250 million sperm
- Prostatic fluid (30%): citric acid, acid phosphatase, magnesium and zinc ions
- Seminal fluid (60%): fructose (energy source for sperm), alkaline
- pH 7.0–8.3
- Volume: 2–6 ml

A few hundred sperm reach the uterine tubes within a few hours of coitus; this first wave of rapid transport probably depends on rhythmic muscular movements of the female reproductive tract. However, muscular activity of the female genital tract does not seem to be essential for fertilization; some sperm will be stored in cervical crypts and then travel in a relatively slow second wave through the cervical mucus, reaching the uterine tube a few days after ejaculation. A chemoattractant, probably present in follicular fluid or released from the follicle, guides the sperm to the ovum.

Capacitation

Ejaculated sperm are unable to fertilize an oocyte immediately. In vitro, there may be a delay of several hours before unprepared sperm can fertilize an oocyte. However, in vivo (and in sperm reclaimed from the uterus) the action of female enzymes and the oestrogen-stimulated high salt concentration of the uterine secretions speed up the preparation of the sperm. These biochemical and functional changes undergone by the sperm in the uterus and uterine tubes are known as capacitation. The changes include removal of adherent seminal plasma proteins from the sperm, reorganization of plasma membrane lipids and proteins, influx of extracellular calcium, increase in cAMP and a decrease in intracellular pH. The modifications alter ion channels in the membrane allowing a transmembrane flux of ions, which direct protein phosphorylation thereby initiating hyperactivation of the sperm. Sperm metabolism changes from oxidative to glycolytic. The hyperactivated sperm tail movements change to become whiplash-like so the sperm thrusts vigorously forward, moving from the isthmus of the uterine tube to the ampulla (Mbizvo 1995). The accentuated lateral head movements generate a boring action, which aids access to the oocyte. The tail is also involved in sperm movement within the oocyte (Van Blerkom et al 1995).

Access to the oocyte

The ovulated oocyte is surrounded by two layers which need to be penetrated by the sperm in order for it to reach the oocyte membrane and to acquire fusibility. The first barrier preventing access of the sperm to the oocyte is the outer layer of cumulus cells, the corona radiata, embedded in an intercellular matrix of carbohydrates, protein and hyaluronic acid. Hyaluronidase, released from the sperm acrosome, breaks down the hyaluronic acid matrix between the follicular cells so sperm can pass through to the zona pellucida. The hyperactive swimming movements of the sperm aid penetration of the corona radiata. The gradual release of sperm from the reservoir of cervical mucus and their activation close to the oocyte means the time limit of fertility is extended.

Binding to the zona pellucida

The oocyte is surrounded by the zona pellucida, which is about 14–15 μm thick. It is an extracellular matrix composed of sulphated glycoproteins that were produced by the growing oocyte. It is permeable to some viruses, immunoglobulins and enzymes. Before ovulation, cytoplasmic processes from the corona radiata cells penetrate the zona pellucida, allowing communication to, and nourishment of, the oocyte via gap junctions. When these are withdrawn in response to the luteinizing hormone (LH) surge, they may leave gaps in the zona pellucida that offer easier access for sperm penetration, thus facilitating fertilization (Familiari et al 1992). The zona pellucida acts as a barrier that allows species-specific sperm–egg interaction.

Human zona pellucida comprises glycoproteins ZP1, ZP2 and ZP3. ZP2 and ZP3 are implicated as sperm receptors; isolated ZP3 binds to sperm and blocks their binding to the zona pellucida (Tulsiani, Yoshida-Komiya & Araki 1997). Penetration through the zona pellucida gives the sperm access to the perivitelline space where interaction with the oocyte membrane can take place. The zona pellucida confers a high degree of species specificity; if it is removed, sperm from a different species are able to fertilize an oocyte, though development will rapidly arrest. This is the basis of the hamster zona-free ovum (HZFO) test or sperm penetration assay (SPA) in which hamster oocytes with their zona chemically removed are used to test the ability of human sperm to penetrate an oocyte.

The zona pellucida is antigenic: anti-zona pellucida antibodies may be the cause of some cases of infertility. The composition of the zona pellucida changes with the cortical reaction after fertilization so it prevents polyspermia but allows secretions of the uterine tube to reach the oocyte during the early stages of cell division. The zona pellucida also has a role in preventing the blastocyst from prematurely implanting into the wall of the uterine tube before it reaches the uterus. It is possible that an excessively thick zona pellucida could cause problems with blastocyst hatching and subsequent implantation.

Interaction of sperm with the zona pellucida seems to occur in two stages (Wasserman 1987). At first, the capacitated sperm loosely and reversibly adhere to the surface of the zona pellucida. Then, the sperm become strongly and irreversibly bound to the zona pellucida. Many sperm bind to the oocyte zona pellucida but usually only one will penetrate and fuse with the oocyte plasma membrane.

The acrosome reaction

After binding to the zona pellucida, the sperm undergo the acrosome reaction (Fig. 6.2). The sperm binding to the ZP receptor is a carbohydrate-mediated event which initiates a signal transduction cascade and raised intracellular calcium concentration. However, the acrosome reaction can also be triggered by follicular fluid and progesterone (Brucker & Lipford 1995). The outer acrosome membrane fuses with the covering plasma membrane of the sperm. Small vesicles containing acrosomal enzymes are pinched off and their contents are released. The inner acrosomal membrane is then exposed. A tunnel is digested through the zona pellucida by acrosin, a serine protease that remains bound to the inner acrosomal membrane, and the acrosomal enzymes released from the vesicles. The lurching movements of the sperm propel it forward through the zona pellucida and the perivitelline space so that its head is in contact with the oocyte vitelline (surface) membrane. Penetration through the zona pellucida requires both hyperactivated sperm and lysis of the zona pellucida.

Gamete fusion

The acrosome reaction triggers changes in the sperm membrane that allow fusion to occur. Adhesion molecules present on the oocyte and sperm membranes are important in sperm–egg fusion (Blobel et al 1992). The surface of the oocyte is covered with microvilli except in the region overlying the meiotic spindle. Oocyte microvilli surround the head of the sperm preceding fusion and then the sperm plasma membrane is

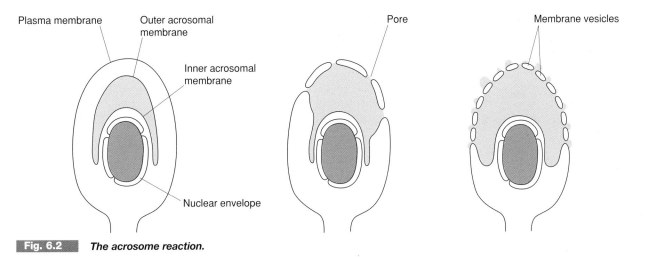

Plasma membrane   Outer acrosomal membrane   Inner acrosomal membrane   Nuclear envelope   Pore   Membrane vesicles

Fig. 6.2   *The acrosome reaction.*

incorporated into the oocyte membrane. Various docking and recognition molecules on both the sperm head and the oocyte are implicated in sperm-oocyte binding and fusion; these include sperm ADAMs (a family of proteins with **a d**isintegrin **a**nd **m**etalloprotease domain) and CD9 and other proteins on oocytes (Kaji & Kudo, 2004). In human fertilization, the sperm tail remains motile and is incorporated into the oocyte (Payne et al 1997). It is thought that any paternal mitochondria entering the oocyte are selectively expelled (Kaneda et al 1995). The zygote and resulting embryo have only maternal mitochondria (Gyllensten et al 1991); the oocyte seems to lose mitochondrial DNA (mtDNA) with increasing maternal age, a factor that may be important in fertility. As well as the male nuclear component, the fertilizing sperm also contributes the centriole and microtubule-organizing centre, from which the first mitotic spindle will develop (Van Blerkom et al 1995). Fertilization takes about 10–20 minutes.

The cortical reaction and block to polyspermia

Oocytes from most mammals develop mechanisms during growth and development to block polyspermia, the entry of more than one sperm. Following fertilization by one sperm, polyspermia is prevented by a sequence of events which modifies the structure of the plasma membrane and/or the zona pellucida. The relative importance to the plasma membrane versus the zona pellucida block to polyspermia varies with species. In most mammalian oocytes, the zona pellucida is thought to provide the most important block to polyspermia. Two events are involved: the cortical reaction and modification of the zona pellucida by enzymes released from the cortical granules (the 'zona reaction'). Failure of either of these steps results in polyspermia. Polyspermia results in non-diploid zygotes which are usually not viable but, in some cases, can develop into tumours such as hydatidiform mole or choriocarcinomas. The incidence of non-diploid zygotes increases with alcohol, drug use, anaesthesia and fertilization of 'aged' oocytes (i.e. aged in terms of hours after ovulation).

The secretion of cortical granules is triggered by a rise in intracellular calcium concentration. When the sperm fuses with the oocyte, there is increased potassium conductivity, which depolarizes the membrane. The changed membrane potential itself may be important in blocking further sperm fusion but it also results in calcium release from intracellular stores, which promotes fusion of the cortical granules with the oocyte membrane (Hoodbhoy & Talbot 1994). The calcium signal starts from the site of fusion and moves as an oscillating wave through the oocyte sequentially activating about 4000 cortical granules (Fig. 6.3). The trigger for this calcium-induced calcium rise seems to be a soluble cytosolic factor released from the fertilizing sperm. This sperm factor is probably a novel phospholipase C (PLC-ζ, or PLC-zeta) which diffuses into the oocyte cytoplasm following fusion of the sperm and oocyte plasma membranes, initiating the calcium release that leads to the appropriate waves or oscillations of calcium (Swann et al 2004). These calcium oscillations may last for several hours (Palermo et al 1997) and act as the signal for the oocyte to activate and begin development. During the intracytoplasmic sperm injection (ICSI) procedure used in IVF

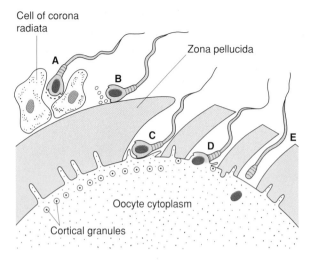

Cell of corona radiata

Zona pellucida

A
B
C
D
E

Oocyte cytoplasm

Cortical granules

Fig. 6.3 *Fertilization. A acrosome reaction; B binding to zona pellucida; C penetration of zona pellucida; D fusion of oocyte and sperm, and cortisol reaction; E fertilization.*

(see below), it is common practice to immobilize the sperm by mechanical damage to the sperm tail just before injecting it into the egg (Yanagida et al 2001). The extensive disruption of the sperm membrane wrought by this damage may help the sperm factor to be released as there is a more rapid onset of calcium oscillations after ICSI.

The secretion of cortical granules is triggered by the rise in intracellular calcium concentration. These calcium oscillations result from the release of calcium from intracellular stores and cause exocytosis of the cortical granule contents into the perivitelline space. The rise in calcium can be visualized with calcium-dependent intracellular probes; it seems to start from the site of fusion and move as a wave through the oocyte, sequentially activating about 4000 cortical granules and subsequently initiating the first division of the embryo

The zona reaction

The contents of the cortical granules (enzymes, such as proteases and peroxidase, and polysaccharides) are released into the perivitelline space and diffuse through the zona pellucida to digest the ZP3 sperm receptors. The zona pellucida loses its ability to bind to sperm and induce the acrosome reaction. The changed texture of the zona pellucida is described as 'zona hardening'. This reaction is known as the zona

reaction. The composition of the oocyte plasma membrane is also altered.

In experimental species used to study fertilization, such as sea urchin eggs, two mechanisms have evolved to reduce the occurrence of polyspermia. Prior to the ubiquitous zona reaction, sperm binding rapidly triggers an influx of sodium ions, leading to depolarization of the oocyte membrane which transiently blocks binding of additional sperm. This is known as the 'fast block to polyspermia' and does not occur in human oocytes.

Events leading to the first mitotic division

Possible benefits of arrested meiosis

The chromosomes of the oocyte had been arrested in metaphase of the second nuclear division (see Fig. 7.11, p. 155). It has been suggested that growth of the oocyte requires a diploid number of chromosomes. Meiotic arrest in the diplotene stage of metaphase means that both maternal and paternal alleles can be expressed during oocyte maturation. Observation of IVF has shown that the human meiotic spindle is unstable and very sensitive to external influences.

As a species, humans have a high frequency of aneuploidy in products of fertilization. This results in zygotes and embryos with the wrong number of chromosomes, for example Down's syndrome with 47 chromosomes (see Table 7.1, p. 156). Down's syndrome is an example of a chromosome complement that is compatible with fetal survival; other examples are thought to be just as likely but may result in failed implantation or failed in utero development. Aneuploidy is mostly due to non-disjunction of bivalent chromosomes in the first meiotic division (see Fig. 7.11) and is associated with pregnancy loss or mental retardation if the fetus survives (Griffin 1996). The frequency of aneuploidy increases with increased maternal age; ageing oocytes seem more prone to errors in meiosis and normal segregation of chromosomes. Other factors have been found to disrupt meiosis such as alcohol abuse, chemotherapy and smoking (Zenzes et al 1995). Arrest in the second meiotic division may help to prevent aneuploidy and the inclusion of an extra or absent chromosome in the oocyte.

Completion of the second meiotic division

The calcium rise that triggers the cortical reaction is also the stimulus for the oocyte to increase its metabolism.

Calcium regulates the cell cycle (Whittaker 1995); it promotes resumption of meiosis, probably via activation of M-phase-promoting factor, and completion of second meiotic division (Fig. 6.4). The increase in oxidative metabolism is preceded by a rise in intracellular pH. The 23 paired chromatids then separate, half being expelled as the second polar body into the perivitelline space. A pronuclear membrane appears around the remaining 23 chromosomes forming the female pronucleus, thus completing the meiotic division.

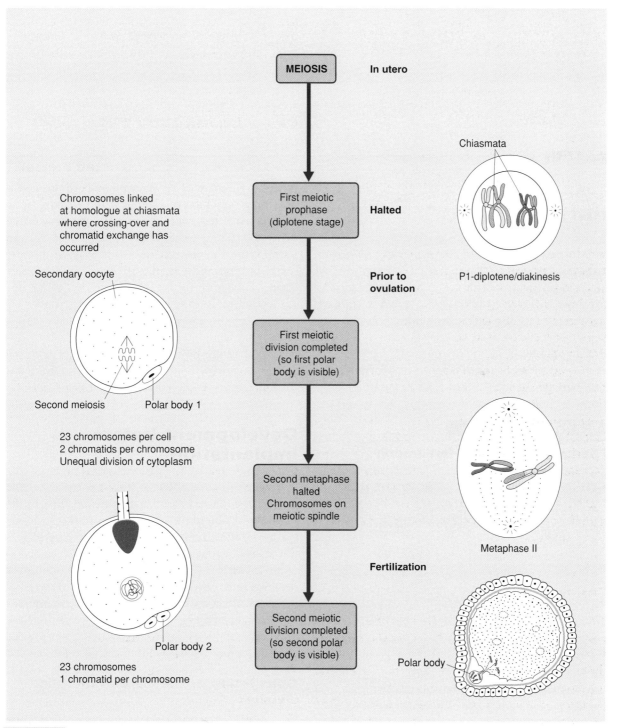

Fig. 6.4   *Fertilization and the generation of the second polar body.*

Decondensation of the sperm nucleus

The chromatin or genetic material of the mature sperm is transcriptionally inert and compacted tightly in the head. After the head of the sperm enters the cytoplasm of the oocyte, it is affected by cytoplasmic factors that cause the chromatin threads of the DNA to decondense and become transcriptionally competent. The decondensation takes place while the sperm pronucleus is moving towards the pronucleus of the oocyte. The centrioles radiate microtubules in a formation known as a sperm aster, which aids the movement of the two pronuclei (Schatten 1994). Then oocyte histones begin to associate with the male chromosomal material (see Ch. 7). As the developing pronuclei near each other in the centre of the cell, they synthesize DNA in preparation for the first mitotic division and the chromosomes replicate into chromatids.

First mitotic division

In the first mitotic division, the two pronuclei membranes first break down and the male and female chromosomes become organized around a mitotic spindle ready for the first cell division. The combination of the male and female chromosomes is called syngamy. Fertilization is complete about 18–24 hours after fusion, and the fertilized oocyte is known as a zygote (the steps of fertilization are summarized in Box 6.2). A cleavage furrow then appears and the zygote becomes two identical cells.

The random assortment of nuclear material in meiosis and the random exchange of nuclear material create new combinations of genes so the gametes are both haploid and genetically unique. Fertilization of one gamete with another results in a unique combination of genetic material in the zygote, which is important in variation of the species (see Ch. 7). Whether the sperm carries an X or Y chromosome will determine the primary sex of the zygote so it will differentiate into either a female or male embryo (see Ch. 5). Fertilization restores the diploid number of chromosomes and initiates the cleavage of the zygote.

The mitochondria contained in the mid-piece of the sperm enter the egg at fertilization but seldom survive beyond 2 or 3 days after fertilization. The mechanism by which sperm mitochondria, but not the mitochondria derived from the oocyte, are selectively destroyed relies on the tagging of spermatozoa with ubiquitin during spermatogenesis, although this label is subsequently masked by disulphide bond formation during maturation and storage in the epididymis. Following fertilization, the glutathione-rich environment of the early embryo exposes the ubiquitin-tagged sperm midpiece which is then lysed and its component mitochondria and their mtDNA are destroyed. The outcome of this efficient destruction of male-derived mitochondria and their mtDNA is that all mtDNA in human offspring is maternally derived. The relatively simple analysis of, for example, buccal smears can therefore establish maternal ancestry (see Ch. 7).

Development before implantation

The zygote spends about 4–6 days travelling to the uterus. It is moved through the uterine tube by the peristaltic action of the smooth muscle and the sweeping movements of the cilia and the fluid produced by the ciliated epithelium. The embryo at first divides approximately every 15 hours; the division time becomes progressively shorter. During the initial cleavage steps, the embryo is enclosed within the restraining zona pellucida and its total mass remains approximately constant. Cytoplasmic factors regulate cleavage, which occurs without net growth (Fig. 6.5) so cell number increases but the cells become progressively smaller.

Initially, the cleavage divisions are synchronous and each cell (blastomere) is identical, but then the cells divide at an independent rate. Later synchrony is lost,

---

Box 6.2

Sequence of steps in fertilization

- Deposition of sperm
- Sperm capacitation in the female reproductive tract
- Penetration of the corona radiata
- Binding of capacitated sperm to the zona pellucida
- Acrosome reaction
- Penetration of zona pellucida
- Fusion of sperm with oocyte plasma membrane
- Cortical reaction and prevention of polyspermia
- Increased respiration and metabolism by the oocyte
- Completion of the second meiotic division of the oocyte
- Extrusion of the second polar body
- Decondensation of the sperm nucleus
- Development and fusion of the male and female pronuclei

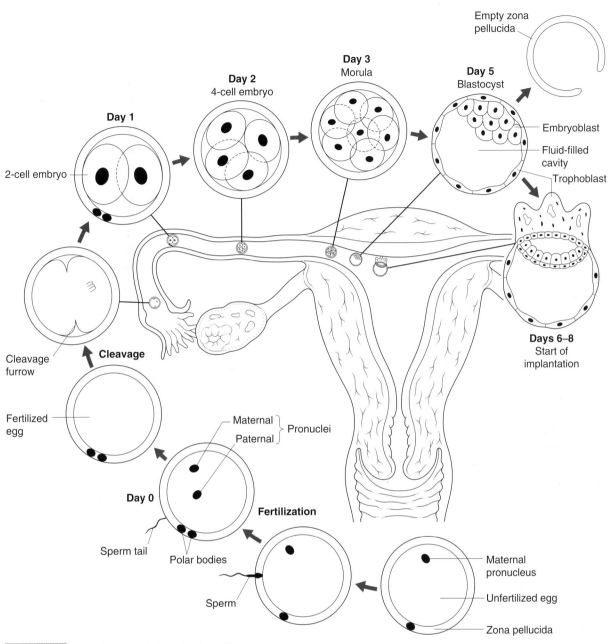

Fig. 6.5 *Development before implantation.*

so the pattern of doubling of cell number is also lost. In humans and mice embryos at the eight-cell stage, each of the cells is totipotent (i.e. is able to generate all types of cell line) and its fate is not irreversible (Hardy et al 1990). Experiments on mouse embryos have demonstrated that each of the cells has the capability of independently developing into an embryo. Cells from different origins can also be combined to form a mosaic or a chimera. In human IVF, a single blastomere can be removed from the blastocyst at this stage for genetic testing using the technique of preimplantation genetic diagnosis (PGD) without prejudicing the outcome for the embryo if it is transferred to the uterus (see Ch. 7).

After the eight-cell stage, the cells change morphologically so some of the cells at the outer edge of the embryo become flatter. About day 4, as it reaches the uterus, the embryo is a mass of cells known as the morula (derived from the Latin word for mulberry). The dividing ball of cells enters a phase called compaction. The inner cells are sealed off by outer cells, which adhere tightly in a sphere, developing a polarity and communicating by gap junctions. A fluid-filled cavity, or blastocoele, forms between the inner and outer cell layers; the embryo is now known as a blastocyst. By the 64-cell stage, the cells of the conceptus are irreversibly differentiated on the pathway to becoming embryonic or extraembryonic tissue. Differentiation into a particular cell type seems to be related to positional information of the cells, which induces particular genes to be expressed. Cells of the blastocyst initially differentiate into two distinct cell lines. Most of the outer layer of cells forms the trophoblast, which will develop into the placenta, chorion and extraembryonic tissue. Most of the cells of the inner cell mass will develop into the embryo, umbilical cord and the amnion (Fig. 6.6).

Parental imprinting

Chromosomes from the oocyte and sperm express different alleles depending on their origin. Both maternal and paternal chromosomes are required for normal zygote formation and development but genes from both chromosomes are not always expressed. This is described as imprinting and is due to gamete-specific patterns of DNA modification such as methylation. This means that, although the pairs of chromosomes carry the same genetic information, this information is expressed differently depending on whether it originates from the oocyte or the sperm. Paternal imprinting favours development of the placenta and inhibits development of the embryo. Maternal imprinting seems to switch off some of the genes involved in placental development. Normally the paternal copy of the X chromosome is preferentially activated in cells derived from the trophoblast. Conversely, in the inner cell mass the paternal and maternal chromosomes are randomly inactivated (see Ch. 7). X-chromosome inactivation is irreversible except in oogonia. Parental genetic imprinting is lost (reordered) on formation of the new gametes, which have new parental imprinting on the new formation of new chromosome sets. Most imprinted genes are expressed in placental tissue and affect growth and development (Miozzo & Simoni, 2002).

In mice embryo cells, removal and replacement of one of the pronuclei with another of opposite sex (so both pronuclei are of the same sex) results in abnormal development. If both the pronuclei are female,

early embryo development appears normal but placental development is impaired. If both pronuclei are male, placental development appears normal but embryonic development is extremely stunted. Hydatidiform mole development in the human occurs as a result of diandric diploids, i.e. when two sperm fertilize an oocyte and the maternal chromosome complement does not participate in development (Jacobs et al 1980). The result is extreme overdevelopment of the placental tissues and extreme underdevelopment of the embryonic tissues. This situation could also arise from the fertilization of an oocyte with a diploid sperm. Digynic triploids (i.e. two maternal and one paternal chromosome sets) can occur if the polar body is retained.

Human oocytes can be induced to undergo spontaneous cleavage in the absence of fertilization by a sperm and develop into parthenotes. Early stages of cleavage, therefore, seem to be maternally imprinted. However, mouse parthenogenic oocytes arrest after the first cleavage divisions, at the time the embryonic genes would be expressed. Some maternal genes are expressed in the blastocyst but overall embryonic genes are required for blastocyst formation. Imprinting causes difficulties in cloning such as premature ageing and increased risk of cancer; the clones may not have DNA which is methylated in the correct places. It is also thought that there is an increased risk of low birthweight in otherwise healthy infants born after assisted reproduction technologies (see p. 136) which may be partially related to different conditions very early in life affecting the imprinting of genes involved in fetal growth (Miozzo & Simoni 2002). Kaguya, a parthenogenic mouse that survived to adulthood (a 'virgin birth'), has been developed (Kono et al 2004) by engineering eggs to produce the normally paternally imprinted growth factor, IGF-2. The method was very problematic and only 2 of 457 reconstructed eggs developed; there is a consensus that cloning of humans would be of little merit and be likely to have major risks for maternal health and offspring development (Mollard et al 2002).

Twins

Throughout history, twinning has fascinated civilizations. The incidence of twins in the UK is 1 in 80 live-births (Hall 2003). Approximately two-thirds of the twins are dizygotic (fraternal or non-identical) and one-third is monozygotic (identical). The rate of

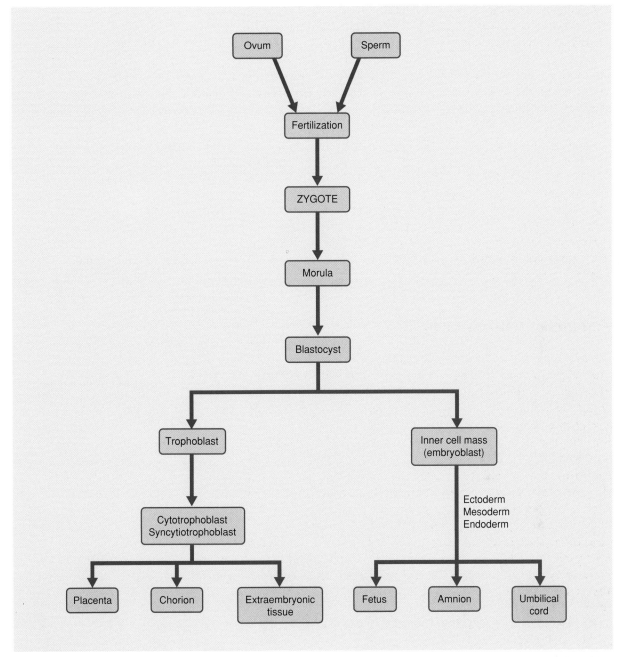

Fig. 6.6   *The pathway of cell division.*

monozygotic twins is fairly constant worldwide but the ratio of monozygotic to dizygotic twins varies markedly from country to country and is affected by season, ethnic origin and parity. Dizygotic twins arise from multiple ovulation and two fertilized oocytes implanting and developing; they have separate placentas and membranes (though sometimes these are fused). Monozygotic or identical twins are derived from one fertilized oocyte; the single embryo divides and then splits. Although it is possible that a two-celled embryo could split and result in twins, most twins in practice result from the subdivision of the inner cell mass at the blastocyst stage (Fig. 6.7). About 75% of monozygotic twins share one placenta; the remainder have separate placentas and membranes.

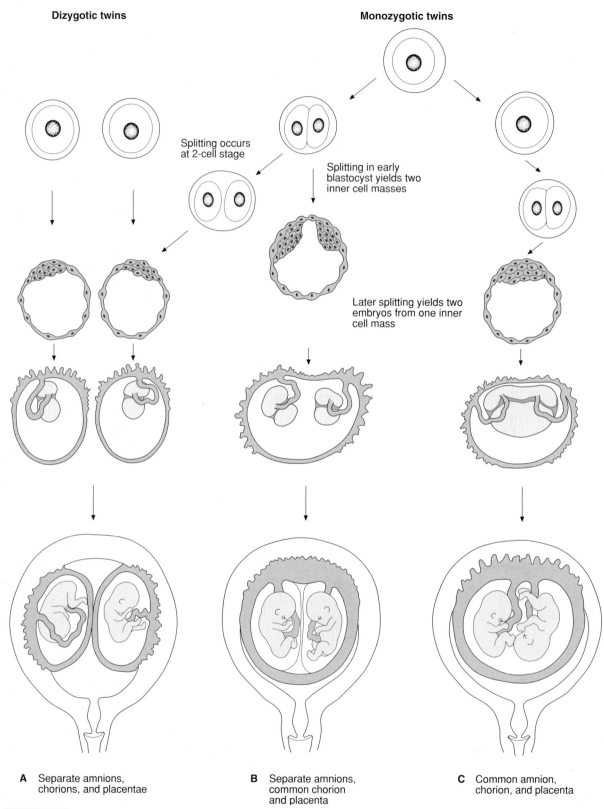

Dizygotic twins

Monozygotic twins

Splitting occurs
at 2-cell stage

Splitting in early
blastocyst yields two
inner cell masses

Later splitting yields two
embryos from one inner
cell mass

A   Separate amnions,
     chorions, and placentae

B   Separate amnions,
     common chorion
     and placenta

C   Common amnion,
     chorion, and placenta

Fig. 6.7   *The pathway of development for dizygotic and monozygotic twins. (Reproduced with permission from Larsen 1997.)*

Implantation

The blastocyst may remain free-floating in the uterine cavity until implantation at day 7. The blastocyst accumulates fluid and expands. This, together with the digestion and thinning of the zona pellucida by uterine enzymes, results in shedding of the zona pellucida described as 'hatching' at about 6–7 days post-fertilization. The disappearance of the zona pellucida allows the cells of the blastocyst to come into contact with the epithelium of the uterus. The blastocyst consists of at least 100 cells, but some programmed cell death (apoptosis) has already occurred even at this very early stage of the lifecycle (Hardy et al 1989). In most blastocysts, there is a degree of degeneration of some trophoblasts and some of the inner cell mass. After hatching, growth is no longer physically restricted and the blastocyst grows in mass as well as cell number. Embedding or nidation of the blastocyst normally occurs in the upper part of the body of the uterus (the fundal region). The blastocyst implants at the embryonic pole, where the inner cell mass lies. The inner cell mass forms the embryonic disc (see Ch. 9).

The outer cells of the blastocyst secrete proteolytic enzymes and collagenase, which break down and destroy some of the cells of the endometrial surface, forming a depression in which the blastocyst lies. Implantation in humans is a very invasive mechanism. Uterine muscle activity is low at this time because secretion of progesterone is high. Once implantation has occurred, the lining of the uterus closes over the blastocyst and the pregnancy is established. The trophoblast cells absorb nourishment from the decidua and secrete human chorionic gonadotrophin (hCG) which stimulates growth and secretory activity of the corpus luteum to produce steroid hormones, which support continued growth of the decidua. Critical amounts of hCG are required for blastocyst survival.

Maternal recognition of the pregnancy

Successful implantation requires cross-talk (reciprocated two-way communication between mother and embryo) (Hill 2001). The menstrual cycle, under the control of ovarian steroids, induces the biochemical, physiological and morphological changes which prepare the uterus for blastocyst implantation. Many signals are involved in the crucial role of maintaining the corpus luteum, regulating uterine vascular permeability and maternal immunosuppression. Not all of the signals have been identified. hCG is involved in maintaining the corpus luteum and its essential endocrine role. hCG is luteotrophic, binding to the LH receptors and stimulating a progressive rise in progesterone and oestrogen secretion. Levels of hCG are abnormally low if implantation is inadequate, if trophoblast cell division is insufficient, if implantation is ectopic or if growth of the corpus luteum is deficient (Check et al 1992). Secretion of hCG from the trophoblast is regulated by trophoblastic gonadotrophin-releasing hormone (GnRH). hCG also binds to the embryonic trophoblast cells and affects the differentiation of cytotrophoblast into syncytiotrophoblast (see Ch. 8). Before it becomes receptive, the uterus contains high levels of the endogenous cannabinoid, anandamine. The concentrations of anandamine fall as receptivity increases, leading to the suggestion that lower birthweight associated with maternal marijuana use occurs because the cannabinoid level is not optimal (Piomelli 2004).

Implantation and the three stages of apposition, adhesion (attachment) and penetration (invasion) require the endometrium to change and to become responsive. The endometrial stroma is modified (see Ch. 8); vascular permeability increases, and the endometrial cells become hypertrophied and produce prolactin. The processes inducing the changes are known as decidualization; the changed uterine lining is called the decidua. The initial changes begin in the luteal phase of the menstrual cycle. The uterine glands become more tortuous, the spiral arteries develop and the endometrium becomes thicker and oedematous. Uterine secretions increase and intercellular spaces develop. The decidua forms a physical barrier to invasive trophoblast cells migration and generates a cytokine environment that promotes trophoblast attachment rather than invasion (Fazleabas et al 2004). The decidualized endometrial cells produce IGF-BP-1 (see p. 80), which modulates interactions at the maternal–fetal interface and is involved in regulating growth.

Effectively, a nidation or implantation window, related to changes in the endometrial epithelium, occurs at about day 20–23 of the cycle (6–8 days after ovulation). The timing of the endometrial changes is mediated by preovulatory increase in 17β-oestriol and subsequent luteal progesterone secretion and has to synchronize with the time the fertilized ovum enters the uterus (Csemiczky et al 1998). Problems with coincident timing can cause infertility or impaired fertility. During this receptive period, tiny hair-like microvilli protruding from the endometrial cells transiently fuse into single smooth flower-like apical membrane protrusions called pinopodes or uterodomes (Nikas & Aghajanova, 2003). The pinopodes form a week after ovulation and are present for only 2 days before regressing. They absorb fluid and molecules from the uterine lumen which tends to decrease the size of the uterine cavity and to increase the chance of apposition between the embryo and the endometrium. The transient absence of cilia may also prevent the blastocyst being swept away from the site of implantation. Progesterone stimulates pinopode formation, as well as increased uterine secretions, increased blood flow and oedema.

The microenvironment of the reproductive tract is influenced by the secretion of maternal proteins which may then be further modified by proteins secreted by the developing embryo. Embryo-derived platelet-activating factor (ED-PAF) influences vasodilatation and oedema of the decidua. It increases vascular permeability, induces thrombocytopenia, regulates prostaglandin synthesis and activates platelets. Prostaglandins are also involved in regulating decidual factors. Other substances thought to be involved in maternal–conceptus cross-talk include chemokines and cytokines (such as interleukins, interferons and tumour necrosis factor), inhibin and other growth factors (see Box 4.3, p. 79), adhesion molecules (such as integrins), angiogenic and apoptotic factors, leptin and vitamin D (Vigano et al 2003). The expression of these proteins and peptides can act as a marker of uterine receptivity. The uterine immune system plays an important role in implantation and trophoblastic growth and development; more than 40% of decidua cells are immune cells, predominantly uterine natural killer (NK) cells.

Artificial fertilization

Infertility is defined as failure to conceive after 12 months of unprotected intercourse in couples wishing to start a family. Subfertility is thought to affect about 15–20% of couples. However, this figure depends on how subfertility is defined as couples may also experience delays in achieving second and subsequent pregnancies. In practice, infertility cannot be cured but may be treated; medical intervention attempts to optimize conditions that will aid conception. The study of

infertility is a relatively new field, open to new research. It involves not just biological aspects of fertility but also social and psychological aspects. Many couples seeking fertility treatment will not succeed. In the UK, fertility treatment is regulated by the Human Fertilisation and Embryology Act 1990 and monitored by the Human Fertilisation & Embryology Authority (HFEA).

If gametes are available, either from the couple themselves or from a donor, assisted conception techniques can be used. Laboratory techniques can be used to prepare the gametes and bring them closer together to enhance fertility (Box 6.3). Such techniques can be utilized in situations where there is damage to the uterine tubes (the site of normal fertilization), endometriosis, which may alter the uterine environment, male infertility (reduced number, motility or fertilizing ability of sperm) or coital dysfunction. They are also used to treat unexplained fertility where they will test the fertilizing ability of the sperm or where preimplantation diagnosis of genetic disorders is advisable.

IVF is now a routine procedure for certain types of infertility. Gamete intrafallopian transfer (GIFT) and zygote intrafallopian transfer (ZIFT) are related procedures, which require patent uterine tubes.

In vitro fertilization

IVF is now a routine procedure for certain types of infertility. There are a number of stages in a cycle of IVF treatment (Box 6.4) (Van Steirteghem, Liebaers & Devroey 1996). The couple may have more than one cause of infertility. IVF can also be used with oocyte donation, for instance, where the woman has ovarian dysfunction (such as premature menopause or Turner's syndrome) or has a high risk of transmitting a serious chromosomal abnormality. Ovarian stimula-

---

Box 6.3

Commonly used assisted-reproduction procedures

- In vitro fertilization and embryo transfer — IVF+ET
- Gamete intrafallopian transfer — GIFT
- Zygote intrafallopian transfer — ZIFT
- Intracytoplasmic sperm injection — ICSI
- Donor insemination — DI
- Intrauterine insemination — IUI

Box 6.4

Stages in an IVF cycle

- Patient selection
- Ovarian stimulation
- Oocyte retrieval
- Semen preparation
- Possible cryopreservation of gametes (variable success rates)
- Insemination
- Assessment of fertilization
- Embryo cleavage
- Embryo replacement
- Cryopreservation of excess embryos
- Detection of pregnancy

tion is used to increase the number of mature oocytes that will be harvested as some are likely to fail to be fertilized. The method is based on suppressing the natural menstrual cycle by inhibiting the LH surge with a GnRH agonist and then stimulating follicular development with hMG (human menopausal gonadotrophin, which contains FSH and LH). Ultrasound techniques can be used for both follicular assessment and the retrieval of oocytes. When several follicles have grown to a particular size (17–18 mm), ovulation is induced with human gonadotrophin. The oocytes are collected at a preovulatory stage so they are not truly mature. Progesterone or hCG is necessary to support the luteal phase. The collected oocytes are then cultured. The semen is prepared by separating the motile sperm from the seminal fluid and allowing them to capacitate. The capacitated sperm are introduced to the oocyte within a few hours of oocyte retrieval. The oocyte is enclosed by the corona radiata. The presence of the first polar body shows that the oocyte is at the metaphase II stage (see Fig. 7.11, p. 155) and ready to be fertilized.

At about 18 hours after insemination, the oocytes are denuded by mechanical removal of the cumulus cells. If fertilization has occurred, two distinct pronuclei, and usually two polar bodies, will be observable under a microscope. Twenty-four hours later, embryonic cleavage is evident and the quality of the embryo can be assessed morphologically for its potential to continue developing by the number of anucleate fragments and the evenness of the cells. Embryos with fragmented or uneven cells rarely continue developing. At the four-cell stage, a blastomere can be removed for preimplantation diagnosis (Handyside et al 1992).

Two or three embryos are then selected for transfer to the uterus about 48 hours after the two-cell stage; morphological scoring systems are used to assess embryo quality and potential viability. The zona pellucida tends to harden in culture and has to be eroded mechanically or by acid digestion to aid hatching prior to the transfer. Multiple births are common with IVF, particularly in younger women, as two to three embryos may be replaced. Successful implantation relies on both embryo quality and endometrial receptivity.

Other procedures

In GIFT, the gametes are collected and prepared as for IVF but they are immediately transferred to the uterine tubes so fertilization occurs in vivo. In ZIFT, the fertilized oocyte is transferred into the uterine tube before cleavage. Excess embryos can be cryopreserved (carefully frozen using protectant fluid and specific rates of freezing and thawing). Increased hCG levels 10–12 days after fertilization confirm a successful pregnancy; levels of hCG usually double every 1.3 days.

Where there is severe male infertility the sperm are unable to fertilize the oocyte. Several techniques have been developed to micromanipulate the gametes to allow the sperm direct access to the oocyte. In PDZ (partial zona dissection) a small hole is made in the zona pellucida to allow the sperm to enter the perivitelline space. In SUZI (subzonal sperm injection) several sperm are injected into the perivitelline space. Both of these techniques have now been superseded by ICSI where a single sperm is injected directly into the oocyte (Palermo et al 1997). The advantage of this method is that it is successful even with very severe sperm dysfunction. Sperm do not need to be motile and can even be harvested from the epididymis by microepididymal sperm aspiration (MESA) or percutaneous epididymal sperm aspiration (PESA). The success rates of ICSI are usually high because the oocyte and endometrium are healthy and apparently not damaged by the procedures (although the cytoplasm of the egg is disrupted during injection so there is a small risk of mechanical injury to the meiotic spindle that could potentially lead to aneuploidy). ICSI bypasses almost all the natural selection mechanisms that challenge the sperm in a normal conception.

It will be important to monitor the health of children born following assisted conception procedures.

For instance, the fertility of male offspring resulting from fertilization with a sperm incapable of normal fertilization may be affected. Also, male offspring born following ICSI from fathers with Y-chromosome deletions may inherit the same deletion (Chandley 1998). Cryopreservation techniques have resulted in increased fertility rates; cryopreserved embryos that are surplus to requirement may be offered to other couples who are either infertile or carry a genetic disease but find antenatal diagnosis and termination of an abnormal pregnancy unacceptable. Embryo donation has many ethical, legal and psychosocial implications. There is an increasing trend for patients facing intensive chemotherapy and other procedures to request gamete retrieval and cryopreservation; a more ethically complex area is requests for gamete retrieval from men who are terminally ill, dead, near-dead (for instance, in a persistent vegetative state) or brain-dead.

Case study 6.2 is an example of artificial fertilization.

Case study 6.2

Elizabeth is a 42-year-old primipara who has been married for 20 years to Thomas. They had never used contraception. After initial investigations at a subfertility clinic, they were told that Thomas had a very low sperm count and that the sperm present were morphologically abnormal and displayed little motility. After eight attempts of IVF, Elizabeth and Thomas were offered ICSI and as a result a pregnancy occurred.

- Should the advice that the midwife gives to Elizabeth and Thomas be any different to that given to a fertile couple?
- What kinds of anxieties and concerns would Elizabeth and Thomas have and how might these be addressed?

Key points

- The male gamete (sperm) is one of the smallest human cells and is motile, whereas the female gamete (oocyte) is one of the largest human cells and is immotile.

- Fertilization is the union of the sperm and the oocyte, resulting in a diploid zygote.

- Coitus requires circulatory and neuronal activity resulting in erection of the penis by increasing blood volume. Sexual arousal causes analogous physiological changes in the female.

- Although sex selection is practised in the husbandry of domesticated animals, there is little evidence to suggest it can be successfully manipulated in humans.

- In order to fertilize the oocyte, sperm undergo a series of changes: (a) development in the testes; (b) maturation in the epididymis and (c) capacitation in the female reproductive tract which alters their tail movements and metabolism and enables them to fertilize the oocyte.

- The acrosome reaction, and release of enzymes, results in digestion of a pathway through the follicular cells and zona pellucida. Interaction between the sperm and the oocyte is mediated by species-specific receptors.

- Fusion of the gametes results in the cortical reaction (which prevents polyspermia), metabolic changes, completion of the oocyte meiotic division, extrusion of the second polar body, DNA replication and initiation of the first mitotic division.

- The embryo or zygote undergoes cell cleavage as it is moved towards the uterus.

- As the number of cells increases, the embryo is described as a morula. The inner and outer cells undergo compaction and differentiate.

- The accumulation of fluid causes the embryo to 'hatch' out of the zona pellucida and it is then described as a blastocyst. The blastocyst has an outer layer of trophoblast cells (the future placenta) and an inner cell mass (the future embryo).

- The trophoblast cells secrete hCG, which promotes the survival and further growth of the corpus luteum.

- Maternal recognition of the pregnancy allows embryonic development and uterine receptiveness to be coordinated.

- Implantation occurs about 7 days after fertilization.

- Assisted fertility techniques have been developed for couples who have subfertility.

Primarily, the midwife is not involved with the treatment of infertility. However, with the advance of technology there are an increasing number of conceptions and successful pregnancies as a result of fertility treatment.

An understanding of the complexities and interventions required to achieve conception is essential in order for the midwife to support women and partners. A knowledge of fertilization is also required in the understanding of contraceptive techniques.

....

Annotated further reading

Balen AH, Jacobs HS 2003 Infertility in practice, 2nd edn. Churchill Livingstone, New York
A practical guide, based on the authors' clinical practice, which provides an overview of human infertility problems, aetiology and evidence-based possible interventions.

Bancroft JHJ 2003 Human sexuality and its problems, 3rd edn. Churchill Livingstone, New York
A comprehensive text of factors determining human sexuality which covers sexual development, anatomy and physiology, biochemistry and endocrinology in addition to sociological and psychological aspects of sexuality. Topics include development of sexual preferences, investigation of sexual dysfunction, marriage, marital therapy, prostitution, AIDS, ageing, sexual abuse and sexual abuse survivors.

Carlson BM 2004 Human embryology and developmental biology, 3rd edn. Mosby, St Louis
An illustrated textbook detailing the development of the human embryo from conception to birth including the molecular and mechanistic basis of normal and abnormal development; provides a particularly good description of control of development at the cellular and molecular level.

Coticchio G, Fishel S 1998 Conception to implantation. In: Chamberlain G, Broughton Pipkin F (eds) Clinical physiology in obstetrics, 3rd edn. Blackwell, Oxford, pp 439–466
A detailed review of this early period of embryo development by authors working in the field of fertility treatment.

Fleming S, King R 2003 Micromanipulation in assisted conception. Cambridge University Press, Cambridge
This is a practical handbook which provides comprehensive and well-illustrated descriptions of the micromanipulation techniques used in IVF laboratories, clearly explaining the procedures and potential difficulties.

Furse A 2001 Your essential infertility companion: a user's guide to tests, technology and therapies. Harper Collins, London
A useful and sensitively written reference on all aspects of human infertility including practical information on the medical help available, the procedures involved, potential side-effects of fertility drugs, self-help, complementary therapies and emotional aspects of fertility treatment.

Gerhart J, Kirschner M 1997 Cells, embryos and evolution. Blackwell, Oxford
This text explores how the origin of phenotypic variation in relation to evolutionary adaptation is achieved in the development of the eukaryotic cell and its processes.

James WH 1997 Sex ratio, coital rate, hormones and the time of fertilization within the cycle. Annals of Human Biology 24:403–409
This article examines the relationship between coital rates, the timing of conception within the menstrual cycle and the sex ratios of the offspring produced.

Johnson MH, Everitt BJ 2000 Essential reproduction, 5th edn. Blackwell, Oxford
An excellent, up-to-date and well-organized research-based textbook that explores comparative reproductive physiology of mammals including anatomy, physiology, endocrinology, genetics and behavioural studies.

Larsen WJ 2001 Human embryology, 3rd edn. Churchill Livingstone, New York
A good introduction to embryology which is clearly written and illustrated, covering the concepts and principles underlying development.

Lee RG, Morgan D 2001 Human fertilisation and embryology: regulating the reproductive revolution. Blackstone Press
A comprehensive review of the regulation of assisted conception including complex moral issues such as abortion, embryo research and cloning.

Lee J, Yap C 2003 Embryo donation: a review. Acta Obstetrica et Gynecologica Scandinavica 82:991–996
A thought-provoking evaluation of the uses of embryo donation that considers the legal and psychosocial issues associated with the technique.

Trounson AO, Gosden RG (eds) 2003 The biology and pathology of the oocyte: its role in fertility and reproductive medicine. Cambridge University Press, Cambridge
This book is about the development, biology and pathology of the oocyte, and the new developments involved in enhancing fertility, overcoming infertility, avoiding inherited diseases, cloning and creating genetically engineered animals.

··

References

Andersson KE, Wagner G 1995 Physiology of penile erection. Physiological Review 75:191–236

Argiolas A, Melis MR 1995 Neuromodulation of penile erection: an overview of the role of neurotransmitters and neuropeptides. Progress in Neurobiology 47:235–255

Baker RR, Bellis MA 1988 Kamikaze sperm in mammals. Animal Behaviour 36:936–939

Blobel CP, Wolfsberg TG, Turck CW, Myles DG, Primakoff P, White JM 1992 A potential fusion peptide and an integrin ligand domain in a protein active in sperm–egg fusion. Nature 356:248–252

Bromwich P 1991 The sex ratio, and ways of manipulating it. Progress in Obstetrics and Gynaecology 7:217–231

Brooker CG 1998 Human structure and function, 2nd edn. Mosby, St Louis, p 477

Brucker C, Lipford GB 1995 The human sperm acrosome reaction: physiology and regulatory mechanisms. Human Reproduction Update 1:51–62

Burnett AL 2003 Neurophysiology of erectile function: androgenic effects. Journal of Andrology 24:2–5

Chandley AC 1998 Chromosome anomalies and Y chromosome microdeletions as causal factors in male infertility. Human Reproduction 13(Suppl 1):45–50

Check JH, Weiss RM, Lurie D 1992 Analysis of serum human chorionic-gonadotropin levels in normal singleton, multiple and abnormal pregnancies. Human Reproduction 7:1176–1180

Csemiczky G, Wramsby H, Johannisson E, Landgren BM 1998 Importance of endometrial quality in women with tubal infertility during a natural menstrual cycle for the outcome of IVF treatment. Journal of Assisted Reproduction and Genetics 15:55–61

DeLamirande E, Leclerc P, Gagnon C 1997 Capacitation as a regulatory event that primes spermatozoa for the acrosome reaction and fertilisation. Molecular Human Reproduction 3:175–194

De Waal FBM 1995 Bonobo sex and society. Scientific American 272(3):82–88

Dey J, Shepherd MD 2002 Evaluation and treatment of erectile dysfunction in men with diabetes mellitus. Mayo Clinic Proceedings 77:276–282

Familiari G, Notola SA, Macchiarell G, Micara G, Aragona C, Motta PM 1992 Human zona pellucida during in vitro fertilization: an ultrastructural study using saponin, ruthenium red and osmium thiocarbohydrazide. Molecular Reproduction and Development 32:51–61

Fazleabas AT, Kim JJ, Strakova Z 2004 Implantation: embryonic signals and the modulation of the uterine environment—a review. Placenta 25:S26–31

Filippi S, Vignozzi L, Vannelli GB, Ledda F, Forti G, Maggi M 2003 Role of oxytocin in the ejaculatory process. Journal of Endocrinological Investigation 26(3 Suppl):82–86

Griffin DK 1996 The incidence, origin and etiology of aneuploidy. International Review of Cytology 167:263–296

Gyllensten U, Wharton D, Josefsson A, Wilson AC 1991 Paternal inheritance of mitochondrial DNA in mice. Nature 352:255–257

Hall JG 2003 Twinning. Lancet 362:735–743

Handyside AH, Lesko JG, Tarin JJ, Winston RML, Hughes MR 1992 Birth of a normal girl after in vitro fertilisation and pre-implantation diagnostic testing for cystic fibrosis. New England Journal of Medicine 327:905–909

Harcourt AH 1991 Sperm competition and the evolution of non-fertilizing sperm in mammals. Evolution 45:314–328

Hardy K, Handyside AH, Winston RML 1989 The human blasto-cyst-cell number, death and allocation during late preimplantation development in vitro. Development 107:597

Hardy K, Martin KL, Leese HJ, Winston RML, Handyside AH 1990 Human preimplantation development in vitro is not adversely affected by biopsy at the 8-cell stage. Human Reproduction 5:708–714

Harlap S 1979 Gender of infants conceived on different days of the menstrual cycle. New England Journal of Medicine 291:1445–1448

Hill JA 2001 Maternal–embryonic cross-talk. Annals of the New York Academy of Sciences 943:17–25

Hoodbhoy T, Talbot R 1994 Mammalian cortical granules: contents, fate and function. Molecular Reproduction and Development 39:439–448

Jacobs PA, Wilson CM, Sprenkle JA, Rosenheim NB, Migeon BR 1980 Mechanism of origin of complete hydatidiform mole. Nature 286:714–717

Kaji K, Kudo A 2004 The mechanism of sperm–oocyte fusion in mammals. Reproduction 127:423–429

Kaneda H, Hayashi JL, Takahama S, Taya C, Lindal KF, Yonekawa H 1995 Elimination of paternal mitochondrial DNA in intraspecific crosses during early mouse embryogenesis. Proceedings of the National Academy of Sciences USA 92:4542–4546

Kono T, Obata Y, Wu Q, Niwa K, Ono Y, Yamamoto Y, Park ES, Seo JS, Ogawa H 2004 Birth of parthenogenetic mice that can develop to adulthood. Nature 428:860–864

Larsen WJ 1993 Human embryology, 2nd edn. Churchill Livingstone, New York, p 481

Levin RJ 1998 Sex and the human female reproductive tract: what really happens during and after coitus. International Journal of Impotence Research 10(Suppl 1):514–521

Matilsky M, Battino S, Ben-Ami M, Gesleivich Y, Eyali V, Shalev E 1993 The effect of ejaculatory frequency on semen characteristics of normozoospermic and oligozoospermic men from an infertile population. Human Reproduction 8:71–73

Master VA, Turek PJ 2001 Ejaculatory physiology and dysfunction. Urologic Clinics of North America 28:363–375

Mbizvo MT 1995 Functional motion changes during sperm transport to the site of fertilization and in vitro applications: a review. International Journal of Andrology 18:1–6

Miozzo M, Simoni G 2002 The role of imprinted genes in fetal growth. Biology of the Neonate 81:271–228

Mollard R, Denham M, Trounson A 2002 Technical advances and pitfalls on the way to human cloning. Differentiation 70:1–9

Nikas G, Aghajanova L 2003 Endometrial pinopods: some more understanding on human implantation? Reproductive BioMedicine Online 4:18–23

Palermo GP, Avrech OM, Colombero LT et al 1997 Human sperm cytosolic factor triggers Ca^{2+} oscillations and overcomes activation failure of mammalian oocytes. Molecular Human Reproduction 3:367–374

Payne D, Flaherty SP, Barry MF, Matthews CD 1997 Preliminary observations on polar body extrusion and pronuclear formation in human oocytes using time-lapse video cinematography. Human Reproduction 12:532–541

Piomelli D 2004 THC: moderation during implantation. Nature Medicine 10:19–20

Schatten G 1994 The centrosome and its mode of inheritance; the reduction of the centrosome during gametogenesis and its restoration during fertility. Developmental Biology 165:299–335

Short RV 1997 The testis: the witness of the mating system, the site of mutation and the engine of desire. Acta Paediatrica Supplement 422:3–7

Stanford JB, White GL, Hatasaka H 2002 Timing intercourse to achieve pregnancy: current evidence. Obstetrics and Gynecology 100:1333–1341

Sullivan ME, Keoghane SR, Miller MA 2002 Vascular risk factors and erectile dysfunction. British Journal of Urology International 87:838–845

Swann K, Larman MG, Saunders CM, Lai FA 2004 The cytosolic sperm factor that triggers Ca^{2+} oscillations and egg activation in mammals is a novel phospholipase C: PLCzeta. Reproduction 127:431–439

Tulsiani DRP, Yoshida-Komiya H, Araki Y 1997 Mammalian fertilization: a carbohydrate mediated event. Biology of Reproduction 57:487–494

Van Blerkom J, Davis P, Merriam J, Sinclair J 1995 Nuclear and cytoplasmic dynamics of sperm penetration, pronuclear formation and microtubule organization during fertilization and early preimplantation in the human. Human Reproduction Update 1:429–461

Van Steirteghem A, Liebaers I, Devroey P 1996 Assisted reproduction. In: Hillier SG, Kitchener HC, Neilson JP (eds) Scientific essentials of reproductive medicine. WB Saunders, Philadelphia, pp 230–241

Vigano P, Mangioni S, Pompei F, Chiodo I 2003. Maternal–conceptus cross talk: a review. Placenta 24:S56–S61

Wasserman PM 1987 The biology and chemistry of fertilisation. Science 235:553–560

Whittaker M 1995 Regulation of the cell division cycle by inositol phosphate and the calcium signalling pathway. Advances in Second Messenger and Phosphoprotein Research 30:299–310

Yanagida K, Katayose H, Hirata S, Yazawa H, Hayashi S, Sato A 2001 Influence of sperm immobilization on onset of Ca(2+) oscillations after ICSI. Human Reproduction 16(1):148–152

Zenzes MT, Wang P, Casper RF 1995 Cigarette smoking may affect meiotic maturation of human oocytes. Human Reproduction 10:3213–3217

7 Overview of human genetics and genetic disorders

Learning objectives

■ To describe the packaging of genes in the chromosome and how they are expressed.

■ To describe the general characteristics of dominant, recessive and X-linked genetic traits.

■ To interpret a pedigree chart and make simple genetic predictions.

■ To discuss the principles of genetic screening.

■ To relate current genetic research to midwifery practice.

■ To discuss evolutionary influences upon human reproduction.

Introduction

Genetics is the science of genes, heredity and the variation of organisms. Although genetics is a component of virtually all areas of biology, it tends to be reductionist in nature. Life is the result of the genetic codes that all living things carry in almost all of their cells. The mechanisms that govern the manner in which genetic information is duplicated, altered, transferred and expressed provide a wealth of information about the biochemical processes of all living organisms. The advent of molecular biology has meant that many problems considered formidable until very recently may now be understood and resolved. Molecular biology has added new dimensions to understanding the origin of the human species, to creating new drugs, and to sequencing of entire genomes of a variety of species, including disease-causing microorganisms, plants and humans.

Within living organisms, the genetic information is usually carried in chromosomes where organization of the DNA provides a gene or 'blueprint' directing protein synthesis and thus the expression of the genes. Characteristics are passed from one generation to the next in the form of genes. In sexually reproducing species, the genes are shuffled and packaged into the gametes. Variations between genes affect survival so the individuals with the best-adapted characteristics to cope with environmental conditions have an advantage. This is described as natural selection.

The study of genetics focuses on inherited characteristics, particularly those that are considered abnormal, how these arise and their effects on the individual. Genetics is a predictive science and its rules are based upon the application of mathematical statistics and probability. Evolutionary effects on genetics may determine the penetration of recessive genetic disorders such as cystic fibrosis into gene pools. The impact of genetics upon antenatal screening is of particular relevance for midwives.

Chapter case study

As part of the routine antenatal care, which Zara is receiving from her midwife at her local maternity unit, Zara is offered a 20-week anomaly ultrasound as part of the screening policy of the local maternity services. This scan examines the physical structures of the baby and enables a skilled ultrasonographer to identify major structural abnormalities of the internal organs and other signs of structural problems such as polyhydramnios, oligohydramnios, placental abnormalities, etc. Often the presence of a number of abnormalities (frequently referred to as a syndrome) could indicate the presence of many possible genetic disorders.

Zara is quite upset because one of her friends has just undergone amniocentesis as her ultrasound scan had revealed cardiac, brain and limb abnormalities. Zara's scan appears to be normal and the baby appears to be growing well but Zara is still concerned that all may not be well and wishes to discuss what further tests are available that would reassure her all is well. How would you, as Zara's midwife, reassure and counsel her and James through this difficult period?

A brief history of genetics

Historically, humans unknowingly but successfully applied genetics to breeding and domestication of animals and plants. However, the first systematic study of genetic interactions is associated with the breeding experiments of Gregor Mendel, an Austrian monk, in the 1860s. Mendel established inheritance patterns of certain traits in pea plants and demonstrated that application of statistics to inheritance could be very useful. Subsequently, more complex forms of inheritance have been identified.

Mendel correctly identified the concept of genes long before the structures of DNA and chromosomes were understood. He proposed that 'particles of inheritance' were transmitted from one generation to the next and defined a concept that he described as an allele. The term 'allele' is now used to describe a specific variant or alternative form of a particular gene occupying a given locus (position) on a chromosome.

The term 'eugenics' was coined by Francis Galton (a cousin of Charles Darwin) who advocated that application of Darwinian theories and selective breeding could improve the quality of entire populations, particularly with respect to talent and intelligence. In the late 19th century, eugenics societies formed in various parts of the world sought to promote such practices as marriage restriction, sterilization and custodial commitment of those thought to have unwanted characteristics and positively encouraging reproduction in those individuals perceived as the best and brightest. The popularity of the eugenics movement was already waning when infamous eugenics programmes of Nazi Germany were revealed at the end of World War II.

Darwin's 'survival of the fittest' theory promoted the concept of natural selection and how environmental conditions determine survival and reproduction of organisms with particular traits. If environmental conditions do not vary much, these traits continue to be adaptive and become more common within the population.

Neo-Darwinism (or 'modern evolutionary synthesis') extends the scope of Darwin's ideas of natural selection by including modern genetic knowledge about DNA and concepts such as speciation, kin selection and altruism. It advocates that survival of a species is not necessarily by the fittest but by those that are most likely to reproduce successfully. This is reflected in the work of Richard Dawkins who asserts that the gene, rather than the organism or species, is the true unit of reproduction and the primary driver and beneficiary of evolution. He provocatively describes genes as 'selfish' because in order to replicate and be successful they use organisms that contain them solely as vehicles to ensure survival (Dawkins 1989). Obviously, reproduction is vital to ensure that this occurs.

This controversial view portrays organisms solely as mechanical methods of survival to pass genes on to as many offspring as possible. However, there are a number of arguments against this view. Organisms are not perfectly adapted; for instance, humans seem to have some non-advantageous genes such as those coding for the vermiform appendix. It could be argued that these genes have not been obliterated because other linked genes are advantageous and effectively protect them. The other important point is that species not only interact with their environment but also positively alter their environment.

The environment interacts with genes (the nature/nurture debate) and has a tremendous influence on how they are expressed, affecting susceptibility and resistance to disease. Genes may act in competition with each other, which may explain certain pathophysiological conditions and their aetiology. Some organisms may use their genes to alter the phenotype of another animal to increase their chances of survival. For example, infection with the trematode parasite causes its snail host's shell to become thicker (Dawkins 1999).

Within the modern medical world there now exist ethical dilemmas surrounding the screening for, detection of and termination of abnormal fetuses. Current research in genetics is not solely medical (Box 7.1) as it can be applied to population studies, such as tracing the origins of human migration movements, and to genealogy, such as tracing the real families of children of the Argentinean 'Disappeared' (Jones 1994) and the route the early Polynesians took to reach New Zealand (Sykes 2001).

Genes and chromosomes

Genes are the units of inheritance. Each gene is a length of DNA on a chromosome that contains the coded information to direct the synthesis of a specific protein chain. The differences between organisms are related to different proteins being synthesized that have different structures and functions. Effectively the genes act as a blue-print, or instruction manual, for the total development of the organism and how it will function and change during its lifetime (Box 7.2). Chromosomes are packages of DNA in the nucleus, on which the genes are linearly arranged. Chromosomes have two arms: a shorter p arm and a longer q arm, with a centromere between them. Chromosomes are impor-

tant in cell replication and the passing of the genetic message from one generation to the next. Usually the DNA, about 180 cm per nucleus, exists as an unstructured mass of threads in the nucleus. However, when the cell is undergoing division the DNA becomes organized and compacted into chromosomes, which can be visualized by microscopy (see Ch. 1). This chromosomal organization allows biologists to identify genes and localize them to a particular chromosome to follow their pattern of inheritance. Each cell has the same genetic information in its nucleus as the original zygote (fertilized ovum) and all of the cells derived from it. Different cells behave in different ways because they express different subsets of information from the DNA.

The structure of DNA and RNA

Watson, Crick, Franklin and Wilkins elucidated the biochemical structure of DNA in 1953. Their description of the helical structure revealed how the molecule was able to replicate itself and thus explained the cellular mechanism of reproduction. DNA is composed of two strands of sugar phosphate molecules that are joined together to form long chains (Fig. 7.1). The strands of DNA are made up of repeating units called nucleotides. The DNA nucleotide has three components: a deoxyribose sugar, a phosphate group and a base. There are four types of bases: thymine and

---

Box 7.2

Genetics as a language

Genetics can be considered as a language based on the DNA molecule. Linguistic development and evolution have a number of similarities. Studies looking at the origins of a particular word and how it has evolved to be slightly different in different languages are similar to the changes in genes (Jones 1994). Genetic mutations are analogous to new words being introduced into the language (such as 'email').

- Language = genetics
- Vocabulary = genes
- Grammar = rules about the arrangement of information
- Literature = the instructions to make a human
- Alphabet = four bases of DNA
- Word = codon (three 'letter' code for an amino acid)

Box 7.1

Areas of genetic research

- Screening for fetal abnormality
- Genetic counselling for parents with a family history of genetic disorders
- Identification of fetal sex in the early (indifferent) embryological phase
- Cloning of whole organisms
- Gene manipulation, not only to eradicate disease, but also to improve existing disease states
- Treatment by gene manipulation in animals to produce human proteins, hormones, etc.
- Genetic modification
- Identification of individuals by genetic 'fingerprinting'

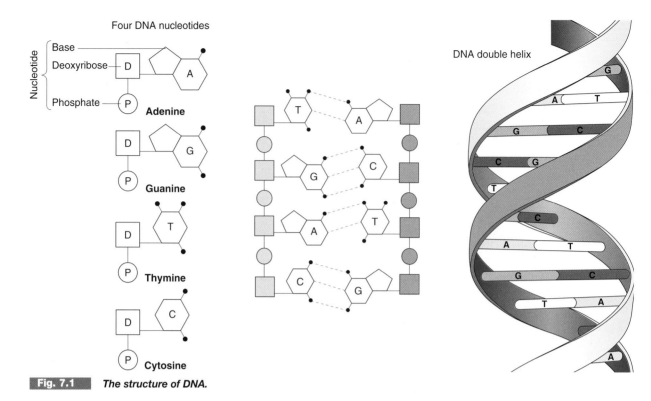

Fig. 7.1 *The structure of DNA.*

cytosine, which have single-ring structures, and adenine and guanine, which have double-ring structures. DNA exists as a double-stranded molecule wound into a helix. The strands are kept together by hydrogen bonding between the bases. The bases are of different sizes and have a different potential number of hydrogen bonds so they always pair in the same ways. Adenine (A) and thymine (T) pair with two hydrogen bonds; cytosine (C) and guanine (G) pair with three. This means that the sequence of the bases is complementary; the sequence of bases on one strand can be deduced from the sequence on the other strand.

DNA replication and cell division

The arrangement of base pairs of the two strands is like the rungs of a ladder or teeth of a zip. When DNA replicates, the strands unwind and the hydrogen bonds holding the base pairs together separate (unzip). Each strand acts as a template for the synthesis of another new strand of complementary DNA bases to form from nucleotides that enter the nucleus through the nuclear pores (Fig. 7.2). So two new DNA double helices are formed, each with one strand of 'old' DNA

and a newly synthesized strand. Thus the replication is described as semiconservative. Replication occurs as part of mitosis, or cell division. Replication of DNA means that the chromosomes have double their nuclear material in preparation for dividing into two separate cells. Therefore the chromosome is formed of two identical chromatids.

Mitosis

The replication of the entire human genome is achieved through the process of mitosis, which is part of the cell cycle (Fig. 7.3). Cellular replication results in growth of tissues through hyperplasia (an increase in the number of cells); each cell has the identical genetic message (DNA content) to its parent cell. Mitotic rates are different for different types of cells. Cells that divide fast (have a high mitotic index) include skin and gut epithelial cells, spermatogonia and tumour cells. With increased age the mitotic rate slows down so skin renewal, for instance, takes longer and the appearance of the skin is more aged. Drugs used to treat cancers also inhibit mitosis so their side-effects are mostly clearly manifested in normal cells with high mitotic rates, causing problems with

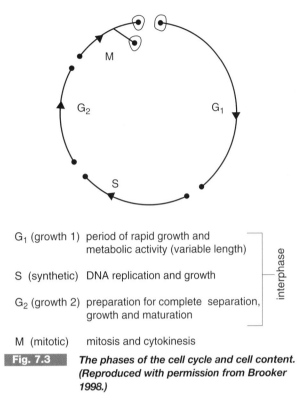

G_1 (growth 1) period of rapid growth and
                    metabolic activity (variable length)

S (synthetic) DNA replication and growth

G_2 (growth 2) preparation for complete separation,
                    growth and maturation

M (mitotic)   mitosis and cytokinesis

interphase

Fig. 7.3   *The phases of the cell cycle and cell content. (Reproduced with permission from Brooker 1998.)*

Fig. 7.2   *DNA replication. (Reproduced with permission from Brooker 1998).*

T, A, G, C nitrogenous bases   T   A   G   C

▲ hydrogen bond
● pentose sugar
■ phosphate

new strand   original strand   original strand   new strand

nutrient absorption and decreasing male fertility. Many cells, such as brain, heart and liver cells, have an extremely slow rate of mitosis and do not regenerate or heal well after injury. Mitosis is a continuous process but for ease of description is traditionally described in distinct phases: prophase, metaphase, anaphase and telophase (Fig. 7.4). Interphase is the name given to the gap between mitotic divisions.

The genetic message

The structure of DNA allows both ease of replication and duplication of the genetic message prior to cell division, and also a method of directing protein synthesis and ultimate cell function. The DNA message is interpreted as a specific protein product. Proteins are synthesized at the ribosomes of the cell whereas the encoded information, in the form of DNA, remains within the nucleus. The information is carried from DNA to the site of protein synthesis by the second type of nucleic acid, RNA. Whereas DNA is a double strand, RNA exists as a single strand of sugar phosphate units, and has ribose sugar units (instead of deoxyribose) and similar complementary base molecules to those found in DNA, except that uracil instead of thymine pairs with adenine. RNA also exists as different forms with different functions. It is messenger RNA (mRNA) that carries the message from the nucleus to the ribosome, as a complementary strand of mRNA is formed using a stretch of unwound DNA as a template.

Transcription

The process starts with the DNA strands separating like a zip pulling open in the middle. This is the reverse process to the way it coils when condensing into chromosomes (Fig. 7.5). Only one strand of DNA, the coding or 'sense' strand, is used as the template; the other is described as non-coding or 'non-sense'. The mRNA chain is built by RNA polymerase enzymes as the

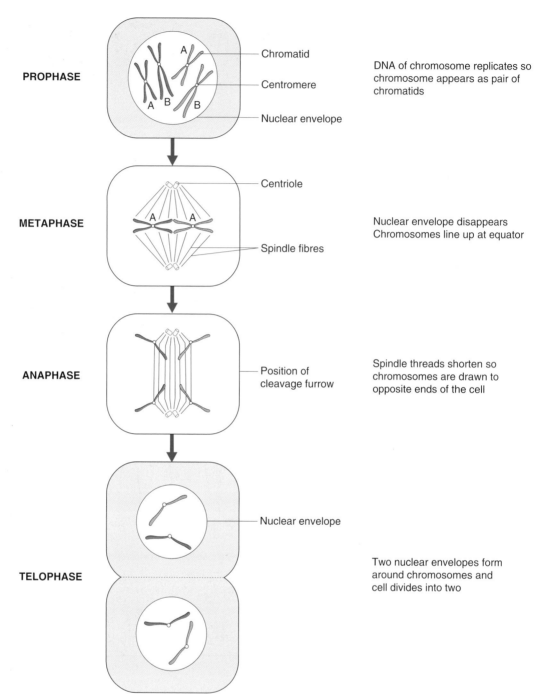

PROPHASE

Chromatid

Centromere

Nuclear envelope

DNA of chromosome replicates so chromosome appears as pair of chromatids

METAPHASE

Centriole

Spindle fibres

Nuclear envelope disappears Chromosomes line up at equator

ANAPHASE

Position of cleavage furrow

Spindle threads shorten so chromosomes are drawn to opposite ends of the cell

TELOPHASE

Nuclear envelope

Two nuclear envelopes form around chromosomes and cell divides into two

Fig. 7.4 *The stages of mitosis. (Reproduced with permission from the Open University 1987.)*

bases pair with the DNA template; this is called transcription (Fig. 7.6).

The whole gene is transcribed but not all of it is used so the primary transcription product mRNA is modified (cut and spliced) into functional mRNA (Fig. 7.7). The parts of the mRNA that are removed have been copied from parts of the gene called introns and those that are retained come from the parts of the DNA known as exons. It is estimated that only about 2–5% of the total genome (genetic code or DNA) is composed of exons and actually codes for protein synthesis. Some of the DNA modulates genetic expression, switching the process of protein synthesis on and off; these control genes are

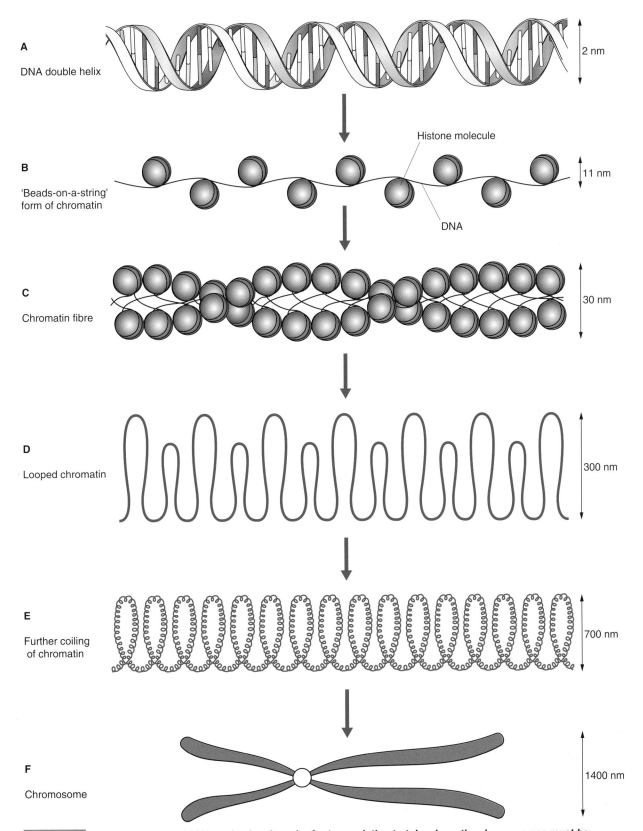

A DNA double helix — 2 nm

B 'Beads-on-a-string' form of chromatin — Histone molecule — DNA — 11 nm

C Chromatin fibre — 30 nm

D Looped chromatin — 300 nm

E Further coiling of chromatin — 700 nm

F Chromosome — 1400 nm

Fig. 7.5 *A–F The stages of DNA packaging; in order for transcription to take place, the chromosomes must be uncoiled and 'unzipped' in the reverse process to that shown. (Adapted with permission from Goodwin 1997.)*

Fig. 7.6   *Transcription.*

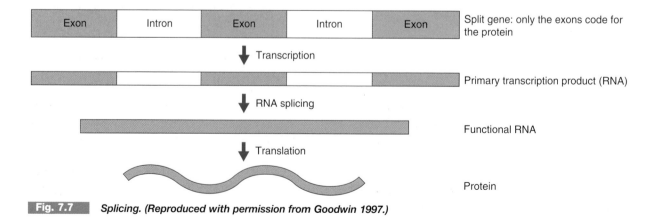

Fig. 7.7   *Splicing. (Reproduced with permission from Goodwin 1997.)*

referred to as operator, regulator and inducer genes. Introns form the majority of the DNA sequence and do not appear to be involved in coding for protein synthesis, although they may allow different proteins to be formed from the same length of DNA. Much of the genome (about 98%) may be composed of redundant genes that are no longer activated and involved in the synthesis of proteins. These unused stretches of DNA are used to compare tissue samples for DNA fingerprinting.

Single nucleotide polymorphisms or SNPs (pronounced *snips*) are DNA sequence variations that occur when a single nucleotide in the genome is altered, often with the substitution of cytosine with thymine. Variations that occur in at least 1% of the population are considered to be SNPs. There are more than 1.4 million SNPs in the human genome, occurring approximately every 100–300 bases and accounting for up 90% of all human genetic variation. These variations in the human genome alter how individuals respond to disease, infection, drugs, etc. SNPs are valuable because they do not change much from generation to generation and can be targeted for biomedical research and developing drugs.

The term 'genome' refers to a complete DNA sequence of one set of chromosomes of an organism. As such, it does not describe the genetic polymorphism (diversity) of a species. To understand how variations in DNA cause particular traits or diseases will require comparison between individual genomes. The Human Genome Project was established in 1993 to map the common human nucleotide sequence of the 3 billion DNA bases. In April 2003, it was announced that 99% of the genome had been sequenced. It is hoped that identification of the 30 000–35 000 genes will accelerate progress to diagnosing, treating and ultimately preventing diseases as well as answer questions about evolution.

Protein synthesis

When transcription and post-transcription modification are complete, the finished functional mRNA strand detaches from the DNA and leaves the nucleus, via a nuclear pore, to go to the ribosomes. Ribosomes are structures formed of two subunits made of protein and another type of RNA, ribosomal RNA (rRNA). mRNA attaches to ribosomes and the sequence of bases of the mRNA is decoded to direct the synthesis of a protein; this step is called translation (Fig. 7.8).

The mRNA sequence is 'read' three bases at a time. A particular sequence of three bases is called a codon; each codon prescribes that a specific amino acid is incorporated into the final amino acid chain of the overall protein structure. There are 20 amino acids; however, as a three-base genetic code allows the potential of $4 \times 4 \times 4 = 64$ permutations, most amino acids are coded for by more than one codon (Fig. 7.9).

Another form of RNA in the cytoplasm, called transfer RNA (tRNA), carries amino acids to the ribosome to be incorporated into the protein chain. There are different types of tRNA, each one with a specific binding site for a particular amino acid at one end and an 'anticodon', which recognizes the codon on the mRNA at the other end. The first amino acid of a new protein is methionine. The next amino acid joins to the carboxyl group of methionine with a peptide bond. Successive amino acids join, forming a chain of amino acids until a 'stop' codon on mRNA signals the end of the chain. The sequence of amino acids determines the primary structure of the protein. The further configuration of the protein is determined by the interactions between different amino acids on the chain, which change the protein shape into a 'folded' structure, the final shape determining its function. Hence the sequence of bases of the gene, or region of DNA, determines the sequence of amino acids, which in turn prescribes the structure and function of the protein.

Mutation

The copying of DNA has to be accurate. If mistakes are introduced into a region of DNA that is expressed as a protein (i.e. into an exon), the altered sequence of amino acids can change the structure of the protein. This permanent and transmissible change in base sequence of DNA is described as a mutation. Mutations can lead to death of a cell or cause cancer. They are considered to be the driving force of evolution; favourable mutations tend to accumulate and less favourable ones tend to be removed by natural selection. It is estimated that mutations occur every half hour in each person but a mutation in a functional gene only occurs once in five generations. A mutation can be described as 'descent with modification'. DNA has regions of 'hotspots' where the mutation rate can be up to 100 times more frequent than normal. New gene mutations are associated with increasing paternal age (above 35 years); it is suggested that new gene mutations are exclusively

CELL

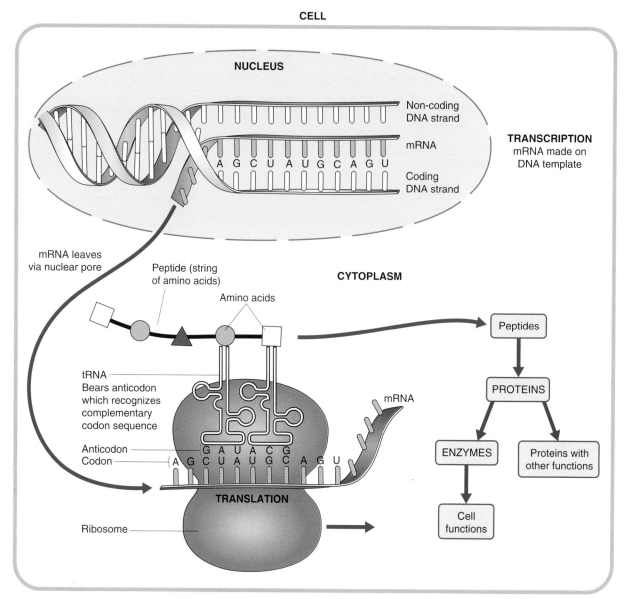

DNA makes RNA (transcription) makes protein (translation)

Fig. 7.8 *The stages of protein synthesis translation.*

inherited from the father and occur during spermatogenesis. All dominant mutations seem to arise in the male germline and may be caused by fragmentation induced by free radical damage (Aitken & Graves 2002). In mitosis, there are accumulated errors in copying the genetic message. Each chromosome has a specialized length of DNA at its end, which gets shorter with each successive division. About four bases seem to be lost with each successive cell division.

A base pair may be spontaneously replaced by a different base pair (a 'point mutation') thus altering the codon and ultimately the amino acid sequence. Age, environmental pressure, radiation and chemicals increase mutation rate. One notable example is haemophilia, the sex-linked genetic condition that afflicted male members of the European Royal Family for several generations. The spontaneous mutation for changed haemoglobin structure may have occurred in one of the gametes forming the zygote that became Queen Victoria. This type of mutation is referred to as a substitution. Mutations may arise as an insertion or deletion of a nucleotide into or from the DNA strand; these mutations could cause a shift in the 'reading frame' of the codons or alter splicing of mRNA thus altering the gene product. Mutations may also occur by the complete insertion of new codons or by the

Second letter

First letter	U		C		A		G		Third letter
U	UUU UUC	Phe	UCU UCC		UAU UAC	Tyr	UGU UGC	Cys	U C
	UUA UUG	Leu	UCA UCG	Ser	UAA UAG	stop stop	UGA UGG	stop Trp	A G
C	CUU CUC	Leu	CCU CCC	Pro	CAU CAC	His	CGU CGC	Arg	U C
	CUA CUG		CCA CCG		CAA CAG	Gln	CGA CGG		A G
A	AUU AUC	Ileu	ACU ACC	Thr	AAU AAC	Asn	AGU AGC	Ser	U C
	AUA AUG	Met	ACA ACG		AAA AAG	Lys	AGA AGG	Arg	A G
G	GUU GUC	Val	GCU GCC	Ala	GAU GAC	Asp	GGU GGC	Gly	U C
	GUA GUG		GCA GCG		GAA GAG	Glu	GGA GGG		A G

The abbreviated names of amino acids are:

Ala = alanine	**Gln** = glutamine	**Leu** = leucine	**Ser** = serine
Arg = arginine	**Glu** = glutamic	**Lys** = lysine	**Thr** = threonine
Asn = asparagine	**Gly** = glycine	**Met** = methionine	**Trp** = tryptophan
Asp = aspartic acid	**His** = histidine	**Phe** = phenylalanine	**Tyr** = tyrosine
Cys = cysteine	**Ileu** = isoleucine	**Pro** = proline	**Val** = valine

Fig. 7.9 *Codons and the amino acids they code for. (Reproduced with permission from the Open University 1988.)*

deletion of a complete codon, thus altering protein structure by introducing or deleting amino acids in the protein. This can be complicated if codons are duplicated and repeated one after the other, for example in fragile X syndrome.

Many mutations occur in the non-coding areas of DNA, so protein structure and function are not affected by the change; these mutations are described as 'silent' as they have no effect. If the mutation results in a different codon that codes for the same amino acid as the original, there will also be no effect. However, a different base, or a missing base, will cause a change in the final sequence of amino acids of the protein, which may have serious effects on protein structure and function. An example is sickle cell anaemia (Box 7.3, Fig. 7.10).

Meiosis

The basic characteristics of meiosis—two cell divisions without intervening DNA replication, halving the chromosome complement of the resulting cells—are conserved in evolution. Each species has a

Box 7.3

Sickle cell anaemia

Most haemoglobin (Hb) in adults is HbA, which has two α-peptide chains and two β-peptide chains forming the haemoglobin molecule. Sickle cell anaemia is an example of a single point mutation where the substitution of one base changes the codon and results in the substitution of one amino acid (Fig. 7.10). Uracil replaces adenine so, instead of glutamic acid, valine is inserted in the protein chain at position 6. Valine has a different charge to glutamic acid so the protein folds differently. The result is that the protein structure of the β-chain of haemoglobin is changed, which affects the molecular shape and oxygen-binding properties. The red blood cells distort into a characteristic sickle shape, particularly at low oxygen tension. Sickle cell anaemia is inherited as an autosomal recessive condition; affected patients have two mutant haemoglobin S genes, one from each parent. The parents are heterozygotes (HbA/HbS) and are thus clinically normal but carry the sickle cell gene. Homozygotes (HbS/HbS) have chronic haemolytic anaemia and are prone to infarction; lifespan is shortened.

Normal (A) β-chain   Sickle (S) β-chain

DNA   C T $\left(\begin{array}{c}T\\C\end{array}\right)$ C A* $\left(\begin{array}{c}T\\C\end{array}\right)$

mRNA   G A $\left(\begin{array}{c}A\\G\end{array}\right)$ G U $\left(\begin{array}{c}A\\G\end{array}\right)$

Amino acid at position 6   Pro-**Glu**-Glu   Pro-**Val**-Glu

Abnormal globin protein

Abnormal haemoglobin

Sickling of red blood cells

↑Destruction   ↑Clumping   ↑Sickle cells in spleen

Anaemia   Tissue damage   Enlarged spleen

Poor physical development   Heart and lung
Weakness   Muscle, joints
Tiredness   Brain
Impaired mental function   Gut
Overactive bone marrow   Kidney

Fig. 7.10 *The sickle cell mutation and its effects.*

characteristic number of chromosomes; humans have 46 chromosomes, arranged as 23 pairs. One chromosome of each pair is maternally derived (from the ovum); the other is paternally derived (from the sperm). (The members of each pair are called homologous; see below.) Human gametes contain only 23 chromosomes, i.e. half the normal number of chromosomes in other human cells. This reduction from the diploid number of chromosomes (46) to the haploid number (23) is accomplished by meiosis. Meiosis is the process whereby a diploid parent cell produces four haploid daughter cells, resulting in gametes, or sex cells, that are not identical to their parent cells.

These gametes are haploid and during meiosis the genetic instructions are randomly assorted, thus generating unique combinations. Meiosis is also described as 'reduction division' because the number of chromosomes is reduced from 46 (i.e. 23 pairs) to 23. It occurs in two successive divisions (meiosis I and II), each of which can be divided into steps (Fig. 7.11). Meiosis II is very similar to mitosis.

In anaphase I, there is random segregation of each member of the chromosome pairs with a maternal and a paternal chromosome randomly going to a particular end of the cell. This would theoretically generate 2^{23} (i.e. 8 388 608) different possibilities of gamete

Division I of meiosis

PROPHASE I

Chromosomes appear, divided into chromatids Red chromosomes have been inherited from the mother, grey chromosomes from the father

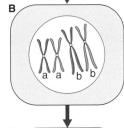

Pair of chromatids

Centromere

Nuclear envelope

Chromosomes pair up: the two chromosomes (a) form one pair, the two chromosomes (b) form another

Division II of meiosis

Chromatids cross over and exchange material

PROPHASE II

Beginning of division II (Only one of the two cells of stage F is shown here – the upper one)

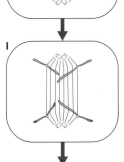

METAPHASE I

Nuclear envelope disappears and chromosomes line up at equator of cell

METAPHASE II

Nuclear envelope breaks down and chromosomes align themselves at the equator

ANAPHASE I

Chromosomes pull away and move to opposite poles of the cell

ANAPHASE II

Centromeres divide and chromatids separate and move to opposite poles

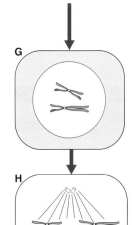

TELOPHASE I

Nuclear envelopes develop around both sets of chromosomes and cell divides into two

TELOPHASE II

New nuclear envelopes enclose the two sets of chromatids (i.e. chromosomes) and cell divides into two

Fig. 7.11 *The stages of meiosis A–J. (Reproduced with permission from Goodwin 1997.)*

combination. However, the crossing over of genetic material between the chromosomes adds far more variation. Meiosis allows the genomes of the parents to be combined to form an individual whose genome is related to their parents and siblings but is unique.

Mammalian oogenesis begins meiotic development during fetal development but arrests in meiosis I and does not complete meiosis I until ovulation; the second division is only completed if the egg is fertilized. Oogenesis, therefore, requires several stop and start signals and, in humans, may last for several decades. The longer an oocyte is immobilized at prophase I the greater is the chance of failure of separation of the homologous chromosomes (non-disjunction). Often genetic abnormalities arise as extra genetic material is incorporated into the genome. If an extra chromosome is inserted, the condition is referred to as trisomic (Table 7.1). Most combinations of trisomy are not seen, but there is no reason to believe that certain chromosomes are more susceptible to failed disjunction. Those seen are probably those that are compatible with fetal survival, although they may cause congenital abnormalities or affect neonatal survival. Sometimes extra chromosomal material may become attached to a chromosome, making it abnormally long. Rarely a condition called triploidy occurs where the chromosomes of the zygote are in triplicate rather than the normal duplicate complement. This condition

Table 7.1 *Examples of chromosome disorders*

Disorder	Example	Incidence	Outcome	Notes
Polyploidy	Triploidy 69 chromosomes (69,XXX, 69,XXY, 69,XYY)	Occurs in 2% of conceptions but early spontaneous abortion is normal	Lethal	Usually arises from fertilization of oocyte by two sperm or from a diploid gamete. 69, XXY is most common. Polyploid cells occur normally in the bone marrow and liver as a stage of cell division
Trisomy	Trisomy 13	1/5000 livebirths	Patau's syndrome	Usually due to non-disjunction of chromosomes or chromatids at anaphase. Trisomy increases with increased maternal age and is sometimes associated with radiation or viral infection. There may be a familial tendency
	Trisomy 18	1/3000 livebirths	Edward's syndrome	Maternal age effect. Incidence at conception much higher—most affected fetuses abort spontaneously. More female fetuses seem to survive
	Trisomy 21	1/700 livebirths	Down's syndrome	Incidence at conception is higher. Maternal age effect; the extra chromosome is maternal in 85% cases. The most serious complications are mental handicap and congenital heart problems
	47, XXY	1/1000 male births	Klinefelter's syndrome	Trisomies involving sex chromosomes usually result in a less serious outcome. Condition is usually diagnosed during investigations for infertility
	47, XYY	1/1000 male births		Often asymptomatic, some effects on IQ. Only XX and XY offspring observed
Monosomy	Monosomy X	1/5000 female births, much higher at conception	Turner's syndrome	Due to non-disjunction in either parent; 80% of affected females have maternal X so it is the paternal chromosome that is missing

Deletion and ring chromosome	Wolf-Hirschhorn syndrome (partial deletion of short arm of chromosome 4) Cri du chat syndrome (partial deletion of short arm of chromosome 5)	Incidence of deletions and/or duplications is 1/2000 births	Chromosome imbalance of autosomes is usually associated with mental retardation and multiple dysmorphic features	A deletion is the loss of part of chromosome. A ring chromosome is due to deletions in both arms of a chromosome and the fusion of the proximal sticky ends. Microdeletions are deletions that can just be detected by light microscopy
Duplication				Duplication is where there are two copies of a segment of chromosome. This is more common and less harmful than deletions
Inversion			The carriers of balanced inversions and translocations are healthy because the cells have all the genetic material but gamete formation is affected so there is a high rate of miscarriage and malformation	A segment of the chromosome is inverted through 180° between breaks Usually does not cause clinical. problems but unbalanced gamete may result
Translocation	Reciprocal			Translocations involve transfer of chromosomal material between chromosomes. Two chromosomes are broken and repaired abnormally or there is recombination between non-homologous chromosomes at meiosis. Reciprocal translocations involve transfer of material between two chromosomes
	Robertsonian (centric fusion)			Robertsonian translocation involves transfer of material, which leaves a large chromosome, and a fragment of a chromosome, which is unable to replicate; most common centric fusion translocations are 13/14 and 14/21. Balanced carriers have 45 chromosomes and are healthy. Gametogenesis is affected

is not compatible with embryo survival but is sometimes found in products of a failed conception (early miscarriage) and is associated with a high incidence of hydatidiform mole (see Ch. 6). Imperfect disjunction also causes conditions where the genome is lacking part or a whole chromosome. For example, there is only one X chromosome present in Turner's syndrome (see Ch. 5) and Wolf–Hirschhorn syndrome is caused by loss of chromosomal tissue from chromosomes 4 and 5.

Autosomes and sex chromosomes

Each gene has a specific location on a specific chromosome, which is referred to as a locus (plural: loci). Each chromosome may have 1000–2000 different genes, each with its own location and function. The visualization of the chromosomes from a cell is described as a karyotype (Box 7.4). Of the 23 pairs of chromosomes that constitute the human genome, 22

Box 7.4

Karyotyping

Karyotyping is the method of visualizing the chromosomes in an ordered display of the chromosomes as they appear in the nucleus of a cell during metaphase of mitosis. For a fetal karyotype, a sample of amniotic fluid is removed. The cells are centrifuged to concentrate the fetal cells. The supernatant can also be used diagnostically for biochemical tests such as investigation of enzyme deficiencies, protein defects and gene alterations. Alternatively, cells may be taken from the chorionic villus. A karyotype of adult cells is usually derived from a sample of venous blood, where the anuclear red blood cells are lysed and the washed remaining cells are, therefore, white blood cells containing nuclei.

The fetal cells or white blood cells are grown in cell culture. The time taken for this depends on the number of cells in the original sample. Contamination of the sample can interfere with the success of the method. Colchicine, a chemical poison, is added to the culture medium to prevent spindle formation. Thus, mitosis in all cells is halted at the metaphase stage when the chromosomes are maximally contracted and well defined as paired chromatids (therefore they take on the typical X-shaped appearance). The cells, all halted at the same stage, can be separated from the culture medium. Exposure of the cells to hypotonic saline causes the nucleus to swell so the chromosomes are spread out. The cells are then fixed and stained. Visualization of the karyotype is done by computer-aided photographic techniques. The chromosomes are ordered according to size with the homologous autosomes being paired together. The chromosomes of pair number 1 are the longest and those of pair number 22 are the shortest. The position of the centromere is also used to sort the chromosomes into order. Stains that bind preferentially to some areas of the chromosome, producing a distinct pattern of bands, can be used to identify the chromosomes. Karyotypes can be used to identify gross abnormalities such as additional or missing chromosomes and missing or duplicated parts of chromosomes. However, a normal karyotype does not reveal the presence of abnormal genes at specific loci. In order to identify such genes, the chromosomes are stained, which produces a pattern or banding enabling an abnormal gene or a marker gene to be identified. A marker gene is a gene that is often found in close proximity to an abnormal gene; the closer the marker gene to the abnormal gene the higher is the association.

Occasionally, results from karyotyping may be complicated by mosaicism. Mosaicism, a different number of chromosomes in different populations of cells, may occur for instance where the chorionic tissue has a different number of chromosomes to the fetus.

pairs of chromosomes can be seen in both sexes; these are referred to as the autosomes and contain the autosomal genes. The 23rd pair of chromosomes comprises the sex chromosomes; these are homologous within the female (i.e. XX) but in the male the XY arrangement consists of a pair of non-homologous chromosomes.

Sex chromosomes

The sex chromosomes provide the mechanism for the determination of sex and the differentiation into male morphology, which is usually dependent on the inheritance of a Y chromosome (see Ch. 5). As well as sex determination and identity, other genetic traits can be inherited on the sex chromosomes (see below).

It is thought that the sex chromosomes originated from a pair of autosomes (see Ch. 7) during the evolution of sex determination (Graves 2002). The X and Y chromosomes are very different in size and sequence compared to the other 22 pairs of autosomes. The Y chromosome is very small in comparison to the X chromosome and is completely different from the X chromosomes except at its tips. These identical regions at the tips, known as the pseudoautosomal regions, contain most of the Y chromosome genes involved in control of growth and allow the pairing of the X and Y chromosome and crossing over during cell division. The X chromosome is about 5% of the total length of a single set of chromosome and bears about 3000–4000 genes, many of which are conserved (identical to those of other placental mammals). The Y chromosome contains only about 50 genes, many of which appear to be non-functional; others are involved with male differentiation and spermatogenesis, implantation and promoting placental growth. It is suggested that the Y chromosome is particularly vulnerable to gene deletions because it cannot retrieve lost genetic information by homologous recombination and that, over the last 300 million years, it has already lost most of its original 1500 genes and continues to deteriorate; at its present rate of decay (losing about five genes per million years), it will self-destruct in about 10 million years (Aitken & Graves 2002). This has already happened in the mole vole, which has lost the Y chromosome and all of its genes from the genome. An alternative view is that the Y chromosome, rather than being 'damaged', is an efficient carrier of male-specific genes, rationalized by evolutionary selection (Craig et al 2004).

Alleles

Each pair of autosomes is homologous; this means that their gene arrangements, although not necessarily the specific gene at each locus, are identical. So although the genes at a specific locus code for a specific physiological feature these features in themselves may vary. For instance, the genes at a particular locus may code for eye colour, but this could be blue eye colour on the chromosome inherited from one parent and brown eye colour on the chromosome inherited from the other parent. Genes that code for the same physical feature but produce variations in that feature are called alleles.

If the genes are identical alleles, then the structure and coding of the pair are referred to as being homozygous. If the genes are differing alleles then the pair is referred to as being heterozygous. If one copy of a gene is required for a trait to be expressed (i.e. for the feature to be 'visible' in the resultant individual), the gene is described as being dominant. If two copies are required, the gene is described as being recessive. Autosomal traits (genetic instructions carried on the autosomes) can be expressed as either dominant or recessive traits. Simple inheritance of these traits can be predicted diagrammatically (see Figs 7.12, 7.16).

Prediction of genetic outcomes

Genetic predictions forecast the chance of an ovum carrying a specific combination of genes being ferti-

PARENT	GENOTYPE	PHENOTYPE
Male	BB	Brown eyes
Female	bb	Blue eyes

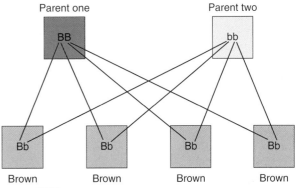

Fig. 7.12 *Combination diagram to illustrate the genetic outcomes of crossing a homozygous male with brown eyes (carrying two dominant genes for brown eye colour, BB) and a homozygous female with blue eyes (carrying two recessive genes for blue eye colour, bb). All the offspring will be heterozygous, carrying one recessive gene and one dominant gene. All the children will have the phenotype of brown eye coloration.*

lized by a sperm carrying a specific combination of genes. The convention is to show the dominant gene as a capital letter. The genetic potential is described as the genotype; how it is expressed is called the phenotype. Combination diagrams and Punnett squares give the same results, predicting the chance of a particular outcome (Figs 7.12, 7.13).

The genetic rules that dictate eye colour follow the traditional form of dominant and recessive interaction (see Box 7.5). However, it is important to realize that, like so many other physiological states, expressed characteristics may be the outcome of multifactorial genes where more than one gene is involved. The environment may also influence the expression of genes. For instance, inheriting genes for tall stature does not

		Parent one Gametes	
		B	B
Parent two Gametes	b	Bb	Bb
	b	Bb	Bb

Fig. 7.13 *Punnett square.*

Box 7.5

Selected examples of recessive and dominant traits

Autosomal trait	Recessive trait
■ Brown eye colour	■ Blue or grey eye colour
■ Curly hair	■ Straight hair
■ Dark brown hair	■ All other colours
■ Near or far sight	■ Normal vision
■ Normal skin pigment	■ Albinism
■ Normal hearing	■ Deafness
■ Migraine headaches	■ Normal
■ A or B antigen (A, B or AB blood group)	■ No A or B antigen (O blood group)
■ Rhesus antigen (Rh+ blood group)	■ No Rhesus antigen (Rh– blood group)

Characteristics of different types of inheritance

Autosomal dominant inheritance

The trait is expressed by a gene on an autosome and is expressed provided that at least one chromosome has the dominant gene. Each person expressing the trait usually has a parent with the trait (Fig. 7.14 shows a pedigree chart for a pattern of autosomal dominant inheritance; the symbols used in these charts are shown in Box 7.6). This means that a particular characteristic or disorder can be traced through several generations if it has little effect on survival. However, a trait occurring in a new generation may be the result of polygamic behaviour (illegitimacy) or a fresh mutation. Autosomal dominant traits also tend to be extremely variable in expression so they may be undetectable and appear to 'skip' a generation. For instance, polydactyly (an extra digit) may be manifest as a tiny pedicle, rather than an extra finger. Autosomal dominant disorders are often caused by defects in structural proteins.

necessarily mean the child will be tall. In the absence of appropriate nutrition at critical times of growth, the genetic potential may not be realized.

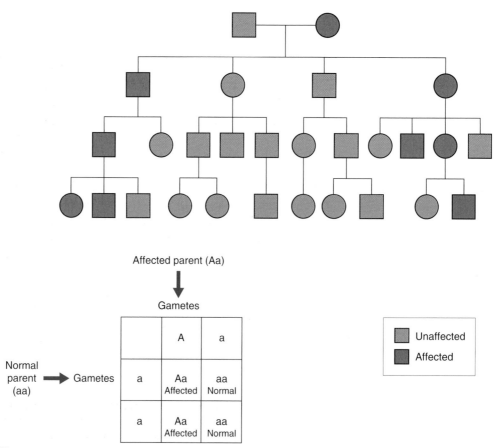

Fig. 7.14   *Inheritance of a dominant trait.*

Box 7.6

Symbols used in pedigree charts

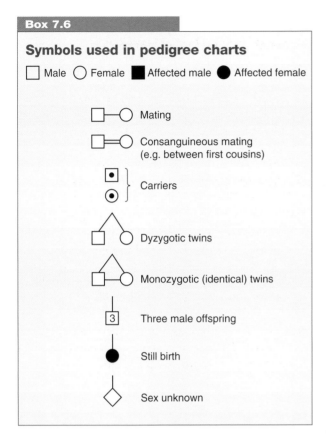

☐ Male ○ Female ■ Affected male ● Affected female

☐—○ Mating

☐—○ Consanguineous mating
(e.g. between first cousins)

⊡
⊙ } Carriers

Dyzygotic twins

Monozygotic (identical) twins

3 Three male offspring

● Still birth

◇ Sex unknown

If an affected person mates with an unaffected person, the chances of any child being affected are one in two (i.e. 50%). Some autosomal diseases or traits do not affect the predicted 50% of offspring. These are described as having incomplete penetrance. Conversely, a highly penetrant gene is expressed regardless of environmental and other factors.

In the UK, the most common dominantly inherited traits are Huntington's disease and achondroplasia (Table 7.2). Huntington's disease, a degenerative neuropsychiatric disorder initially characterized by spasmodic movements of the body and limbs and ultimately dementia, is usually not expressed until the third or fourth decade when the person affected is likely to have reproduced. The age at onset and progression of the disease is linked to the number of polyglutamine sequence repeats in the disease protein (coded by CAG bases in the gene).

A complication occurs in the case of inherited achondroplasia (dwarfism) (note that 80% of cases of achondroplasia are caused by new mutations in the offspring of parents of normal height). Humans exhibit selective rather than random mating, often being attracted to partners of similar height, intelligence and other physical attributes. In consequence, individuals with achondroplasia partner each other with a higher frequency than expected by chance. If two people with achondroplasia mate, there is an expected prediction of a one in four chance of a child having normal stature (Fig. 7.15). However, homozygosity (two genes for achondroplasia) results in the fetus having lethal respiratory problems, which are incompatible with survival. Hence the actual ratio of newborn children is one in three. (Arguably, achondroplasia could be viewed as a recessively inherited respiratory condition that confers dwarfism on the heterozygote.)

Autosomal recessive inheritance

As with autosomal dominant inheritance, this type of inheritance can affect both sexes equally. However, the recessive trait is expressed only if the gene is present on *both* alleles, which means it has been inherited from both parents. If the parents are heterozygotes, each carrying one recessive gene for the trait and one normal dominant gene, they express the dominant gene and are described as 'carriers' of the recessive gene. In some conditions, the carriers may exhibit mild signs of a disease or have an unusual level of certain biochemical markers that can be measured in genetic testing.

Most inherited enzyme disorders are recessive. Another characteristic of recessive disorders is that they show a variation in birth frequency among different

Table 7.2 *Examples of autosomal dominant diseases*

Trait	Incidence
Familial hypercholesterolaemia	1/500 births
von Willebrand disease	1/20–30 000
Huntington's disease	1/18 000
Achondroplasia	1/26 000

	A	a
A	AA	Aa
a	Aa	aa

Expected outcome might be 25% chance of child with normal height, but AA is lethal lung deformity so observed outcome is 2:1 chance of achondroplasia:normal height.

Fig. 7.15 *Inheritance of achondroplasia.*

populations (Table 7.3). It is suggested that the reason some recessively inherited disorders reach such a high incidence within a population is because advantages are conferred on the heterozygotes. For example, it is recognized that carriers of the gene for sickle haemoglobin (see Box 7.3), namely HbS or C, have a resistance to malaria falciparum, the most dangerous form of malaria (but not to other types). Obviously, such an advantage will selectively increase the number of people within the population who carry the gene. The inci-

dence of malaria and the inheritance of other forms of altered haemoglobin, such as β-thalassaemia, can be mapped to the same parts of the world.

In the Caucasian population, the most common autosomal recessive condition is cystic fibrosis. The carrier rate within the population is about 1 in 25 people. This means that there is a one in 25 chance that any person might be heterozygous for (i.e. carry) the cystic fibrosis gene. The chance, therefore, of two carriers mating is one in 625 (25 × 25) (Fig. 7.16). If two heterozygous parents have children, there is a one in four chance that any child will be affected and a one in two chance that any child will be a carrier of the gene themselves. The livebirth rate of children with cystic fibrosis is about one in 2500 (625 × 4). Because of the relatively high incidence of the disease, parents who already have an affected child or those whose family history has a strong incidence of the disease will be offered genetic counselling. Carriers of the cystic fibrosis gene appear to have resistance to gastrointestinal conditions, tuberculosis and cholera, and to have increased fertility. Cystic fibrosis is a condition which has the potential to be treated by gene therapy (Box 7.7).

Table 7.3 *Examples of recessively inherited diseases*

Trait	Carrier frequency
β-thalassaemia	1 in 6 Cypriots
Cystic fibrosis	1 in 25 Northern Europeans
Phenylketonuria	1 in 10 000 Europeans
Sickle cell anaemia	Varies amongst Mediterranean, Middle Eastern and Afro-Caribbean races
Tay-Sachs disease	1 in 30 Ashkenazi Jews

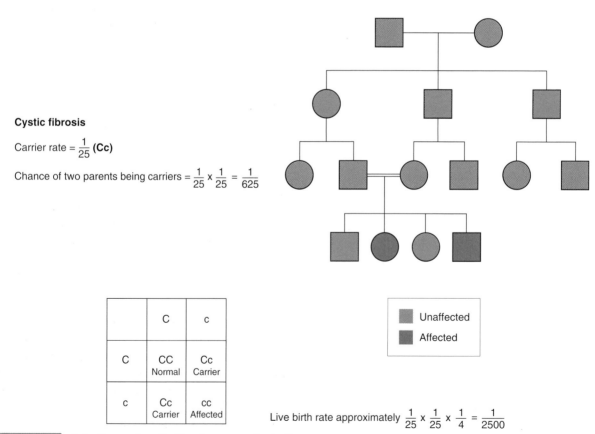

Cystic fibrosis

Carrier rate = $\frac{1}{25}$ **(Cc)**

Chance of two parents being carriers = $\frac{1}{25}$ x $\frac{1}{25}$ = $\frac{1}{625}$

	C	c
C	CC Normal	Cc Carrier
c	Cc Carrier	cc Affected

Unaffected

Affected

Live birth rate approximately $\frac{1}{25}$ x $\frac{1}{25}$ x $\frac{1}{4}$ = $\frac{1}{2500}$

Fig. 7.16 *Inheritance of cystic fibrosis, a recessive trait.*

Box 7.7

Advances in gene therapy

Recent advances in gene therapy have led to techniques to insert normal genes into human cells and tissues which express abnormal genes. Gene therapy aims to supplement a defective allele with a functional allele and focuses on single gene defects such as cystic fibrosis, muscular dystrophy, sickle cell anaemia and haemophilia. This is achieved by using a modified virus that acts as a vehicle by which the normal gene is carried into and thus incorporated into the genome. The altered virus is unable to replicate and so causes no harm to the recipient. In treatment of cystic fibrosis, the cells of the nasal passages and lining of the lungs are exposed to the virus in the form of an inhaled spray. So far, all human gene therapy has targeted at somatic (body) cells; germline engineering (altering stem cells or gametes) remains controversial.

Table 7.4　*Examples of sex-linked recessive disorders*

Trait	UK freq./10 000 males
Red–green colour blindness	800
Haemophilia A (factor VIII)	2
Haemophilia B (factor IX)	0.3
Duchenne muscular dystrophy	3
Fragile X syndrome	5

Sex-linked inheritance

The sex chromosomes not only determine the sex of the embryo but also have other structural genes. Very few genes appear to be carried on the Y chromosomes so sex-linked inheritance usually relates to X-linked inheritance. Most genes carried on the X chromosome are recessive. The effects of a recessive X-linked gene are usually masked in the female by the presence of the paired normal gene upon the other X chromosome. However, should such a woman carry an abnormal gene, she may pass it on to her sons. Males inherit only one of the paired X chromosomes, therefore if they acquire the abnormal gene on the X chromosome the disease will automatically be manifest because the Y chromosome lacks the corresponding allele of the other X chromosome that is found in the female. Also, if a female inherits two abnormal genes, one on each X chromosome, the condition is usually incompatible with life and the embryo is lost at a relatively early stage. X-linked recessive disorders therefore affect many more males than females. Very few sex-linked abnormalities are inherited as dominant traits which affect would both male and female offspring. One example is vitamin D-resistant rickets.

Most sex-linked diseases (Table 7.4) involve a female carrier partnered with a trait-free man (Fig. 7.17). There is a one in two chance that any male offspring will inherit and express the disorder and a one in two chance that any female offspring will carry the trait. An affected man cannot pass the disorder to his sons because they will receive a Y chromosome only, but all of his daughters will be carriers of the disease.

The Y chromosome is small and contains very little active genetic coding. However, it does contain the *SRY* (sex-determining region of the Y chromosome) gene, which, when activated, directs male embryonic development (see Ch. 5). The male, however, still requires the presence of an X chromosome as this contains many genes that are vital for normal development to occur.

The female inherits two X chromosomes but evidence suggests that only one of the chromosomes is activated within the cell. On examination of the cell nucleus, one chromosome is always contracted, forming a characteristic Barr body at the outskirts of the nucleus. The number of Barr bodies is one of the tests used in determining the sex of a baby born with ambiguous genitalia. The contracted Barr body chromosome was assumed to be inert, but a small number of genes appear to remain active and expressed.

There are examples of mosaic phenotypes where a heterozygous woman has a mix of dominant and recessive expression. For instance, in X-linked ectodermal dysplasia, affected males have smooth skin with no sweat glands. Female carriers may have patches of normal skin interspersed with patches of dysplasic skin. Similarly, females who are heterozygous for ocular albinism may have a mosaic pattern of pigmentation in their irises. There also seems to be some form of dosage compensation, as the inheritance of two X chromosomes does not result in twice the amount of proteins coded for by genes on the X chromosome. The explanation is that, early in embryonic development, a process called X-inactivation or

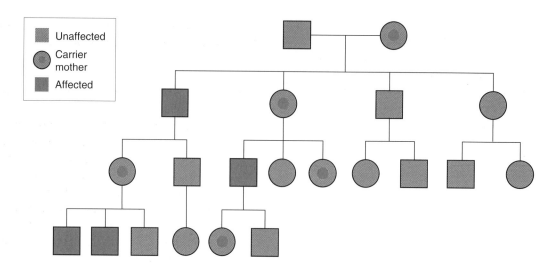

Fig. 7.17 *Inheritance of a sex-linked trait.*

'Lyonization' occurs in which one of the X chromosomes is permanently inactivated (Box 7.8, Fig. 7.18). As random chromosomes are selected for inactivation, different regions of the adult body have different chromosomes inactivated.

The three main types of inheritance are summarized in Box 7.9.

Other types of inheritance

Blood groups A and B are inherited as co-dominant genes, whereas the gene for blood group O is recessive (Fig. 7.19, Box 7.10). Some disorders are inherited via the mitochondria. The mitochondria of the zygote and subsequent cells are exclusively derived from the oocyte (see Ch. 6); therefore no paternal mitochondria are passed on to the next generation. Disorders of mitochondrial metabolism are passed from mother to child but never from father to child. The unique matrilineal transmission of mitochondrial DNA (mtDNA) has been particularly useful for the study of population genetics and evolutionary biology. This has been

Box 7.8

X-inactivation or Lyonization

X-chromosome inactivation or Lyonization (named after Dr Mary Lyon, who first proposed the hypothesis in 1961) occurs at approximately 15 days into the gestation. In humans, the cell mass of the embryo at around this stage is approximately 5000 cells (Fig. 7.18). The female embryo randomly inactivates all but one X chromosome on each cell; once inactivated, all the cells descending from each parent cell retain their pattern of either paternal or maternal inactivation. In some animals, such as marsupials, it is always the paternally derived X chromosome that is deactivated but in mammals it appears that either one of the pair is inactivated. Random inactivation would predict that 50% of female cells would have an active paternal X and 50% have an active maternal X; however, skewed patterns of inactivation can arise which means that the X chromosomes from one parent may be predominantly inactivated so the X chromosomes from the other parent will then be expressed. This could lead to the dominant proportion of expressed X chromosomes carrying a disorder that can be expressed. The inactivated chromosome appears as a sex chromatin body (Barr body) and is identified as it always divides late in mitosis. However, not all the chromosome is totally inactivated: the pseudoautosomal region of the short arm as well as other loci remain active to prevent the manifestation of Turner's syndrome in all normal genotypical women.

particularly useful in determining family lineage, such as the notable case of Anastasia, the Russian princess. DNA analysis showed that the mtDNA of members of the present Royal Family was different to that of the person who claimed to be Anastasia (Sykes 2001). Determining patterns of inheritance can be complicated, however, where different inherited disorders apparently cause the same effect, such as blindness.

The presence of 23 pairs of normal chromosomes indicates a normal karyotype (see Box 7.4).

Chromosomal abnormalities

Changes within the genetic message, for instance those due to mutation, may involve large parts of the chromosome (Box 7.11). If the changes can be seen by light microscopy, they are termed gross aberrations and can be detected from an examination of the karyotype. Chromosomal abnormalities can be classified as numerical or structural, affecting either the autosomes or the sex chromosomes. These types of abnormality are easier than a single gene abnormality to detect.

Numerical abnormalities

The loss or gain of one or more chromosomes is described as aneuploidy (wrong number of

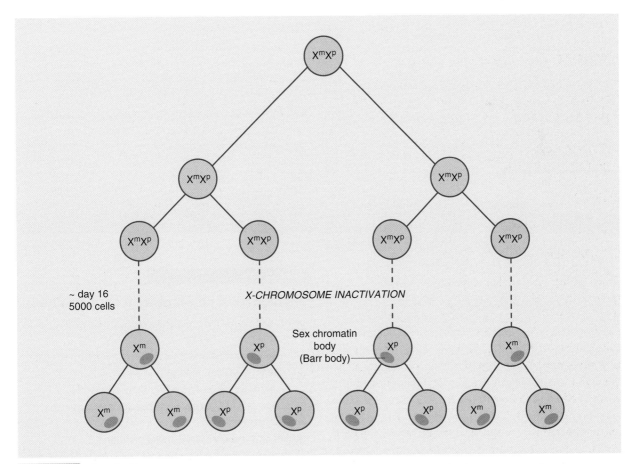

Fig. 7.18 *Lyonization.*

Characteristics of different types of inheritance

Autosomal dominant inheritance

- Effects are manifest in heterozygotes
- Affected person + unaffected person: half of offspring are affected
- Unaffected persons do not transmit condition
- Fresh mutation may produce abnormal genes
- An affected person usually has an affected parent
- Traits are often variably expressed and may not be penetrant (an individual can have the mutant gene but have a normal phenotype)
- Often structural, receptor or carrier proteins are affected and clinical effects tend to be less severe than those due to recessively inherited traits

Autosomal recessive inheritance

- Effects are manifest in homozygotes
- Affected person receives genes from both parents
- Heterozygote = 'carrier'
- Heterozygote parents:
  —one in four chance that offspring will be affected
  —one in two chance that offspring will be carriers
  —one in four chance that offspring will be unaffected
- Variation in birth frequency
- Recessive traits usually result in enzyme defects

Sex-linked inheritance

- Sex chromosomes carry genes *and* determine sex
- Sex-linked = X-linked
- Most conditions are rare
- Genes involved are usually recessive
- Female carrier:
  —one in two chance that male offspring will be affected
  —one in two chance that female offspring will also be carriers
- Affected male:
  —all sons will be normal
  —all daughters will be carriers

PHENOTYPES OF PARENTS		PHENOTYPES OF POSSIBLE	OFFSPRING IMPOSSIBLE
A	A	A, O	B, AB
A	B	A, B, AB, O	none
A	AB	A, B, AB	O
A	O	A, O	B, AB
B	B	B, O	A, AB
B	AB	A, B, AB	O
B	O	B, O	A, AB
AB	AB	A, B, AB	O
AB	O	A, B	AB, O
O	O	O	A, B, AB

Antigens A and B are inherited as dominant traits whereas O is inherited as a recessive trait.

Fig. 7.19   *Inheritance of ABO blood groups*

Erythrocyte surface antigens: blood group classifications

The reason for the evolution of differing blood groups in humans remains a mystery except that at some point during evolutionary history they may have been advantageous to ensure overall survival of the population. Other animals do not have the same number or type of blood groups. The more common human blood cell antigens give rise to the blood groups A, B, AB and O (Table 7.5).

Other surface antigens commonly found in practice are Duffy, Rhesus D, C, E and Kell. The presence of other antigens explains why, even with closely matched blood, recipients can react to the blood of the donor. The Rhesus antigen, which is present in approximately 85% of the population, has implications for fetal survival (see Ch. 10).

Incidence of chromosomal abnormalities

- Incidence of major chromosomal abnormality:
  —about 1 in 200 livebirths
  —about 1 in 20 perinatal deaths (stillbirths and early neonatal deaths)
  —about 1 in 2 early spontaneous abortions
- About 1 in 100 births: single-gene (unifactorial) disorder
- About 1 in 50 births: + major congenital abnormality

chromosomes) whereas cells with the correct number of chromosomes are euploidic. It is estimated that 10–25% of all human fetuses are aneuploidal, predominantly due to non-disjunction in maternal meiosis (Hunt & Hassold 2002), although trisomy 18 most often results from non-disjunction in meiosis II. Aneuploidy occurs more frequently in humans than in other species which is probably the reason for such a

Table 7.5 *ABO blood groups*

Blood type	A	B	AB	O
Antigen on RBC (agglutinogen)	A	B	A + B	None (universal donor)
Antibody in plasma (agglutinin)	b	a	None (universal recipient)	a + b
Can donate to	A and AB	B and AB	AB	All
Can receive from	A and O	B and O	All	O
Distribution in UK (%)	42	9	3	46
Genotype	AA, AO	BB, BO	AB	OO
Phenotype	A	B	AB	O

RBC = red blood cell.

high rate of miscarriage in humans. Aneuploidy is usually due to non-disjunction in the formation of the gametes resulting in a zygote that does not have 46 chromosomes. Monosomy describes the loss of a complete chromosome and trisomy the addition of a single chromosome, as in Down's syndrome (trisomy 21) (see Table 7.1, p. 156). Monosomy and triploidy (an extra complete set of 23 chromosomes) are usually lethal. Most autosomal trisomies are also lethal except those involving chromosomes 13, 18 or 21 but these, and the sex chromosome trisomies, are the main cause of mental retardation and developmental disability. It is interesting to note that chromosomes 13, 18 and 21 carry the fewest genes. Abnormal numbers of sex chromosomes have a less serious effect on development; for instance a missing sex chromosome can result in a Turner's syndrome monosomy (45,X0). Although it might be possible that paternally derived aneuploidies are preferentially eliminated, it is more likely that more errors occur in maternal meiosis and/or that the mechanisms for detecting and correcting or eliminating them are less stringent. The most likely reason for non-disjunction is age-related deterioration of the meiotic spindle and the motor proteins which move chromosomes along it.

Down's syndrome

Down's syndrome is the most common chromosomal anomaly at birth affecting about one in 700 livebirths. The conception rate is much higher but it is associated with a high incidence of spontaneous abortion and stillbirth. Either the ovum or the sperm carries the extra chromosome 21. Although non-disjunction is associated with older maternal age, there is evidence to suggest that

older men, perhaps because of a lower incidence of coitus, also have an increased rate of non-disjunction in their sperm formation. There is also a slight increase in the incidence of Down's syndrome in teenage pregnancies which may reflect a tendency to non-disjoin in early ovarian cycles (Hassold & Hunt 2001).

Affected children have typical stigmata of Down's syndrome (Box 7.12). Their life expectancy tends to be shorter because of increased susceptibility to infection, congenital heart disease and leukaemia. It is also hypothesized that individuals with Down's syndrome have increased oxidative damage to neurons, which results in accelerated brain ageing similar to that of Alzheimer's disease.

Over half of the conceptions with trisomy 21 fail, suggesting that the extra copy of chromosome 21

Box 7.12

Down's syndrome: clinical features

- Slanting palpebral fissure, almond-shaped eyes
- A roundish head and flat facial profile
- Small nose
- Low-set ears
- Simian crease (single palmar crease) in 50% of cases
- Folds of redundant skin around neck
- Clinodactyly (inwardly curved little finger) in 50% of cases
- Usually mentally retarded with IQ < 60
- Congenital heart malformations occur in 40% of cases
- Prone to presenile dementia in fifth decade

interferes with intrauterine development. Although males with Down's syndrome are infertile, females with Down's syndrome can reproduce; theoretically half the ova will have an extra copy of chromosome 21 but the effects on uterine development mean the livebirth rate does not correlate with the conception rate. Amniocentesis for cytogenetic screening is offered to all mothers over 35 years of age and the triple test is available to all women in the UK regardless of their age (see p. 171). Some women may also be offered ultrasonography screening.

About 4% of babies with Down's syndrome have 46, rather than 47, chromosomes. The extra chromosomal material from a chromosome 21 is attached to another chromosome (Robertsonian or balanced translocation; see Table 7.1). Usually, one of the parents is a carrier of Down's syndrome and has the translocation in a balanced form; 45 chromosomes with the extra copy of chromosome 21 attached to another chromosome (Fig. 7.20). This means that the translocation carrier is not directly affected but will produce a proportion of gametes with an unbalanced complement of chromosomes. There is frequently an associated his-

tory of recurrent spontaneous abortion due to lethal arrangements of chromosomes in the gametes.

Case study 7.1 looks at concerns related to Down's syndrome.

Case study 7.1

Josie is 48 years old and has four children between 14 and 24 years of age. She attends the midwives' clinic in a state of shock as her doctor has just informed her she is 8 weeks' pregnant.

- What advice would the midwife need to give to Josie in relation to antenatal screening?

Josie attends her local maternity unit at 12 weeks' gestation for a nuchal translucency scan and is given an estimated risk of a one in six possibility of a Down's syndrome baby.

- What further investigations could be offered to Josie and how can the midwife best support her during this period of investigation?

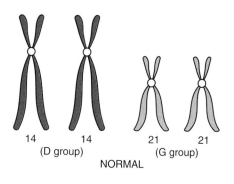

14   14   21   21
(D group)   (G group)
NORMAL

14   14/21   21
14; 21 ROBERTSONIAN TRANSLOCATION
(45 chromosomes)

GAMETES

14   21
1 Normal

14/21
2 Carrier

14/21   21
3 Down's syndrome
(46 chromosomes)

14
4 Monosomy
(lethal)

Fig. 7.20 *Robertsonian translocation.*

Structural abnormalities

Autosomal abnormalities

Structural chromosomal abnormalities include translocations, where material is exchanged between chromosomes, inversions, where a segment of the chromosome is rotated through 180°, and deletions, where segments of chromosomes are lost (Fig. 7.21). Cri du chat syndrome is associated with deletion of the short arm of chromosome 5. Deletions leave the affected chromosomes with fragile sites that adhere to each other, forming ring chromosomes. In inversions, a parent may have the correct amount of chromosomal material and therefore no clinical problem, but

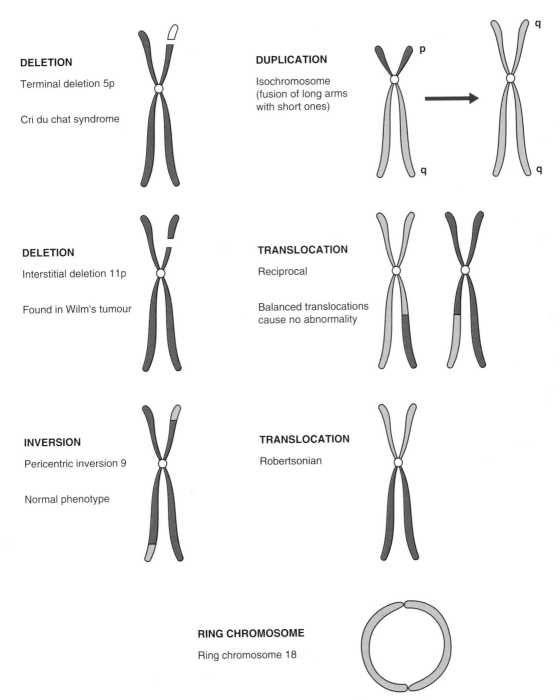

DELETION

Terminal deletion 5p

Cri du chat syndrome

DUPLICATION

Isochromosome
(fusion of long arms
with short ones)

DELETION

Interstitial deletion 11p

Found in Wilm's tumour

TRANSLOCATION

Reciprocal

Balanced translocations
cause no abnormality

INVERSION

Pericentric inversion 9

Normal phenotype

TRANSLOCATION

Robertsonian

RING CHROMOSOME

Ring chromosome 18

Fig. 7.21 *Gross chromosome aberrations: deletions, inversion, duplication, translocation.*

the chromosomes align inappropriately in meiosis so gamete formation is affected. Many chromosomal disorders affect fertility.

Sex chromosome abnormalities

Sex chromosome anomalies are relatively common but produce fewer ill-effects than autosomal anomalies. Generally, the greater the number of extra sex chromosomes the higher is the degree of mental retardation. Many sex chromosome anomalies also affect reproductive performance (see Ch. 5).

An example of an X-chromosome abnormality is fragile X syndrome (Box 7.13).

Genetic imprinting

Genetic imprinting is the suppression or silencing of certain alleles on the chromosomes depending on parental origin. Following fertilization, some alleles only become active if they were inherited from the mother (maternally imprinted genes) and others only if they were inherited from the father (paternally imprinted genes). The switching on and off of genes can be achieved by DNA methylation (adding a methyl group to a cytosine residue of DNA), phosphorylation or by modification of histone proteins. Normal development requires genes to be inherited from both parents. Imprinting prevents embryonic development where both sets of chromosomes come from the same parent; it has created challenges in animal cloning experiments and in human ovarian tissue cryopreservation. Some genetic diseases are due to abnormal imprinting, such as Präder–Willi syndrome (PWS) and Angelman syndrome (AS). These syndromes both result from either a maternal or a paternal deletion on chromosome 15 but the resulting syndrome depends on the parental origin of the chromosomes; only paternal deletions occur in PWS and

---

Box 7.13

Fragile X syndrome

Fragile X syndrome is one of the commonest causes of mental retardation in males. It is inherited as an X-linked trait, affecting one in 1000 male babies. The fragile site on the X chromosome is on the long arm. Affected males often have a large head, prominent chin and ears and may develop large testes at puberty. A significant proportion of carrier women are mentally retarded.

---

only maternal deletions in AS. In PWS both copies of chromosome 15 are inherited exclusively from the mother and none from the father; the situation is reversed in AS.

Genetic screening

The detection of abnormal genetic conditions such as cystic fibrosis (e.g. Case study 7.2) has been the focus of much ongoing research. There are three particular areas in which genetic investigation can be used to assess risk factors and confirm diagnosis of genetic disorder: parental screening, preimplantation screening and antenatal assessment.

Parental screening

Individuals from families with a known prevalent genetic disorder may be tested to confirm whether or not they carry the abnormal gene. The findings form the basis of genetic counselling in which both the risks of passing on the abnormal gene and the possible consequences for a child are discussed. Frequently, this follows the delivery of an affected baby, especially if there is no family history. The condition may have arisen by spontaneous mutation and so the chances of it re-occurring in subsequent pregnancies may be much smaller than if the parents were actually carrying the defective gene.

Preimplantation genetic diagnosis

Preimplantation genetic diagnosis (PGD) is a technique which allows screening for genetic and chromosomal disorders in an embryo before pregnancy is established (Sermon et al 2004). With the development of in vitro fertilization techniques (see Ch. 6), it has become possible to detect some genetic abnormalities by removing and analysing a polar body or a single cell from the 3-day-old embryo thus allowing selection of normal embryos for subsequent implantation. PGD utilizes molecular techniques such as fluorescent in situ hybridization, DNA analysis and polymerase chain reaction (PCR; see Box 7.14) to detect single-gene disorders, such as thalassaemias or cystic fibrosis, or to screen for structural or numerical chromosome disorders. PGD offers an alternative to prenatal diagnosis and selective termination of an

Case study 7.2

Tania has a brother who was diagnosed as having cystic fibrosis some years ago. Tania has been identified as being a carrier. Tania presents herself at the midwives' clinic with an unplanned pregnancy at 8 weeks' gestation. Her partner, Paul, has no family history of cystic fibrosis.

- What reassurance and advice can the midwife give to Tania?
- What referrals should the midwife make and how should this be explained to Tania?

affected pregnancy, which may be important for couples who cannot contemplate termination of a pregnancy. The identification and selection of euploid embryos also has a positive effect on the clinical outcome of assisted reproductive technologies (see Ch. 6) as chromosomal abnormalities are one of the major causes of spontaneous abortion and implantation failure.

Box 7.14

Molecular detection of abnormal genes

Molecular genetics studies human variations and mutations at the level of the gene and is important for understanding and identifying genetic diseases. Application of molecular genetic methods allows DNA diagnosis from very small amounts of tissue.

Fluorescent in situ hybridization (FISH)

This involves the use of a genetic probe, which attaches to the target gene that it is designed to detect. The probe has a fluorescent label and so the abnormal gene can be visualized. FISH is used to identify microdeletions, aneuploidy and translocations.

Polymerase chain reaction (PCR)

A small fragment of DNA is selectively amplified (at least a million times) by enzymatic procedures to produce large quantities of the relevant restriction fragments. These fragments can then be visualized by electrophoresis through an agarose gel, which is stained with a fluorescent dye. PCR is used to identify single gene disorders such as fragile X syndrome, Huntington's disease and muscular dystrophy. PCR can be used for any condition for which gene sequencing, and therefore the information required to design primers for selective amplification, is available.

Antenatal assessment

It is common throughout the UK for the screening for certain genetic disorders to be offered to all women. Currently two types of screening programmes are available: nuchal translucency (ultrasound) and the double/triple/Bart's test.

Nuchal translucency

At around 12 weeks' gestation, the nuchal fat pad at the back of the fetus's neck is measured using ultrasound assessment. Nuchal translucency (NT) increases with crown–rump length so the findings combined with maternal age and fetal size (crown–rump length) indicate a higher or lower risk of the fetus having Down's syndrome. The detection rate is about 83%. If the NT is raised, but the karyotype is normal, the fetus may be checked later for other physiological conditions such as cardiac abnormalities.

An increased NT (thicker fat pad) indicates an increased risk of a genetic or physical abnormality being present. Abnormal NT is also associated with other trisomies and fetal abnormalities (Souka et al 1998). It is not clear why such conditions result in a thicker NT but this may be related to oedema due to cardiac conditions, or failure of the neck lymphatic structures to develop at the right time, or both. Each case has to be assessed on an individual basis taking into consideration the maternal age and fetal size, although measurements less than 1.9 mm are probably normal, whereas those greater than 3 mm are probably abnormal.

The double/triple/Bart's test

The risk of Down's syndrome can also be estimated by a combination of blood tests, such as the levels of hCG (human chorionic gonadotrophin, which is usually raised in singleton Down's syndrome pregnancies) and AFP (alpha-fetoprotein, which is usually low in a Down's syndrome pregnancy) at around 16 weeks in combination with maternal age (Table 7.6). These tests have various formats and are often referred to as double, triple or Bart's test, etc. Trisomy becomes more common with an increase in maternal age and is linked to an increasing failure of the division of the oocyte to be completed normally. The results from the biochemical indicators are combined with the maternal age risk and compared with normal values, adjusted for gestational age, to establish the likelihood ratio (probability or risk) of the pregnancy being affected.

Table 7.6 *Combination test screening for chromosomal abnormalities*

Indicator	Source	Rationale	Considerations
Alpha fetoprotein (AFP)	Amniotic fluid Maternal serum (MSAFP—levels about 1000 times less than amniotic fluid)	MSAFP levels are reduced in pregnancies affected by trisomy 21 and other trisomies. AFP leaks from exposed capillaries into amniotic fluid in fetuses with NTD and some other malformations	The results are interpreted using appropriate standards for ethnic background: MSAFP is lower in Asian women and higher in Black women. Levels are reduced in mothers with insulin-dependent diabetes
Human chorionic gonadotrophin (hCG)	Maternal serum	Values are higher in trisomy 21 and lower in trisomy 18	Free β-subunit may be measured
Unconjugated oestriol (E$_3$)	Maternal serum	Values are lower in trisomy 21	
Pregnancy-associated plasma protein A (PAPP-A)	Maternal serum	Values are lower in trisomy 21	PAPP-A increases with gestation. PAPP-A measurement may be used in first-trimester screening

Ultrasound

All pregnant women in the UK are currently offered an ultrasound scan at approximately 20 weeks' gestation. The scan entails the detailed examination of the gross anatomical structures, such as internal organs, head, limbs and spine, and assessment of fetal growth. Many physical abnormalities, such as cardiac defects and limb length, are markers which may indicate the presence of a genetic abnormality. The more abnormal the ultrasound findings, the higher the risk of fetal aneuploidy. Abnormalities include structural malformations, increased nuchal thickness, short ear length, short femur or humerus, an extra vessel in the umbilical cord, a wide space between the toes and increased bowel echogenicity (Ott & Taysi 2001). This has led to the development of ultrasound scoring systems to identify fetuses at risk and support to the suggestion that ultrasound alone may be an alternative method of detecting genetic abnormalities in women who are reluctant to undergo amniocentesis.

Amniocentesis and chorionic villus sampling

Diagnosis of the above disorders can be confirmed only with more invasive procedures such as chorionic villus sampling (CVS) and amniocentesis (withdrawal of amniotic fluid) (Fig. 7.22). Both of these procedures enable the karyotype of the fetus to be examined, enabling fetal sexing, the identification of a trisomy or the presence of markers indicating the presence of abnormal alleles. Other invasive techniques are fetoscopy and cordiocentesis (fetal blood sampling) and biopsy. These procedures carry a slightly increased risk of procedure-related loss; however, the spontaneous abortion rate is higher in pregnancies with chromosomal abnormalities.

The fetal cells in the amniotic fluid or villus sample are grown in culture to produce enough cells for testing. The time taken for a result depends on the number of cells in the original sample and their growth rate, which can be affected by contamination with blood or maternal cells. The cell sample is greater in CVS so results are usually quicker. Occasionally, results can be complicated by chromosomal mosaicism where an individual has two or more cell lines, each with different chromosome numbers, derived from one zygote. For example, 1% of people with Down's syndrome are mosaics with both trisomic cells and normal cells; the clinical outcome is much better in these cases but if the abnormal cells are in the gonads there may be a high risk of producing abnormal gametes.

Amniocentesis and CVS are both invasive methods of prenatal diagnosis with inherent risks for the pregnancy. Alternative less-invasive methods of obtaining fetal cells and DNA are being studied. The placenta is not a totally impermeable barrier. Some, albeit very few, fetal cells transfer to the maternal circulation (see microchimerism, p. 242); there is approximately one fetal cell per millilitre of maternal blood. These intact fetal cells can be separated from maternal cells by flow cytometry (automated cell sorting equipment) as the

(A)

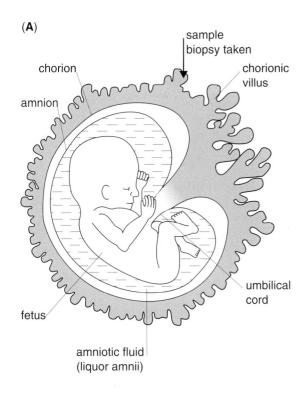

chorion

amnion

sample biopsy taken

chorionic villus

umbilical cord

fetus

amniotic fluid (liquor amnii)

(B)

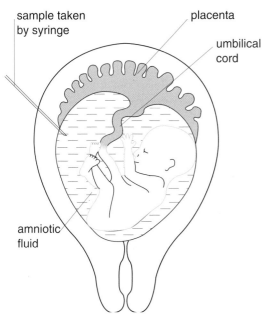

sample taken by syringe

placenta

umbilical cord

amniotic fluid

Fig. 7.22   *A Amniocentesis; B transvaginal chorionic villus sampling (CVS). (Reproduced with permission from Brooker 1998.)*

cells have different morphological characteristics. Developments in molecular biology mean that PCR amplification assays (see p. 171) can be used for pre-natal screening and genetic diagnosis. The discovery that fetal cell-free DNA (probably derived from the placenta) can also be extracted from the maternal blood has potential widespread clinical applications (Bianchi 2004).

Table 7.7 summarizes the prenatal diagnostic procedures and Box 7.14 describes the techniques for molecular detection of abnormal genes.

Evolution

Evolution is the study of genetic variation within populations and how this variation allows populations to evolve in response to changes within the environment in which they live. The variation of genes within a defined population is referred to as the gene pool. Charles Darwin's famous book 'On the Origin of the Species by Means of Natural Selection, or the Preservation of Favoured Races in the Struggle for Life' (known as 'The Origin of the Species') (1859) presented the argument that all organisms descended from a common ancestor and advocated natural selection as the mechanism of evolution. The mechanism of evolution is still contested, particularly how other mechanisms such as random genetic drift have contributed to evolution and the effects of gradual accumulation of small genetic changes rather than fewer large ones.

As described earlier in this chapter, many disease processes have their aetiology in the physical expression (phenotype) of an abnormal gene (genotype). They are normally recessive, so the effects of the abnormal gene are masked by the presence of a normal gene. The physical effects of recessive genes are only seen when there are two recessive genes present in the genome, for instance, in cystic fibrosis (see also in Case study 7.3, which looks at the Rhesus-negative blood type). Some abnormal genes may be partially expressed or modified by the presence of a normal gene. Many heterozygous, partially expressed genetic conditions may, in the right environment, impart a beneficial effect on the individual. An example is the sickle cell trait HbA/HbS or HbA/HbC (see Box 7.3, p. 153). If one recessive gene is present, the anaemia condition is expressed in a minor form. Whilst this can cause problems for individuals in periods of stress and physiological change, such as pregnancy, the symptoms are usually not life-threatening; on the contrary,

Table 7.7   *Prenatal diagnostic procedures*

Procedure	Gestation at which test is performed (weeks)	Conditions screened for or diagnosed
Non-invasive techniques		
NT measurement by ultrasound scan	12	Screen for trisomic conditions and other abnormalities
AFP test	16	Screen for neural tube defects
Triple/double/Bart's test	16	Screen for Down's syndrome
Ultrasound scan	20	Diagnosis of gross physical defects
Invasive techniques		
CVS	10–12	Diagnosis of chromosomal abnormality
Amniocentesis	16	Diagnosis of chromosomal abnormality
Fetoscopy		Diagnosis of chromosomal abnormality
Cordocentesis (removal of fetal blood from the umbilical cord)		Diagnosis of metabolic disorders Assessment of antibody status in haemolytic disease Detection of fetal infection
Organ biopsy (liver, skin, etc.)		Metabolic disorders Hereditary disorders

in the malaria zones of the world the sickle cell trait is beneficial to heterozygotes as it affords some protection from the malaria parasite. This is because entry of the parasite into the red blood cell causes the cell to die before the parasite has time to reproduce. In the major form of the disease when the individual inherits two abnormal genes, one from each parent, the haemoglobin configuration is abnormal. The erythrocytes are sickle-shaped and fragile which leads to severe complications of blood cell lysis and coagulation. Hence, although the homozygous form has implications for the survival of the affected individual, the abnormal gene is maintained within the gene pool because its partial form confers advantage in the gene pool of the population by increasing resistance to falciparum malaria. The absence of the Duffy surface antigen, which is usually present on the erythrocyte cell membrane, also affords protection against malaria as the malarial parasite attaches itself to this particular antigen to enable it to enter the cell.

The environment is ever changing and so the process of evolution as a result continues to facilitate adaptation to such changes. The process of evolution itself may then complicate our own understanding of human physiological processes. More than one regulatory system may develop at different times within our evolutionary progression. Different prevailing environmental conditions would thus influence the evolution of changes within the regulation mechanisms to match the change within the environment. Human physiological processes can be described as being in two evolutionary states that are either progressing or declining. Our reproductive physiology may still be influenced by processes that evolved to cope with the Pleistocene environment, in which it is believed that the genus *Homo* first evolved, even though these may now be in a state of evolutionary decline. In contrast, it is believed that our physiological processes may be responding to 'younger' evolutionary influences and therefore be in a state of

Case study 7.3

Jane is a 30-year-old woman expecting her second baby. Her first baby was born 3 years ago in rural Africa. She has now returned to this country at 36 weeks' gestation. The blood group results from her first antenatal visit show that Jane's blood group type is O, Rhesus negative.

■ What are the implications of this?
■ If it is known that her partner has the same blood group, what are the risks of the pregnancy being affected?
■ If Jane's first baby was Rhesus positive, what risk is there to the current fetus and how does it depend on its own blood group?
■ If a baby is affected by haemolytic disease of the newborn, what clinical symptoms are likely to be evident and how can they be treated?
■ If the first baby had been born in England, how would Jane have been treated?

evolutionary progression. Depending on the external (exogenous) and internal (endogenous) conditions present, the response to either of these evolutionary types may still be initiated.

Application to practice

It is important to realize that the genetic diversity of a population drives the process of evolution and adaptation to changes in the external environment.

Many genes are labelled as abnormal but they may be essential variants that may at least contribute to the survival of the population as a whole.

The focus of antenatal screening of the fetus is based upon the detection of the abnormal using tests that are both invasive, such as CVS, and non-invasive such as ultrasound scanning. In many situations, the conditions being screened for have a genetic cause or dysfunction. Knowledge of this is essential for the midwife to be able to understand and explain what the tests actually involve and what the results may indicate.

Midwives have an increasing role in the care of women suffering from pregnancy loss for whatever reasons, so an in-depth knowledge of fetal abnormalities is essential in providing care for the women.

Key points

- Genetics is a reductionist science that uses mathematical probability to predict the risk of inheriting certain characteristics, usually of medical relevance. Techniques such as combination diagrams and Punnett squares can be used to predict the probability of inheriting single-gene traits.

- DNA is the 'blueprint' of the organism, which is organized into chromosomes within the cell nuclei. A gene is a unit of a chromosome, or length of DNA, that codes for a particular instruction. Humans have 23 pairs of chromosomes: 22 pairs of autosomes and a pair of sex chromosomes (XX in females and XY in males).

- The structure of DNA facilitates its semiconservative replication prior to cell division, thus each cell of an organism has the same DNA.

- Mitosis is normal cell division producing daughter diploid cells with 23 pairs (i.e. 46) of chromosomes. Meiosis is a specific cell division in gamete formation that results in the number of chromosomes being reduced to 23 (the haploid number).

- DNA controls protein synthesis by acting as a template for the formation of mRNA (transcription); mRNA induces protein synthesis by directing the incorporation of amino acids into the protein (translation).

- There are accumulated errors in replicating DNA, which may manifest as mutations causing proteins with abnormal structure and function to be formed.

- A trait that is dominantly inherited is expressed if the individual has at least one copy of the gene, whereas a recessively inherited trait is expressed only if the individual inherits the gene from both parents. Sex-linked traits affect males more than females, who may be carriers.

- Chromosomal abnormalities may be numerical or structural and have serious clinical implications for those affected.

- Detection of fetal abnormalities is a routine part of antenatal care, which has developed screening programmes to assess risk and tests to confirm diagnosis.

Annotated further reading

Connor JM, Ferguson-Smith MA 1997 Essential medical genetics, 5th edn. Blackwell, Oxford
A well-written text that introduces the basic principles and clinical applications of genetics with a focus on the molecular mechanisms involved in genetic disorders and diseases. Also covers the genetics of common diseases and cancer, prenatal screening and gene therapy.

Dennis C, Gallagher R 2001 The human genome. Palgrave Macmillan
This book, written by editors of Nature, is an illustrated description of the human genome project for the general reader. It provides a reprinting of the Nature paper describing the first analysis of the first human genome sequence, an introduction to the underlying biology and the techniques used, together with an outline of the history of the human genome project and a discussion of its implications.

Emery AEH, Mueller RF, Young ID 2001 Emery's elements of medical genetics, 11th edn. Churchill Livingstone, New York
A comprehensive textbook which is divided into three parts. Section A focuses on genetic principles, risk prediction and factors influencing inheritance. Section B covers medical aspects of genetics including genetic diseases and genetic factors in diseases. Section C deals with clinical

applications, including genetic counselling, ethical issues, screening and diagnosis.

Hartl DL, Jones EW 2002 Essential genetics, 3rd edn. Jones & Bartlett
A popular and well-illustrated textbook, suitable for beginners, which clearly explains genetic concepts from the principles of hereditary to molecular genetics.

Kingston HM 2002 ABC of clinical genetics, 3rd edn (revised). BMJ, London
A slim, well-illustrated volume, targeted at clinicians, which describes genetic mechanisms, diseases and diagnosis.

Maynard Smith J, Szathmary E 2000 The origins of life: from the birth of life to the origin of language. Oxford Paperbacks
The authors present their hypothesis on the origin of life and alternative views of evolution focusing on seven transitions from the beginning of life on earth, the chemistry of molecular cycles and the origins of language.

Riccardi VM 1997 The genetic approach to human disease. Oxford University Press, Oxford
A clear and concise book which covers a variety of issues surrounding clinical genetics, including the ethical and moral aspects.

Ridley M 2004 Nature via nurture: genes, experience and what makes us human. Harper Collins, New York
A readable discourse about the effects of environment on genetics which covers historical and social facets as well as biological aspects of various topics such as child development, schizophrenia and the experience of twins.

Russell PJ 1998 Genetics, 5th edn. Harper Collins, New York
A weighty but clearly presented and well-organized genetics textbook covering fundamentals of genetics using a problem-solving approach. Includes experimental data, problems and worked examples.

Suzuki D, Knudtson P 1990 Genethics: the clash between new genetics and human values. Harvard University Press, Boston

A good review of the development of genetic engineering and gene manipulation with a balanced discussion of ethical issues.

....

References

Aitken RJ, Graves JAM 2002 The future of sex. Nature 415:963

Bianchi DW 2004 Circulating fetal DNA: its origin and diagnostic potential—a review. Placenta 25:S93–S101

Brooker CG 1998 Human structure and function, 2nd edn. Mosby, St Louis, pp 8, 20, 514

Craig IW, Harper E, Loat CS 2004 The genetic basis for sex differences in human behaviour: role of the sex chromosomes. Annals of Human Genetics 68:269–282

Darwin C 1859 On the origin of the species by means of natural selection. John Murray, London

Dawkins R 1989 The selfish gene, 2nd edn. Oxford University Press, Oxford

Dawkins R 1999 The extended phenotype: the long reach of the gene, revised edn. Oxford University Press, Oxford

Goodwin B 1997 Health and development: conception to birth. Open University, Milton Keynes

Graves JAM 2002 The rise and fall of SRY. Trends in Genetics 18:259–264

Hassold T, Hunt P 2001 To err (meiotically) is human: the genesis of human aneuploidy. Nature Reviews Genetics 2:280–291

Hunt PA, Hassold TJ 2002 Sex matters in meiosis. Science 296:2181–2183

Jones S 1994 The language of the genes: biology, history and evolutionary future. Flamingo, London

Open University 1987 Inheritance and cell division. Unit 20 in: Science foundation course (S102). Open University, Milton Keynes, p 48

Open University 1988 DNA: molecular aspects of genetics. Unit 24 in: Science foundation course (S102). Open University, Milton Keynes, pp 14, 36

Ott WJ, Taysi K 2001 Obstetric ultrasonographic findings and fetal chromosomal abnormalities: refining the association. American Journal of Obstetrics and Gynecology 184:1414–1421

Sermon K, Van Steirteghem A, Liebaers I 2004 Preimplantation genetic diagnosis. Lancet 363:1633–1634

Souka AP, Snijders RJM, Novakov A, Soares W, Nicolaides KH 1998 Defects and syndromes in chromosomally normal fetuses with increased nuchal translucency thickness at 10–14 weeks of gestation. Ultrasound in Obstetrics & Gynecology 11:391–400

Sykes B 2001 The seven daughters of Eve. Transworld Publishers, London

....

8 The placenta

Learning objectives

- To describe the development of the placenta, membranes and umbilical cord.
- To understand the role of the placenta.
- To discuss how abnormal placental development might affect fetal development and the outcome of the pregnancy.
- To describe methods for monitoring placental function.
- To outline the development of the placenta in twin pregnancies.

Introduction

The development of the placenta is critical for fetal survival because of the importance of the placenta in maternal–fetal transfer. It has a range of functional activities (Table 8.1), including complex synthetic capabilities, which are essential to the development of a normal term baby. The placenta flourishes in an immunologically foreign environment and has an important role in the immunological acceptance of the fetal allograft (see Ch. 10). Essentially the placenta acts as a vascular parasite, depending on maternal blood for oxygen and nutrients. The structure of the placenta means that, although optimal diffusion gradients are established, maternal and fetal blood never actually mix.

The placenta and the chorion (outer membrane) are derived from the trophoblast layer of blastocyst cells (see Fig. 6.6, p. 133). Other extraembryonic tissues develop from the inner cell mass. These include the amnion (inner membrane), the yolk sac, the allantois (a largely vestigial structure in humans) and the extraembryonic mesoderm. The umbilical cord and the blood vessels of the placenta are derived from the extraembryonic mesoderm.

The human placenta is haemochorial, which means that maternal blood comes into contact with the placental trophoblast cells. The uteroplacental unit is made up of both fetal and maternal components. The placenta as seen at delivery is just the fetal component or chorionic plate. The maternal component or basal plate is the underlying placental bed and the uteroplacental circulation that vascularizes it. Between the chorionic and basal plates is the intervillous space where the maternal–fetal exchange occurs. Abnormal placental function is strongly associated with fetal complications, but study of the human placenta, particularly the maternal component, is not easy. Placentation in the human is unique, which means that observations from other species can be applied to humans only with caution. Placental reserve needs to exceed fetal requirements (otherwise the fetus could be compromised under conditions of hypoxia). It might be expected that placental size would increase in parallel with increased fetal size; however, the placental:fetal weight ratio actually decreases during gestation (Kingdom et al 1993). Instead, placental efficiency is enhanced by an increase in both the number of carrier proteins involved in the transport of substances across the placenta and the placental perfusion.

Chapter case study

At Zara's 20-week scan the ultrasonographer documented in her report that the placenta was situated on the anterior wall of the uterus with the majority of the placental body situated in the middle and lower pole of the uterine body with the lateral edge of the placenta approximately 2 cm from the internal cervical os. What are the possible complications that could arise from this situation? How do you think the midwife should discuss these possible complications with Zara and how they could be recognized? Why is it common for women with this situation to have vaginal bleeding around 34 weeks of pregnancy?

Differentiation into cytotrophoblast and syncytiotrophoblast

There are two distinct cell layers in the blastocyst (see Ch. 6): the inner cell mass and the outer sphere of trophoblast cells. It is this outer layer that rapidly proliferates and develops into placental tissue. The morula enters the uterus about 4 days after fertilization. It may float freely in the uterus before it hatches out of the protective zona pellucida (Kingdom & Sibley 1996). About 7 days after fertilization, the blastocyst hatches and comes into contact with the endometrium. The blastocyst orientates itself so that the embryonic pole implants first; this is the part of the blastocyst where the inner cell mass is located. Uterine contact stimulates the trophoblastic cells to undergo rapid mitosis and proliferate. Signals between the embryo and endometrium also cause endometrial changes, or decidualization, whereby the stromal cells under the endometrial epithelium accumulate lipid and glycogen and become known as decidual cells. The stroma thickens and blood flow increases. Decidualization promotes changes in the endometrium that make it receptive to implantation. Synchronous development and communication between the maternal endometrium and the embryonic tissue are required for successful establishment of pregnancy. Whereas mammalian embryos have

Table 8.1 *Summary of placental functions*

Function	Placental role
Respiration	Maternal oxyhaemoglobin dissociates in the intervillous spaces. O_2 diffuses through the walls of the villi where it binds to fetal haemoglobin forming fetal oxyhaemoglobin. Transfer is increased by the higher affinity of fetal haemoglobin for O_2 (see Ch. 15). The lower CO_2 level facilitates transfer of CO_2 in the reverse direction in pregnancy (see Ch. 11)
Nutrition	Active transport of glucose, iron and some vitamins and passive transport of other nutrients. The placenta can metabolize proteins, fats and carbohydrates into simple molecules. Fats cross the placenta with less ease so the fat-soluble vitamins (A, D, E and K) cross slowly. The placenta stores glycogen, which can be converted to glucose when required
Excretion	Waste products of metabolism, CO_2 and heat cross from the fetus to the mother
Protection	The placenta acts as a barrier against most bacteria (such as cocci and bacilli). However smaller microorganisms (such as the syphilis bacterium) and viruses (including rubella, varicella-zoster, cytomegalovirus, coxsackie and HIV) can cross the villi. The placenta transfers IgG antibodies (see Ch. 10) and Rhesus antibodies to the fetus. Drugs including teratogens (see Ch. 9), anaesthetics and carbon monoxide (from smoking) can cross the placenta
Endocrine role	Initially, the trophoblast produces hCG, which maintains the corpus luteum and its production of steroid hormones. From the 3rd month onwards, oestrogen and progesterone are produced in large quantities by the placenta. hPL is produced from the syncytiotrophoblast. The placenta also produces a broad range of other hormones including corticosteroids, ACTH, TSH, IGFs, prolactin, relaxin, endothelin and prostaglandins
Immunological role	The trophoblast has unique immunological properties that render it immunologically inert so a maternal antigenic response does not occur (see Ch. 10)

intrinsic invasive potential and can initiate implantation-type reactions in many different tissues, the endometrium protects itself from implantation except for the limited duration of the implantation window (Bischof et al 2000). The interaction between the endometrium and the developing trophoblast is facilitated by a number of cytokines, metalloproteinases, surface integrins and growth factors, including insulin-like growth factors and their binding proteins, which create a specific microenvironment which modulates trophoblast function.

The trophoblast differentiates into two layers: the outer syncytiotrophoblast and the inner cytotrophoblastic layer. Some of the proliferative cells lose their cell membranes and coalesce to form a syncytium (a united mass of fused cellular material): the syncytiotrophoblast. Human chorionic gonadotrophin (hCG) enhances differentiation of cytotrophoblasts into the syncytiotrophoblast. Electron microscopy reveals the syncytiotrophoblast to be a mass of cytoplasm containing remnants of intercellular membrane, evenly dispersed nuclei and a few intermediate cells. This syncytial organization of cells is unusual; other than the trophoblast, multinucleated cells are seen only in some tumour cells and inflammatory giant cells (Chard 1998). Interestingly, a range of tumour cells appears to secrete hCG (Iles & Chard 1991) but at lower concentrations than those characteristic of trophoblast cells; these tumours usually affect individuals late in life.

The cytotrophoblasts, which form the inner monolayer of cells, are large clear discrete cuboidal cells each with a single nucleus and a well-defined cell membrane. These cells have marked mitotic activity and DNA synthesis. The syncytiotrophoblast increases in volume throughout the second week as cells detach from the proliferating layer of cytotrophoblast and fuse with the mass of syncytiotrophoblast. The syncytiotrophoblast secretes enzymes, which attack the endometrium, and hormones, which sustain the pregnancy. It is also involved in absorption of nutrients. The syncytiotrophoblast is aggressively invasive; between 6 and 9 days postfertilization the embryo becomes completely implanted into the endometrial stroma. The hydrolytic enzymes produced cause breakdown of the extracellular matrix between the cells of the endometrium thus eroding a pathway. The surface of the syncytiotrophoblast has tiny processes extending from it that penetrate between the endometrial cells, pulling the conceptus into the uterine wall. As implantation progresses, the expanding syncytiotrophoblast gradually envelops and encircles the blastocyst. The endometrial epithelium regenerates over the site of implantation, forming the decidua capsularis (Fig. 8.1). By 9 days, a thick layer of symmetrical syncytiotrophoblast within the endometrial wall encloses the entire blastocyst, apart from a small region at the embryonic pole. Implantation is complete by about 10 days after fertilization. A plug of a cellular material called the coagulation plug or operculum seals the small hole at the point of implantation (Fig. 8.2).

In the first week of development, as the free-floating embryo or conceptus moves towards the uterine cavity propelled by the cilia movement and muscular contraction of the uterine tube, the cells can obtain nutrients from secretions of the uterine tubes and endometrium and eliminate waste products by simple diffusion. It is thought that endometrial secretions of lactate and pyruvate and possibly some amino acids may be important in the nutrition of the embryo for up to 8 weeks (Burton et al 2001). The nutrients and oxygen are taken up by the syncytiotrophoblast; this is known as histiotrophic nutrition. By the end of the first trimester, there is a transition to haemotrophic nutrition from the uteroplacental circulation which provides a system in which the maternal and fetal circulation come into close contact to facilitate transfer of substances from one system to the other.

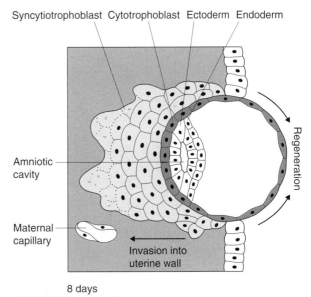

Fig. 8.1 *Regeneration of endometrium over the site of implantation.*

Uterine gland / Amnioblasts (future amniotic membrane) / Amniotic cavity / Syncytiotrophoblast

Trophoblastic lacuna (space filled with maternal blood) / Bilaminar embryonic disc / Coagulation plug (operculum) / Endometrial wall

Fig. 8.2 *Implantation of blastocyst into the endometrial wall at 9 days postfertilization.*

Syncytiotrophoblast / Extraembryonic mesoderm

Secondary villus

Amniotic cavity

Cytotrophoblast / Lacuna / Embryonic disc / Primary yolk sac / Secondary yolk sac / Extraembryonic coelom

Fig. 8.3 *Formation of extraembryonic mesoderm.*

As the syncytiotrophoblast invades the uterine wall, it comes into contact with the maternal endometrial capillaries. Fragments of these are engulfed within the syncytiotrophoblast forming trophoblastic lacunae (literally 'little lakes'), which are the precursors of the intervillous spaces. As maternal blood vessels are progressively invaded, the lacunae fill with maternal blood. Maternal capillaries near the syncytiotrophoblast expand to form maternal sinusoids which rapidly anastomose with the trophoblastic lacunae. As this development continues, the lacunae become separated by columns of syncytiotrophoblast, or trabeculae, which effectively form a framework on which the villous tree develops. The trabecular columns project radially from the blastocyst. The cytotrophoblast at the core of the columns proliferates locally to form extensions, which grow into the columns of syncytiotrophoblast. The growth of these protrusions is induced by the newly formed extraembryonic mesoderm (Fig. 8.3). The result is the primary stem villus, an outgrowth of cytotrophoblast covered by syncytiotrophoblast, which penetrates into the blood-filled lacuna (Fig. 8.4).

Extravillous cytotrophoblast and remodelling of the uterine vessels

Cytotrophoblast migration and invasion

Some cytotrophoblast cells migrate from the villi beyond the leading edge of syncytiotrophoblast into the stroma, forming the extravillous cytotrophoblast. From about 12 days postfertilization, these cells invade the maternal capillaries and spiral arteries of the decidua. The extravillous cytotrophoblast cells initially block the lumen of the maternal vessels that have been invaded and subsequently replace the endothelium of these vessels. Plugging of the lumen of the invaded maternal blood vessels prevents bleeding and is achieved by day 14, which coincides with the expected date of the next menstrual period. If the maternal vessels are not plugged adequately during implantation and early development then vaginal bleeding may occur, which is associated with an increased risk of spontaneous miscarriage (sometimes haematomas can be seen on ultrasound investigation).

The plugs prevent flow of maternal blood into the intervillous space in early pregnancy but allow a slow seepage of plasma (Jauniaux et al 2003) so the lacunar spaces enclosed by the syncytiotrophoblast initially contain exudate from maternal vessels rather than blood. The developing placenta forms an effective barrier between the mother and developing embryo that persists up to 10 weeks' gestation when intervillous blood flow is established (Jauniaux et al 1992). It is at this time that peak hCG secretion occurs (Meuris et al 1995). Doppler ultrasound shows there is no intervillous blood flow in normal pregnancies before this period and oxygen electrodes have demonstrated that an oxygen gradient exists across the placenta and decidua. This means that embryogenesis occurs in a relatively hypoxic environment. In fact, maternal–placental blood flow has been observed in the first trimester in a number of non-viable pregnancies but it is not clear whether this is a cause of the pregnancy failure or an effect (Kingdom & Sibley 1996). The developing embryo is thought to be particularly vulnerable to damaging oxygen free radicals during the sensitive period of organogenesis and the first-trimester placenta has limited antioxidant capacity; thus, limiting fetal exposure to oxygen may be protective.

Placental remodelling

Between the 4th and 16th week of gestation, villus growth and considerable remodelling of the placenta occur, including remarkable changes to the maternal blood vessels underlying the fetal placenta. In the early weeks, some of the cytotrophoblastic cells (described as extravillous cytotrophoblast) move from the tips of the anchoring villi to colonize the decidua and myometrium of the placental bed. It is this invasion of extravillous cytotrophoblast cells into the maternal blood vessels that promotes maternal recognition of the fetus and the subsequent production of blocking antibodies (see Ch. 10), which are important for the survival of the pregnancy. The extravillous cytotrophoblast cells are involved in the destruction and remodelling of the endothelium of the maternal spiral arteries, which is completed by the end of the first trimester. After an apparent rest phase of a couple of weeks (weeks 14–16), there is a resurgence of the endovascular trophoblastic migration. The second wave of cytotrophoblast cells moves down the myometrial segments of the spiral arteries to their

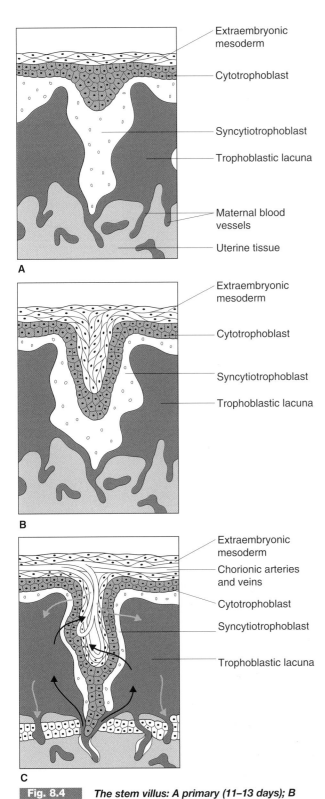

A

- Extraembryonic mesoderm
- Cytotrophoblast
- Syncytiotrophoblast
- Trophoblastic lacuna
- Maternal blood vessels
- Uterine tissue

B

- Extraembryonic mesoderm
- Cytotrophoblast
- Syncytiotrophoblast
- Trophoblastic lacuna

C

- Extraembryonic mesoderm
- Chorionic arteries and veins
- Cytotrophoblast
- Syncytiotrophoblast
- Trophoblastic lacuna

Fig. 8.4 *The stem villus: A primary (11–13 days); B secondary (16 days); C tertiary (21 days).*

origin at the branching from the radial arteries. The syncytiotrophoblast cells are involved with the replacement of the endothelium, destruction of the musculoelastic tissue and a change in the vessel wall vasoresponsiveness. The result is conversion of the thick-walled muscular spiral arteries to compliant dilated sac-like uteroplacental vessels that have low impedance to blood flow (Fig. 8.5). Insufficient remodelling of the spiral arteries is associated with growth restriction and pre-eclampsia (Box 8.1).

The remodelled vessels can passively dilate and accommodate a greatly increased blood flow (about 30% of maternal cardiac output) but they are not responsive to vasoactive agents. The effect of this interaction between the trophoblastic cells and the maternal blood vessels is that a low-pressure, high-conductance vascular system is established, which provides an adequate maternal blood flow to the placenta and thus a plentiful provision of oxygen and nutrients to the fetus. The maternal uteroplacental

circulatory system is mostly complete by mid-gestation. In contrast, the fetal villous tree continues to branch and develop throughout the pregnancy, ensuring that the capacity of the placenta matches the growth of the fetus.

As the maternal cardiac output increases by about 40% (see Ch. 11), the net effect is to increase the uteroplacental blood flow by about 10-fold to over 500 ml/min (Kingdom & Sibley 1996). Doppler ultrasound flow velocity waveforms provide diagnostic and prognostic information about maternal vessels, placental circulation and fetal vessels together with implications for both mother and fetus (Harman & Baschat 2003). Flow in the uterine arteries gives a picture of the maternal vascular effects of the invading placenta, predicting likely pre-eclampsia and intrauterine growth restriction. Umbilical artery Doppler ultrasound depicts placental vascular resistance, which correlates with intrauterine growth restriction and effects of placental deficiency. Before pregnancy and in the

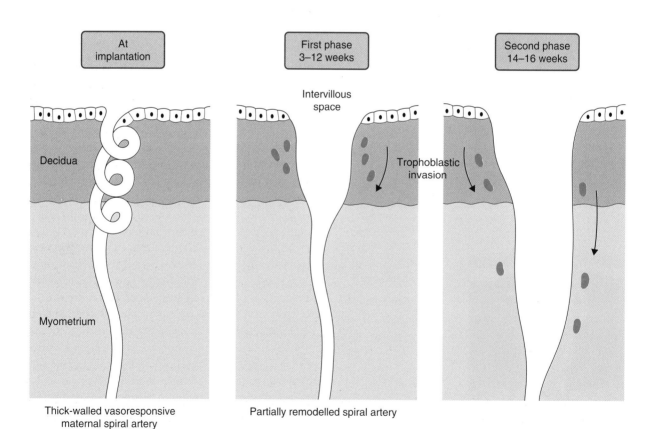

Fig. 8.5 *Conversion of spiral arteries into uteroplacental arteries. The maternal spiral arteries have thick muscular walls and are responsive to vasoactive substances. They are remodelled by the trophoblastic cells in two waves, ultimately forming non-responsive dilated vessels. Where remodelling is inadequate, a proportion of the vessels retain the structure of preimplantation or partially remodelled vasoresponsive vessels.*

Box 8.1

Pre-eclampsia

Pre-eclampsia is a placental condition; it can occur in the absence of a fetus in a molar pregnancy. One of the theories about the aetiology of pre-eclampsia is that it is due to partial failure of placentation resulting in inadequate blood flow to the placenta and fetus. This leads to placental hypoxia, oxidative stress and possibly infarction. In normal pregnancies, all spiral arteries in the placental bed are invaded by cytotrophoblast cells. In pre-eclampsia, it seems that only a proportion of the maternal vessels are invaded and that a significant number of vessels show complete absence of physiological changes. The second wave of arterial invasion may be the stage that is most compromised owing to the endovascular trophoblast failing to reach the intramyometrial portion of the vessels. This means that the spiral arteries are not completely transformed to uteroplacental vessels. Maternal uteroplacental blood flow is therefore restricted, which results in placental abnormalities and fetal complications such as intrauterine growth retardation (IUGR). The effect is compounded by the persistence of vasoresponsiveness of the spiral arteries, which retain the ability to constrict and limit placental perfusion, like the spiral arteries of a non-pregnant uterus. There are serious maternal complications of pre-eclampsia which have been attributed to an as-yet unidentified placentally derived 'factor X' which is released into the maternal circulation; possible candidates include inflammatory cytokines from the syncytiotrophoblast, products of placental oxidative stress and placental debris such as syncytiotrophoblast microfragments (Fig. 8.6).

and folate and hyperhomocysteinaemia are risk factors for these placenta-mediated diseases (Ray & Laskin 1999). Smoking is associated with poorer outcomes of pregnancy including low birthweight, spontaneous abortion and placental abruption. Nicotine, cadmium and polyaromatic hydrocarbons in cigarette smoke adversely affect fertility, oocyte development and oestrogen synthesis (Shiverick & Salafia 1999). Effects of these compounds on trophoblastic invasion and proliferation are thought to account for the increased miscarriage rate of women who smoke; however, smoking seems to reduce the incidence of pre-eclampsia possibly because smoking reduces endothelium sensitivity. Severe placental dysfunction is more common with a male fetus (Edwards et al 2000); this may be the cause of the male:female ratio decreasing from 164:100 soon after conception to 106:100 at birth. Placental pathologies may be due to defective trophoblast function and/or impaired maternal decidualization.

Vascularization of the placental villi

Fetal blood cells are derived from blood islands in the extraembryonic mesoderm surrounding the yolk sac (see Ch. 9). The blood vessels that perfuse the placenta also develop in this tissue. In the 3rd week postfertilization, the extraembryonic mesoderm associated with the cytotrophoblast penetrates into the core of the primary stem villi transforming them into secondary stem villi. This mesoderm develops into the blood vessels and connective tissue of the villi. It forms at the same time as the embryonic vasculature with which it will eventually connect. Haemangioblast cells (precursors of blood cells) appear and capillaries form. The linking of the blood vessels of the villi with the vessels of the embryo results in a circulating blood system so the villi begin to be perfused by the fetal circulation at about 28 days after fertilization. The fetal red blood cells containing embryonic haemoglobin allow oxygen transfer at low partial pressures of oxygen and low pH. The villi containing differentiated blood vessels are described as tertiary stem villi. By the end of the 4th week after fertilization, these villi cover the entire blastocyst surface forming a spherical shell of villi projecting outwards into the maternal tissue (Fig. 8.8). It is possible to remove a sample of the developing placental villi for genetic testing (Box 8.2). The placental barrier now effectively limits diffusion of gases,

first trimester, the uterine arterial waveform has a low end-diastolic flow velocity and early dichrotic notch during diastole. By 18–20 weeks' gestation, successful trophoblastic invasion alters this pattern to one showing a high diastolic flow velocity and loss of the dichrotic notch. If the dichrotic notch and low end-diastolic velocity persist, this indicates that the uterus still has high impedance to blood flow, which is predictive of intrauterine growth retardation (IUGR) and severe pre-eclampsia (Fig. 8.7).

A number of pathologies including placental infarction or abruption, pre-eclampsia and recurrent pregnancy loss are associated with defects within the placental vascular bed. Deficiencies of vitamin B_{12}

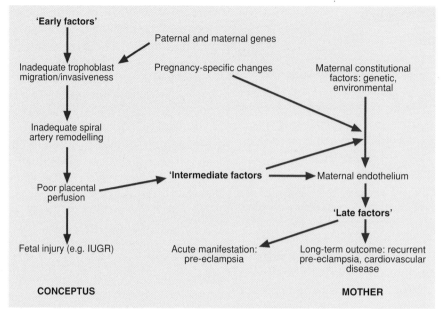

Fig. 8.6   *Interactions between the conceptus and the mother in the development of pre-eclampsia. (Reproduced with permission from Lala & Chakraborty 2003.)*

nutrients and waste materials. There are four layers: the endothelium lining the villus capillary, the connective tissue in the villus core, a layer of cytotrophoblast cells and a maternal-facing layer of syncytiotrophoblast (Fig. 8.9). By mid-gestation, most of the cytotrophoblast layer of many villi disappears and the placental barrier becomes very thin. The syncytiotro-

phoblast may even come into direct contact with the fetal capillary so the maternal and fetal blood may only be about 2–4 μm apart.

Development of the discoid placenta and chorionic membrane

From the 4th week to the 16th week, the villus growth over the entire surface of the blastocyst is remodelled. Most of the villi orientated towards the uterine cavity degenerate and regress, leaving behind an area that develops into the typical placental structure and shape seen at delivery. As the embryo starts to enlarge, the uterine wall where it has implanted starts to protrude into the uterine cavity (Fig. 8.10). The protruding portion of the embryo is covered by the decidua capsularis, a thin layer or capsule of endometrium. The layer of decidua under the embryonic pole of the embryo is the decidua basalis. The remaining areas of the decidua are described as the decidua parietalis.

In the 3rd month, as the fetus enlarges and grows to fill the uterus, the thin rim of decidua capsularis covering the bulge gradually thins and disappears so the chorion comes into contact with the decidua

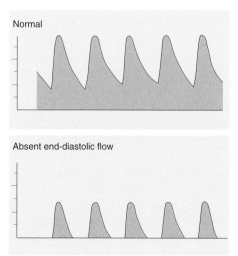

Fig. 8.7   *Doppler ultrasound waveforms showing diastolic flow and dichrotic notch. (Reproduced with permission from Miller & Hanretty 1998.)*

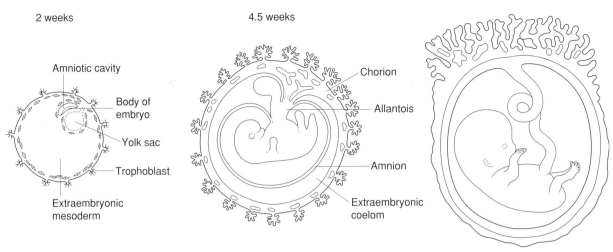

2 weeks

4.5 weeks

Amniotic cavity

Body of embryo

Yolk sac

Trophoblast

Extraembryonic mesoderm

Chorion

Allantois

Amnion

Extraembryonic coelom

Fig. 8.8 *Early villus formation occurs in a sphere-like organization around the whole of the enlarging conceptus; eventually most of the villi will degenerate leaving only the ovoid development of the fetal placenta.*

Box 8.2

Chorionic villus sampling (CVS)

In the CVS procedure, 20–40 mg of placental tissue can be obtained from a villus for genetic diagnosis of trisomy 21 for instance, or of a single-gene abnormality such as cystic fibrosis or β-thalassaemia. After 10 weeks' gestation, the tissue can be extracted transabdominally by needle aspiration or transcervically using curved biopsy forceps. The collected trophoblast cells, which divide very rapidly, can be cultured for 24 hours and then the chromosome number can be determined (see Ch. 7). Because of the problems associated with mosaicism (see Ch. 7), a more accurate determination of chromosome number and structure is obtained by using fibroblast cells taken from the vascular core of the villus. These cells grow more slowly so they have to be cultured for 2 weeks before being stained and examined (which means the results of the test take longer). As fibroblast cells are derived from the mesoderm, they originate from the inner cell mass and are embryonic rather than the trophoblast-derived cells from the outer layers of the villus. Placental mosaicism is associated with increased fetal loss and IUGR. There is a 1–2% procedure-related loss in CVS, although it should be remembered that the procedure is being performed because there is already a concern about the pregnancy. Pregnancies associated with genetic abnormality have a much higher risk of spontaneous failure.

parietalis of the opposite wall of the uterus. Before the trophoblastic shell comes into contact with the uterine wall on the opposite side, cells of fetal origin can enter the uterine cavity and can be collected by flushing or aspiration from the endocervical canal (Kingdom et al 1995). This is potentially a route of non-invasive prenatal diagnosis, particularly for newer testing procedures that require fewer cells. The size of the chorionic, or embryonic, sac can be used to determine the gestational age of the embryo.

The uterine cavity is obliterated by 12 weeks' gestation. The enlarging blastocyst compresses the trophoblastic layer, distal to the entry pole, and limits nutrient supply and further growth by the villi in this region of the decidua capsularis. The underlying villi slowly degenerate and regress so by the 5th month this region becomes devoid of villi and smoother. This flattened surface forms the chorion laeve, the uteroplacental membrane, which is also known as the chorionic membrane or bald chorion. Effectively the chorion is extraplacental trophoblast with similar immunological properties; it may also be an important source of hCG, particularly in early pregnancy. The portion of the trophoblastic tissue associated with the decidua basalis implants further and receives a plentiful supply of nutrients so it continues growing. This area of the chorion, therefore, retains villi that proliferate and progressively arborize forming the chorion frondosum ('frondosus' is Latin for leaf), which ultimately develops into the definitive discoid fetal placenta. The placenta is a union

Fig. 8.9 *Exchange of substances across the placenta occurs across a barrier consisting of four layers of tissue: syncytiotrophoblast, cytotrophoblast, mesoderm and fetal blood vessel wall. (Reproduced with permission from Miller & Hanretty 1998.)*

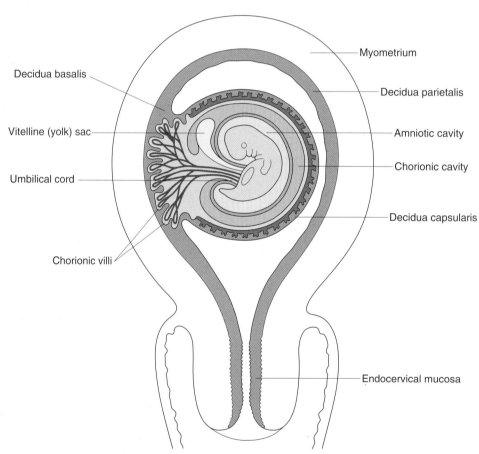

Fig. 8.10 *Protrusion of the developing conceptus into the uterine cavity and formation of the decidua capsularis.*

between the chorion frondosum derived from the fertilized ovum and the decidua basalis (basal plate) formed from the maternal uterine wall. It is anatomically complete by the end of the first trimester but continues to grow throughout the pregnancy.

Development of the amnion (inner membrane)

The amniotic cavity first appears at about day 7. The primitive ectoderm cells enclosing the cavity become flattened forming aminoblasts, cells which become the fetal-facing amniotic membrane. These cells secrete amniotic fluid, thus the embryo is enclosed in the fluid-filled amniotic sac. The outer surface of the amnioblast cell layer becomes covered with mesoderm. As the embryo expands, the amnion comes into contact with the chorion. The chorionic cells are lined with mesoderm cells on the inner side. When the amnion and chorion meet, the two layers of mesoderm loosely fuse. The fetal membranes protect the fetus and secrete factors into the amniotic fluid which affects amniotic fluid activity and also can influence the maternal uterine physiology.

Amniotic fluid

Amniotic fluid has an important role in protecting the fetus, cushioning it from external impact and stresses. It also allows symmetrical fetal growth and movement, preventing fetal parts from adhering together or to the amnion. Amniotic fluid has bacteriostatic properties and is also important in maintaining a constant body temperature. In the first half of gestation, before skin keratinization takes place, fluid and electrolytes can diffuse freely across the skin (Jauniaux & Gulbis 2000). Although the amnioblasts actively secrete amniotic fluid, the composition of the fluid at this time is similar to that of fetal tissue fluid. After 20 weeks, the skin becomes keratinized and transudation from maternal and fetal blood vessels contributes less to the amniotic fluid. Fetal urine and lung secretions are also important. Fetal swallowing and exchange across the amnion mean that turnover of fluid is rapid, particularly close to term. The fetus may swallow 20 ml of fluid per hour; the extra water crosses the gut, enters the fetal circulation and can then cross the placenta. By term, the normal volume of amniotic fluid is 500–1000 ml. Polyhydramnios is an excess amount of fluid (over 2000 ml), which is usually associated with multiple pregnancies or fetal swallowing problems. A deficiency of amniotic fluid (less than 500 ml) is classified as oligohydramnios, a condition often associated with impaired fetal renal function.

Amniotic fluid provides a useful tool to monitor fetal development and well-being. A small amount of amniotic fluid can be removed in amniocentesis for measurement and testing. Amniotic fluid contains many maternal and fetal proteins and fetal cells, which can be used for genetic testing (see Ch. 7). If the fetus has a neural tube defect (see Ch. 9), concentrations of AFP (alpha-fetoprotein, derived from spinal fluid) in the amniotic fluid are very high. Levels of AFP are low in Down's syndrome (trisomy 21) and are measured as part of the triple test (see Ch. 7). It has been proposed that this could be due to the persistence of extra-embryonic coelom or related to interferon receptor levels (Chard 1998).

Growth and maturation of the placental villi

The placental villi continue to grow for most of the pregnancy. There is a widely held belief that the placenta ages during the pregnancy and that at term it is about to decline into functional senescence. Instead, the continuous morphological changes should perhaps be viewed as an increase in functional efficiency rather than ageing. Placental efficiency is favoured by the attenuated maternal–fetal barrier and reduced diffusion distance rather than by an increase in weight. Although the rate of placental growth does decline in the later part of gestation, this decrease in growth rate is not irreversible or inevitable. If the maternal environment becomes unfavourable, for instance because of maternal anaemia or increased altitude, fresh villus growth will ensue and the placenta will expand its surface area and continue branching past term. In all placentas, total placental DNA levels continue to increase linearly beyond the 40th week of gestation.

Later growth of the placenta (see Fig. 8.4, p. 181) can be divided into three stages. Earlier in pregnancy, the villi proliferate and form new generations of villi. Later on, more lateral branches develop and the layers forming the placental barrier become more refined. In the 9th week, the tertiary stem villi lengthen to form mesenchymal villi. These originate from the trophoblastic sprouts of the syncytiotrophoblast with a similar cross-section to the primary stem villi. By the 16th week, the terminal extensions of the tertiary stem villi reach their maximum length. At this stage, the villi are described as immature intermediate villi. The cells of the cytotrophoblast layer become more dispersed within the villi creating gaps in the cytotrophoblast layer of the villus wall. Near the end of the second trimester, the tertiary stem villi form numerous side-branches and are described as mature intermediate villi. The earliest mature intermediate villi finish forming by about week 32 and then begin to produce small nodule-like secondary branches characteristic of the terminal villi. This is the final structure of the placental villous tree. The terminal villi are not formed by active outgrowth of the syncytiotrophoblast but by coiled and folded villus capillaries that bulge against the villus wall and expand by unfurling. Two types of chorionic villi can be identified: deep villi anchor the placenta to the decidua basalis; shorter villi extend into the intervillous spaces and have a nutritive role.

The blood-filled intervillous space into which the villi project is formed from the trophoblastic lacunae that grow and coalesce. Therefore, the intervillous space is lined on both sides with syncytiotrophoblast. The maternal face of the placenta is the basal plate, which consists of syncytiotrophoblast lining plus a supporting layer of decidua basalis. The fetal side is formed of the layers of chorion of the chorion plate.

The functional unit within the placenta is the placentome, a villous tree arising from the chorionic plate within the intervillous space, which is perfused by a spiral artery. There are about 50–100 such units within the placenta. The villous tree has rami (major branches) and smaller ramuli. The terminal villi have little impedance to flow and therefore an increased fetoplacental flow; they are probably the major sites of nutrient and gaseous exchange in late gestation. The progressive development and branching of the placental tree structure is important for fetal growth and development. For instance, in IUGR pregnancies requiring elective preterm delivery, there are fewer terminal villi, which seem to have an abnormal extravillous cytotrophoblast structure.

The placenta is subdivided into cotyledons by wedge-like placental septa, which appear in the 3rd month. The placental (decidual) septa grow into the intervillous space from the maternal side of the placenta, separating the villi into 15–20 cotyledons. The placental septae do not fuse with the chorionic plate so maternal blood can flow freely from one cotyledon to another. This means that the villi are bathed in a lake of maternal blood which is constantly exchanging; this organization of placental perfusion is described as haemochorial. Haemochorial placentation is efficient because the trophoblast is in contact with maternal blood optimizing maternal–fetal transport of gases, nutrients, water and ions. The trophoblast can also endocytose the immunoglobulin IgG. In addition, hormones produced by the fetoplacental unit can easily access the maternal circulation. There are, however, some costs to the haemochorial arrangement; bleeding may be extensive at parturition and cells can be transferred between mother and fetus, for instance, resulting in microchimerisms (see Ch. 10) or erythro-

blastosis fetalis (haemolytic disease of the newborn due to Rhesus incompatibility).

Placental blood flow

The fetal blood reaches the placental blood system via the two umbilical arteries which spiral around the umbilical vein (Fig. 8.11). On reaching the chorion, the vessels usually each supply half of the placenta. The arteries (which are vessels carrying blood away from the fetal heart and therefore carry deoxygenated blood) divide repeatedly to form a branching network of smaller arteries and capillaries running through the intervillous space. The fetal blood flow through the placenta is about 500 ml/min, propelled by the fetal heart. Smooth muscle fibres contracting in the villi may help to pump blood back from the placenta to the fetus.

The maternal blood enters the intervillous space via about 50–100 of the remodelled spiral arteries. There is a pressure gradient from the maternal arteries to the intervillous space to the maternal veins. The blood leaves the intervillous space via the endometrial veins. Most organs have a progressive decrease in arterial diameter as the blood nears its target tissue. In the uteroplacental vessels, the remodelled spiral arteries increase in diameter as the vessels approach the intervillous space. Therefore, the intervillous space is a low-pressure system; the blood gently flows through and washes over the fetal placental tissue. The placenta has little resistance to maternal blood flow and a high vascular conductance so there is little fall in pressure across the intervillous space. The main determinant of the rate of maternal blood flow is the vascular resistance in the myometrial arteries. Myometrial contractions can decrease or stop afferent blood flow to the intervillous space. This effect is probably due to the compression or occlusion of the veins draining this space. During a contraction, the space distends so the fetus is not totally deprived of oxygen.

Intrauterine growth retardation and 'placental insufficiency'

Fetal hypoxia, IUGR or fetal death are often attributed to 'placental insufficiency'. A proportion of those babies with a low birth weight (less than 2.5 kg) probably failed to achieve their growth potential because

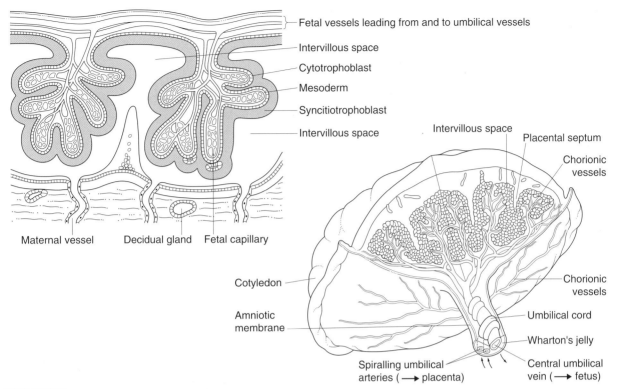

Fetal vessels leading from and to umbilical vessels
Intervillous space
Cytotrophoblast
Mesoderm
Syncitiotrophoblast
Intervillous space
Maternal vessel
Decidual gland
Fetal capillary

Intervillous space
Placental septum
Chorionic vessels
Cotyledon
Amniotic membrane
Chorionic vessels
Umbilical cord
Wharton's jelly
Spiralling umbilical arteries (⟶ placenta)
Central umbilical vein (⟶ fetus)

Fig. 8.11 *The umbilical cord and the circulation through the placenta.*

placental transfer of oxygen and nutrients was inadequate. However, the fetal placenta is rarely insufficient. Like all essential organs, it has a considerable physiological reserve. It has been estimated that the placenta could lose 30–40% of its villi (and therefore surface area) without affecting its function.

Placental insufficiency really describes inadequate maternal uteroplacental blood flow, which is probably due to incomplete conversion of the spiral arteries during the early stages of pregnancy. Studies suggest the uteroplacental perfusion is greatly reduced because of a failure of the trophoblast invasion into the myometrium and subsequent remodelling of the spiral arteries (Brosens et al 2002) which results in fewer terminal villi and other placental abnormalities affecting blood vessels and membranes involved in diffusion. It is possible that some small-stem arterioles may be occluded by fetal platelets (Wilcox & Trudinger 1991). Measurement of abnormal oxygen and amino acid levels in the umbilical vein blood suggests a defect in placental transport mechanisms (Cetin et al 1990). However, it is not established whether these changes are causative or adaptive. Compensatory mechanisms exist in the fetus, which result in redistribution of blood to the fetal brain at the expense of the lower body. This is

supported by the finding that amniotic fluid volume is decreased presumably because blood flow to the kidneys is reduced (Kingdom & Sibley 1996). Substances that cause vasoconstriction, such as cocaine and alcohol, are implicated in preterm labour, possibly because they cause a decrease in blood flow to the placenta affecting uterine contractility and sensitivity.

Case study 8.1 details an example of a small baby.

Case study 8.1

Polly was diagnosed as carrying a small-for-dates baby. She spontaneously delivered Thomas at 39 weeks, and although he weighed only 2.4 kg he appeared healthy and vigorous. The midwife noted that the third stage appeared complete but failed to identify that the placenta appeared relatively large.

- Do you think that there is any need to weigh placentas and to compare the placental and birth weights?
- Are there any situations where the weight and condition of the placenta may be used as a possible indicator for disease states in later life?

Fetoplacental blood flow

Blood leaving the right atrium is diverted into the ductus arteriosus, into the aorta and down to the lower body (see Ch. 15). At term, about 40–50% of the fetal cardiac output goes to the placenta via the umbilical arteries. Blood flow from the aorta to the umbilical arteries is high because the resistance to flow in these vessels is low compared with the systemic circulation of the lower body. The vessels of the fetoplacental circulation lack autonomic innervation but a variety of substances can affect the smooth muscle of the stem villous arteries. Of particular importance are paracrine agents, which have a local effect on the fetoplacental circulation. Both prostacyclin and nitric oxide (NO), which have vasodilatory and anticoagulant effects, are produced from the vessel endothelium. It is suggested that flow-mediated release of NO may have an important role (Learmont et al 1994). Diffusion of NO into the intervillous space affecting maternal uteroplacental vessels may also be important (Myatt et al 1993). The heterogeneous cells of the placental vessel endothelium also produce endothelin-1 (a potent vasoconstrictor), substance P, serotonin, ATP, atrial natriuretic peptide (ANP) and neuropeptide Y (NPY) (Cai et al 1993, Myatt et al 1992); whether these substances have a physiological role is yet to be established.

Optimal placental exchange requires adequate vascularization of the placental bed by the maternal arteries matched by circulation of fetal blood to the placenta. The fetus does not appear to have a mechanism to increase umbilical flow in response to hypoxia or volume depletion. It has a limited ability to increase cardiac output. Therefore, the fetus adapts to hypoxia or decreased nutrient availability by decreasing oxygen consumption and growth rate. The cardiac output is redistributed to the heart, brain and adrenal glands at the expense of the flow to the body and gut. Hypoxia and acidosis cause cerebral vasodilatation and constriction of the pulmonary and femoral vessels. Blood flow to the liver is high when oxygen and nutrients are plentiful but the hepatic circulation is bypassed if placental exchange is compromised.

It is hypothesized that perfusion of the placental vessels is controlled to match the maternal perfusion of the uteroplacental vessel in a similar way to the perfusion–ventilation matching in the neonatal or adult pulmonary system (see Ch. 1). If an area of the placenta is underperfused by the maternal blood flow, hypoxia ensues. The endothelium of the placental vessels responds by vasoconstricting (by decreasing NO synthesis and increasing endothelin-1 production) so fetoplacental blood flow is diverted to a better-perfused villous tree.

Placental exchange

Many substances are transported from the maternal blood in the intervillous space to the fetal blood in the capillaries of the villi and vice versa. By term, most exchange occurs in the terminal villi, which have a high surface area and small diffusion distance, perhaps of only a few micrometres in some areas. The surface area of the placenta is calculated to be 5 m^2 at 28 weeks, increasing to about 11 m^2 at term (Carlson 1994). The precise mechanisms of placental transport for many substances are not clear. Diffusion depends on the concentration gradient, the placental permeability and the surface area; however, passive diffusion alone is not likely to be adequate for fetal requirements for nutrients. Lipophilic substances (soluble in lipid) are soluble in cell membranes so their transport depends on the concentration gradient and the relative rates of maternal and fetal blood flow. Diffusion of hydrophilic substances (soluble in aqueous solutions) is limited by the diffusion distance and the membranes of the placental barrier. The fetal capillary endothelium probably limits transport of large proteins (such as albumin, IgG and AFP). Transport studies of the syncytiotrophoblast suggest that it is much more permeable than was previously believed and probably offers a route continuous with, and containing, extracellular fluid (Kingdom & Sibley 1996), which allows the diffusion of large proteins. The transfer of substances across the placenta occurs in both directions, to and from the fetus.

There are specific transport proteins on the placental plasma membrane involved in the efficient transfer of metabolically important substances. Some of these proteins form channels and others act as shuttles. Glucose demands are high and are estimated to be 4–8 mg/kg/min (Aldoretta & Hay 1995). Glucose transport is predominantly carried out by the facilitative–diffusion glucose transporter GLUT1 and also by GLUT3 (Knipp et al 1999). Glucose transport by GLUT1 is concentration-dependent, bi-directional and independent of insulin. GLUT1 expression is higher on the maternal side of the syncytiotrophoblast which favours mother-to-fetus transfer and protects glucose being transported from the fetus during maternal hypoglycaemia. GLUT1 expression is down-regulated by hyperglycaemia so fetal development is partially protected if there is maternal hyperglycaemia. GLUT3 is not the major facilitator of glucose transport to the developing fetus but may be important during periods of maternal hypo- or hyperglycaemia.

Some substances, such as certain amino acids and calcium, are transported by active (energy-dependent) transport against their electrochemical gradients. Fatty acids, particularly the long-chain polyunsaturated fatty acids (LCPUFA), are important for synthesis of phospholipids and cell membranes, and growth and development of the brain and nervous system. The fetus is dependent on placental transfer which is mediated by specific fatty acid binding and transfer proteins and preferentially transports LCPUFA. The placenta nucleoside transporters enable the fetus to meet its high demands for nucleosides to synthesize nucleotides; transport of adenosine is decreased by ethanol. There are additional mechanisms for the transport of some very large molecules such as receptor-mediated pinocytosis for IgG (see Ch. 10). There is a net flux of water to the fetus, mostly across the placenta.

Steroid hormones cross the placenta but peptide hormones seem to be poorly transferred. Gas transfer occurs by diffusion and is probably limited by blood flow. As well as oxygen and carbon dioxide, the placenta permits diffusion of other gases such as carbon monoxide and inhalation anaesthetics. The placenta itself has a high rate of oxygen consumption; much of this oxygen is used for oxidative phosphorylation of glucose. The consequent production of ATP is used mainly for synthesis of peptide and steroid hormone and for transport of nutrients.

The placenta has a protective function and limits transfer of some xenobiotic substances to the fetus. The placenta expresses cytochrome P450 enzymes which metabolize and detoxify a number of drugs. There are also export pumps in the syncytiotrophoblast which reduce placental transfer of potentially toxic substances. However, some bacteria (such as the one that causes syphilis), some protozoa (such as the parasite that causes toxoplasmosis) and a number of viruses (including HIV, cytomegalovirus, rubella, polio and varicella) can cross the placenta and affect outcome.

Placental hormone production

Placental hormones have a role in adjusting maternal physiology to provide the optimal environment for fetal development (see Ch. 11); however, roles for all of the placental products have not yet been elucidated. Concentrations of placental protein hormones are higher in the maternal blood than in the fetus because the fetal circulation limits the transfer of large molecules (Firth & Leach 1996). Conversely, levels of steroid hormones are about 10 times higher in the fetal circulation (Chard 1998). Although the levels of placental protein hormone fluctuate randomly, a true circadian rhythm of placental secretion has never been demonstrated (Chard 1998). This includes secretion of hCG, which is not higher in urine specimens collected in the morning (Kent, et al 1991).

The placenta has a broad endocrine capacity and diversity, producing many hormones that other endocrine organs also produce. The syncytiotrophoblast is probably the source of most placental products, although the cytotrophoblast may also produce hCG, human placental lactogen (hPL), inhibin, relaxin and placental releasing hormones (Chard 1998). The major steroids produced are progesterone and oestrogens (oestriol). The production of oestrogens requires both maternal and fetal precursors, so monitoring maternal oestrogen levels during the pregnancy is a useful indicator of fetal well-being. Cholesterol from maternal low-density lipoprotein (LDL) is mostly used as the precursor for steroid hormone production. Oestriol synthesis requires 16α-hydroxydehydroandrosterone sulphate derived from the fetal liver and adrenal gland. Most of the steroid hormones produced enter the mother's circulation, affecting her physiology (see Ch. 11). The placenta also produces neuropeptides (although it has no nerves), which may regulate placental hormone production, leptin, growth factors and cytokines.

hCG and steroids

Embryo development requires progesterone to maintain uterine quiescence. Initially hCG from the trophoblast rescues the corpus luteum from atresia (see Chs 4 and 6) thus maintaining the production of oestrogen and progesterone. Release of hCG from the trophoblast seems to begin about 7 days after fertilization (Chard 1998). However, levels of hCG and luteal steroid hormones are not directly related in normal pregnancies (Hamilton-Fairley & Johnson 1998). Hormone levels fall following in vitro fertilization (IVF) despite increasing levels of hCG (Johnson et al 1993a). The relationship between hCG and steroid hormone production is stronger in anembryonic pregnancies (Johnson et al 1993b), where embryonic development has failed, suggesting that the embryo itself takes over the control of steroid hormone production by the corpus luteum. The corpus luteum becomes redundant at about 7 weeks after fertilization when steroid hormone production is taken over by the placenta. The change in site of production is described as the luteoplacental shift; a relative progesterone and oestradiol deficiency can develop and lead to abortion (Schindler 2004). Inadequate hormone production by the corpus luteum early in pregnancy before this shift, or insufficient placental development, are also thought to be responsible for early miscarriages.

hCG can be detected in maternal blood about 10 days postfertilization once implantation has occurred and secretions from the trophoblast can enter the maternal vessels. hCG is composed of two subunits; the α-subunit is common to all glycoprotein hormones such as LH (luteinizing hormone), FSH (follicle-stimulating hormone) and TSH (thyroid-stimulating hormone). Dissociated α- and β-subunits of hCG, as well as the intact dimer (the complete hCG molecule formed of two subunits), are measurable in pregnancy (Kingdom & Sibley 1996). The concentration of α-subunits progressively increases throughout the pregnancy reaching maximal levels at about 36 weeks. The concentration of free β-subunits parallels the concentration of intact dimer, reaching a peak about 10 weeks after fertilization, and then declines to a plateau. It is thought that the cytotrophoblast produces α-subunits and the more differentiated syncytiotrophoblast produces both α- and β-subunits (Kingdom & Sibley 1996). Raised levels of β-subunits of hCG are associated with Down's syndrome, reflecting abnormal formation of the syncytiotrophoblast (Spencer et al 1992). Levels of the hormone are also significantly higher in cases of severe pre-eclampsia (see Box 8.1, p. 183) and IUGR (Wenstrom et al 1994). The role of hCG in maintaining hormone production by the corpus luteum is clearly established. However, the peak of hCG production is reached after the function of the corpus luteum has already started to decline, suggesting other roles for the hormone. hCG levels appear to be associated with fetal testosterone production and so may be involved with male sexual differentiation (see Ch. 5).

Human placental lactogen

hPL is also a product of the syncytiotrophoblast. Levels of hPL increase throughout gestation and cor-

relate well with placental syncytiotrophoblast mass so it can be used clinically to evaluate placental function. By term, 1–3 g of hPL are produced per day. hPL affects maternal metabolism, erythropoietin activity, fetal growth, mammary gland development and ovarian function; it induces insulin resistance and carbohydrate intolerance and is important in the provision of fatty acids for the fetus. Lower hPL levels are associated with pre-eclampsia, aborting molar pregnancy (hydatidiform mole), choriocarcinoma and placental insufficiency. Higher than normal hPL levels are associated with multiple pregnancies, placental tumours, intact molar pregnancy, diabetes and Rhesus incompatibility. However, there are reports of women with abnormally low or absent levels of hPL having completely normal pregnancies (Kingdom & Sibley 1996). hPL is also known as human chorionic somato-mammotrophic hormone.

Placental growth hormone

PGH is synthesized by the syncytiotrophoblast. It has high sommatogenic (growth) activity and low lactogenic activity. It gradually replaces pituitary growth hormone in the maternal circulation (Evain-Brion & Malassine 2003). It is secreted continuously (whereas pituitary growth hormone has a pulsatile secretory pattern) and is important in facilitating maternal metabolic adaptation to pregnancy and the provision of fetal glucose.

The allantois and yolk sac

The allantois and yolk sac are semivestigial structures that have a more important role in other species, such as birds and reptiles, where the yolk sac is important in nutrition of the maternally isolated eggs and the allantois has a respiratory and excretory role. The allantois forms from a pocket of the hindgut embedded within the umbilical cord, which is incorporated into the developing urinary system. Blood cells develop in the wall of the allantois during weeks 3–5 and its blood vessels become the vessels of the umbilical cord. The yolk sac develops on the ventral side of the embryonic disc and is important in nutrition of the embryo while the uteroplacental circulation is forming. The primordial germ cells (see Ch. 5) and the blood islands develop in the tissue of the yolk sac. The yolk sac becomes thin and elongated and is incorporated into the umbilical cord and primitive gut. Its role in haematopoiesis is taken over by the liver in the 6th week of development.

The placenta at term

The mature placenta is an oval/round disc about 18–20 cm across and 2–3 cm thick in the middle, petering out towards the edges. The margins of the placenta are continuous with the fetal membranes. On average, a placenta weighs about one-sixth of the weight of the fetus, about 500 g. The amniotic membrane is smooth so the fetal aspect of the placenta appears shiny and grey. The maternal side is grooved and lobed with a dull red coloration, often flecked with blood clots. The chorion retains the ridged appearance owing to the regression of the early villi. The umbilical cord gets progressively longer with the duration of the pregnancy. At term, the umbilical cord is normally between 50 and 60 cm long. If the cord is abnormally short, it can cause bleeding problems. If it is long, it may prolapse through the cervix or entangle with the fetus, possibly forming knots that could impede fetal circulation during delivery, causing potentially fatal anoxia. Abnormal cord length is clinically used as a marker of undetected intrauterine events (Calvano et al 2000). Short cords are associated with prenatal exposure to alcohol and drugs such as cocaine. Most umbilical cords are twisted but true knots occur in about 1% of births (Moore & Persaud 1998). The vessels of the cord, two arteries carrying blood from the fetus and one vein carrying blood to the fetus, are embedded in Wharton's jelly. This jelly is a connective tissue that protects the vessels of the cord.

Examination of the placenta

Examination of the placenta, membranes and umbilical cord at delivery is an important responsibility of the attendant midwives. The vessel number in the cord is checked. There are usually two arteries and a vein. An abnormal number of cord vessels, such as a single umbilical artery, occur in about 1% of births and are associated with an increased frequency of fetal and chromosomal abnormalities, particularly of the renal or cardiovascular systems (Benirschke 1994). Sometimes more vessels are present because the initial pair of veins has failed to fuse. Although an abnormality in the number of vessels is associated with congenital abnormalities, it is not clear whether the wrong number of vessels is a cause or a result of the abnormality.

The cord appearance is also examined. Macrosomic babies of diabetic mothers tend to have thick oedematous cords whereas thin delicate cords are associated with IUGR. The cord can be inserted into the placental bed in different ways. Insertion of the cord is usually central but may be lateral. Abnormal insertion of the cord can create problems at delivery (Table 8.2). If the cord is ruptured, it indicates that there may have been some fetal blood loss during labour.

The membranes are easier to examine if the placenta is held up by the cord. Usually the two membranes hang down in a neat uniform way. The placenta is continuous with the chorion but the amnion should be able to be separated from the chorion up to the base of the cord. If the membranes are ragged and torn, some parts of the membrane may be retained in the uterus, which can impede uterine involution and staunching of blood loss.

Table 8.2	*Placental abnormalities*
Condition	**Description and cause**
Abruptio placentae	Separation of normally situated placenta from site of implantation after 24th week of gestation, but before delivery of the fetus. More common in women with high parity and history of obstetric problems. May cause uterine tenderness and tetany, and variable bleeding. Complications may include disseminated intravascular coagulation (DIC), postpartum haemorrhage (PPH) and shock. It is essential to avoid vaginal examination until placenta previa has been excluded
Placenta previa	Abnormally implanted placenta, positioned partially or totally (over the os) in the lower segment, which obstructs normal delivery. More common in multigravidae, particularly those of high parity and with multiple pregnancy. Usually causes painless vaginal bleeding. Factors that cause damage and scarring of the endometrium increase risk. Possibly due to deficient decidua in fundus at implantation. The placenta is likely to be large and may have succenturiate lobes (see below)

Continued

Table 8.2 *Placental abnormalities—Cont'd*

Condition	Description and cause
Abnormal insertion of cord	Vasa previa is a rare condition that may occur with velamentous insertion of cord where some of the umbilical vessels cross the internal os. Velamentous insertion occurs in 1% of singleton pregnancies. The cord is attached to the membranes outside the placental boundary
Abnormal conformation of placenta	Placentation may be extrachorial, where the surface area of the chorionic plate is less than the basal (maternal) area. A circumarginate placenta has a flat ring at the transition from placenta to chorion. A circumvallate placenta has a raised rolled ring at the transition and is associated with increased incidence of growth retardation
Succenturiate (accessory) lobes	Variations in shape and number of lobes do not normally affect the outcome of the pregnancy. The placenta may have accessory lobes or be completely bi-lobed. This may cause problems in determining whether the placenta has been completely expelled at delivery
Hydatidiform mole and choriocarcinoma	Abnormal placental development where the embryo is absent or non-viable. Related to abnormal fertilization and survival of paternal chromosomes only (see Ch. 7). Hydatidiform mole is a non-invasive chorionic development and choriocarcinoma is a malignant tumour derived from trophoblast tissue, possibly from a hydatidiform mole. The villi are not vascularized in either case (as extraembryonic mesoderm is derived from the inner cell mass)
Abnormal adherence of chorionic villi	In placenta accreta, the villi adhere to the uterine wall, which has an abnormal decidual layer. In placenta percreta, the villi penetrate right through the myometrium to the perimetrium. The placenta fails to separate properly in the third stage of labour and maternal haemorrhage is likely

A healthy placenta is normally rounded and uniform. An excessively large or oedematous placenta is associated with maternal diabetes, hydrops or cardiac abnormalities. The placenta is also examined for abnormal numbers of lobes (Table 8.2) or missing areas of the maternal surface, which could indicate that a lobe has been retained, potentially causing serious postpartum bleeding. Depending on whether twins are monozygotic or dizygotic, the placenta may be shared or regions fused (Box 8.3).

Case study 8.2 details an example of placental abnormality revealed by inspection.

Case study 8.2

Following what appeared to be a normal delivery, the midwife inspected the placenta and membranes. She discovered a hole in the membranes that had blood vessels leading to it, radiating out from the main body of the placenta.

- What do you think the midwife concluded from these findings?
- What care and observation will the woman require?
- How will this be explained to the woman and what information might she require?

Box 8.3

The placenta in multiple pregnancies

Dizygotic (non-identical) twins and monozygotic (identical) twins resulting from early splitting of the blastocyst prior to implantation can have separate placentas and membranes. However, if the two blastocysts implant in close proximity, the placentas and chorion may fuse. If monozygotic twins arise from division of the inner cell mass, they usually have separate amnions but share the placenta and chorion. The vascular systems within the placenta may remain separate but can fuse. If the vascular systems fuse within the placenta, twin-to-twin transfusion syndrome may occur where the twins have an unequal blood supply. This condition, which occurs in 10–15% of monozygotic twins (thus affecting 1 in 400 pregnancies, 1 in 1600 babies) with a shared placenta, can threaten the survival of both twins because the donor twin is anaemic and the recipient twin is polycythaemic and prone to cardiac hypertrophy and heart failure. Modern treatments have increased the survival of twins but the survivors are at increased risk of brain injury and neurodevelopment consequences.

Application to practice

The placenta has an important physiological role in supporting and maintaining pregnancy. Dysfunctioning of the placenta and its development result in abnormal conditions, which may be observed in pregnancy.

Knowledge of the gross anatomy and the variants in the placental structure is essential in the postnatal examination of the placenta and membranes.

. . . .

Annotated further reading

Benirschke K, Kaufmann P 2000 Pathology of the human placenta, 4th edn. Springer, New York

A comprehensive reference text, which covers the structure of the placenta at birth, types of placenta, early development and cellular details.

Gude NM, Roberts CT, Kalionis B, King RG 2004 Growth and function of the normal human placenta. Thrombosis Research 114(5–6):397–407
A recent review of placental development which also covers placental functions and transport mechanisms.

Kaufmann P, Mayhew TM, Charnock-Jones DS 2004 Aspects of human fetoplacental vasculogenesis and angiogenesis. II. Changes during normal pregnancy. Placenta 25(2–3):114–126
The second of a series of three excellent well-illustrated reviews presenting an in-depth description of placental vasculogenesis (de novo formation of blood vessels) and angiogenesis (creation of new blood vessels from preexisting vessels).

Kingdom J, Jauniaux E, O'Brien S 2000 The placenta: basic science and clinical practice. Royal College of Obstetricians and Gynaecologists, London
A comprehensive handbook covering scientific and clinical aspects of placental structure and function, placental pathology including growth restriction and pre-eclampsia), placental infection, preterm labour, placental malignancy, clinical assessment of the placenta and placental complications in labour.

Redman CW, Sargent IL 2003 Pre-eclampsia, the placenta and the maternal systemic inflammatory response: a review. Placenta 24(Suppl A):S21–S27
An excellent review which contends that a maternal systemic inflammatory response is a normal feature of the third trimester which may have evolved to promote insulin resistance and divert glucose from skeletal muscle to the fetus. The authors argue that pre-eclampsia is the extreme end of this continuum, which is common to all pregnancies.

Wee LY, Fisk NM 2002 The twin–twin transfusion syndrome. Seminars in Neonatology 7(3):187–202
A review of twin-to-twin transfusion syndrome covering pathogenesis, possible effects on donor and recipient twins, various treatments and their outcomes.

. . . .

References

Aldoretta PW, Hay WW Jr 1995 Metabolic substrates for fetal energy metabolism and growth. Clinics in Perinatology 22(1):15–36

Benirschke K 1994 Obstetrically important lesions of the umbilical cord. Journal of Reproductive Medicine 39:226

Bischof P, Meisser A, Campana A 2000 Paracrine and autocrine regulators of trophoblast invasion: a review. Placenta 21(Suppl A):S55–S60

Brosens JJ, Pijnenborg R, Brosens IA 2002 The myometrial junctional zone spiral arteries in normal and abnormal pregnancies: a review of the literature. American Journal of Obstetrics and Gynecology 187(5):1416–1423

Burton GJ, Hempstock J, Jauniaux E 2001 Nutrition of the human fetus during the first trimester: a review. Placenta 22(Suppl A):S70–S77

Cai WQ, Bodin P, Sexton A, Loesch A, Burnstock G 1993 Localization of neuropeptide Y and atrial natriuretic peptide in the endothelial cells of human umbilical blood vessels. Cell and Tissue Research 272:175–181

Calvano CJ, Hoar RM, Mankes RF, Lefevre R, Reddy PP, Moran ME, Mandell J 2000 Experimental study of umbilical cord length as a marker of fetal alcohol syndrome. Teratology 61(3):184–188

Carlson BM 1994 Human embryology and developmental biology. Mosby, St Louis

Cetin I, Corbetta C, Sereni LP et al 1990 Umbilical amino acid concentrations in normal and growth-retarded fetuses sampled in utero by cordocentesis. American Journal of Obstetrics and Gynecology 162:253–261

Chard T 1998 Placental metabolism. In: Chamberlain G, Broughton Pipkin F (eds) Clinical physiology in obstetrics, 3rd edn. Blackwell, Oxford, pp 419–436

Edwards A, Megens A, Peek M, Wallace EM 2000 Sexual origins of placental dysfunction. Lancet 355:203–204

Evain-Brion D, Malassine A 2003 Human placenta as an endocrine organ. Growth Hormone & IGF Research 13(Suppl A):S34–S37

Firth JA, Leach L 1996 Not trophoblast alone: a review of the contribution to the fetal microvasculature to transplacental exchange. Placenta 17:89

Hamilton-Fairley D, Johnson MR 1998 The ovary. In: Chamberlain G, Broughton Pipkin F (eds) Clinical physiology in obstetrics, 3rd edn. Blackwell, Oxford, pp 396–416

Harman CR, Baschat AA 2003 Comprehensive assessment of fetal wellbeing: which Doppler tests should be performed? Current Opinion in Obstetrics & Gynecology 15(2):147–157

Iles RK, Chard T 1991 Human chorionic gonadotrophin expression by bladder cancers: biology and clinical potential. Journal of Urology 145:453

Jauniaux E, Gulbis B 2000 Fluid compartments of the embryonic environment. Human Reproduction Update 6(3):268–278

Jauniaux E, Jurkovic D, Campbell S, Hustin J 1992 Doppler ultrasonographic features of the developing placental circulation: correlation with anatomic findings. American Journal of Obstetrics and Gynecology 166:585

Jauniaux E, Gulbis B, Burton GJ 2003 The human first trimester gestational sac limits rather than facilitates oxygen transfer to the foetus: a review. Placenta 24(Suppl A):S86–S93

Johnson MR, Bolton VN, Riddle AF et al 1993a Interactions between the embryo and corpus luteum. Human Reproduction 8:1496–1501

Johnson MR, Riddle AF, Irvine R et al 1993b Corpus luteum failure in ectopic pregnancy. Human Reproduction 8:1491–1495

Kent A, Kitau MJ, Chard T 1991 Absence of diurnal variation in urinary chorionic gonadotrophin excretion at 8–13 weeks gestation. British Journal of Obstetrics and Gynaecology 98:1180

Kingdom J, Sibley C 1996 The placenta. In: Hillier SG, Kitchener HC, Neilson JP (eds) Scientific essentials of reproductive medicine. Saunders, Philadelphia, pp 312–318

Kingdom JCP, Awad H, Fleming JEE, Bowman AW 1993 Obstetrical determination of relative placental size. Placenta 14:A36

Kingdom JCP, Sherlock J, Rodeck CH, Adinolfi M 1995 Detection of trophoblast cells in transcervical samples collected by lavage and cytobrush. Obstetrics and Gynecology 86:283–288

Knipp GT, Audus KL, Soares MJ 1999 Nutrient transport across the placenta. Advances in Drug Delivery Reviews 38(1):41–58

Lala PK, Chakraborty C 2003 Factors regulating trophoblast migration and invasiveness. Placenta 24(1):575–587

Learmont JG, Braude PR, Poston L 1994 Flow induced dilation is modulated by nitric oxide in isolated human small fetoplacental arteries. Journal of Vascular Research 31(Suppl 1):26

Meuris S, Nagy AM, Delogne-Desnoeck J, Jurkovic D, Jauniaux E 1995 Temporal relationship between the human chorionic gonadotrophin peak and the establishment of the inter-villus blood flow in early pregnancy. Human Reproduction 10:947

Miller AWF, Hanretty KP 1998 Obstetrics illustrated, 5th edn. Churchill Livingstone, New York, pp 12, 99

Moore KL, Persaud TVN 1998 Before we are born: essentials of embryology and birth defects, 5th edn. Saunders, Philadelphia

Myatt L, Brewer AS, Brockman DE 1992 The comparative effects of big endothelin-1, endothelin-1, and endothelin-3 in the human fetal–placental circulation. American Journal of Obstetrics and Gynecology 167:1651–1656

Myatt L, Brockman DE, Eis ALW, Pollack JS 1993 Immunohistochemical localization of nitric oxide synthase in the human placenta. Placenta 14:487–495

Ray JG, Laskin CA 1999 Folic acid and homocyst(e)ine metabolic defects and the risk of placental abruption, pre-eclampsia and spontaneous pregnancy loss: a systematic review. Placenta 20(7):519–529

Schindler AE 2004 First trimester endocrinology: consequences for diagnosis and treatment of pregnancy failure. Gynecological Endocrinology 18(1):51–57

Shiverick KT, Salafia C 1999 Cigarette smoking and pregnancy I: ovarian, uterine and placental effects. Placenta 20(4):265–272

Spencer K, Coombes J, Mallard SA, Ward MA 1992 Free beta human chorionic gonadotrophin in Down's syndrome screening: a multicentre study of its role compared to other biochemical markers. Annals of Clinical Biochemistry 29:506–518

Wenstrom KD, Owen J, Boots LR, DuBard MB 1994 Elevated second trimester human chorionic gonadotropin levels in association with poor pregnancy outcome. American Journal of Obstetrics and Gynecology 171:1038–1041

Wilcox GR, Trudinger BJ 1991 Fetal platelet consumption: a feature of placental insufficiency. Obstetrics and Gynecology 77:616–621

9 Embryo development and fetal growth

Learning objectives

- To describe the formation of the bilaminar and trilaminar embryonic discs in week 2 and week 3 of development.
- To outline the events involved in folding of the embryonic disc into the characteristic shape of the human embryo.
- To define key embryological terms: gastrulation, neurulation, primitive streak, somites and notochord.
- To outline events in development in the first 8 weeks.
- To describe developmental characteristics of the fetal organ systems.
- To discuss factors affecting fetal growth and the implications these have for future health.
- To relate the timing of development with sensitive periods and to appreciate the developmental factors limiting survival of a preterm baby.

Introduction

During pregnancy, the single cell of the zygote divides to produce 6 billion cells of the mature fetus. On average, an adult cell is the product of about 47 cell divisions from the zygote, at least 40 of which occur before birth. The first 3 weeks of development are often described as the pre-embryonic period when the cells differentiate into germ layers from which all organs and tissues develop. This stage is similar in all sorts of animals, including *Drosophila* (fruitfly), nematodes, amphibians and birds as well as mammals. The embryonic stage lasts from week 4 to week 8 in the human. During this time the organ systems are established and the embryo develops distinct human characteristics. The fetal stage, from week 9 to birth, is largely a period of growth, during which time the systems become more refined and mature, ready to function at birth. Fetal age is timed from fertilization whereas pregnancy is dated from the first day of the last normal menstrual period. This means that the timing of the pregnancy is 2 weeks more than the true fetal age. The average length of pregnancy is 280 days (40 weeks) when the fetus is 266 days old (38 weeks). Understanding fetal development is important in monitoring the well-being of the fetus. Pregnant women are also obviously interested in knowing how their baby is changing during the duration of the pregnancy. (Development in the 1st week after fertilization is described in Chapter 6.)

Chapter case study

Zara is 5 feet and 2 inches tall (155 cm) and, prior to pregnancy, wore size 8 clothes; she wears size 3 (European size 35.5) shoes. Her husband, James, is 6 feet tall (180 cm) and has quite a broad, muscular frame and has size 11 feet (European size 46). Zara has frequently discussed with her midwife her concerns that she will have a big baby and problems in labour because James is tall and has a large frame. How can the midwife reassure Zara that the baby's growth is unlikely to be disproportionate to her size and what physiological measurements and observations can be made to support this? If Zara was found to be carrying a large baby how would the midwife be able to recognize this and what could be the possible explanations for this?

Week 2

By the end of the 1st week, the blastocyst has entered the uterine cavity, hatched out of the zona pellucida and started the process of implantation into the endometrial wall. Two types of cells are evident: the outer trophoblast (see Ch. 6) and the inner cell mass (or embryoblast). The inner cell mass gives rise to tissues of the embryo, and also contributes towards some of the extraembryonic membranes. The undifferentiated cells from the blastocyst are called stem cells and have some potential therapeutic uses (see Box 9.1). At about day 7 after fertilization, the cells of the inner cell mass start to proliferate and differentiate rapidly. The inner cell mass becomes flattened into a bilaminar embryonic disc with the cells forming two distinct layers (Fig. 9.1). The cells adjacent to the blastocyst cavity appear distinctly cuboidal. These form the hypoblast or primary endoderm layer, which gives rise to the future gut and its derivatives. The upper layer of cells is formed of columnar epiblast cells, which will differentiate into the ectodermal layer. Some of the epiblast cells spread laterally to form the amniotic membrane that encloses the amniotic cavity. Cells from the hypoblast layer migrate forming a membrane called the exocoelic membrane or Heuser's membrane which lines the cytotrophoblast so the blastocyst cavity is also enclosed. This is the cavity that will become the primitive (primary) yolk sac. There are two waves of endoderm cell remodelling of the blastocyst cavity, which form initially the primary yolk sac and then, at the beginning of the 5th week, the

Box 9.1

Stem cells

Stem cells are cells that are not terminally differentiated, therefore they can potentially be directed to become any cell and used to treat various diseases. There are three categories of stem cells: totipotent (capable of becoming a whole organism), pluripotent (capable of becoming any cell in the body) and multipotent (or unipotent; capable of becoming a particular type of cell such as blood cells). There are a number of sources of stem cells. Umbilical cord and cord blood cells are a good source; in some countries, parents are asked whether they would like to have their baby's cord blood cells frozen in case they can be used later in life to treat a disease such as acute lymphocytic leukaemia. The blood is taken from the umbilical vein of the cleaned cord once the baby has been delivered; it is checked for infectious agents, tissue-typed and then stored in liquid nitrogen. Stem cells can be used either autologously (for the same person they came from) or as allogenic treatment where the donor and recipient are different individuals.

Stem cells can be taken from adults, such as bone marrow cells which are undifferentiated blood cells; these can be differentiated into liver, kidney, muscle and nerve cells as well as blood cells. There is evidence that skin dermis cells are pluripotent and can be transdifferentiated into many types of tissue including neurons, smooth muscle cells and fat cells. It is possible that brain cells could be harvested from dead organ donors. However, embryonic stem cells have the most potential because they are totipotent and could grow into any of the 200+ cell types in the body. Embryonic stem cells can be obtained from a cloned embryo which would make them genetically compatible with the recipient. However, collection and use of embryonic stem cells requires the destruction of the embryo, which generates controversial and ethical decisions. The ethical debate is complicated because embryologists apply the term 'embryo' to any stage of development beyond fertilization. In addition, the general public is thought to find the pace of scientific advance too fast for full consideration of ethical and other issues (Gardener 2002).

definitive (secondary) yolk sac (Fig 9.2). The formation of the definitive yolk sac creates the chorionic cavity and the extraembryonic mesoderm, which gives rise to the vascular structures of the placenta (see

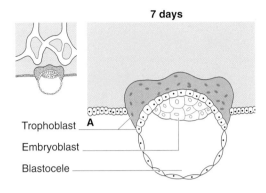

7 days

Trophoblast   **A**

Embryoblast

Blastocele

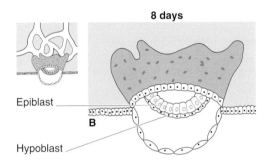

8 days

Epiblast

B

Hypoblast

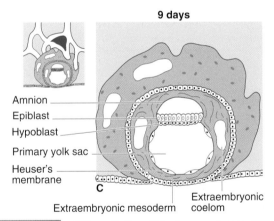

9 days

Amnion

Epiblast

Hypoblast

Primary yolk sac

Heuser's membrane

C

Extraembryonic mesoderm

Extraembryonic coelom

Fig. 9.1   *Differentiation of the inner cell mass into the bilaminar disc: A 7 days; B 8 days; C 9 days. (Reproduced with permission from Fitzgerald & Fitzgerald 1994.)*

Ch. 8). The definitive yolk sac synthesizes several proteins including alpha-fetoprotein (AFP). The bilaminar disc lies between two fluid-filled cavities: the amniotic cavity on the epiblast (ectoderm) side and the yolk sac cavity on the hypoblast (endoderm) side. (The primitive yolk sac will shrink away from the cytotrophoblast in the 4th week, creating a new cavity called the chorionic cavity or extraembryonic coelom, which fills with fluid and becomes the largest cavity in the developing conceptus.)

Fig. 9.2   *First-trimester gestational sac about 3 weeks postfertilization, showing chorionic plate (CP) surrounding entire sac, extraembryonic coelom (ECC), amniotic cavity (AC) and embryo (E) with its secondary yolk sac (SYS) providing nutrients. (Reproduced with permission from Jauniaux et al 2003.)*

At the end of the 2nd week, a region of endodermal cells starts to thicken and become columnar, forming the prochordal plate (Fig. 9.3). This marks the cranial region (head end) and is the site of the future mouth. The prochordal plate is also important in influencing further development of the cranial region.

By the 2nd week, according to the 'rule of twos' (Larsen 1993), the following have taken place:

- two germ layers have formed: the endoderm and the ectoderm
- two trophoblastic layers have formed: cytotrophoblast and syncytiotrophoblast
- two waves of remodelling have occurred: that of the blastocyst into the primary and then the definitive yolk sac
- two novel cavities have formed: the amniotic cavity and the chorionic cavity
- two layers have formed from the extraembryonic mesoderm.

Week 3

At this stage, when the woman may first realize she is pregnant, embryo development is rapid. A line of epiblast cells, starting from the caudal region (tail end) at the other side from the prochordal plate, undergoes very rapid cell division, forming the primitive streak in the midline (see Fig. 9.3). The cells of the primitive streak form a groove and then invaginate (move inwards) to spread between the epiblast and hypoblast layers. The bilaminar disc is therefore converted into a trilaminar disc consisting of three germ layers (ectoderm, mesoderm and endoderm), which give rise to specific tissues of the body (Fig. 9.4). The middle layer is the mesoderm, from which connective tissue, smooth muscle, the cardiovascular system and blood, the skeleton and the reproductive and endocrine systems develop (Fig. 9.5). The epiblast becomes the ectoderm, which will develop into the epidermis, central and peripheral nervous systems and the retina. Therefore the ectoderm, which will give rise to the skin, is in contact with the amniotic cavity. The hypoblast becomes the endoderm, from which epithelial linings and some glandular structures will form. The three germ layers interact, generating signals that cause structural alterations and more complex interactions.

The endodermal prochordal plate is fused to the ectoderm forming the oropharyngeal membrane (future mouth). Below the primitive streak, there is another area of fusion between the ectoderm and endoderm; this is the cloacal membrane (the future anus). Some mesoderm cells migrate towards the prochordal plate forming a cord of adhesive cells (Fig. 9.6). This is the notochordal process, which develops a lumen forming the notochord canal. The notochord evolves into a cellular rod-like tube, which gives the trilaminar disc a degree of rigidity and defines the central head–tail axis of the embryo. If identical twins are going to develop, there are two parallel notochords. If there are two notochords that cross, conjoined (Siamese) twins will result. The notochord establishes the development of the axial skeleton (bones of head and spinal cord) and the neural

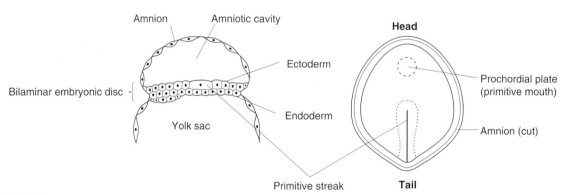

Fig. 9.3 *Formation of the prochordal plate (future mouth) and primitive streak on the bilaminar and trilaminar embryonic discs.*

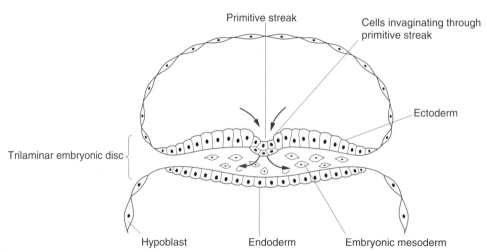

Fig. 9.4 *The invagination of cells of the primitive streak between the ectodermal and endodermal layers creates a trilaminar embryonic disc. (Reproduced with permission from Fitzgerald & Fitzgerald 1994.)*

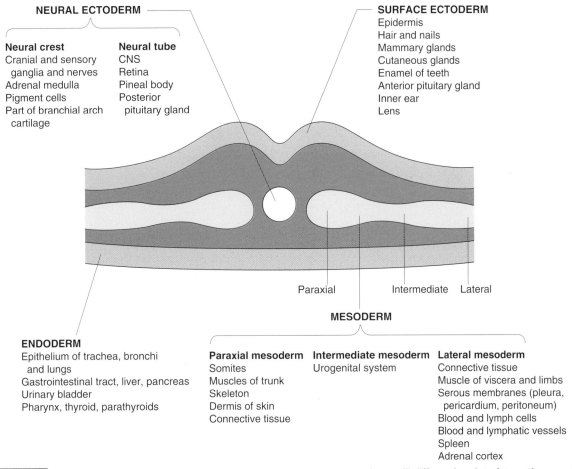

NEURAL ECTODERM

Neural crest
Cranial and sensory
 ganglia and nerves
Adrenal medulla
Pigment cells
Part of branchial arch
 cartilage

Neural tube
CNS
Retina
Pineal body
Posterior
 pituitary gland

SURFACE ECTODERM
Epidermis
Hair and nails
Mammary glands
Cutaneous glands
Enamel of teeth
Anterior pituitary gland
Inner ear
Lens

Paraxial   Intermediate   Lateral

MESODERM

ENDODERM
Epithelium of trachea, bronchi
 and lungs
Gastrointestinal tract, liver, pancreas
Urinary bladder
Pharynx, thyroid, parathyroids

Paraxial mesoderm
Somites
Muscles of trunk
Skeleton
Dermis of skin
Connective tissue

Intermediate mesoderm
Urogenital system

Lateral mesoderm
Connective tissue
Muscle of viscera and limbs
Serous membranes (pleura,
 pericardium, peritoneum)
Blood and lymph cells
Blood and lymphatic vessels
Spleen
Adrenal cortex

Fig. 9.5   *The neural and surface ectoderm, the endoderm and the mesoderm will differentiate into future tissues of the body.*

plate, which gives rise to the primitive nervous system. The vertebral column forms around the notochord and the notochord induces neurulation, the formation of the neural tube and early nervous system (see below). During the 3rd week, aggregates of mesoderm on either side of the notochord form pairs of bead-like blocks called somites, which direct the segmented structure of the body and induce the overlying ecto-derm to form structures of the nervous system.

The formation of the primitive streak, the three germ layers, the prochordal plate and the notochord are described as gastrulation. Gastrulation marks the beginning of morphogenesis, the emergence and deve-lopment of body form and structure. It begins with the appearance of the primitive streak at day 14. The primitive streak defines the time when experimental manipulation of human embryos is legally obliged to stop under the terms of the UK Human Fertilisation and Embryology Act of 1990. During the 3rd week of

development, as well as gastrulation, the primitive nervous system and cardiovascular system begin to develop.

Box 9.2 is a summary of the events taking place in weeks 1–3.

Weeks 4–8: organogenesis

During this period of embryonic development, the tri-laminar disc folds into a C-shaped cylindrical embryo and all the major structures and organ systems are established. However, apart from the cardiovascular system, few of the systems function. Organogenesis, the development of the organ systems, is a critical period during which the processes are susceptible to external influences that can cause disruption and sub-sequent serious congenital abnormalities. By the end of the 8th week, the embryo becomes known as the

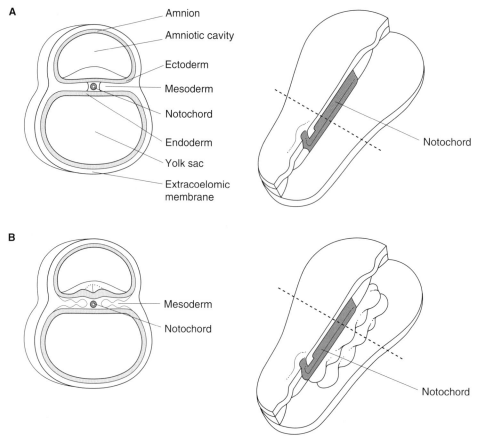

A

- Amnion
- Amniotic cavity
- Ectoderm
- Mesoderm
- Notochord
- Endoderm
- Yolk sac
- Extracoelomic membrane

Notochord

B

- Mesoderm
- Notochord

Notochord

Notochord

Fig. 9.6 *Notochord formation: A 17 days; B 18 days. (Reproduced with permission from Goodwin 1997.)*

fetus and has a distinct human appearance (Fig. 9.7). Human development can be crudely classified as three types (Moore & Persaud 1998a):

- growth: cell division
- morphogenesis: development of form, which involves movement of sheets and masses of cells
- differentiation: maturation of cells forming tissues and organs capable of specialized function.

Growth is achieved by hyperplasia (cell division) and hypertrophy (increase in cell size). Initially the cells are stem cells which are similar and not differentiated or specialized into any particular cell type. They differentiate into one of the 350 different types of cell found in the body in two phases. Before differentiation occurs, there is a stage of determination during which the cell becomes restricted in its capability to develop along different pathways. As the cells differentiate fully, they develop specific morphological and functional characteristics.

Differentiation is often orchestrated by the establishment of a signalling centre or polarizing region in a small bud of undifferentiated cells, as occurs in the development of the vertebrate limb. This process in which cells in one place influence the surrounding cells to develop in a specific way is known as induction. Induction involves the surrounding cells to produce cellular signals which have an effect on the responding cells via cell receptors. Differentiation can allow some plasticity. Branching morphogenesis is the formation of branched epithelial tubules which is essential to the development of several tissues including the kidneys, lungs, breasts and salivary glands.

One of the cornerstones of embryology is the concept that germ cells in the developing embryo migrate to the final destinations (Horwitz & Webb 2003). The migrating cells are thought to be polarized (have a front and back), to sense chemical signals and 'home' towards them by amoeboid movement. In gastrulation, cell migration leads to the formation of the three

Summary of pre-embryonic period: weeks 1–3

Week 1: fertilization to produce zygote

- Cleavage of zygote while travelling in uterine tube
- Cell division without increase in mass to form morula
- Fluid accumulation: hollow blastocyst formed
- 'Hatching' out of zona pellucida
- Blastocyst cells differentiate into trophoblast and inner cell mass
- Implantation in decidual wall

Week 2: inner cell mass forms bilaminar embryonic disc of hypoblast and epiblast

- Trophoblast differentiates into dividing cytotrophoblast and invasive syncytiotrophoblast (see Ch. 8)
- Lateral movement of cells from epiblast layer encloses yolk sac, forming the extraembryonic mesoderm
- Prochordal plate (mouth) develops at caudal end
- Day 14: primitive streak develops

Week 3: gastrulation

- Cells from primitive streak invaginate and migrate between the epiblast and the hypoblast forming the mesoderm
- Trilaminar disc of three germ layers: ectoderm (epiblast), mesoderm and ectoderm (hypoblast)
- Notochord forms, inducing development of the neural plate and giving rise to axis of development
- Somites become evident
- Neurulation begins

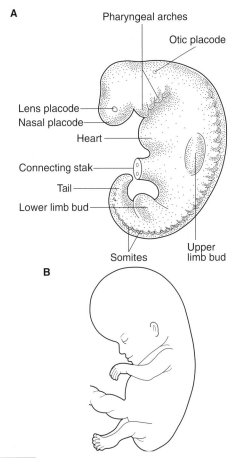

Fig. 9.7 *A 4-week-old and B 8-week-old fetus. (A reproduced with permission from Fitzgerald & Fitzgerald 1994.)*

layers of the trilaminar disc which then migrate to targets where they differentiate. The muscle precursor cells migrate from the somites to their targets in the limbs. Failure of cells to migrate at all or to the correct location is thought to result in abnormalities or to have life-threatening consequences; for instance, congenital defects in brain development leading to mental disorders are ascribed to defects in neuronal migration. Cell migration also occurs in postnatal life and is central to homeostasis such as effective immune responses and repair of injured tissues in the wound healing process. Migration can also occur in pathological processes, including vascular disease and tumour metastasis, where some tumour cells migrate to new sites where they form secondary tumours.

However, recent research has questioned whether germ cells do actually migrate at all during ontogeny (Freeman 2003).

Apoptosis or programmed cell death is another mechanism important in embryonic development. Apoptosis involves the cells effectively autodestructing in a precisely timed manner. Embryogenesis also involves cell recognition and adhesion.

Folding

The disc-like arrangement of the germ layers is converted into a recognizable vertebral embryo by folding in the 4th week of development. Folding is due to a differential rate in growth of the different parts of the embryo. The embryo is in a contained space so as it grows, it curves and ridges of tissues form. The embryonic disc grows rapidly particularly in length, because of the growth of the brain and tail, so it has to fold. Although this is a momentous stage of development, relatively little is known about it. The yolk sac does not grow and, as the outer rim of the endoderm is attached to the yolk sac, the embryo becomes convex. Folding occurs at the cephalic (head) and lateral regions on day 22 and at the caudal (tail) end of the embryo on day 23 (Fig. 9.8). The cephalic, lateral and caudal edges of the embryonic disc are brought into apposition and the layers fuse along the midline, which converts the endoderm into the gut tube. Initially the foregut and the hindgut fuse, leaving the midgut open to the yolk sac.

The folds cause a constriction between the embryo and yolk sac. The yolk sac gives rise to the primitive gut. The amnion expands, enveloping the connecting stalk and neck of the yolk sac, forming the umbilical cord. Folding is precisely coordinated and is controlled. The developmental pattern involves synchronized tissue communication and interaction. Adjacent tissues induce changes in the movement and behaviour of neighbouring cells. Signals integrating genetic and environmental influences control cell proliferation, migration and apoptosis (Bard & Weddon 1996). These signals, which may be diffusible molecules or direct

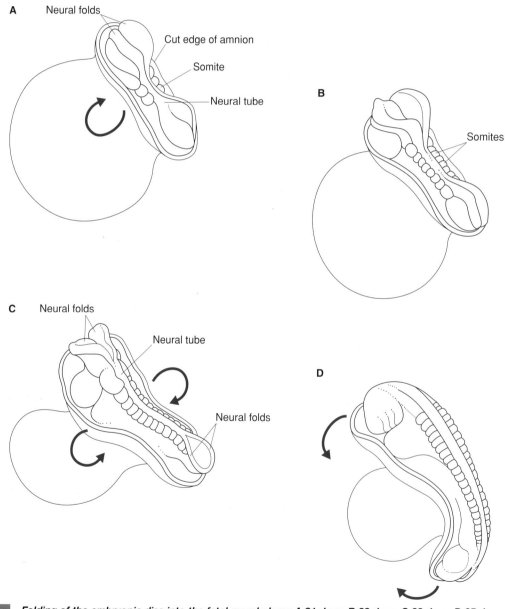

Fig. 9.8   *Folding of the embryonic disc into the fetal morphology: A 21 days; B 22 days; C 23 days; D 25 days. (Reproduced with permission from Goodwin 1997.)*

physical contact, direct the expression of particular genes in the responding cells (Moore & Persaud 1998b). Although all cells have the same DNA in their nuclei, depending on the signal received, some will express certain genes but not others. So, for instance, a skin cell expresses the genes that control the behaviour of a skin cell because they are switched on by the signals skin cells receive. A liver cell has the same genes as the skin cell but expresses different genes.

The organization of the basic body plan

Techniques and concepts used to study molecular genetics (how the genetic code is expressed) in bacteria and *Drosophila* can be applied to mammalian embryogenesis, including human development. The DNA in the nucleus sets up a basic body plan, which establishes the pattern of the early embryo. The genes that control the basic body plan are the same in very diverse species. A highly conserved region of about 180 base pairs of DNA, known as the homeobox, is found in the genes that regulate development in almost all species studied (Murtha et al 1991). The homeobox encodes a protein domain called the homeodomain which can bind DNA specifically. Homeobox genes encode transcription factors which switch on cascades of other genes, for instance all the ones needed to make a particular body part. Other morphogenic agents, signals and growth factors activate the homeobox genes. Hox genes are a particular subgroup of homeobox genes which are found in a special gene cluster, the HOX cluster. Hox genes determine the patterning of the body axis. They direct the identity of particular body regions, determining where limbs and other body segments will develop in the fetus. There appears to be a series of three sequential steps in the conversion of the oval trilaminar embryonic disc into the cylindrical configuration with the endoderm on the inside, the ectoderm on the outside and the mesoderm in between (Fig. 9.9) (Carlson 1994). These steps result in segmentation of the embryo. Gap genes subdivide the embryo into broad regional domains. Pair-rule genes are involved in the formation of individual body segments and segment-polarity genes control the anterior–posterior organization of each segment (De Robertis et al 1990). As the embryo develops, the segmental plan becomes less evident; remnants can be seen in the arrangement of the

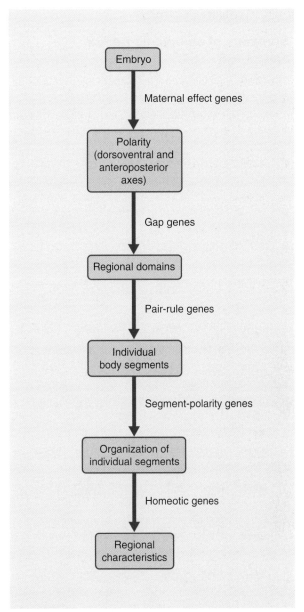

Fig. 9.9   *Organization of the vertebrate body plan: three steps in the conversion.*

backbone and ribs and in the organization of the spinal nerves.

Box 9.3 summarizes the events taking place during weeks 4–8.

Ninth week to birth: fetal period

During this period, the body grows rapidly and the tissues and organs differentiate and mature (see below).

Box 9.3

Summary of embryonic period: weeks 4–8

4th week

- Neural tube fusing but neuropores open at rostral (anterior) and caudal ends
- Folding produces characteristic C-shaped curved embryo
- Otic pits present (primitive ear)
- Optic vesicles formed
- Upper limb buds appear, then lower limb buds
- Three pairs of brachial arches present
- Beating heart prominent
- Forebrain prominent
- Attenuated tail
- Rudiments of organ systems established
- Rostral neuropore, then caudal neuropore, close
- Crown–rump length 4–6 mm

5th week

- Rapid brain development and head enlargement (cephalization)
- Facial prominences develop
- Upper limb buds become paddle-shaped
- Lower limb buds are flipper-like
- Mesonephric ridges denote position of mesonephric (interim) kidneys
- Crown–rump length 7–9 mm

6th week

- Joints of upper limbs differentiate
- Digital rays (fingers) of upper limbs evident
- External ear canal and auricle (pinna) formed
- Retinal pigment formed so eye is obvious
- Head very large, projects over heart prominence
- Reflex responses to touch
- Crown–rump length 11–14 mm

7th week

- Notches between digital rays partially separate future fingers
- Liver prominent
- Rapidly growing intestines herniate out of small abdominal cavity into umbilical cord
- Crown–rump length 16–18 mm

8th week

- Digits of hand separated (but still webbed)
- Notches visible between digital rays of feet
- Stubby tail disappears
- Purposeful limb movements occur

- Ossification begins in lower limbs
- Head still disproportionately large (about half of total embryo length)
- Eye lids closing
- Ears are characteristic shape but still low-set
- External genitalia evident (but not distinct enough for sexual identification)
- Crown–rump length 27–31 mm

The head growth rate becomes relatively slower so, by birth, the length of the head is about a quarter of the total length. Growth rate can be used to determine embryonic or fetal age (Box 9.4) and ultrasound examination can be used to examine developmental details (Box 9.5). With expert care, a fetus can be viable and may survive from 22 weeks.

Box 9.6 is a summary of the changes during the fetal period.

Box 9.4

Estimation of embryonic/fetal age

- Greatest length (GL) is used to measure embryos of about 3 weeks, which are straight
- Crown–rump length (CRL) is sitting height, used to measure older, curved embryos
- Carnegie embryonic staging system uses external characteristics to estimate developmental stage
- Number of somites
- Fetal head measurements, such as biparietal diameter (BPD) and head circumference
- Abdominal circumference
- Femur length and foot length

Note that it is suggested that CRL should be abandoned and replaced by GL for all embryos because GL is simpler to measure accurately.

Box 9.5

Ultrasound examination

- Estimation of size and age of embryo
- Detection of congenital abnormality
- Evaluation of growth rate
- Investigation of uterine abnormality or ectopic pregnancy
- Guidance for CVS (chorionic villus sampling)

Box 9.6

Summary of changes in the fetal period

9–12 weeks
- Growth in body length and limbs accelerates
- Ears are low-set, eyes are fused
- Primary ossification centres develop in skeleton, notably skull and long bones
- Intestines return to abdominal cavity and body wall fuses
- Erythropoiesis (formation of red blood cells) decreases in liver and begins in spleen
- Urine formation begins
- Fetal swallowing of amniotic fluid

13–16 weeks
- Rapid growth
- Coordinated limb movements (not felt by mother)
- Active ossification of skeleton
- Slow eye movements
- Ovaries differentiated and contain primordial follicles
- External genitalia recognizable
- Eyes and ears closer to normal positions

17–20 weeks
- Growth slows down
- Limbs reach mature proportions
- Fetal movements felt by mother ('quickening')
- Skin covered with protective layer of vernix caseosa, held in position by lanugo (downy hair)
- Brown fat deposited

21–25 weeks
- Fetus gains weight
- Skin wrinkled and translucent, appears red–pink
- Rapid eye movements begin
- Blink–startle responses to noise
- Surfactant secretion begins but respiratory system immature
- Fingernails are present
- May be viable if born prematurely

26–29 weeks
- Lungs capable of breathing air
- Central nervous system can control breathing
- Eyes open
- Toenails visible
- Fat (3.5% body weight) deposited under skin so wrinkles smooth out
- Erythropoiesis moves from spleen to bone marrow

30–34 weeks
- Pupillary light reflex
- Skin pink and smooth, limbs chubby
- White fat is 8% of body weight
- From 32 weeks, survival is usual

35–38 weeks
- Firm grasp
- Orientates towards light
- Circumference of head and abdomen are approximately equal
- White fat is about 16% of body weight, 14 g fat gained per day
- Skin appears bluish-pink
- Term fetus is about 3400 g, crown–rump length is about 360 mm

Development of organ systems

The central nervous system

Neurulation is the formation of the neural plate and neural folds and the closure of these folds to form the neural tube, which is the precursor of the brain and spinal cord. The neural tube is completed by the end of the 4th week. The developing notochord induces the overlying ectoderm to thicken forming the neural plate, a raised slipper-like plate of neuroepithelial cells. This will give rise to the central nervous system (brain and spinal cord) and other structures such as the retina. In the middle of the 3rd week, the neural groove appears in the centre of the neural plate (Fig. 9.10). To each side of the groove are neural folds, which enlarge at the cranial end as the start of the developing brain. Marked development of the brain is a characteristic of embryonic development in primates; human brain growth exceeds that of other species, continuing into adulthood. At the end of the 3rd week, the neural folds start to fuse forming the neural tube, which separates from the surface ecto-derm. The neural crest cells, which detach from the lateral edges of the neural folds, give rise to the spinal ganglia and ganglia of the autonomic system as well as a number of other cell types (Box 9.7). The paraxial mesoderm, closest to the notochord and developing neural tube, differentiates to form prominent paired blocks of tissue, or somites. The first somites appear from day 20. There are about 30 pairs of somites by

A

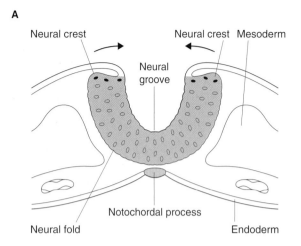

Neural crest

Neural crest Mesoderm

Neural
groove

Notochordal process

Neural fold

Endoderm

B

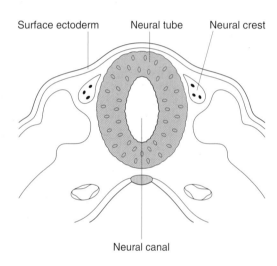

Surface ectoderm Neural tube Neural crest

Neural canal

C

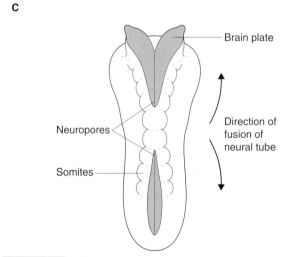

Brain plate

Direction of
fusion of
neural tube

Neuropores

Somites

Fig. 9.10 *The neural groove and neural tube fusion: A 21 days; B & C 23 days.*

day 30 increasing to a total of 44 pairs, but the cranial ones begin differentiation as new somites are added at the caudal end. The somites differentiate into sclerotomes, myotomes and dermatomes, which give rise to the axial skeletal bones, skeletal muscles and the dermis of the skin, respectively. The number of somites indicates the age of the embryo. The limbs carry with them the nerves from the somites from which they developed. The somatic pattern of development is important in understanding referred pain (see Ch. 13).

Neural tube defects (NTD) are one of the most common congenital abnormalities (see Ch. 12), resulting from the failure of the neural tube to close during embryogenesis. Neurulation is very sensitive to disturbances such as teratogenic drugs or lack of folate, which is required for DNA synthesis of the rapidly dividing cells (see Ch. 7). Most neurons are formed between 10 and 18 weeks; this is therefore the critical window for brain development. Undernutrition or other insults in the first trimester often result in microcephaly (James & Stephenson 1998). In later gestation, undernutrition may result in blood flow being redistributed to the brain at the expense of other tissues. As brain size in humans is proportionately larger, the effects of protecting the brain from undernutrition may be exaggerated compared with other species (Barker 1998). Glial cells begin to develop at about 15 weeks. In the second half of pregnancy, the glial cells hypertrophy and the axons and dendrites undergo marked growth. This rapid nervous system growth spurt continues until the second postnatal year, and at a slower rate for at least the first decade, and is unique to humans (Johnson 2001). The fetal response to impaired nutrition tends to 'spare' the brain at the cost of somatic growth, hence the asymmetric (disproportionate) growth patterns of babies born after intrauterine growth retardation (IUGR) where their heads seem disproportionately bigger. However, neither brain function nor neurology is perfectly protected; neuronal number tends to be reduced and myelination disturbed (Gluckman & Pinal 2003). The IUGR brain also seems more vulnerable to asphyxia.

Human brain size is enormous compared to other primates. Bite muscles of the jaw are very strong and enclose the skull in non-human primates. It is suggested that early humans developed a single gene mutation that resulted in weaker jaw muscles (Stedman et al 2004). The slacker jaw muscles relaxed their grip on the skull, allowing the human brain to grow and expand. Alternative explanations suggest that environmental changes forced humans to invent tools and develop manual dexterity or that natural selection favoured bigger brains because they permitted more complex and supportive societies. Impaired nutrition, particularly early in development, permanently affects brain size and cell number (assessed by head circumference); neurodevelopmental abnormalities occur at increased frequency in IUGR children.

Fetal sensory organs develop around the middle of gestation. At 24 weeks, the fetus responds to noise. As gestation progresses, the fetus exhibits increased sensitivity and responds to an increased range of sound frequencies. Babies are thought to enjoy being carried and cuddled because they can hear sounds of their mother's heart and digestive system, which they became accustomed to in utero.

Gastrointestinal system

The gut begins as a single tube running from mouth to anus. The mouth and anus are fused areas of endoderm and ectoderm (see above). The tube is therefore fixed at both ends so that when it grows it convolutes and loops (Fig. 9.11). Some parts of the tube dilate, such as the stomach and colon, and the gut rotates around other structures such as the developing liver. Between the 6th and 8th week of development, the proliferation of the epithelial cells lining the gut obliterates the lumen, which is then gradually recanalized. Early growth of the gut is extremely rapid so it extrudes into the amniotic cavity. If it is not withdrawn at about 10 weeks, the abdominal wall fails to close and the baby is born with exomphalos or gastroschisis. Normal fusion of the lateral body folds occurs at the linea nigra, the abdominal line that becomes pigmented in pregnancy (see Ch. 11). Normal growth of the gut depends on fetal swallowing. A fetus swallows about a third of the total volume of amniotic fluid per hour by the 16th week of development. Not only does amniotic fluid provide about 10% of the fetal protein requirements, but it also seems to be associated with effective development of the gastrointestinal mucosa, liver and pancreas and promotion of growth.

The digestive enzymes are present from about 24–28 weeks, with the exception of lactase (see Ch. 16). Peristaltic coordination of the fetal gut is evident from the 14th week of development. By 34 weeks

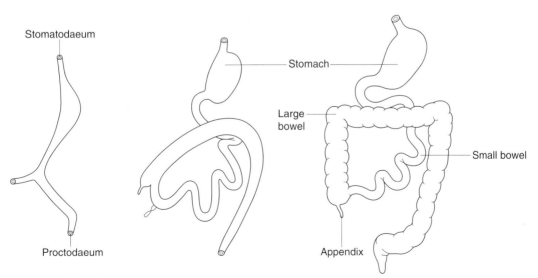

Fig. 9.11　*Convolution of the primitive gut. (Reproduced with permission from James & Stephenson 1998.)*

there is coordination of sucking, swallowing and peristalsis. As the gut matures, it produces mucus, which will eventually be required to lubricate the passage of food and faeces during transit. The mucus accumulates in the fetal gut as meconium. Adrenaline, produced in response to fetal distress, stimulates contractions of the gut, and can lead to meconium-stained amniotic fluid. The liver reaches metabolic maturity relatively late in gestation, storing glycogen in the last 9 weeks. Inadequate placental transfer of amino acids will affect tissues with high protein turnover, such as the liver (James & Stephenson 1998). The placenta is extremely metabolically active and extracts 40–60% of glucose and oxygen from the maternal circulation (Gluckman & Pinal 2003), some of which transfers from maternal to fetal circulation and then is re-extracted from the fetal circulation. In IUGR, the rate of placental extraction from the fetal circulation increases and can lead to loss of lean body mass from the fetus and wasting. There is a hierarchy: the fetus may become catabolic to nourish the placenta and both fetus and placenta may be compromised in attempting to sustain maternal requirements. As hepatic stores of glycogen and fat are mobilized in IUGR, the liver is the first organ affected so the head:abdomen ratio is an important indicator of IUGR.

Case study 9.1 is an example of developmental abnormality of the gut.

The face

The face is formed between weeks 5 and 12 from the brachial arches. The nose grows downwards as a

---

Case study 9.1

At 11 weeks of gestation, Julie has an ultrasound scan. She is asked to return for a further scan in 2 weeks as her unborn baby appears to have some gut tissue herniating into the umbilical cord. Julie seeks advice from her midwife.

- Is this normal?
- How might you reassure Julie that the ultrasonographer was just being cautious?
- If there were a pathological condition present, what two conditions are most likely?
- How would they be further investigated before Julie is advised upon the prognosis?

---

pillar of tissue (Fig. 9.12). The eyes, which are formed from a combination of nervous tissue and specialized ectoderm, are initially in a lateral position but move medially. The ears are initially low-set. Below the nose, maxillary processes extend to form the floor of the nose and the roof of the mouth. The upper lip is formed from processes that extend to meet centrally. Inadequate fusion of the maxillary processes causes congenital malformations of the mouth, such as cleft lip or palate. Palatal fusion is complete by the 11th week.

The skull

The skull develops from mesenchymal tissue around the brain. It is formed from the neurocranium, which protects the brain, and the viscerocranium, which forms the skeleton of the face. Each of these elements of the skull has membranous and cartilaginous components. Ossification is of the membrane rather than of cartilage and begins from the base of the skull (Larsen 1993).

The bones of the calvaria (cranial vault) have not completed development at birth. In the fetus, the flat bones of the calvaria are held together by soft fibrous sutures made of dense connective tissue, which allows some flexibility. The fetal head can mould to the shape of the maternal pelvis and distort as it passes through the birth canal. During delivery, the frontal bone becomes flat, the occipital bone is drawn out and the parietal bones overlap. The head usually returns to a normal shape a few days after delivery. Six large membranous fontanelles are formed where the sutures meet (see Ch. 13). The posterior fontanelles close at about 3 months after birth and the anterior ones close when the infant is about 18 months old. Raised intracranial pressure can be detected by palpating these fontanelles; a depression indicates dehydration.

The fetal skull is relatively large compared with the skeleton. The newborn skull has relatively thin bones compared with those in later life. The face is relatively small and has a characteristic neonatal roundish shape because the jaws are small. The paranasal sinuses (which give the individual shape of the face and resonance of the voice) are virtually absent and the facial bones are underdeveloped (Moore & Persaud 1998b). After birth, brain growth is rapid so the calvaria increases markedly during the first 2 years. The calvaria continues to grow until the child is about 16 years old; the skull bones then thicken.

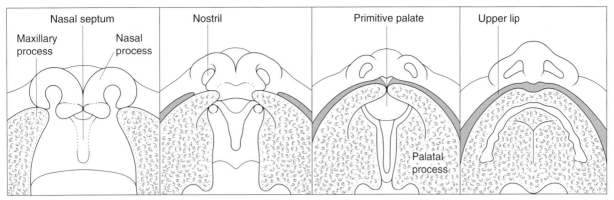

Fig. 9.12 *Growth of the palate and nose between the 6th and 9th week. (Reproduced with permission from James & Stephenson 1998.)*

The cardiovascular system

This is one of the first systems to develop; its function is important extremely early in development, unlike some of the other systems that do not have to achieve full function until after birth. This is because, as the embryo becomes larger, diffusion of oxygen and nutrients is no longer adequate.

The primordial vascular system develops by vasculogenesis (new vessel formation); later development is by angiogenesis (new vessels branching off the existing vessels and remodelling). A few cells in the mesoderm of the yolk sac lose adherence and start to move, forming clusters called blood islands (Fig. 9.13). The haemocytoblasts (or haemangioblasts), the precursors of both blood cells and blood vessel endothelial cells, are nucleated and start to synthesize primitive forms of haemoglobin. The outer cells of the blood islands, angioblasts, develop characteristics of endothelial cells, the cells that line blood vessels. The blood islands fuse, forming vascular channels that eventually amalgamate to form a primitive vascular network with identifiable routes. The organization of the routes across the yolk sac is similar to the geographical organization of river deltas where little streams meander and combine, taking the route of least resistance. Pericytes and smooth muscle cells are recruited. Expansion and elastic resistance of the vessel walls, which become rhythmic generating a peristaltic pattern, propel the blood cells. Blood vessel differentiation and growth is orchestrated by a range of signals including cell adhesion molecules, transcription factors and angiogenic growth factors and their receptors (Breier 2000).

The primitive heart develops from a horseshoe area of embryonic mesoderm, anterior to the prochordal plate. It forms two tubes, one on each side of the foregut, which fuse to form a single heart tube. The primitive atrium forms where the flow from the umbilical veins from the placenta joins with the blood vessels from the head, generating the greatest volume

Fig. 9.13 *Formation of the first blood vessels: A appearance of blood islands; B vessels at 24 days (A reproduced with permission from Fitzgerald & Fitzgerald 1994; B reproduced with permission from Goodwin 1997.)*

Continued

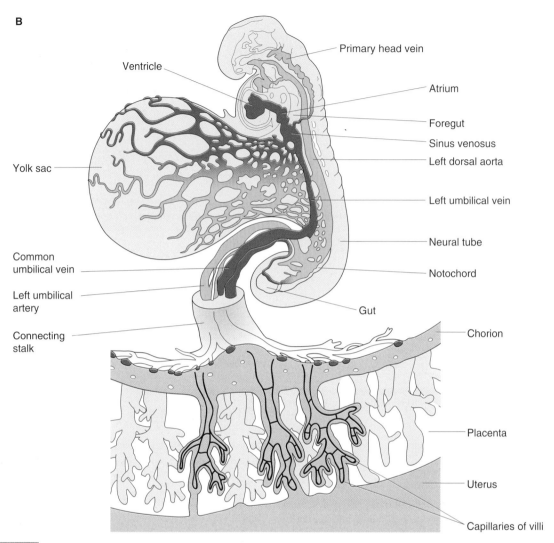

B

Ventricle

Primary head vein

Atrium

Foregut

Sinus venosus

Left dorsal aorta

Yolk sac

Left umbilical vein

Neural tube

Common umbilical vein

Notochord

Left umbilical artery

Gut

Connecting stalk

Chorion

Placenta

Uterus

Capillaries of villi

Fig. 9.13   Cont'd

of blood. The swirling vortex of blood leaving the primitive atrium induces the development of the primitive ventricle, which becomes the main source of pumping activity. The characteristic shape of the heart is generated by the flow of blood cells within the vascular channels; this causes the heart tube to form an S-shaped loop that will eventually take on the configuration of the heart (Fig. 9.14). By 21 days after fertilization, the cells surrounding the heart have become differentiated as myocardial cells capable of eliciting an organized response, so the heart, which consists of four chambers in series, begins beating.

The development of the outer layers of the vessel walls is stimulated by stress (Martyn & Greenwald 1997). In areas where there is more turbulence, the vessel wall responds by developing more elasticity. Therefore, the heart and arterial structures develop thicker and more elastic walls. The mature organization of the chambers of the heart is achieved by the ingrowth of the septa towards the central atrioventricular cushion in the centre (Fig. 9.14). The growth of the fetal heart partially depends on afterload. If afterload is increased by factors leading to peripheral vasoconstriction or high placental impedance, the likely outcome is a growth-restricted baby with an enlarged heart (Veille et al 1993). If the fetus receives less than adequate nutrition or oxygenation during its development then blood flow is diverted to the brain and heart. The decreased flow to the peripheral vessels results in the development of less elastic tissue, which is the hypothesis underlying the association of poor maternal nutrition with an increased risk of cardiovascular disease in adult life (Barker et al 1993). The initial response to impaired nutrition is to increase

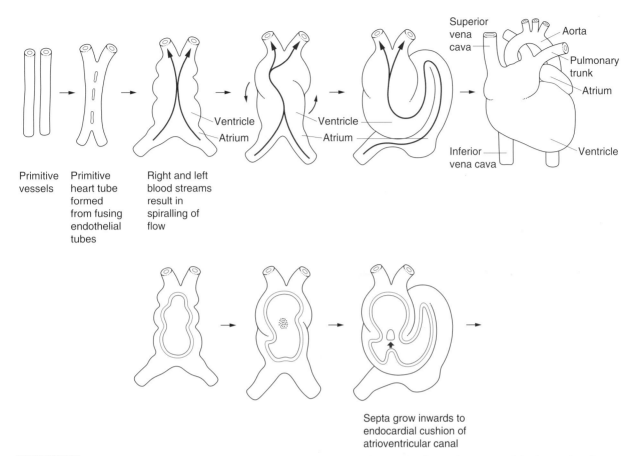

Superior vena cava · Aorta · Pulmonary trunk · Atrium · Inferior vena cava · Ventricle

Primitive vessels

Primitive heart tube formed from fusing endothelial tubes

Right and left blood streams result in spiralling of flow

Ventricle
Atrium

Ventricle
Atrium

Septa grow inwards to endocardial cushion of atrioventricular canal

Fig. 9.14 *Formation of the heart from bending of the cardiac tube (21–35 days), and formation of the heart chambers.*

placental growth; if this is not adequate, blood flow is diverted to the brain (and other essential organs such heart, adrenal glands and placenta). Therefore adults who were small at birth, but with relatively large placentas, have an increased risk of developing hypertension because less elastic tissue was established in their blood vessels during fetal development (Fig. 9.15). It is argued that impaired fetal nutrition also leads to fewer tissue stem cells being formed which leads eventually to early exhaustion of organ function and the development of chronic adult disease (Cianfarani 2003).

The respiratory system

The trachea and major bronchi develop as outpouches of the alimentary tract. The development depends on interaction between the endodermal bud from the developing foregut and the splanchnic mesoderm it invades at about day 22. The bud bifurcates between day 26 and day 28. In the 5th week of development, three secondary buds develop on the right branch and

two on the left; these are the primitive lobes of the lung. There are four stages in the development of the respiratory system: the embryonic phase from weeks 3 to 7, the pseudocanalicular phase from 7 to 16 weeks, the canalicular phase from 16 to 24 weeks and the terminal sac phase from 24 weeks until birth (Fig. 9.16). One of the most critical stages in development is the production of surfactant from the type II pneumocytes, allowing efficient inflation and gas exchange following birth and therefore postnatal survival. Although the cells can be identified at about week 22, production of surfactant increases significantly after 30 weeks. The diaphragm starts to develop high in the neck and descends as the lungs and heart develop. This is the reason why diaphragmatic pain is often felt as referred pain in the shoulder.

Fetal breathing movements (FBM) are a feature of normal fetal life and are used to assess fetal well-being. FBM oppose lung recoil and maintain the level of lung expansion that is essential for normal growth and structural maturation of the fetal lungs (Harding & Hooper 1996). Normal development of the fetal lungs

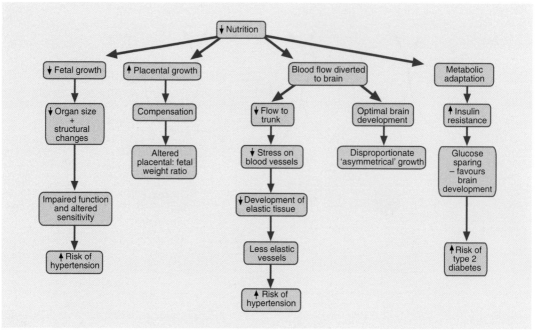

Fig. 9.15 *The fetus adapts to suboptimal nutrition with strategies for survival. The slower growth rate reduces use of nutrients but affects final organ size and function. The redistribution of blood to the brain affects development of the blood vessels and predisposes to later hypertension. Altered metabolism and peripheral insulin resistance favours glucose availability for the developing brain but the 'thriftiness' predisposes to insulin resistance, obesity and type II diabetes if the individual experiences good or over-nutrition in later life.*

is very important as there is limited capacity for later recovery. FBM are inhibited by fetal hypoxaemia, hypoglycaemia, maternal alcohol consumption, maternal smoking, intra-amniotic infection and maternal consumption of sedatives or narcotic drugs. The absence of FBM is associated with lung hypoplasia, premature rupture of fetal membranes and oligohydramnios. Decreased amniotic fluid volume causes decreased lung growth and expansion whereas tracheal occlusion, which prevents expulsion of lung fluid, can cause overgrowth of lung tissue (Nardo et al 1998). At term, the infant has about 50 million alveoli, half the adult number; these continue to increase in the first 8 years of life.

The urinary system

The urinary and genital systems both develop from the intermediate mesoderm and are closely associated (see Ch. 5 for a description of genital development). During embryonic folding, urogenital ridges appear each side of the primitive aorta (Fig. 9.17). The nephrogenic ridge develops into the renal system of kidneys, ureters, bladder and urethra. Abnormalities

of the kidneys and ureters affect 3–4% of newborn infants. Most of the abnormalities are harmless, such as variation in blood supply, abnormal position or shapes, and urinary tract duplications. However, unilateral renal agenesis (one kidney failing to develop) affects one in 1000 liveborn babies. Bilateral renal agenesis or Potter's syndrome (inadequate development of both kidneys) affects one in 3000 fetuses and is incompatible with life. It is usually associated with oligohydramnios. Three pairs of kidneys develop during fetal development: the pronephroi, the mesonephroi and the metanephroi (singular: pronephros, mesonephros and metanephros). The pronephroi are transient non-functional structures that exist for only a few weeks. When they degenerate, their ducts are utilized in the next stage. The mesonephroi appear in the 4th week and function as intermediate kidneys until the end of the embryonic period, disgorging waste products into the remnants of the yolk sac. They degenerate and disappear in the 8th week, although parts of their structure persist as mesonephric or Wolffian ducts in males (see Ch. 5).

The permanent kidneys, or metanephroi, develop from the 5th week and begin to function about 4 weeks later. The kidneys start development in the pelvis and

A

Pharynx

B

Trachea

C

Right stem bronchus

Lateral bronchus

Right upper lobe primordia

Left upper lobe primordia

Right middle lobe primordia

Left lower lobe primordia

Right lower lobe primordia

Lung buds

D

Columnar epithelium

Bronchus

Bronchiolar bud

Mesenchyme

E

Ciliated cuboidal epithelium

Terminal bronchiole

Respiratory bronchiole

F

Alveolar sac

Capillary

Fig. 9.16 *Respiratory system development: A pharyngeal pouches (4 weeks); B 32 days; C 35 days; D pseudocanalicular phase (17 weeks); E canalicular phase (17-26 weeks); F terminal sac phase (26 weeks).*

appear to migrate upwards. In fact, this observation is due to continued downward growth of the embryo. As the kidneys 'ascend' out of the pelvic area, new arteries at successively higher levels supply them. During fetal life, the kidney is subdivided into lobes, which disappear in infancy as the nephrons grow. The main increase in size is due to elongation of the proximal convoluted tubules and loops of Henle. Disruption of renal branching during development leads to renal dysplasia, the major cause of renal failure in children (Piscione & Rosenblum 2002). Functional maturation of the kidneys occurs after birth.

Until 20 weeks' gestation, the skin is not keratinized so fluid can move through this semipermeable membrane. Essentially the outer barrier is the amnion. As the skin matures and lays down keratin, the rate of transudation decreases and the outer barrier of the fetus becomes the skin. The urine then becomes an important source of amniotic fluid. The fetus produces up to 600 ml of urine per day. Amniotic fluid is also produced by the amniotic membrane and the fetal lungs. The fetus swallows most of the amniotic fluid; the rest diffuses through the amniotic membranes to the maternal circulation.

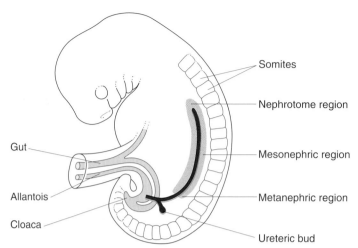

The development of the renal system from the urogenital ridges.

The epidermis of the skin develops from the ecto-derm, which is colonized from melanocytes from the neural crest and Langerhans cells from the bone marrow. The dermis is derived from the embryonic meso-derm.

The muscles and limbs

The first muscles to develop are the back muscles from the paired somites. Bone formation is closely associated with muscle growth and the nervous connections from the spinal cord. The limbs become evident as buds or bulges associated with particular somites in the 4th week of development. The limb buds are formed from migration of muscle cells from the myotomes. The cells form pairs of muscle masses. Adhesive cells form a compacted region between the two muscle masses, which differentiates into cartilage. Cartilage is stiff but flexible whereas bone is stronger but more brittle and able to fracture. Ossification, the conversion to bone structure, begins from about 8 weeks but is still not complete by birth. This preponderance of cartilage in the skeleton aids flexibility at delivery. The arms are slightly ahead of the legs in development because the fetal circulatory system gives an advantage to the upper body (see Ch. 15). Bones and muscles closest to the body develop first so the humerus and femur develop before the distal regions of the limbs. The differential timing of development means that drugs such as thalidomide affect different limbs and parts of the limbs depending on time of exposure of the fetus to the teratogens (Box 9.8). By 41 days, the fingers and toes develop from paddle-like plates. The sculpting of the digits is due to apoptosis of the tissue between the digital rays. A common minor congenital defect observed at birth is a failure of separation of the digits. By 9 weeks, the body skeleton is almost complete, although the skull bones are still forming.

Fetal growth

At 4 weeks, the crown–rump length is about 4 mm and increases by 1 mm per day up to 30 mm (Beck 1996). Thereafter, between weeks 8 and 28, the growth increases markedly, to about 1.5 mm per day,

---

Box 9.8

Thalidomide

Thalidomide was marketed as 'Contergan' in 1957. Congenital malformations of the limbs and ears rose in parallel with sales of the drug with a lag of 7–8 months (Lenz 1962, McBride 1961). The drug was withdrawn in November 1961; 5850 infants were affected, of whom 40% died, leaving 3900 survivors. Thalidomide disturbs cartilage formation and the establishment of the nerve connections to muscles. It is teratogenic 20–36 days after fertilization. Limb development begins at 24 days. Early exposure to thalidomide caused absence of arms; later exposure successively affected development of ears, legs and thumbs. Different species metabolize the drug differently; fetal development in the rodent test species (rats and mice) was not affected.

so this period is recognized as the fetal growth period. The organs and tissues continue to grow and mature. Although growth is most rapid during this period (compared with any other time in life), factors affecting growth may have their origins earlier. In fact, environmental insults regulating growth appear to last for several generations. Fetal growth is due to interaction between the genetic drive for growth and the nutritional supplies in pregnancy to support it, which involves a dynamic interaction between fetus, placenta and mother.

There are characteristic differences between the different phases of growth during development (James & Stephenson 1998). Growth in the first trimester is principally through increased cell number. In the second trimester, cell division continues albeit at a slower rate and the cells increase in size. In the third trimester, cell division slows further and the increase in cell size continues. There is little variation in fetal growth up to about 16 weeks of gestation (Gluckman & Pinal 2003), after which genetic and environmental influences have a marked effect on outcome. Fat deposition, determined by nutrient availability and insulin levels, plays an important contribution in the final weight. There are 42 successive cell divisions between fertilization and birth, but only five more from birth to adult size (excluding mitotic cell division to replace dead cells).

All low-birth weight infants are potentially at some health risk. Low birth weight is traditionally defined as being less than 2500 g at birth. Low birth weight remains one of the great challenges to modern health care services; small size at birth can affect susceptibility to infection, rate of postnatal growth and neurocognitive development. Low birth weight is associated with increased fetal mortality as well as higher neonatal and infant morbidity and mortality with the most adverse outcomes arising in the most immature infants. A number of chronic adult diseases originate in utero as a result of fetal adaptation to optimize survival (Godfrey & Barker 2000), including glucose intolerance, insulin resistance and type II diabetes mellitus, heart disease, hypertension, obstructive lung disease, hyperlipidaemia, hypercholesterolaemia, hypercortisolaemia, renal disease, obesity and reproductive disorders.

The use of low birth weight as the outcome measure of the success of a pregnancy is very widespread and it can be measured with precision and validity (Kramer 1998). Infant mortality increases exponentially with lower birth weight. However, birth weight is a function of two factors (gestational length and rate of fetal growth) which have different aetiologies and different prognoses. The simple definition of a low birth weight infant as one who weighs less than 2500 g at birth does not differentiate between infants who are growth-restricted (small at term) and infants who are born prematurely. Prematurity is often complicated by IUGR. Some small-for-gestational age (SGA) infants are constitutionally small rather than growth-restricted or growth-retarded.

Birth weight is a crude outcome measure of optimal intrauterine growth and development; suboptimal maternal body composition and nutrient intake can have a long-term effect on the offspring without necessarily affecting size at birth (Godfrey 2001). Birth weight does not identify effects of nutrition on body composition and development of specific tissues and organs; a similar birth weight can be attained with different growth trajectories. Birth weight may not identify growth restriction. For instance, if an infant does not reach its potential birth weight but is born above 2500 g, it will not be classified as growth-restricted. Conversely, an infant with 'normal' birth weight, such as 3.4 kg, may be growth-retarded and have long-term health risks if it was destined to be bigger under optimal intrauterine conditions. Most infants born of low birth weight in developed countries are born prematurely rather than growth-restricted; in most cases, the cause(s) of preterm delivery is not known. Rates of low birth weight babies are higher in areas with a higher level of socioeconomic deprivation; birth weight is also related to income level and accessibility to healthcare, education and housing.

A variety of factors affect fetal growth (Box 9.9). Chromosome and genetic disorders often cause fetal growth retardation; excluding these, the dominant cause of growth retardation is due to an inadequate supply of nutrients and oxygen (Gluckman & Pinal 2003) related either to maternal supply or to placental transfer capacity.

Fetal factors

Male offspring are on average heavier than female offspring. The ovaries have limited capability to synthesize steroid hormones whereas the testes produce testosterone, which has anabolic effects. Studies suggest that the Y chromosome positively promotes growth (James & Stephenson 1998). Multiple pregnancies tend to result in smaller babies, probably

Factors affecting fetal size

- Fetal factors
- Maternal size (lean body mass): maternal genetic effects
- Maternal weight gain and nutrition in pregnancy
- Maternal age extremes
- Maternal behavioural factors such as smoking, recreational drug use
- Multiple pregnancy
- Fetal oxygenation: affected by maternal anaemia, etc.
- Maternal medical conditions such as hypertension, heart disease, infections, diabetes
- Placental sufficiency affected by pre-eclampsia, uterine blood flow, etc.
- Growth hormones such as insulin and insulin-like growth factors (IGFs)

because of the limited haemodynamic support in late gestation, although overcrowding is also implicated. Aneuploidy is also a risk factor for IUGR (see Ch. 7). First-born infants tend to be slightly lighter than subsequent siblings.

Maternal size

The classic experiments on horses showing that the size of offspring of hybrid crosses between small Shetland ponies and large carthorses was most closely related to maternal size demonstrated that maternal size is a critical determinant of birth weight (Walton & Hammond 1938). However, final adult size is also affected by paternal genetics to different degrees in different species; in humans about 5% of the variability in size is attributed to paternal influences (Robinson & Owens 1996). In the past, pregnant women were asked for their shoe size, which correlates with their pelvic size, and their husband's hat size, which was found to be related to the size of the baby; the relationship of the two sizes was used to predict the likelihood of difficulties in delivery (Moore, Peters & Frame 1984). A small maternal size appears to impose a constraint on fetal growth, although factors such as immaturity, social circumstances, maternal behaviour (such as smoking and alcohol consumption), diseases and psychological stress all affect the outcome of the pregnancy. Shorter maternal stature is positively correlated with lower socioeconomic status, malnutrition, chronic disease, increased levels of stress and large family size. The cycle of deprivation tends to repeat, as there is a correlation between maternal height and birth weight and between birth weight and adult size, which is not solely due to genetic influences.

Half-siblings who share the same mother have similar birth weights (Gluckman & Harding 1994). The birth weights of babies born after ovum donation are more strongly related to the weight of the recipient mother than to that of the donor woman (Brooks et al 1995). These findings suggest that birth size is more strongly influenced by uterine environment than by genetics.

It is suggested that there is a conflict between the maternal and paternal genes governing fetal size (Moore & Haig 1991). Paternal genes favour fetal growth and the transfer of nutrients to the parasitic fetus; if this happens at the expense of maternal health, the male can choose a different mate. Maternal genes limit transfer to the fetus to optimize survival of the mother and her children. The father's birth weight influences placental size. Birth weights of mothers correlate with their children's birth weights and even with their grandchildren's birth weights, suggesting that the maternal constraint on fetal growth is set very early (Barker 1998). The paternal effect on the fetal growth trajectory is permitted by the lifting of the maternal constraint on growth. Therefore fetal growth rate responds to, and is appropriate for, the prevailing nutrient availability. Maternal constraint is also a mechanism for limiting fetal growth to maternal pelvis size. Constraint of growth by maternal factors is important in preventing fetal overgrowth and dystocia which is risky for mother and infant (and survival of the species).

Growth hormones

It has been suggested that growth in children from fetus through infancy and childhood to puberty follows a mathematical model on which three growth curves are imposed, forming a sigmoidal curve (Fig. 9.18) (Karlberg et al 1994). Phase 1, the infancy growth rate, begins in fetal life with a rapid deceleration until about 3 years of age. This is the phase of growth that seems to be regulated by insulin-like growth factors (IGFs) (see Ch. 4); the effect of poor nutrition on growth may be mediated by IGFs. The childhood phase begins in the 1st year of life and is

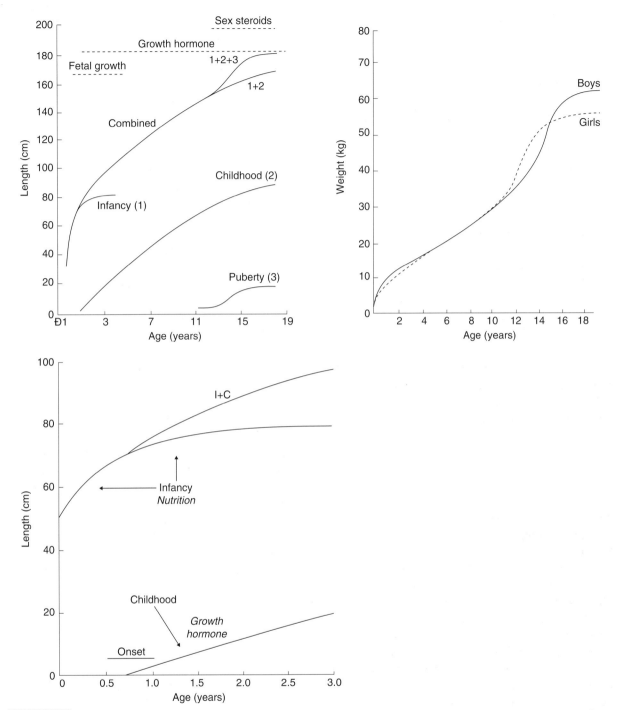

Fig. 9.18 *Karlberg's model of growth: A sigmoidal curve from a combination of three growth curves; B the curve of weight increase; C the curve of increase in length. (Reproduced with permission from Karlberg et al 1994.)*

due to the effect of growth hormone (GH; see Ch. 3) provided thyroid hormone secretion is normal. During this period most of the growth is localized in the lower body (particularly leg length), as the long bones are very sensitive to GH. Children who have deficiency of GH or who are encephalic have normal birth weight

and early infant growth; the deficiency usually becomes apparent only after 6 months of age. The final component of growth is the pubertal growth spurt, which is stimulated by the interaction of sex hormones with GH. Although levels of GH in the fetus are high, GH receptors are expressed at low levels in fetal tissues so GH has little effect. This is supported by observations that GH-deficient fetuses or young infants have almost normal linear growth. Fetal growth seems to be controlled rather by IGFs and their receptors (Robinson & Owens 1996).

IGFs are mitogens (i.e. they stimulate cell division and differentiation) and are modulated by binding proteins, which control growth before and after birth (see Ch. 15). This mechanism can explain both the interaction of genetic drive and nutrient supply and the effects of maternal and paternal size. IGF-II is the primary growth factor influencing embryonic growth, whereas IGF-I, produced by the fetal liver and amniotic membranes, regulates growth in late gestation. IGF-I increases the efficiency of the placenta so fetal weight increases without a corresponding increase in placental weight. Fetal insulin, driven by fetal glucose availability, is the main regulator of IGF-I; IGF-I is very sensitive to maternal nutrition. IGF-I is also involved in fetal gut maturation. Both IGF-I and IGF-II have anabolic effects via the type I receptor. IGF-II also binds to the type II receptor, which effectively competes with the type I receptor for available IGF-II. IGF-II is paternally imprinted and expressed and promotes growth via the IGF-I receptor, whereas the type II receptor, which is hypothesized to be maternally imprinted, limits or controls growth by clearing or 'mopping up' the free IGF-II (Harding & Johnston 1995). Overexpression of IGF-II leads to the Beckwith–Weidemann overgrowth syndrome. Fetal hyperinsulinaemia appears to inhibit the production of IGF-I-binding protein, thus lifting the restriction on IGF-I and contributing to macrosomia (Wang & Chard 1992). Nutrient availability may promote IGF-I levels and fetal growth. Thus, a balance can be achieved between paternal genes promoting growth and maternal genes restricting and regulating growth.

Insulin itself has a growth-promoting effect in the fetus; it is a growth-promoting hormone which signals nutrient plenty. Its sommatogenic (growth-promoting) actions are mediated via IGF-I but it has a direct effect on fat deposition. Maternal hyperglycaemia causes increased placental transfer of glucose to the fetus. The higher concentration of glucose stimulates the fetal pancreas to produce insulin, which facilitates cellular uptake of glucose, stimulating anabolic metabolism and fetal growth. Babies of diabetic mothers are often macrosomic owing to particularly large fat stores. Fetal insulin deficiency, which is rare, can occur with nutrient deprivation or pancreatic agenesis, and results in fetal growth retardation (symmetrical IUGR)

and decreased levels of body fat and muscle development (Robinson & Owens 1996).

Glucocorticoids affect fetal growth and maturation by altering production and secretion of hormones, regulating receptor density and altering the activity of enzymes involved in activating and deactivating hormones (see also Ch. 15). The fetus is usually protected from maternal glucocorticoids because they are inactivated by the placental enzyme 11β-hydroxysteroid dehydrogenase which effectively acts as a barrier. However, maternal undernutrition down-regulates this enzyme so the fetus is exposed to increased glucocorticoids (Gluckman & Pinal 2003) which leads to fetal growth maturation. However, the higher levels of cortisol enhance maturation of the lungs and other organs, promoting survival of the IUGR infant; premature delivery frequently accompanies IUGR. Thyroid hormones promote fetal development and signal energy availability.

Maternal nutrition

Fetal growth is related to maternal size (reflecting nutrient level during her own fetal development), maternal body composition (which indicates nutrient supply), nutrient availability in pregnancy and placental efficiency. If periconceptual maternal nutrition sets the growth trajectory early in gestation, the fetal growth rate is more likely to be accommodated by nutrient availability when its demands are high in later gestation. The fetus is able to adapt metabolically to undernutrition in pregnancy by altering its growth rate and sparing nutrients for certain tissues, like the brain. This can lead to disproportionate organ development and fetal growth patterns; fetal adaptations to undernutrition tend to be permanent (Barker 1998).

Maternal nutrition stores correlate with birth weight. Pregnant women exposed to conditions of starvation during the famines during World War II were particularly susceptible to nutrient deficiency in the first half of their pregnancies. Not only was the size of their babies significantly smaller, but the prenatal growth of their grandchildren was also affected (Lumey 1992). Nutrient deprivation later in pregnancy affected birth weights, but the lengths of the neonates were not affected so much and the babies appeared to regain normal weights after birth. However, the metabolic adaptation in those fetuses exposed to nutrient deprivation late in gestation is associated with persistent insulin resistance and a marked trend to develop glucose intolerance and non-insulin-dependent diabetes mellitus (NIDDM) later in life (Phillips 1996).

In humans, dietary intervention studies have had disappointing results, producing improvement in fetal growth only in severely undernourished women (see Ch. 12). Part of the problem may be the methodology and ensuring that supplements intended for pregnant women are not used as alternative sources of nutrition or to feed other members of the family. The timing of the nutritional supplements may also be important, as fetal growth trajectories may be set before the nutritional status of the mother is improved by the intervention. Women experiencing marginal diets and seasonal famine for generations appear to have evolved strategies to conserve energy by suppressing metabolic rate and acquiring little fat during the pregnancy (Durnin 1987). The energy cost of pregnancy in affluent countries where food is plentiful may be met with little or no increase in energy intake, although economies in energy expenditure may offset the increased requirements (see Ch. 12). Prepregnant size (body fat levels) may direct the trajectory that sets fetal growth via leptin, the product of the *ob* gene (Rink 1994). Appropriate conditions during pregnancy can then fulfil the requirements for this trajectory to be achieved. In experimental animals, the effect of moderate maternal malnutrition over a number of generations is decreased birth weight, which is maintained for a few further generations even when food supply is restored to a good level (Stewart et al 1980). A plentiful food supply imposed after generations of malnutrition in these animals is associated with obstructed labour and poor fetal outcome.

Acute undernutrition in late gestation can cause premature delivery by stimulating prostaglandin release, which promotes cervical ripening and uterine contractility (see Ch. 13). Macronutrient balance at different stages of pregnancy may affect fetal growth (see Ch. 12). Micronutrient availability can affect the somatotrophic and insulin regulation of growth; zinc deficiency is associated with IUGR. Vitamin E and vitamin A affect insulin sensitivity and GH secretion, respectively. Folate status affects gene imprinting and methylation.

Maternal nutrition could also exert an effect on fetal growth even before fertilization. The nutritional support of follicular development prior to ovulation and fertilization may affect the growth trajectory of the embryo (see above). Nutrition of the embryo prior to implantation may be important, as demonstrated by in vitro fertilization (IVF). Sheep and cattle embryos from IVF that are cultured for a few days before being replaced in the uterus grow into significantly larger fetuses (James & Stephenson 1998). It is not clear whether IVF affects human birth weight. However, some 'unexplained infertility' in humans appears to be related to an inadequately developed endometrial lining. Couples with a previous history of 'unexplained infertility' have a high rate of small-for-dates infants, which may be associated with poor conditions for implantation (Wang et al 1994).

Maternal behaviour

Differences in birth weight across different socioeconomic groups may be largely attributable to differences in cigarette smoking. The birth weight appears to fall by about 14 g multiplied by the average number of cigarettes smoked per day. Smoking is associated with a poorer diet and level of healthcare, although effects on oxygen transfer are probably compensated for by 2,3-bisphosphoglycerate (2,3-BPG), which improves the efficiency of oxygen–haemoglobin dissociation (see Ch. 1). Smoking causes nicotine-induced vasoconstriction of the uterine vessels, carbon monoxide inhibits oxygen diffusion and cyanide affects enzyme systems (James & Stephenson 1998). Improving fetal oxygenation in conditions of maternal hypoxia has achieved an improved fetal outcome (Battaglia et al 1992) but there is controversy about the effect of maternal iron deficiency on pregnancy outcome (Godfrey et al 1991). Alcohol consumption in excess of 40 ml/day is associated with effects on growth; one of the common effects of fetal alcohol syndrome is growth retardation (Hannigan & Armant 2000). The use of hard drugs, such as heroin and cocaine, in pregnancy is associated with low birth weight babies but again it is difficult to dissociate the use of the drugs from the other variables. Caffeine, whether from coffee or other sources such as soft drinks, has an effect on fetal growth (see Ch. 12).

Other factors affecting fetal growth

Medical complications of pregnancy or pre-existing maternal diseases can affect fetal growth. Mild maternal hypertension does not restrict growth but severe hypertension is associated with low birth weight particularly if it is complicated with renal disease.

Pre-eclampsia is a major cause of low birth weight; it has been suggested that IUGR of unknown cause may be due to undiagnosed pre-eclampsia (see Ch. 8). Severe respiratory and cardiovascular problems and chronic renal disease are also associated with growth retardation. Fetal growth retardation has also been observed in women with congenital uterine abnormalities.

Fetal malformations, especially those due to chromosomal abnormality, are strongly correlated with impaired growth rates. Trisomies and Turner's syndrome have a marked effect on birth weight (James & Stephenson 1998). CVS (chorionic villus sampling) indicates that in 1–2% of conceptuses tested there is a degree of confined placental mosaicism (where one or more types of placental cells have nuclei with an abnormal number of chromosomes). Placental mosaicism is associated with an increased frequency of IUGR (Robinson & Owens 1996).

Maternal and fetal infections, such as rubella and cytomegalovirus, also detrimentally affect growth. It is not clear whether HIV affects fetal growth as coexisting problems cannot be dissociated. In developing countries, malaria infection causes placental disease and affects fetal growth. Placental supply of amino acids is close to the minimum required to support fetal protein synthesis. It is possible that the adverse circumstances limiting fetal growth do so by increasing levels of catabolic hormones, such as catecholamines, cortisol and β-endorphin (Robinson & Owens 1996) or by altering the expression of the receptor for IGF-II (Haig & Graham 1991).

Box 9.10

Complications associated with SGA

- Increased mortality
- Short- and long-term pulmonary morbidity
- Intrapartum hypoxia
- Hypothermia
- Hypoglycaemia
- Necrotizing enterocolitis
- Ophthalmic morbidity
- Neurological morbidity
- Delayed psychomotor development
- Polycythaemia
- Infection
- Pulmonary haemorrhage
- Sudden infant death syndrome
- Adult-onset cardiovascular and metabolic disease

Complications associated with SGA

Babies who are small for gestational age (SGA) have an increased risk of perinatal complications (Box 9.10). Although some catch-up growth may occur postnatally, some of the effects of IUGR may be irreversible (Barker 1998).

Case study 9.2 details the example of a baby with low birth weight.

Case study 9.2

Razia gives birth to a healthy female infant at term. The baby appears healthy and chubby although she weighs only 2.6 kg.

- Is the midwife right to assume that Asian babies are normally smaller than Western babies?
- What reasons would you give to argue for or against this assumption?

Key points

- During the 2nd week of development, the inner cell mass differentiates into the bilaminar disc, consisting of two germ layers: the epiblast and the hypoblast. The definitive yolk sac is created and the amniotic and chorionic cavities are evident. The differentiated cells migrate and adhere and the genes are switched on and off.

- The embryonic period consists of cell growth (increased cell number and size), differentiation, organogenesis (organization of tissues into organs) and morphogenesis (development of shape). This is the period that is most susceptible to teratogens, which can cause major morphological abnormalities.

- Gastrulation is the major event of the 3rd week. It begins with the appearance of the primitive streak, results in the conversion of the bilaminar disc into a trilaminar disc, consisting of ectoderm, mesoderm and endoderm, and establishes the axis for further embryonic development. The neural tube, precursor of the nervous system, and the somites also appear in the 3rd week.

- The trilaminar disc is converted into the characteristic vertebral structure by differential growth of the cell layers causing folding and fusion.

- Weeks 4–8 are the period of organogenesis, differentiation of the major organ systems.

■ Fetal growth is influenced by genes and the environment, but limited by nutrient and oxygen supply. Paternal genes tend to favour fetal growth whereas maternal genes tend to constrain fetal growth to a growth trajectory that may be set by environmental influences prior to fertilization.

■ The fetus can adapt to undernutrition by altering metabolism and blood flow to protect the brain, albeit at the expense of other organs.

Application to practice

■ An understanding of fetal development is required in the explanation of congenital conditions.

■ Many things, some of which can be affected by advice and guidance of the midwife, for example in regards to smoking, affect fetal growth.

■ As pregnancy progresses, most women are keen to know how their baby is developing, so the midwife should be able to describe fetal development and growth in an appropriate way.

Annotated further reading

Barker DJP 1998 Mothers, babies and health in later life, 2nd edn. Churchill Livingstone, New York
Epidemiological studies link a number of adult diseases with fetal development. This book examines the evidence that fetal adaptation to undernutrition irreversibly alters anatomic, physiological and metabolic development, and links the fetal origins hypothesis to health policy.

Carlson BM 2004 Human embryology and developmental biology, 3rd edn. Mosby, St Louis
A well-illustrated textbook which covers the molecular basis of development, cellular aspects, developmental anatomy and the progression of development. Includes recent research findings, case studies, timeline information, review questions and useful end-of-chapter summaries.

Copp AJ, Greene ND, Murdoch JN 2003 The genetic basis of mammalian neurulation. Nature Reviews Genetics 4(10):784–793
An excellent up-to-date-review covering mammalian neurulation in depth, including the underlying developmental mechanisms, how mutant genes disrupt neurulation and the mechanisms by which folic acid prevents neural tube defects.

Gluckman PD Hanson MA 2004 The fetal matrix: evolutions, development and disease. Cambridge University Press, Cambridge
Written by two of the world experts in this field, this book covers fetal programming, evolutionary mechanisms that promoted survival of our hunter–gatherer ancestors, the implications of nutritional transition and directions for future research and treatment.

Larsen WJ, Sadler TW 2003 Langman's medical embryology, 9th edn. Churchill Livingstone, New York
An up-to-date text (with accompanying compact disc) which covers stages of human development in detail with timelines and sections on the interaction between genetics and human development. Links molecular aspects and experimental principles to clinical applications.

McLachlan J 1994 Medical embryology. Addison-Wesley, New York
This book describes human development, focusing on developmental mechanisms, providing a basis for understanding the aetiology of congenital defects. It includes evolutionary aspects, methods of monitoring development, prenatal diagnosis and the ethical problems that arise from the calculation of risk.

Moore KL, Persaud TVN 2003 Before we are born: essentials of embryology and birth defects, 6th edn. Saunders, Philadelphia
This book covers normal and abnormal human development week by week from fertilization through the development of the major organs and physiological systems to birth.

Moore KL, Persaud TVN 2003 The developing human: clinically orientated embryology, 7th edn. Saunders, Philadelphia
This book is a more detailed description of embryological development, targeted at clinicians, which covers new research findings and their clinical applications. It includes aspects of molecular biology, effects of teratogens and detection of fetal defects.

Spencer R 2002 Conjoined twins: developmental malformations and clinical implications. Johns Hopkins University Press, Baltimore
This book provides a comprehensive guide to the different types of this rare phenomenon.

References

Bard JBL, Weddon SE 1996 The molecular basis of mammalian embryogenesis. In: Hillier SG, Kitchener HC, Neilson JP (eds) Scientific essentials of reproductive medicine. Saunders, Philadelphia, pp 261–273

Barker DJP 1998 Mothers, babies and health in later life, 2nd edn. Churchill Livingstone, New York

Barker DJP, Gluckman PD, Godfrey KM, Harding JE, Owens JA, Robinson JS 1993 Fetal nutrition and cardiovascular disease in adult life. Lancet 341:938–941

Bassett J 1986 Nutrition of the conceptus: aspects of its regulation. Proceedings of the Nutrition Society 45:1

Battaglia C, Artini PG, Dambrogio G, Galli PA, Sgre A, Genazzani AR 1992 Maternal hyperoxygenation in the treatment of intrauterine growth retardation. American Journal of Obstetrics and Gynecology 167:430–435

Beck F 1996 Human embryogenesis. In: Hillier SG, Kitchener H, Neilson JP (eds) Scientific essentials of reproductive medicine. Saunders, Philadelphia, pp 274–281

Breier G 2000 Angiogenesis in embryonic development: a review. Placenta 21(Suppl A):S11–S15

Brooks AA, Johnson MR, Steer PJ, Pawson ME, Abdalla HI 1995 Birth weight: nature or nurture? Early Human Development 42:29–35

Carlson BM 1994 Human embryology and developmental biology. Mosby, St Louis

Cianfarani S 2003 Foetal origins of adult diseases: just a matter of stem cell number? Medical Hypotheses 61(3):401–404

De Robertis EM, Oliver G, Wright CVE 1990 Homeobox genes and the vertebrate body plan. Scientific American 263(1):46–52

Durnin JVGA 1987 Energy requirements of pregnancy: an integration of the longitudinal data from the five-country study. Lancet ii:1131–1133

Fitzgerald MJT, Fitzgerald M 1994 Human embryology. Baillière Tindall, London, pp 23, 24, 37, 42

Freeman B 2003 The active migration of germ cells in the embryos of mice and men is a myth. Reproduction 125(5):635–643

Gardner RL 2002 Stem cells: potency, plasticity and public perception. Journal of Anatomy 200(Pt 3):277–282

George DK, Cooney TP, Chiu BK, Thurlbeck WM 1987 Hypoplasia and immaturity of the terminal lung units (acinus) in congenital diaphragmatic hernia. American Review of Respiratory Disease 136:947–950

Gluckman PF 1989 Fetal growth: an endocrine perspective. Acta Paediatrica Scandinavica Supplement 349:21–25

Gluckman PF, Harding JE 1994 Nutritional and hormonal regulation of fetal growth: evolving concepts. Acta Paediatrica Supplement 399:60

Gluckman PD, Pinal CS 2003 Regulation of fetal growth by the somatotrophic axis. Journal of Nutrition 133(5 Suppl 2): 1741S–1746S

Godfrey KM 2001 The 'gold standard' for optimal fetal growth and development. Journal of Pediatric Endocrinology & Metabolism 14(Suppl 6):1507–1513

Godfrey KM, Barker DJP 2000 Fetal nutrition and adult disease. American Journal of Clinical Nutrition 71(5):1344S–1352S

Godfrey KM, Redman CW, Barker DJ, Osmond C 1991 The effect of maternal anaemia and iron deficiency on the ratio of fetal weight to placental weight. British Journal of Obstetrics and Gynaecology 98:886–891

Goodwin B 1997 Health and development: conception to birth. Open University, Milton Keynes, pp 203–205, 209

Haig D, Graham C 1991 Genomic imprinting and the strange case of the insulin like growth factor II receptor. Cell 64:1045–1046

Hannigan JH, Armant DR 2000 Alcohol in pregnancy and neonatal outcome. Seminars in Neonatology 5(3):243–254

Harding R, Hooper SB 1996 Regulation of lung expansion and lung growth before birth. Journal of Applied Physiology 81(1):209–224

Harding JE, Johnston BM 1995 Nutrition and fetal growth. Reproduction, Fertility and Development 7:539–547

Horwitz R, Webb D 2003 Cell migration. Current Biology 13(19):R756–R759

James DK, Stephenson T 1998 Fetal nutrition and growth. In: Chamberlain G, Dewhurst J, Harvey D (eds) Clinical physiology in obstetrics, 3rd edn. Gower Medical, London, pp 467–497

Jauniaux E, Gulbis B, Burton GJ 2003 The human first trimester gestational sac limits rather than facilitates oxygen transfer to the foetus: a review. Placenta 24(Suppl A):S86–S93

Johnson MH 2001 Functional brain development in humans. Nature Reviews Neuroscience 2(7):475–483

Karlberg J, Jalil F, Lam B, Low L, Yeung CY 1994 Linear growth retardation in relation to the three phases of growth. European Journal of Clinical Nutrition 48(Suppl 1):S25–S44

Kramer MS 1998 Maternal nutrition, pregnancy outcome and public health policy. Canadian Medical Association Journal 159(6):663–665

Larsen WJ 1993 Human embryology. Churchill Livingstone, New York

Lenz W 1962 Thalidomide and congenital abnormalities. Lancet i:45

Lumey LH 1992 Decreased birthweights in infants after maternal in utero exposure to the Dutch famine of 1944–1945. Paediatric Perinatal Epidemiology 6:240–253

Martyn CN, Greenwald SE 1997 Impaired synthesis of elastin in walls of aorta and large conduit arteries during early development as an initiating event in pathogenesis of systemic hypertension. Lancet 350:953–955

McBride WG 1961 Thalidomide and congenital abnormalities. Lancet ii:1358

Moore T, Haig D 1991 Genomic imprinting in mammalian development: a parental tug of war. Trends in Genetics 7:45–49

Moore KL, Persaud TVN 1998a Before we are born: essentials of embryology and birth defects, 5th edn. Saunders, Philadelphia

Moore KL, Persaud TVN 1998b The developing human: clinically orientated embryology, 6th edn. Saunders, Philadelphia

Moore J, Peters A, Frame S 1984 The relevance of shoe size to obstetric outcome. In: Thomson A, Robinson S (eds) Research and the midwife: proceedings of conference held in the Great Hall, Sparshott House, Manchester Royal Infirmary, November 1983. Department of Nursing, University of Manchester, pp 53–68

Murtha MT, Leckman JF, Ruddle FH 1991 Detection of homeobox genes in development and evolution. Proceedings of the National Academy of Sciences USA 88:10711–10715

Nardo L, Hooper SB, Harding R 1998 Stimulation of lung growth by tracheal obstruction in fetal sheep: relation to luminal pressure and lung liquid volume. Pediatric Research 43:184–190

Phillips DIW 1996 Insulin resistance as a programmed response to fetal undernutrition. Diabetologia 39:1119–1122

Piscione TD, Rosenblum ND 2002 The molecular control of renal branching morphogenesis: current knowledge and emerging insights. Differentiation 70(6):227–246

Rink TJ 1994 In search of a satiety factor. Nature 372:406–407

Robinson JS, Owens JA 1996 Control of fetal growth In: Hillier SG, Kitchener HC, Neilson JP (eds) Scientific essentials of reproductive medicine. Saunders, Philadelphia, pp 329–341

Stedman HH, Kozyak BW, Nelson A et al 2004 Myosin gene mutation correlates with anatomical changes in the human lineage. Nature 428:415–418

Stewart RJC, Sheppard H, Preece R, Waterlow JC 1980 The effect of rehabilitation at different stages of development of rats marginally malnourished for ten to twelve generations. British Journal of Nutrition 43:403–411

Veille JC, Hanson R, Sivakoff M, Hoen H, Ben-Ami M 1993 Fetal cardiac size in normal, intrauterine growth retarded, and diabetic pregnancies. American Journal of Perinatology 10:275–279

Walton A, Hammond J 1938 The maternal effects on growth and conformation in Shirehorse–Shetland pony crosses. Proceedings of the Royal Society of London B 125:311–335

Wang H, Chard T 1992 The role of insulin like growth factor-1 and insulin like growth factor binding protein-1 in the control of fetal growth. Journal of Endocrinology 132:11–19

Wang JX, Clark AM, Kirby CA et al 1994 The obstetric outcome of singleton pregnancies following in vitro fertilization/gamete intrafallopian transfer. Human Reproduction 9:141–146

10 Overview of immunology

Learning objectives

- To review the immune system, identifying the roles of innate and specific immunity.
- To recognize how pregnancy affects the maternal immune system.
- To outline the effects of human immunodeficiency virus (HIV) infection on the functioning of the immune system.
- To discuss the reasons why the fetus is not rejected.
- To appreciate the importance of placental transfer of immunoglobulins.
- To demonstrate an understanding of Rhesus incompatibility and how it is prophylactically treated.
- To appreciate the immunological immaturity of the neonate and why this is relevant to midwifery practice.
- To describe the principles of neonatal immunization.

Introduction

Knowledge of the immune system is important in midwifery for several reasons. First, implantation and the nurture of an immunologically foreign fetus present some interesting questions as to the functioning of the immune system in pregnancy. Some causes of infertility may be related to the immunological rejection of the sperm or fetus. During pregnancy, the maternal immune system alters so the fetus is not attacked, but maternal defences against disease still function. Pregnant women have enhanced immunological responses to bacterial infections. However, they seem to develop increased susceptibility to viral infections and human immunodeficiency virus (HIV)-related problems may increase during pregnancy. Some immunology-related conditions improve during pregnancy and some conditions worsen. Maternal immune adaptations in pregnancy also seem to prepare for possible pathogenic contamination of the placental wound site, during the vulnerable period of the puerperium. Blood group incompatibility and the resulting immune response can compromise the well-being of the developing fetus. The neonate is born immunologically immature but receives some passive immunity, both during pregnancy and neonatally in breast milk.

The immune system is a complex network of specialized cells and chemical signals, which interact providing a defence against infectious organisms. A number of microorganisms are associated with the body. Some, described as commensals, exist within or on their host without causing any harm. Others are beneficial, or symbiotic, like those inhabiting the skin and the gut. However, some organisms, including microbes (bacteria, viruses, fungi) and larger organisms like tapeworms, are potentially damaging and are described as pathogens because they cause disease. The immune system of the human has evolved to detect and eradicate these pathogenic organisms. Pathogens are diverse and numerous and have a rapid rate of replication and therefore are constantly evolving their own mechanisms to combat the host's defence.

The role of the immune system becomes clearly evident when it is compromised such as in acquired immune deficiency syndrome (AIDS) when HIV causes breakdown of the immune system (Fig. 10.1). However, under less extreme conditions both infections and poor nutrition can overwhelm the immune system. To some extent, both the pregnant woman and the neonate are immunocompromised.

As part of their preparation to work in Africa both Zara and James underwent in-depth medical screening to ensure that they were fit enough to undertake this work. Zara has the blood group O rhesus negative and James has the blood group AB negative. As they are both rhesus negative then rhesus incompatibility is not going to occur but what possible complications could arise in the pregnancy as a result of these different blood groups, how could they be recognised and what are the possible treatments that may be required?

The evolution of the immune system

The detection of the presence of pathogens initiates the immune response in the host, stimulating a cascade of interactions, which culminates in a counter-attack on the pathogen. There are two types of immunity: innate immunity and adaptive immunity.

Innate (natural) immunity pre-exists in an organism before any contact with pathogens; it is a collection of genetically encoded responses to foreign pathogens which does not change throughout the lifespan. Innate

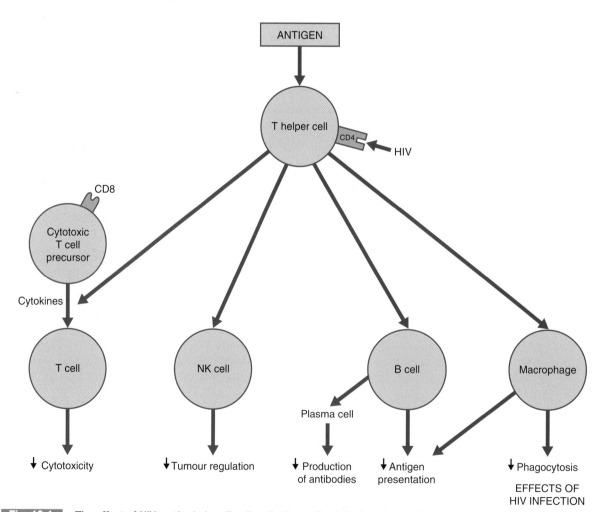

Fig. 10.1 *The effect of HIV on the helper T cell and other cells of the immune system.*

immunity occurs throughout the animal kingdom, occurring in mammals, birds, sponges and worms. It evolved early and is particularly effective against bacteria, probably the earliest form of life on earth. It mounts an immediate non-specific response to an invading microorganism.

The second type of immunity, adaptive immunity, is a mechanism that adapts to the presence of pathogens and becomes more effective with each exposure. As organisms became more complex and colonized new habitats they were vulnerable to a broader range of more recently evolved pathogens such as viruses. Adaptive or acquired immunity occurs exclusively in higher multicellular organisms that have evolved relatively recently such as mammals, birds and some fish. It has evolved in response to increased pressure on survival and augments innate immunity; it is specific and effective at eliminating infection. The adaptive immune system means that, if an animal survives an initial infection by a pathogen, it is usually immune to further illness caused by the same pathogen; this response is utilized in medical vaccination programmes. Although the innate and adaptive systems operate differently, there are many common mechanisms and components. It has been hypothesized that the innate system, though more 'primitive', plays a critical role in viviparity and toleration of the fetal allograft (Sacks, Sargent & Redman 1999).

Overview of the immune system

Innate immunity

Innate immunity is inherent and does not require contact with a pathogen for responses to occur. The responses are mobilized quickly and activated by receptors that respond to a broad range of pathogens. The first line of defence can be considered to be the physical and chemical barriers of the respiratory, reproductive and gastrointestinal systems and skin (Brostoff et al 1991) (Fig. 10.2). Included in this first line of defence are chemical protective mechanisms (such as that provided by lysozyme), the complement system, interferons and phagocytotic activity of the white blood cells (Table 10.1).

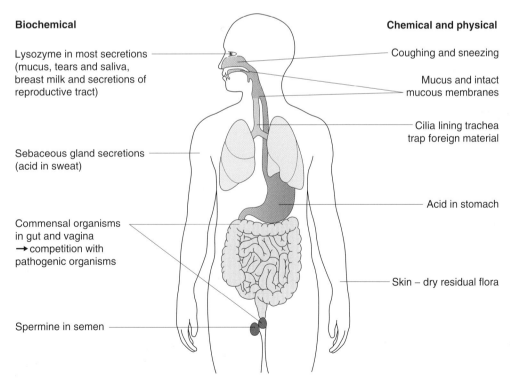

Biochemical

Lysozyme in most secretions (mucus, tears and saliva, breast milk and secretions of reproductive tract)

Sebaceous gland secretions (acid in sweat)

Commensal organisms in gut and vagina → competition with pathogenic organisms

Spermine in semen

Chemical and physical

Coughing and sneezing

Mucus and intact mucous membranes

Cilia lining trachea trap foreign material

Acid in stomach

Skin – dry residual flora

Fig. 10.2 *The main physical and chemical barriers to infection (the 'first lines of defence'). (Reproduced with permission from Brostoff et al 1991.)*

Table 10.1 *Defensive activity of the innate immune system*

Phagocytosis	Neutrophils and macrophages adhere to the surface of the target organism. Adherence is enhanced by opsonins, which form a bridge between the pathogen and the phagocyte. The phagocytic cells produce pseudopodia facilitating the engulfing of the pathogen into a cellular vesicle. Lysosomes fuse with the phagosome and degrade it
Cytotoxicity	Eosinophils and NK cells adhere to targets (opsonins increase efficiency). Eosinophils secrete chemicals, which damage the target cell membrane, causing cell death, and an inflammatory response, which is particularly effective against parasites. NK cells attack body cells expressing viral proteins in their membranes and some tumour cells. The NK cells adhere and release perforin, which penetrates the cell membrane causing cell death
Inflammation	The sequence of events is that the trigger (such as a bacteria signal) stimulates vasodilation and increased blood flow and delivery of blood cells (redness, heat and pain). Vascular permeability (swelling) occurs, which increases exudation and extracellular fluid (oedema), phagocyte invasion, promotion of fibrin wall enclosing infection and tissue repair

Lysozyme

Lysozyme, which is sometimes described as 'the body's own antibiotic', is an enzyme that attacks the unique polysaccharide structure of bacterial cell walls. It is an abundant component of body secretions such as blood, sweat, tears, nasal secretion, breast milk and the mucous secretions of the reproductive tract.

The complement system

The complement system involves over 30 interacting proteins and receptors which form an amplification cascade of defence leading to cytolysis of bacteria, chemotaxis, opsonization and inflammation. As in the blood coagulation cascade, the components of the complement cascade exist in an inactive form that can be triggered and activated. There are three pathways of activation: the classic pathway, which involves antibodies (or immunoglobulins), the alternative pathway, where the complement cascade is activated by the unique composition of an organism's cell wall (activator surfaces), and the mannan-binding lectin pathway. The outcome of complement activation is the formation of a cylindrical assembly of proteins that form a tube that perforates the surface of target cells. The perforation permits fluid to enter cells by osmosis so the bacterial cells swell and burst. The complement cascade stimulates the release of histamine and kinins from mast cells and enhances phagocytosis. The complement system may be a factor in a number of diseases such as multiple sclerosis, asthma, Alzheimer's disease and autoimmune diseases such as systemic lupus erythematosus.

Interferons

Interferons carry out non-specific defence against viruses, bacteria, parasites and tumour cells. They are cytokine proteins produced by cells that have been infected by a virus. Viruses replicate by 'hijacking' the mechanism of protein synthesis in the cells that have been infected. Therefore, the cell is diverted to make viral mRNA, which is translated into viral proteins and assembled as viral particles. Interferons interfere with the production of new proteins; they damage the viral mRNA and inhibit protein translation, not just in the infected cells but in neighbouring uninfected cells, subsequently creating a barrier around the viral infection, which prevents the viral replication. Interferons also stimulate macrophages and natural killer (NK) cells. Interferons produced by genetic engineering are used therapeutically.

Leukocytes and lymphocytes

The cells of the immune system are leukocytes and lymphocytes. Although they are described as white blood cells, some of the cells spend very little time in the circulation whereas others never enter the vascular system at all and remain in the lymphatic system, spleen or other tissues. Blood cells are derived from a single population of stem cells in the bone marrow. These precursor cells have the potential to divide extremely rapidly and can differentiate into several types of end cell. After radiation for cancer treatment, the destroyed stem cells have to be replaced by a bone marrow transplant; very few cells need to be transplanted for regeneration of a mature population of cells.

Phagocytes

Neutrophils and macrophages are phagocytic white blood cells that can engulf and digest foreign cells and unwanted matter through the processes of phagocytosis, cytotoxicity and the generation of an inflammatory response. The cells that mediate the innate immunity are the granulocytes: neutrophils, monocytes, eosinophils and basophils. Neutrophils, also known as polymorphonuclear leukocytes, are the most numerous white blood cells, forming about 40–70% of the circulating white blood cells. On entering the circulation, neutrophils, which have a lifespan of a few days, cease cell division. Neutrophils are motile and exhibit chemotactic behaviour, moving through a concentration gradient towards chemical messengers, such as those released from dividing bacteria or activated platelets, towards the site of infection. Neutrophils have multilobed nuclei, which aids diapedesis (the amoeboid movement of the cells through the gaps between the capillary endothelial cells). Neutrophils usually reach the site of infection and begin phagocytosis within about 90 minutes of the initial stimulation; they generate a vigorous and lethal respiratory burst which kills them and the engulfed pathogen

Adherence of the phagocyte to the target cell can be increased by opsonization. Opsonins are chemical tags that have specific binding sites for the phagocyte and the pathogen, thus increasing the efficiency of recognition and adherence of the phagocyte. Effectively, the opsonin acts as a bridge between the pathogen and the phagocyte, so promoting phagocytosis. Monocytes circulate for a short time in the bloodstream and then migrate to tissues and organs where they differentiate into macrophages and exhibit characteristics specific to their host tissue. Less than 7% of circulating white blood cells are monocytes, but macrophages are abundantly distributed in the body tissues and are particularly dense around blood vessels, the gut walls, the genital tract and lungs. Monocytes are the largest white blood cell and have a characteristic horse-shaped nucleus. They are also phagocytes and have a longer lifespan than neutrophils. Circulating monocytes respond more slowly than neutrophils, reaching the site of infection within about 48 hours, but they have a greater capacity for phagocytosis, engulfing more material than neutrophils.

Natural killer cells

Natural killer (NK) cells are lymphocytes which attack infected cells and cells that might be cancerous. They alter the target cell's plasma membrane so water and ions diffuse in; consequently the cell swells and lyses.

Acquired or specific immunity

Lymphocytes, which constitute about a third of the circulating white blood cells, coordinate the adaptive immune responses. These small lymphocytes have relatively little cytoplasm, few organelles and no granules. B lymphocytes are responsible for humoral activity, mediated by immunoglobulins (antibodies) which attack bacteria and viruses in body fluids. T lymphocytes are responsible for cell-mediated immunity (see Ch. 1). Small lymphocytes also circulate in the lymphoid system and spend much of the time resident in the organs of the lymphoid system. The lymphoid system is the main site of the adaptive immune responses. Fluid leaks out of the blood capillaries into the intercellular spaces. Some of the fluid re-enters the blood capillary (see Ch. 1) but some enters the lymphatic capillaries. This lymph fluid, therefore, has a similar composition to plasma, except that the protein component of plasma is retained within the blood vessels so lymph fluid has a low protein content. Ultimately the lymph fluid is transported through lymph vessels to the thoracic duct and back into the bloodstream. The small lymphocytes burrow out of the small veins as they pass through the lymph nodes and so enter the lymphoid tissue. Each lymphocyte spends minutes in the bloodstream compared with hours residing in the lymphoid system.

Antigen recognition

The classical view is that cells of the immune system differentiate between self and non-self, identifying foreign cells and pathogens and attacking them. It has been hypothesized that the immune system differentiates between dangerous and non-dangerous rather than between self and non-self or infectious or non-infectious (Gallucci & Matzinger 2001). The surface of a pathogen is embedded with a unique combination of atoms and charges that can be recognized by the immune cells, almost like an insignia or signature of 'foreignness' or non-self. The whole cell that engenders an immune response is described as an antigen, although the antigenic cluster itself is called the epitope. The antigen generates an immune response against itself. An antigen is often the pathogenic cell itself but can also be a substance secreted by a pathogen, for instance bacterial toxins, or substances from non-pathogenic sources, such as plant pollens, resulting in allergic responses, or chemicals such as synthetic vaccines. Only certain parts of the entire antigen are immunogenic; these parts bind antibodies and activated lymphocytes. Most naturally occurring antigens have numerous antigenic determinants that can mobilize several different lymphocyte populations. Large chemically simple molecules (such as plastics) have little immunogenicity. Antigenicity depends on the ability of the host to identify the substance as an antigen; there are variations in individual responses.

Small lymphocytes have high-affinity surface receptors that specifically recognize antigens presented on the surface of foreign cells and pathogens. Each small lymphocyte has a single type of specific antigen receptor, unlike the cells of the non-specific immune system, which have many different types of receptor on each cell. However, there are many types of small lymphocyte, thus as a population they can recognize and bind to a diverse range of antigens. There are over 100 million pathogenic epitopes. Each person has, at birth, a population of small lymphocytes consisting of clones, each of a few cells. A clone is a few identical small lymphocytes each of which has many copies of the same antigen receptor on its surface. The population of lymphocytes has the capability, described as its repertoire of receptors, to respond to a vast number of antigens, most of which are unlikely to be encountered in a lifetime. Initially the number of cells expressing cells for any particular antigen is small and this clone will remain small unless the antigen reacts. So one of the first steps in mounting an effective immune response is to expand the clone by increasing the number of cells expressing the same antigen.

There are far more antigen receptors than there are human genes encoded for by DNA (about 100 million epitopes and only 100 000 different human genes). It is hypothesized, therefore, that each antigen receptor site is coded for by five or six randomly selected genes. As there are several hundred possible genes involved, the random selection of a few genes that can be cut and spliced (somatic recombination) can produce enough combinations to make all the 100 million epitope-binding sites. However, in this random production of antigen receptors, some lymphocytes will possess receptors for the body's own antigens. In the fetal thymus, clonal deletion takes place, which results in the destruction of self-reactive T lymphocytes. Any T lymphocyte binding to specialized cells presenting self-epitopes on the surface will be stimulated to undergo apoptosis. Self-reactive B lymphocytes do not need to be destroyed because they require a signal from a T lymphocyte (helper T cell) before they can function. It is important that the immune system has self-tolerance and does not harm cells or molecules that are not recognized as antigenic otherwise the host would be damaged (as happens in autoimmune diseases).

Clonal selection and immunological memory

The immune response to a second and subsequent exposure to the antigen is faster and more effective than the first exposure (Fig. 10.3). The primary adaptive response, on the first exposure, is slow to develop, perhaps taking 7–14 days, and then builds slowly to a peak about 2 weeks later. The time for the response to become evident is termed the 'incubation period'. Then symptoms become apparent until the immune response has become effective. The secondary adaptive response, when the host subsequently encounters the antigen, develops sooner, lasts longer and is more effective so signs of infection or symptoms may be prevented. On first exposure, the small numbers of lymphocytes binding the antigen are stimulated to undergo rapid cell division. A single lymphocyte can divide fast enough to produce 64 000 daughter cells in 4 days. As the new cells, also bearing receptor sites specific to the stimulating antigen, are produced they mature and differentiate. Some members of the new population of lymphocytes are active in attacking the cells bearing the antigen. Most clone cells become antibody-secreting cells. Others become memory cells, which have a long life and continue to circulate as a permanently enlarged clone of lymphocytes capable of recognizing specific antigens and mounting an immediate response. Effectively, the initial immune response is boosted by repeated exposure.

Individuals have immunity to an antigen if their immune system can mount a fast and effective specific response to that antigen. The role of a vaccine is to stimulate the immune response and increase the clonal size without causing the illness. Effective vaccines can be in the form of killed whole organisms, harmless organisms, substances with similar epitopes, synthetic epitopes or inactivated toxins (Table 10.2). Some antigens are more effective at triggering clonal expansion, such as rubella (German measles) virus, which is highly antigenic; thus after primary exposure the host rarely acquires the infection again. Other pathogens, such as *Neisseria gonococcus* (causing gonorrhoea) and *Treponema pallidum* (causing syphilis), are only weakly antigenic; therefore there are no effective vaccines available.

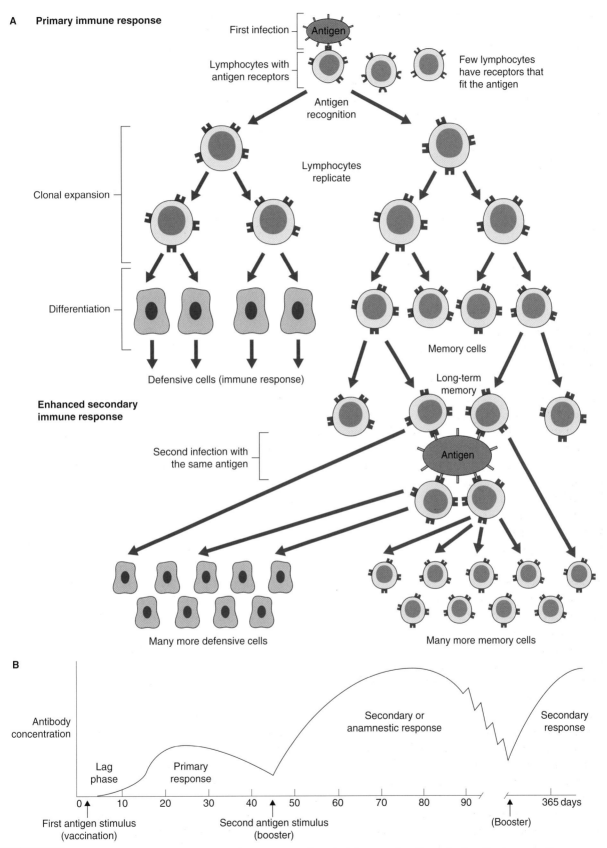

A   Primary immune response

First infection — Antigen

Lymphocytes with antigen receptors

Few lymphocytes have receptors that fit the antigen

Antigen recognition

Lymphocytes replicate

Clonal expansion

Differentiation

Defensive cells (immune response)

Memory cells

Long-term memory

Enhanced secondary immune response

Second infection with the same antigen

Antigen

Many more defensive cells

Many more memory cells

B

Antibody concentration

Lag phase

Primary response

Secondary or anamnestic response

Secondary response

0   10   20   30   40   50   60   70   80   90   365 days

First antigen stimulus (vaccination)

Second antigen stimulus (booster)

(Booster)

Fig. 10.3   *A The enhanced secondary immune response after clonal expansion; B graph of antibody production following exposure to antigen. (A reproduced with permission from Stewart 1997.)*

Table 10.2 *Types of acquired immunity*

Active Natural	Artificial	Passive Natural	Artificial
Clinical or subclinical disease	Vaccines: dead or extract attenuated toxoids	Congenital (across placenta) Colostrum	Antiserum Antitoxin Gamma globulin

---

Case study 10.1

Melanie is expecting her first baby. She attends the midwives' clinic at 11 weeks' gestation concerned over the welfare of her unborn baby. Her 3-year-old nephew, Michael, whom she sees regularly, has German measles.

- What factors would the midwife need to consider in advising Melanie over her concerns?
- Would there be any specific investigations to carry out?

Passive immunity

Resistance to a specific pathogen, acquired by previous exposure or deliberate immunization resulting in clonal expansion, is active immunity. However, sometimes, the effect of infection can be disastrous before the immune system has time to mount a response. Passive immunization can overcome this by providing temporary resistance in the form of products from a donor source. Passive immunization causes destruction of the pathogenic cells without creating clonal expansion so its effects are not permanent. An individual who has no prior immunity but is exposed to antigens or a potentially dangerous disease is given antibodies. Examples include treatment following a bite from a rabid dog or anti-D immunization following potential exposure to Rhesus-incompatible antigens (see below). The transfer of placental antibodies to the fetus and consumption of antibodies in colostrum and breast milk by the neonate are also examples of passive immunity.

Case study 10.1 looks at an example of exposure to German measles.

Lymphocytes

There are two types of lymphocytes: those that mature in the bone marrow, called B lymphocytes, and those that mature in the thymus, called T lymphocytes.

B lymphocytes

On binding to an antigen, B lymphocytes undergo clonal expansion producing two types of daughter cells: memory cells and plasma cells. The plasma cells synthesize and secrete large amounts of antibodies (immunoglobulins), which are specialized glycoproteins. Antibodies enable other components of the immune system to attack the precise organism bearing the antigen fast and effectively. There are five classes of antibody (Table 10.3); these differ in the structure of the 'Y'-shape of the tail, which affects whether the antibodies bind in groups or singly (Fig. 10.4). The antigen receptor on B lymphocytes is a surface immunoglobulin (sIg) closely resembling the structure of the antibody-binding site that will bind to the same antigen. The binding of the B cell to the epitope is relatively straightforward in that the antigen is intact or native, whereas T lymphocytes bind only to processed antigens. However, antigen binding by a B lymphocyte usually requires helper T-cell activity before clonal expansion can take place.

T lymphocytes

T lymphocytes stimulate other B and T lymphocytes and are involved in the response to viral infection, graft rejection and suppression of hypersensitivity reactions. There are three subsets of T lymphocytes: helper T cells, suppressor T cells and cytotoxic T cells. Molecules on the cell surface, which are involved in mediating cell function, can be identified using monoclonal antibodies and used to differentiate subpopulations of cells. The system of nomenclature is based on the cluster of differentiation (CD) system. Cytotoxic and suppressor cells express CD8 protein markers in the plasma membrane; these cells recognize and destroy infected cells which express specific antigens.

T helper cells express CD4 proteins, and are sometimes called CD4 cells. Helper T cells interact with macrophages and produce cytokines, which activate and regulate other components of the immune system. Cytokines are soluble polypeptides with a short range and lifespan that are also synthesized by lymphocytes and macrophages. They can induce fever, stimulate lymphocytes, stimulate antigen expression and potentiate the destruction of tumour cells. Cytokines include interleukins, interferons, tumour necrosis factor (TNF) and some colony-stimulating factors.

Table 10.3	Classes of antibodies
Antibody	**Role and characteristics**
IgG	Most abundant antibody (85% circulating antibody), found in blood and all fluid compartments including cerebrospinal fluid. Produced in large amounts at secondary adaptive response, therefore represent 'history' of past exposure to pathogens. Long lasting. Can diffuse out of bloodstream to site of acute infection and can cross placenta. Act as powerful opsonins bridging phagocyte and target cell. Important in defence against bacteria and activation of the complement system via the classic pathway
IgM	IgM molecules join in groups of five 'IgM pentamers', therefore tend to aggregate antigens into a clump that is a target for phagocytes and NK cells. Large molecules so cannot diffuse out of bloodstream. Very powerful activators of complement, important in immune responses to bacteria. First antibody produced when the body is confronted by a new antigen
IgA	Mostly in secretions such as saliva, tears, sweat and breast milk, especially colostrum. Link in groups of two to three. Protects body by adhering to pathogen and preventing its adherence to body cavity. Cannot activate complement or cross placenta
IgE	Tail binds to receptor on mast cells so involved in acute inflammation, allergic responses and hypersensitivity. Binding sites for antigens on larger parasites such as worms and flukes. Some people have IgE for common harmless environmental proteins such as pollen, fur, house dust mite and penicillin
IgD	Rarely synthesized; little is known about its functions. Large, found only in blood. May be involved in antigen stimulation of B cells

Helper T cells induce proliferation of lymphocytes, stimulate antibody production by B lymphocytes and enhance the activity of cytotoxic T lymphocytes.

The receptor for HIV is the CD4 protein expressed not only by T cells but also by macrophages and possibly other cells. HIV reduces the number of helper T cells by inducing apoptosis so none of the immune mechanisms work effectively. Infection of macrophages shifts the profile of cytokines produced, which contributes to wasting and acute respiratory distress syndrome. Macrophages can act as a reservoir of the virus.

There are at least three forms of T helper cells: Th0, Th1 and Th2 cells, which are classified on the basis of their cytokine secretion. The dendritic cells present the antigen to T helper cells and direct them to differentiate into either Th1 or Th2 cells. When the resting T helper cells are initially activated, they become Th0 cells which have characteristics of both Th1 and Th2 cells; Th0 cells are then further activated and differentiate into either Th1 or Th2 cells depending on the type of threat. This pathway of differentiation is controlled by the cytokine secretion of the dendritic cell. Secretion of interleukins IL-12 and IL-10 by the dendritic cell drives the differentiation of Th1 and Th2 cells, respectively (Fig 10.5).

The Th1 response tends to be initiated by viruses, cancer, yeasts and intracellular bacteria (e.g. *Mycoplasma pneumoniae* or *Chlamydia*). The outcome of the Th1 response is a cell-mediated response and the secretion of gamma-interferon (INF-γ), IL-2, lymphotoxin and granulocyte–macrophage colony-stimulating factor (GM-CSF) which activate cytotoxic T cells and NK cells. Other bacteria, parasites, toxins and allergens predominantly trigger a Th2 response and secretion of IL-3, IL-4, IL-5, IL-6, IL-10 and IL-13 which activate eosinophils, leukocytes and B lymphocytes (which produce antibodies). The Th1 and Th2 systems suppress each other; the Th1/Th2 balance is important. For instance, some viruses produce proteins that mimic IL-10 and drive the differentiation of TH0 cells into Th2 cells which are less effective at attacking viruses so viral survival is enhanced. In pregnancy, the Th1/Th2 balance shifts in favour of Th2; this down-regulation of Th1-induced cellular immunity and enhancement of Th2-induced humoral responsiveness in the maternal immune system in pregnancy is mediated by progesterone effects and is important in preventing fetal rejection (see below).

Suppressor T cells limit the activity of the immune cells and prevent damage to the body's own cells. Cytotoxic T cells produce toxic and perforating substances that kill any of the body's own cells that have been infected; effectively they turn the immune response off when the antigen has been eliminated.

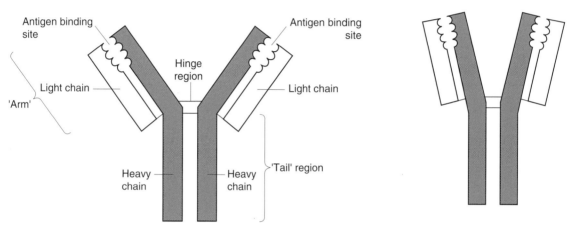

A B-cell surface immunoglobulins are receptors for antigens; B the antibody molecule is a hinge-like structure that allows binding to two antigens. (Reproduced with permission from Stewart 1997.)

T lymphocytes have antigen receptors on their surface, formed of two peptide chains that contain the binding site for a specific epitope. However, the T lymphocyte cannot bind to an epitope unless it is has been processed and presented to the T lymphocyte by one of the host's own cells. Antigen-presenting cells (APCs) are dendritic cells, B lymphocytes and macrophages that bind the antigen and phagocytose it, degrading its protein. The resulting epitope fragments are displayed in the cleft of the major histocompatibility complex (MHC) molecule (Box 10.1) on the surface of the APC (Fig. 10.6). Helper and suppressor T lymphocytes bind only to epitopes processed in this manner. Cytotoxic T cells recognize the epitopes of intercellular pathogens, such as viruses, that are incorporated into the cell membrane during cell replication of an infected cell harbouring the virus.

Interaction of B and T lymphocytes

B lymphocytes and T lymphocytes interact (Fig. 10.7). The B lymphocyte binds to the native (intact) antigen via the sIg receptors on its cell surface. The antigen is then internalized by the B lymphocyte and processed so fragments appear on its cell surface associated with the MHC molecule. In this form, the T lymphocytes can recognize it so helper T cells are activated, producing the signal that allows the B lymphocyte to start cell division and differentiation.

Interaction of the innate and adaptive immune systems

The innate system is an integral part of the immune response. It initiates an immune response by the

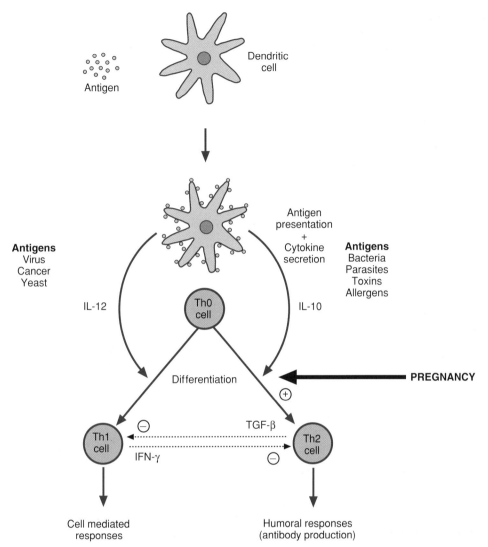

Fig. 10.5 *The differentiation of T helper cells into either Th1 or Th2 cells depends on the type of antigen presented by the dendritic cells and the pattern of cytokine secretion. The outcome of the Th1 response is predominantly cell-mediated, whereas the Th2 response facilitates production of antibodies. The Th1 and Th2 responses are mutually suppressive. In pregnancy, the Th2 response is enhanced, which is important in preventing fetal rejection.*

macrophages processing an antigen in association with the MHC and presenting it to lymphocytes; this is called signal 1. The full response requires adjuvants, such as endotoxin, which produce signal 2, proinflammatory cytokines or co-stimulatory surface molecules. This signal conveys the biological significance of the antigen and effectively instructs the adaptive system to respond (or not). Signals 1 and 2 stimulate T cells to become effector Th1 or Th2 cells. Macrophages secrete cytokines which activate other macrophages, NK cells and granulocytes.

Acceptance of the fetus

Humans are 'outbred'. The genetic diversity resulting from sexual reproduction means that the fetus is phenotypically unique and immunologically distinct from both of its parents. The fetus has a unique combination of histocompatibility antigens. The fetus is classified as an allograft: foreign tissue from the same species but with different antigenic make-up. There is a marked antigenic difference between the maternal tissues and the paternally inherited antigens expressed

The major histocompatibility complex

Each person has a unique configuration of MHC antigens or molecules on the surface of their cells (except monozygous twins who have identical MHC). MHC molecules are a marker of 'self' and are synonymous with human leukocyte antigen (HLA). MHC molecules present the antigens to T cells. There are different classes of MHC molecules, which present antigens with different effectiveness. MHC molecules restrict helper T cells to interact with immune cells that have already bound to the epitope for which the T cell also has an antigen receptor. It is these cells that are involved in rejection of transplanted tissue, as all MHC molecules are different. Tissue grafts have increased survival if there is some similarity in MHC structure between the donor and recipient (hence the need for tissue typing) and if drugs are used to suppress the immune response.

Antigen processing by the APC. (Reproduced with permission from Stewart 1997.)

by the fetus. If tissue from the offspring is grafted on to its mother, a strong maternal immune response is mounted and the tissue is rejected. It seems surprising therefore that the mother does not reject the fetus because of its foreign antigens. Medawar (1953) proposed several possibilities to explain why the fetus is not rejected: as fetal tissue is antigenically immature it may not express normal antigens, the uterus may be a privileged site (or not in contact with fetal tissue), or pregnancy may affect the maternal immune system and normal immune responses.

Fetal antigen expression

Fetal tissue does express antigens and immunocompetence from an early stage (Manyonda 1998). MHC antigens, albeit in smaller amounts, are present on embryonic cells from the time of implantation throughout the pregnancy. Paternal antigens are apparent at the eight-cell stage of the cleavage and major histocompatibility antigens become present later in cell division. The zona pellucida and early trophoblast have glycoprotein coatings, which may limit the cell-mediated immune responses. Immunological problems are usually not a problem prior to implantation because the endometrium secretes immunosuppressive factors.

The uterus as a privileged site

Both the mother and other individuals reject grafts of fetal tissue because fetal tissue expresses antigens. Maternal responses to transplanted tissue remain competent in pregnancy; a pregnant mammal rejects tissue from the father of the fetus and tissue from the fetus grafted to areas other than the uterus. Some tissues, such as parts of the eye and brain, lack components required in immune responses or are not accessible to them (Niederkom 1990). These sites are immunologically privileged and can accept transplanted tissue with fewer problems. However, the uterus is not a privileged site as was suggested (Billingham 1964); the development of ectopic pregnancies shows that the uterus is not a uniquely immunoprivileged site. The increased vascularization of the pregnant uterus allows efficient delivery of lymphocytes and other maternal immune cells so non-fetal allogenic tissue transplanted in the uterus is rejected

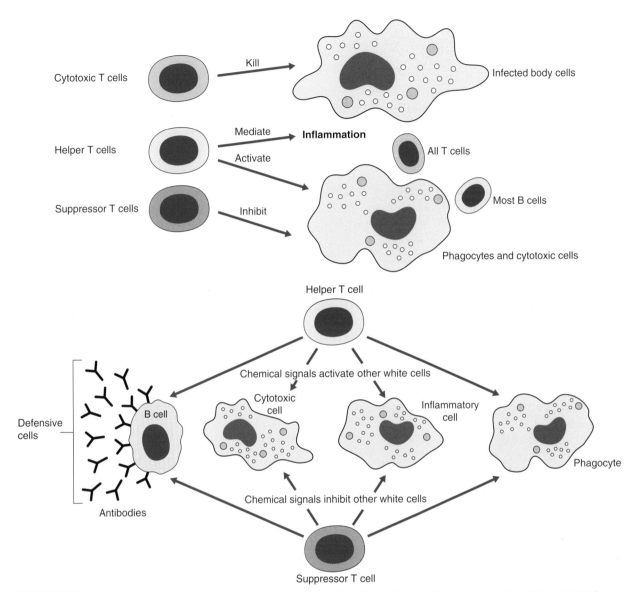

(Beer & Billingham 1974). Maternal and placental tissue are closely situated and in close proximity.

The chorion and trophoblast as a barrier

The fetus is separated from the mother by the placenta and fetal membranes. It is suggested that the chorionic membranes are resistant to maternal rejection and can protect the fetus from maternal antibodies and immune cells. The placenta and chorion originate from cells derived from the fertilized zygote, which are therefore genetically and antigenically different to the

maternal cells. Maternal blood bathes the chorionic villi (see Ch. 8) and is therefore in close contact with tissues derived from the zygote with non-maternal antigens. This means that maternal blood containing immunologically responsive cells is in apposition with the syncytiotrophoblast (outer layer of non-mitotic cells; see Ch. 8).

Some cytotrophoblast cells (the dividing cells underlying the syncytiotrophoblast) penetrate the syncytiotrophoblast layer to form the cytotrophoblast columns, which anchor the villi to the maternal tissue. During implantation and placental development, other invasive trophoblast cells and fragments break away from the mass of placental tissue and enter the uterine veins and maternal venous system. It is this extravillous (non-villous) trophoblast that remodels the uterine spiral arteries to allow increased maternal blood flow to the intervillous space (see Ch. 8). This extravillous trophoblast layer of cells therefore makes extensive contact with the maternal tissue. Some of the cells breach the trophoblast and invade the maternal blood system, forming minute emboli which lodge in the pulmonary circulation where they are destroyed. However, even within the maternal circulation, the extravillous trophoblast cells do not appear to provoke a normal inflammatory or immune response (Johnson & Christmas 1996). So the trophoblast appears to provide an insulating barrier, protecting the fetus from the immunologically responsive maternal cells.

The trophoblast cells do not express MHC class I molecules (HLA-A and HLA-B) or class II molecules (Sacks et al 1999) so they are not recognized by cytotoxic T lymphocytes. Non-trophoblastic placental cells, such as macrophages and stromal cells, do express fetal HLA antigens but are separated from the maternal cells by the HLA-negative trophoblastic barrier. Placental macrophages seem to have diminished ability to present antigens. Effectively, the trophoblastic tissue is presented to the mother's immune system as antigenically neutral. However, the expression of non-classical HLA-G antigen on the trophoblast cells protects the tissue from cytotoxic T lymphocyte activity and inhibits NK cells which recognize and lyse cells that are deficient in class I HLA expression.

The mother's immune response

The mother does respond immunologically to fetal antigens on the trophoblast or entering the maternal circulation; the placenta seems to be a site of active tolerance. Both lymphocytes and antibodies that recognize fetal antigens are present in maternal blood in pregnancy. In fact, an immune reaction by the mother to the paternal histocompatibility antigen seems to be essential for a successful outcome of pregnancy. The maternal recognition of fetal antigens stimulates the generation of blocking antibodies (Johnson & Christmas 1996). The blocking antibodies mask the antigenic sites preventing maternal cells from binding to the antigens (Singal et al 1984). They bind fetal cells in the maternal circulation so they do not interact with maternal lymphocytes or cross the placenta to bind to antigenic sites.

It is suggested that a lack of maternal immune response to the fetus could be harmful. The success of fertility and pregnancy is enhanced when the parents are genetically dissimilar (a concept described as 'hybrid vigour'). The incidence of pregnancy where the parents are closely related, as in incest, is far less frequent, thus heterozygosity is promoted within the population. A close relationship between the parents means that the fetal antigens will be more similar to the maternal antigens so the maternal immunological response will be less.

Conversely, embryo implantation into a surrogate mother, where the embryo is less related to the mother than in a normal implantation, has a higher success rate. It has been suggested that unexplained recurrent spontaneous abortion (RSA; more than three consecutive early pregnancy miscarriages) may be due to a failure of maternal immunological adaptation (Fraser et al 1993). Other known causes of RSA include chromosome and endocrine abnormalities, anatomical problems and infections of the mother's reproductive system. It was controversially hypothesized that increased similarities of antigens between parents (described as HLA parental sharing) would result in the fetus having a high degree of antigen similarities with its mother. The mother would then not produce such a strong immune response to fetal cells, with perhaps fewer blocking antibodies, which would prejudice the outcome of the pregnancy. However, immunotherapy treatment for RSA where women are immunized with paternal cells has not been successful (Fraser et al 1993).

Fetal lymphocytes inhibit replication of stimulated lymphocytes in both the mother and unrelated individuals. This may account for the increased number and increased severity of maternal viral infections, especially in the later part of gestation. Trophoblastic cells express high levels of three membrane-bound complement-regulatory proteins that thwart potential complement-mediated damage to the trophoblast by either the classic or alternative pathways (Rooney et al 1993).

The placenta is in contact with fluids containing high concentrations of progesterone, corticosteroids and hCG (human chorionic gonadotrophin), which may act as local immunosuppressants and inhibit the effectiveness of immune cells. The uterine endometrium has extensive numbers of white blood cells, constituting up to a third of endometrial cells (Bulmer 1989). From early pregnancy, numbers and activity of monocytes and granulocytes progressively increase. The macrophages are highly activated and secrete substantial amounts of interleukin and IgE, which may play a vital role in immunosuppression and rapid non-specific anti-inflammatory activity. T lymphocytes are present but B lymphocytes are uncommon. Cytotoxic activity and interferon production by NK cells decreases but uterine large granular leukocytes (U-LGL) activity increases. These U-LGL cells seem to be hormonally regulated as they occur in decidualized tissue in extrauterine ectopic pregnancies. They have low cytolytic activity and are probably not involved in removal of damaged embryonic cells or regulating trophoblastic invasion. However, they do produce cytokines, which are important in immunosuppression and growth regulation. IgA, secreted from the cells lining the uterine tubes, may also be important in protecting the uterine environment. It is suggested that a pregnancy-specific adjuvant, signal P produced by the placenta, has opposing effects, activating components of the maternal innate immune system and suppressing the adaptive responses (Sacks et al 1999). Signal P may also be responsible for the remission of autoimmune disease, such as rheumatoid arthritis and multiple sclerosis, in pregnancy. However, suppression of T-cell activity increases susceptibility to viral infections and to specific intracellular pathogens such as *Listeria*.

In summary, human pregnancy is a unique immunological situation. It takes place in the specialized environment of the uterus protected by the decidua. The immunological challenge intensifies very gradually and is moderated by hormones and cellular signals from maternal and fetoplacental sources which, together with fetal cells and DNA, can access the maternal compartment. The fetus avoids rejection because the trophoblast does not express MHC class I or II molecules and the maternal adaptive immune responses are suppressed.

Effects of pregnancy on the immune system

The maternal immune response is affected by pregnancy. The number of white blood cells, particularly neutrophils, increases and the cells respond more readily to challenges. hCG stimulates neutrophil production and response (Barriga et al 1994). The high levels of oestrogen and progesterone decrease the number of helper T cells and increase the number of suppressor cells. Yeast infections increase in preg-

nancy, possibly because of the effect of oestrogen on the flora of the reproductive tract.

Local concentrations of corticosteroids around the fetus and placenta suppress phagocytic activity, especially in response to Gram-negative bacteria. This means that pregnant women have a decreased ability to respond to Gram-negative infections of the reproductive tract such as gonococcal infection (Gibbs & Sweet 1994) and *Escherichia coli*. Components of the complement cascade increase from the end of the first trimester so chemotaxis and opsonization are enhanced. Changes like this, which do not occur at the beginning of pregnancy, may be delayed to protect the fetus during implantation.

NK cells and cytokines

NK-cell activity around the uterus is suppressed by local increased concentrations of prostaglandin E_2 (Daunter 1992). This suppression of NK cells may be important in preventing rejection of the fetus. However, maternal resistance to intracellular pathogens such as *Toxoplasma* and *Listeria* may also be reduced (Wegmann et al 1993). The relative proportions of cytokines change in pregnancy. The association between chorioamnionitis and premature rupture of membranes may be related to cytokine-mediated stimulation of proteolytic enzyme released from neutrophils.

Theoretically, the fetus could be perceived by the maternal immune system as a tumour. The conceptus may secrete cytokines, which affect tissues locally, promoting trophoblast growth and fetal survival (Wegmann et al 1993). Concentrations of cytokines that attack tumours, such as TNF, and stimulate NK cell activity, such as IL-2, are suppressed. Local secretion of such cytokines may be important in protecting the fetus without compromising maternal immune function.

Antibodies and B lymphocytes

The levels of most antibodies do not change during pregnancy. However, IgG concentrations may fall. This fall may be due to haemodilution, increased loss in urine or placental transfer of IgG in the third trimester and it can increase the risk of streptococcal infection. Fetal secretion of cytokines may suppress cell-mediated immunity and enhance humoral responsiveness (Wegmann et al 1993). Systemic lupus erythematosus (SLE), an autoimmune condition causing tissue damage in the joints and kidneys, has an increased 'flare-up' frequency in pregnancy, which may be related to enhanced activity of B lymphocytes. This enhanced responsiveness by B lymphocytes may compensate for decreased T lymphocyte activity. B lymphocytes may also produce blocking antibodies which protect the fetus from attack by maternal T lymphocytes.

T lymphocytes

T lymphocytes are involved in graft rejection and could therefore pose a serious threat to the fetus. However, T-cell function is suppressed in pregnancy, especially in the first trimester (Nakamura et al 1993). Circulating numbers of T lymphocytes are lower and they have decreased ability to proliferate, to produce IL-2 and to kill foreign cells. Ratios of helper and suppressor cells change and the Th1/Th2 balance is shifted in favour of Th2, generating non-inflammatory responses that are compatible with trophoblast growth and survival of the fetus. A Th1 reaction in the placenta generates inflammatory responses and is correlated with miscarriage; the cytokines secreted from Th1 cells are harmful in pregnancy as they inhibit embryonic and fetal development (Wegmann et al 1993). Trophoblastic production of cytokines promotes the change in Th1/Th2 balance as does progesterone and the decidual production of leukaemia inhibitory factor. Rheumatoid arthritis, a cell-mediated autoimmune disease, frequently goes into remission during pregnancy, because of the suppression of T lymphocytes. The amelioration of symptoms in pregnancy led to the identification of glucocorticoids as anti-inflammatory agents (Hench 1952). Hormonal changes in pregnancy may augment the suppression of T lymphocytes. As T lymphocytes are involved in the responses to viral infection, pregnant women are at increased risk of viral infections and may experience more severe viraemia.

A number of the immune cells utilize and metabolize tryptophan. The syncytiotrophoblast produces indoleamine 2,3-deoxygenase, an enzyme which catabolizes tryptophan and indirectly suppresses maternal T-cell activity by local tryptophan deprivation, thus optimizing maternal tolerance of the fetus (Thellin et al 2000).

Susceptibility to infection

As maternal immune responses are suppressed in pregnancy and the Th1/Th2 balance altered to favour acceptance of the fetus, pregnant women may have increased susceptibility to infection. Historically, pregnant women were observed to contract smallpox and poliomyelitis more readily. Today, viral hepatitis infections, particularly in developing countries, pose a major threat to pregnant women, who have 10 times the infection rate of non-pregnant women and experience higher morbidity and mortality rates. Women who lack immunity and are exposed to primary cytomegalovirus have an increased susceptibility to infection in pregnancy, which is associated with fetal congenital abnormalities. Pregnant women have an increased susceptibility to listeriosis, influenza, varicella (chickenpox), herpes, rubella (German measles), hepatitis and human papillomavirus. In addition, a number of latent viral diseases and other infections may be of greater severity. These include malaria, tuberculosis (TB), Epstein–Barr virus and HIV-associated infections (Wegmann et al 1993), which can be reactivated in pregnancy. Pregnancy-induced suppression of helper T-cell numbers may be permanent so pregnancy can cause a progression of HIV-related disease. Pregnant women appear to have increased immunological responses to bacterial infection. However, increased incidences of urinary tract infections are probably related to anatomical changes rather than to altered immunological responses.

Microchimerism

Microchimerism is the presence of a tiny number of cells within an individual that have come from another individual. The most common cause of microchimerism is trafficking of fetal cells in pregnancy; fetal cells have been demonstrated to persist in their mother's blood for decades after delivery (Sarkar & Miller 2004). It has been suggested that the higher incidence of autoimmune diseases in women is related to microchimerism inducing a graft versus host disease. Diseases thought to be associated with microchimerism include scleroderma, Graves' disease and SLE. This hypothesis is applicable to men, children and women who have never been pregnant because microchimerism can result from other sources such as transplantation and blood transfusion, cells from a twin or maternal cells as trafficking of cells in pregnancy is bi-directional.

Fetal and neonatal passive immunity

The neonate's immune system is augmented by maternal transfer of immunoglobulins across the placenta to the fetus and in breast milk. The profile of immunoglobulins transported across the placenta and secreted into breast milk depends on specific transport mechanisms for the different classes of immunoglobulin (see Table 10.3). Maternal IgG crosses the placenta into the fetal circulation via a specific active transport mechanism, which is effective from around 20 weeks' gestation but markedly increases in activity from 34 weeks. The mother will produce an immune response to antigens she encounters by producing IgG, which can cross the placenta. Even if maternal levels of IgG are low they will be transported across the placenta. This means that the fetus will receive passive immunization against prevalent pathogens likely to be in the environment from birth. This passive immunity provides essential temporary protection postnatally until the neonate's own immune system matures and produces its own antibodies. Preterm babies are at risk of transient hypoglobulinaemia because they receive less IgG and they are born with immune systems that are less mature than a term infant's. Placental dysfunction limits the transfer of IgG, therefore SGA (small for gestational age) babies have lower levels of IgG. IgA, IgM and IgD do not cross the placenta but are supplied in high concentrations in the colostrum.

As well as beneficial IgG, potentially harmful IgG can cross the placenta. Maternal antibodies to fetal HLA will be generated as the maternal immune system encounters a few fetal cells. The maternal anti-fetal HLA antibodies will cross the placenta but do not cause any damage as they bind to non-trophoblastic cells in the placenta, which bear fetal HLA and can sequester maternal IgG (Johnson & Christmas 1996). In autoimmune diseases, however, pathogenic maternal antibodies can be transferred across the placenta. For instance, antiplatelet antibodies can cross the placenta into the fetus of a mother with autoimmune thrombocytopenic purpura (Johnson & Christmas 1996). The passive transfer of autoimmune antibodies may affect fetal growth and development and can potentially cause at least transient symptoms of the disease in the neonate. The resulting increased risk of

haemorrhage in babies born to mothers with thrombocytopenia means that traumatic procedures, such as fetal blood sampling and instrumental delivery, are avoided.

Preterm babies are at a higher risk of vertical infection of group B streptococci if their mothers are group B streptococcus-positive because they do not gain passive immunity from the placental transfer of immunoglobulins until after 34 weeks' gestation. Term babies do have some degree of protection from group B streptococci and this can be extended if the infant is breastfed. The use of antibiotics in the intrapartum period does reduce the number of group B streptococcal infections in the neonate and so any mother who is found to be group B streptococci positive at any time, not just during the pregnancy, should be offered antibiotic therapy in labour. The antibiotics reduce the bacterial load and so the risk of infection is less although a small number of neonatal infections may still occur (Royal College of Obstetricians and Gynaecologists 2003).

The Rhesus factor and Rhesus incompatibility

In the last trimester, the placental transfer of maternal IgG will include IgG antibodies directed against the fetus's own antigens. Most of these are thought to bind to non-trophoblastic cells bearing fetal antigens within the placental villous tissue so they do not reach the fetal circulation. However, antibodies to the Rhesus antigen can cause severe complications. People who express the Rhesus antigen on their own red blood cell surface do not make antibodies against the Rhesus antigen. These people are described as Rhesus positive (Fig. 10.8). A mother who is Rhesus negative does not have the Rhesus antigen on her own red blood cell surface and her immune system has the capability of making Rhesus antibodies.

The Rhesus antibody is not preformed (existing from birth) like the antibodies of the ABO blood grouping system. Rhesus antibodies are produced if the immune system is given the opportunity to recognize the Rhesus antigen as a foreign protein. In practice, this means that a Rhesus-negative mother could produce antibodies to the Rhesus antigen (which would recognize and attack the red blood cells of a Rhesus-positive fetus) if her immune system encountered it. The immune response can be generated from exposure to red blood cells bearing the Rhesus antigen, for instance

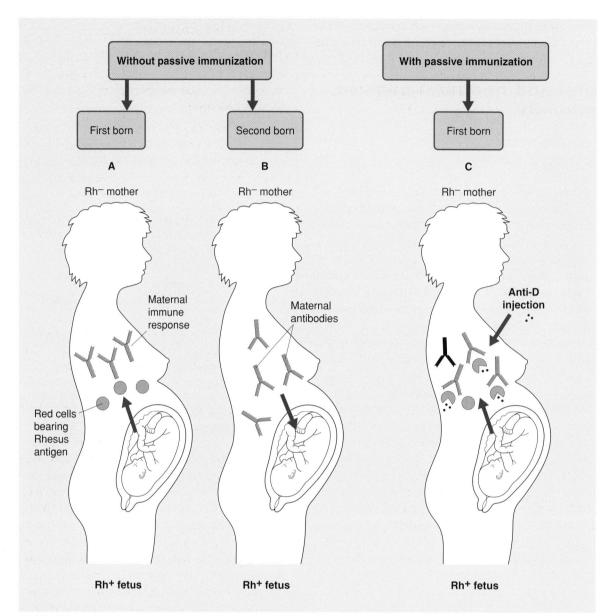

Fig. 10.8   *A Rhesus-negative woman can be sensitized when red cells from a Rhesus-positive fetus cross the placenta into her circulation. B Response comes after delivery of first fetus but in subsequent pregnancies, maternal antibodies can cross placenta and damage fetus. C Anti-D gamma-globulin given to mother immediately at delivery results in fetal Rhesus-positive cells not being recognized by maternal immune systems, so antibodies are not produced to endanger subsequent pregnancy.*

from transplacental leakage of Rhesus-positive fetal cells (following delivery or miscarriage) or in rare instances from a Rhesus-positive blood transfusion.

The occasion when Rhesus isoimmunization is most likely to occur is at the time of the third stage of labour. During placental separation, there is the potential for a small amount of fetal blood (perhaps half a millilitre) to cross into the maternal circulation. If this blood is Rhesus positive, it could stimulate the maternal immune cells to respond by clonal expan-

sion, developing the capacity to produce large quantities of IgG. Once a woman makes antibodies to Rhesus antigens, she is isoimmunized for life. These IgG antibodies can then be transported across the placenta to the fetal circulation late in gestation of a subsequent pregnancy. The binding of maternal Rhesus antibodies to the Rhesus antigen on the surface of the fetal blood cells stimulates lysis of the red blood cells. Severe Rhesus incompatibility is a cause of miscarriage, intrauterine death or hydrops fetalis (abdominal ascites, generalized oedema, polyhydramnios and enlarged placenta). In the neonate, Rhesus incompatibility can result in haemolytic disease of the newborn, where profound haemolysis causes anaemia, increasing the risks of heart failure, hyperbilirubinaemia (jaundice) and kernicterus (see Ch. 15).

Treatment

Prophylactic treatment has been practised since 1967 (Box 10.2) and severe Rhesus D alloimmunization is now rarely seen. Giving passive immunization prevents primary sensitization of the mother and the formation of cells that can produce IgG anti-Rhesus antibody. Although there is actually a complex system of Rhesus antigens, controlled by three pairs of genes (*Cc*, *Dd* and *Ee*), the Rhesus D antigen predominates in incompatibility between mother and fetus.

In accordance with national guidelines (see Annotated Further Reading), the majority of Rhesus-negative women are offered routine anti-D administration at 28 and 34 weeks' gestation. Following delivery of the baby to a Rhesus-negative woman, the Rhesus status of the infant has to be determined. If this proves to be Rhesus positive, then a second test is performed to estimate the amount of fetal blood in the maternal system (Box 10.3) as amounts greater than 4 ml may require more than the standard anti-D dose of 500 international units (i.u.). Although if both parents were Rhesus negative anti-D would not be required, the guidelines do not recommend testing of the father to identify his Rhesus status because it is recognized

---

Box 10.2

Prophylactic anti-D immunoglobulin treatment

- Delivery of Rhesus-positive baby
- Spontaneous abortion
- Therapeutic termination of pregnancy
- Threatened abortion
- Antepartum haemorrhage
- Following external cephalic version of breech presentations
- Following CVS (chorionic villus sampling), amniocentesis or other invasive intrauterine procedure

---

Box 10.3

Maternal and cord blood tests

When a mother is Rhesus-negative, a sample of the baby's blood is obtained from the umbilical cord. Two tests are performed:

1. The baby's blood group and Rhesus factor are identified; if the baby is Rhesus-negative there is no possibility of maternal antibodies forming so the mother does not require anti-Rhesus-D antiserum (known as 'anti-D') administration

2. If the baby is Rhesus-positive or there is another maternal/fetal antibody/antigen incompatibility, then the direct Coombs' test would also be performed. The Coombs' test enables differentiation between normal neonatal haemolysis and abnormal haemolysis caused through the action of maternal antigens. It is based on three variables and is positive when there is reduced haemoglobin in conjunction with an increased reticulocyte count and raised bilirubin levels.

Maternal blood is also taken so that the Kleihauer test (Kleihauer, Hildergard & Bethe 1957) can be performed. The test is based upon the resistance of fetal blood cells to be destroyed by acid (acid elution test). Not only does the test allow the presence of fetal erythrocytes to be detected but the amount of fetal blood transfused into the maternal circulation can be estimated as well. The test is not as accurate if there are maternal haemoglobinopathies present as abnormal maternal erythrocytes (such as sickle cell disease) are also resistant to acid destruction. The test may also be falsely negative if there is an A/B incompatibility as the maternal anti-A and/or anti-B antigens quickly destroy the fetal erythrocytes, especially if the Kleihauer test is delayed, so it should be conducted within half an hour of delivery of the third stage.

It is estimated that a fetal–maternal blood transfer occurs in approximately 50% of pregnancies (Zipursky et al 1959). Usually the amount of blood is small, less than 0.5 ml. However, in 8% of pregnancies it may be in the range of 0.5–40 ml and in 1% it may well exceed 40 ml. In most cases 500 i.u. of anti-Rhesus-D antiserum is enough to eradicate the misplaced fetal erythrocytes. However, if a large transfusion is suspected then larger doses will be administered.

Continued

Maternal and cord blood tests—cont'd

If an exceptionally large transfusion is suspected following the administration of anti-Rhesus-D antiserum the Kleihauer test should be repeated and if fetal cells are still detected then further doses of anti-Rhesus-D antiserum would be administered.

that the apparent father might not be the biological father which may create a difficult situation to manage. It is difficult to justify routine anti-D administration if the father is certain he is Rhesus negative; however, it is prudent to observe the infant for signs of early and excessive jaundice in case the conception occurred outside of the pair bond.

If a small volume (less than 4 ml) of fetal blood has entered the maternal circulation at delivery, the exogenous antibodies ('anti-D') will bind to the fetal Rhesus D antigen and cause cell lysis before the maternal lymphocytes have the opportunity to recognize the antigen and undergo subsequent clonal expansion. ABO compatibility exacerbates Rhesus isoimmunization so ABO incompatibility offers a degree of protection against Rhesus sensitization. If the fetal blood transfused is of a different ABO grouping, the existing natural maternal IgM anti-A or anti-B antigens will rapidly eliminate the fetal blood cells before an immune response can be mounted against the Rhesus D antigen.

Other antibodies

Most antibodies in the ABO system are IgM type so they do not cross the placenta. However, in successive ABO-incompatible pregnancies in group O mothers, a degree of neonatal haemolysis, causing mild neonatal jaundice, may occur. Haemolytic disease can potentially occur with other blood group incompatibilities such as Kell and Duffy. However, the density of these minor antigens on fetal red blood cells is so low that maternal IgG antibodies usually do not elicit a cytolytic effect. Women who require or have had multiple blood transfusions are at risk of developing antibodies to surface antigens which could potentially put their unborn babies at risk.

Vulnerability of the neonate

Neonates are born immunocompromised and are susceptible to infection. The natural flora colonizes and protects the external surfaces of the body, and those membranes that appear internal but come into contact with external pathogens, such as the upper respiratory tract, gut and urinary system. The natural flora may protect by competing with pathogenic microorganisms for resources or by altering the local environment making it less hospitable to pathogens. The fetus in the uterus is sterile because there is no route for colonization. Colonization takes about 6–8 weeks, which is similar to the time it takes for the resident flora of non-pathogenic bacteria to repopulate in NASA astronauts, who are made bacteriologically sterile before a space flight. As the bowel flora produces much of the body's vitamin K requirements, neonates have an increased risk of vitamin K deficiency until the resident flora is established. Colonization processes can be disrupted, for instance, by disinfectant swabs or antibiotic use. Colonization of the neonate begins at birth, with transfer of organisms from the mother's vagina, skin of her hands and breasts and the respiratory tracts of the baby's carers.

Neonatal skin is delicate and easily damaged, thus it can offer a route for opportunistic infection. The umbilical cord, which becomes necrotic, presents a locus for possible infection and offers a potential pathway to the liver. The neonatal defence mechanisms are further compromised by procedures such as blood sampling or insertion of endotracheal or nasogastric tube or intravenous cannulas.

Infants have less efficient immune systems, especially if they are born prematurely or are small at birth. The cells of the immune system are immature and do not function as efficiently in early life; for instance, T lymphocytes have decreased responses and cytolytic function. The phagocytes exhibit decreased phagocytosis and bactericidal activity. Their function in severe illness, such as respiratory distress syndrome or meconium-aspiration pneumonia, is further limited. The complement cascade components at birth are 50–80% of the adult levels.

Active immunization

The immature immune system of the neonate is supported by natural passive immunization from placental transfer of IgG and breast milk provision of IgA. It is also supported by programmes of deliberate immunization. Active immunization requires administration of an antigen in a form that is inactivated and does not produce a disease (Box 10.4). IgG levels start to increase by 3 months so immunization is delayed after birth. However, some protection is required before the immune system is mature. Therefore, immunization programmes are often started when the baby is 3 months old. At about this age, many babies receive the 'triple' vaccine, of pertussis, diphtheria and tetanus antigens presented appropriately. Diphtheria and tetanus elicit strong antigenic responses despite the infant's immature immune system, whereas children are given further doses of pertussis vaccine. Live polio vaccine is given orally at the same time as the 'triple' vaccine. Although theoretically only one dose is required, there are at least three strains and the immune response may not be produced the first time. Measles vaccine is usually delayed until the infant is about 1 year old as maternal IgG, which is present for the first 6–9 months of life, tends to destroy the attenuated organisms of the vaccine before the infant's immune system has time to recognize and respond to them.

Immunization using viral vaccines may be ineffective if the individual has had a recent viral infection, such as a cold. Levels of interferon persist after a viral infection so the virus in the vaccine preparation may not be able to reach concentrations adequate to stimulate the immune system. Therefore, immunization may not be effective until 2–3 weeks after a viral infection. Oral doses of vaccines may be ineffective if their absorption is compromised, for instance with diarrhoea or vomiting. High levels of steroids suppress the immune response, so steroid therapy or overactive adrenal glands can limit the effectiveness of a live vaccine and compromise the immune response. Allergic reactions can occur, especially to vaccines prepared in tissue culture or containing whole cells. Problems with allergic reactions are often associated with vaccines grown in egg-based tissue culture preparations or to which antibiotics have been added. Obviously, a severe reaction to a vaccine precludes its further use. Administration of live vaccines is not recommended in pregnancy. Immunization programmes benefit the health of the population, unfortunately at the expense of the few individuals who may have an extreme reaction to a vaccine with irreversible effects.

Other immunological aspects of pregnancy

Antisperm antibodies in either the male or female partner have been implicated in the causes of infertility (Manyonda 1998). Antisperm antibodies could inhibit spermatogenesis or fertilization. However, the Sertoli cell protects the developing sperm and seminiferous tubules from antibodies and suppressor T cells secrete immunosuppressive cytokines in the epididymis. Some are coated with glycoproteins and lactoferrin, which may be why some antigen sites are evident only after capacitance. Seminal fluid has potent immunosuppressive properties and can inhibit a range of immune responses (James & Hargreave 1988). The presence of antisperm antibodies in the secretions from the genital tracts, rather than in the blood, seems important particularly in male infertility.

Box 10.4

Principles of immunization

Adjuvants
For example, aluminium hydroxide or phosphate. Increases antigenic properties of a vaccine that would otherwise produce only a weak immune response, e.g. triple vaccine of diphtheria, tetanus and pertussis toxins

Toxoid
Bacterial exotoxin treated so it does not cause a disease but still stimulates the immune cells. Examples include treatment of diphtheria and tetanus toxin with formalin

Killed vaccine
Dead organisms such as pertussis, typhoid and paratyphoid. As with toxoid preparations, two or three doses and booster doses are required as only a small number of antigens are introduced each time

Attenuated vaccines
Live organisms that have been cultured to produce non-pathogenic strains. Very effective as organisms multiply within body mimicking a natural infection. Therefore only one dose is required for full immune response (lifetime immunity), e.g. smallpox, poliomyelitis, measles, rubella, TB

The risk of developing antisperm antibodies is increased with exposure to sperm that is excessive, as in prostitutes, or in an inappropriate site, as in homosexual men (Johnson & Christmas 1996). Generation of antisperm antibodies may reflect a lack of immunosuppressive factors in the seminal fluid. It has also been proposed that exposure to semen can positively affect the maternal immune responses (Robertson & Sharkey 2001). Insemination might present a 'priming' event which induces maternal tolerance to paternal antigens in the semen, many of which will also be expressed by the developing conceptus.

Endometriosis, which is deposition of endometrial tissue at non-uterine sites, can be very painful if the tissue becomes inflamed. Severe endometriosis can cause infertility but many women have extrauterine endometrial tissue that neither causes pain nor affects fertility. The cause of endometriosis is not known but an autoimmune aetiology has been proposed.

Pre-eclampsia, inadequate placental development following inadequate remodelling of the spiral arteries, is also suggested to have an immune component (see Ch. 8). The incidence of pre-eclampsia is higher in first pregnancies and in subsequent pregnancies with a new partner, which suggests an immunological mechanism.

The effects of HIV and AIDS in pregnancy are detailed in Box 10.5 and Case study 10.2.

- HIV infection causes decreased numbers of helper T cells, which affect the organization of all the immune responses so the risk of opportunistic and pathogenic infection increases
- In Britain, women usually acquire HIV from sexual exposure and intravenous drug use
- Pregnancy can mask some of the non-specific symptoms of HIV infection, such as fatigue, anaemia and dyspnoea
- HIV can remain latent for years (estimated to be an average 11 years) before AIDS becomes evident
- Progression to symptom development may be accelerated by pregnancy
- HIV can be transmitted to the baby via the placenta, from exchange of body fluids at birth or from the breast milk
- Mothers with HIV may be advised to breastfeed their babies if the risk of fatal malnutrition is considered to be higher than the risk of HIV infection

---

Box 10.5

HIV and AIDS in pregnancy

- HIV (human immunodeficiency virus) causes AIDS (acquired immune deficiency disorder)
- HIV is a retrovirus, which invades cells expressing CD4, including helper T cells, monocytes and neural cells
- A retrovirus contains a single strand of RNA, which is incorporated into the host cell's DNA by an enzyme called reverse transcriptase
- When the infected cell is activated it will produce viral proteins, which can be released and infect other cells

---

Case study 10.2

Mary is 16 weeks' pregnant. She has no fixed abode and has not previously been seen by a health professional in relation to her pregnancy. Mary attends the local hospital antenatal clinic in a state of distress. She informs the midwife that she is an intravenous drug abuser and her best friend has just died from an AIDS-related illness.

- How prepared would you be, as the midwife, to counsel and advise Mary?
- What referrals and expert advice would you seek on her behalf?
- What considerations are needed in relation to the unborn child, in relation to both HIV transmission and Mary's general situation?

- Pregnancy enhances humoral immunity and suppresses cell-mediated immunity so responses to bacterial infection are enhanced but there may be increased susceptibility to viral infections.

- Histoincompatibility, such as the differences in fetal and maternal antigen expression, would normally lead to tissue rejection.

- The trophoblast cells lack classic HLA antigens, which prevent an anti-fetal response, but express HLA-G, which prevents non-specific cytolysis.

- Fetal cells entering the maternal circulation are important in the generation of blocking antibodies, which block any immune response that does occur.

- Maternal IgG is transferred to the fetus late in gestation, which provides the neonate with passive immunization during the period of immunological immaturity. Harmful antibodies against fetal antigens are sequestered by non-trophoblastic tissue in the placenta.

- The birth of a Rhesus-positive baby to a Rhesus-negative woman can initiate an immune response. Prophylactic administration of anti-Rhesus-D immunoglobulin is therefore given after possible or actual exposure.

- The neonate is immunocompromised at birth. Immunization programmes seek to address this lack of immunity.

Application to practice

Pregnancy results in an alteration of the immune system, so normal non-pregnant white cell counts cannot be applied in pregnancy. An understanding of changes within the immune system will enable the midwife to explain the consequences of such changes to the pregnant women.

Midwives may be involved in the administration of some vaccines such as rubella and TB so an understanding of the immune system is required. The interaction of the maternal immune system and the baby is an important aspect of lactation and breastfeeding.

Annotated further reading

Kassianos GC 2001 Immunization: childhood and traveller's health, 4th edn. Blackwell, Oxford
A useful reference source which covers immunization theory and mechanisms together with practical aspects. Each vaccine is considered separately with detailed notes about dosage, use, precautions and side-effects.

Playfair JHL 2000 Immunology at a glance, 6th edn. Blackwell, Oxford
Covers a wide range of immunological topics using clear, well-labelled diagrams to summarize and simplify the mechanisms of immunological processes together with succinct written explanations on facing pages.

Roitt IM, Delves PJ, Rabson A 2004 Really essential medical immunology, 2nd edn. Blackwell, Oxford
A concise version of the origin best-selling textbook Essential Immunology; includes recent developments in immunology such as cellular signalling and hormonal regulation of the immune system.

Royal College of Obstetricians and Gynaecologists 2002 Use of anti-D immunoglobulin for Rh prophylaxis. Clinical guideline. RCOG, London
National Institute for Clinical Excellence 2002 Guidance on the use of routine antenatal anti-D prophylaxis for RhD-negative women. NICE
These two clinical guidelines form the basis of the current use of anti-D in the UK and provide a comprehensive and referenced guide to the use of anti-D.

Royal College of Obstetricians and Gynaecologists 2003 Prevention of group B streptococcus in the neonate. RCOG, London
This evidence-based guideline provides a framework for the management of women who are group B streptococcus positive in order to reduce vertical transmission in the peripartum period.

Sompayrac LM 2003 How the immune system works. Blackwell, Oxford
Clearly explained textbook, illustrated with useful diagrams, which covers progressive development of immune concepts.

Staines N, Brostoff J, James A 1993 Introducing immunology, 2nd edn. Mosby, St Louis
A small volume which introduces the basic concepts of immunology, with sections on immunity, hypersensitivity,

interaction of nutrition and immunity, cancer and transplantation.

Wood P 2001 Understanding immunology (Cell & molecular biology in action series), 2nd edn. Wiley, Chichester
A clear, well-illustrated introductory text which is written for students with little prior knowledge of immunology.

....

References

Barriga C, Rodriguez AB, Ortega E 1994 Increased phagocytic activity of polymorphonuclear leukocytes during pregnancy. European Journal of Obstetrics, Gynecology and Reproductive Biology 57:43–46

Beer AE, Billingham RE 1974 Host responses to intra-uterine tissue, cellular and fetal allografts. Journal of Reproduction and Fertility 21:49

Billingham RE 1964 Transplantation immunity and the materno-fetal relation. New England Journal of Medicine 270:720

Brostoff J, Scadding GK, Male D, Roitt IM 1991 Clinical immunology. Gower Medical, London

Bulmer JN 1989 Decidual cellular responses. Current Opinion in Immunology 1(6):1141–1147

Daunter B 1992 Immunology of pregnancy: towards a unifying hypothesis. European Journal of Obstetrics, Gynecology and Reproductive Biology 43:81–95

Fraser EJ, Grimes DA, Schulz KF 1993 Immunization as therapy for recurrent spontaneous abortion: a review and meta-analysis. Obstetrics and Gynecology 82:854–859

Gallucci S, Matzinger P 2001 Danger signals: SOS to the immune system. Current Opinion in Immunology 13:114–119

Gibbs RS, Sweet RL 1994 Clinical disorders. In: Creasey RK, Resnik R (eds) Maternal-fetal medicine: principles and practice, 3rd edn. Saunders, Philadelphia, pp 639–703

Hench PS 1952 The reversibility of certain rheumatic and non-rheumatic conditions by the use of cortisone or of the pituitary adrenocorticotrophic hormone. Annals of Internal Medicine 36:1

Hunt JS 1992 Immunobiology of pregnancy. Current Opinion in Immunology 4:591–596

James K, Hargreave TB 1988 Immunosuppression by seminal plasma and its possible significance. Immunology Today 5:357

Johnson PM, Christmas SE 1996 Immunology in reproduction. In: Hillier SG, Kitchener HC, Neilson JP (eds) Scientific essentials of reproductive medicine. Saunders, Philadelphia, pp 284–291

Kleihauer E, Hildergard B, Bethe K 1957 Demonstration von fetlem Hamoglobin in den Erythrocyten eines Blutausstrichs. Klinische Wochenschrift 35:637

Kovats S, Main EK, Librach C, Stubblebine M, Fisher SJ, DeMars R 1990 A class I antigen, HLA-G, expressed in human trophoblasts. Science 248:220–223

Ljunggren H-G, Karre K 1990 In search of the 'missing self': MHC molecules and natural killer cell recognition. Immunology Today 11:237–244

Manyonda IT 1998 The immune system. In: Chamberlain G, Broughton Pipkin F (eds) Clinical physiology in obstetrics, 3rd edn. Blackwell, Oxford, pp 129–163

Medawar P 1953 Some immunological and endocrinological problems raised by the evolution of viviparity in vertebrates. Symposia of the Society for Experimental Biology 11:320–338

Nakamura N, Miyazaki K, Kitano Y, Fujisaki S, Okamura H 1993 Suppression of cytotoxic T-lymphocyte activity during human pregnancy. Journal of Reproductive Immunology 23:119–130

Niederkom JY 1990 Immune privilege and immune regulation in the eye. Advances in Immunology 48:191

Robertson SA, Sharkey DJ 2001 The role of semen in induction of maternal immune tolerance to pregnancy. Seminars in Immunology 13:243–254

Rooney IA, Ogelesby TJ, Atkinson JP 1993 Complement in human reproduction: activation and control. Immunological Research 12:276–294

Sacks G, Sargent I, Redman C 1999 An innate view of human pregnancy. Immunology Today 20:114–118

Sarkar K, Miller FW 2004 Possible roles and determinants of microchimerism in autoimmune and other disorders Autoimmunity Reviews 3:454–463

Singal DP, Butler L, Liao S-K, Lui K 1984 The fetus as an allograft: evidence for anti-idiotypic antibodies induced by pregnancy. American Journal of Reproductive Immunology 6:145

Staines NA, Brostoff J, James A 1993 Introducing immunology, 2nd edn. Mosby, St Louis

Stewart M 1997 Growing and responding. Open University, Milton Keynes, pp 185, 188–191, 193, 200

Thellin O, Coumans B, Zorzi W, Igout A, Heinen E 2000 Tolerance to the foeto-placental 'graft': ten ways to support a child for nine months. Current Opinion in Immunology 12:731–737

Wegmann TG, Lin H, Guilbert L, Mosmann TR 1993 Bi-directional cytokine interactions in the maternal–fetal relationship: is successful pregnancy a TH2 phenomenon? Immunology Today 15:15–18

Zipursky A, Hull A, White FD, Israels LG 1959 Foetal erythrocytes in the maternal circulation. Lancet i:451

....

11 Physiological adaptation to pregnancy

Introduction

During the 279 days (40 weeks) of an average pregnancy (measured from the last menstrual period), maternal physiology changes remarkably to support the development of the fetus and to prepare the mother for labour and lactation. The changes begin in the luteal phase of the menstrual cycle, before fertilization and implantation, as progesterone secretion from the corpus luteum is initiated. If fertilization is successful, levels of progesterone and oestrogen progressively increase. Together, they orchestrate many of the changes to the maternal physiology in pregnancy.

Chapter case study

Zara is now in the third trimester of her pregnancy. She informs her midwife that she is not sleeping well, and James prefers to sleep in the spare room as Zara's loud snoring and frequent waking disturbs him. When Zara does sleep, she experiences vivid dreams that cause her to wake suddenly. Her sleeping is not helped by the fact she often wakes up feeling hungry and thirsty and is having to make increasingly frequent visits to the toilet. Zara has now stopped working and finds that the only way she can cope is to a have a rest in the afternoon. She often falls asleep sitting in front of the television for 3–4 hours and says this afternoon sleep is less disturbed than the night time. What physiological changes could account for these changes in Zara's sleep pattern and what reasons would you give to reassure Zara that this is normal? Why do you think Zara is able to sleep more peacefully in the afternoon? Are there any advantages in these behavioural changes and might they be preparing Zara to care for her newborn baby?

Endocrine changes in pregnancy

The physiological changes of pregnancy are controlled by an alteration in hormone secretion. The trophoblastic cells produce human chorionic gonadotrophin (hCG), which stimulates secretion from the corpus luteum, increasing ovarian steroid hormone production. As the placenta develops, it also produces oestrogen and progesterone. However, placental endocrine function is much broader as the placenta synthesizes a range of hormones and releasing factors that are similar to those originating from the hypothalamus and other maternal endocrine organs (see Ch. 8). Placental products may reach both the maternal and fetal circulation, thus regulating maternal physiology and fetal development.

Steroid hormones

Steroidogenesis depends on interaction and cooperation between the mother, placenta and fetus. The mother is the source of precursors for placental progesterone production and the fetus is the source of precursors for placental oestrogen production. Placental progesterone is used for fetal synthesis of testosterone, corticosteroids and mineralocorticoids. Progesterone is known as the hormone of pregnancy; it stimulates respiration, relaxes smooth muscle (of blood vessels, uterus and gut), increases body temperature, increases sodium and chloride excretion, and may act as an immunosuppressant in the placenta (Picciano 2003). Progesterone levels increase gradually at first (Fig. 11.1). There is little change in progesterone concentration between the 5th and 10th week, but after the 10th week the levels increase more markedly as the placenta becomes the main site of steroid hormone synthesis. By the end of the first trimester, levels of progesterone are 50% higher than luteal levels and by term the levels have increased three-fold. The syncytiotrophoblast uses maternal cholesterol as a substrate for progesterone synthesis. Placental production of progesterone is adequate by 5–6 weeks. A primate pregnancy can survive ovariectomy (oophorectomy, removal of ovaries), although the corpus luteum is essential in other mammalian pregnancies (Johnson & Everitt 2000). Human corpus luteal production of 17α-hydroxyprogesterone decreases from 6 to 9 weeks as placental production increases. Measurement

of the different progesterone metabolites can be used to assess placental function.

The primary oestrogen of pregnancy is oestriol. Early in pregnancy, oestrone and oestradiol levels increase but oestriol levels do not begin to rise until the 9th week when the fetal adrenal glands begin to synthesize the precursor dehydroepiandrosterone sulphate (DHEAS) from placental pregnenolone; DHEAS is the substrate for placental production of oestriol (see Ch. 3). Maternal and placental steroids are conjugated in the fetal liver and adrenal glands into water-soluble, and thus biologically inactive, forms (so the fetus is protected from the effect of the steroids' precursors). As the 16-hydroxyl precursor originates only from the fetal liver, production of oestriol indicates fetal well-being. In 'at risk' pregnancies, decreased oestriol may indicate fetal distress and the need to induce premature delivery, although as an index of placental function and fetal well-being it has largely been replaced by Doppler investigation and biophysical profiling. Oestriol measurement is part of the Bart's (triple) test for Down's syndrome (see Ch. 7). Oestrone and oestriol levels increase about 100 times and oestradiol levels about 1000 times during the course of the pregnancy (Blackburn 2003). The oestrogens promote the growth of the endometrium and breasts, enhance myometrial activity, increase sensitivity to carbon dioxide, increase pituitary prolactin secretion, promote myometrial vasodilation, stimulate fluid retention, alter the composition of connective tissue and increase the sensitivity of the uterus to progesterone in late pregnancy.

Human chorionic gonadotrophin

The main function of hCG is to maintain production of steroid hormones from the corpus luteum in early pregnancy until the placenta can take over. hCG has a very similar structure to that of luteinizing hormone (LH)—as well as follicle-stimulating hormone (FSH) and thyroid-stimulating hormone (TSH)—and acts on the LH receptors, prolonging the life of the corpus luteum. hCG is produced initially by the outer cells of the blastocyst which are the cells that differentiate into trophoblast cells and subsequently into the placenta. The syncytiotrophoblast, which evolves from the trophoblast (see Ch. 8), continues to produce hCG. It is secreted, and can be detected before implantation, in vaginal secretions and in the maternal circulation (see

Fig. 11.1 *Increasing concentrations of oestrogen and progesterone during pregnancy.*

Fig. 11.1). As the lacunae begin to be formed by the invading syncytiotrophoblast, the hCG diffuses into the maternal blood and significant levels can be detected. Measurable urine values are present 2 weeks after fertilization; home pregnancy tests are very sensitive and specific. The presence of hCG confirms successful fertilization as, apart from very rare production by certain gut tumours, it is not produced by other tissues (Iles & Chard 1991). hCG is produced by hydatidiform moles (see Ch. 8); following evacuation of a molar pregnancy, urinalysis for the presence of hCG is continued for 2 years to exclude choriocarcinoma.

Production of hCG is maximal at 8–10 weeks and then falls to a low plateau level that is maintained throughout the pregnancy. hCG levels, therefore, reflect the placental transformation from an organ of invasion to one of transfer. Persistently low levels of hCG are associated with abnormal placental development or ectopic pregnancy. If hCG is given to non-pregnant women, the corpus luteum is maintained and progesterone secretion rises. Alternatively, antibodies to hCG given to a pregnant woman cause the corpus luteum to regress. hCG, rather than LH, is used to induce ovulation in fertility treatment. By 4–5 weeks, the placenta and fetus are synthesizing significant amounts of steroid hormones and can assume endocrine control of the pregnancy. hCG has thyroid-hormone-stimulating properties, affecting appetite and fat deposition, and also affects thirst, release of antidiuretic hormone (ADH) and other osmoregulatory changes (Davison et al 1990). It also promotes myometrial growth and inhibits myometrial contractility (Kornyei, Lei & Rao 1993). The effects of hCG are summarized in Box 11.1.

Human placental lactogen

As hCG levels fall, there is increased secretion of human placental lactogen (hPL). The levels of hPL increase in parallel with the size of the placenta and correlate well with fetal and placental weight. hPL has a similar structure and properties to growth hormone and prolactin; it is a single polypeptide chain and is lactogenic and stimulates growth of both maternal and fetal tissues. hPL appears to protect the fetus from rejection, and low levels of hPL are associated with pregnancy failure and spontaneous abortion. hPL is antagonistic to insulin, resulting in increased maternal metabolism and utilization of fat as an energy sub-

> **Box 11.1**
>
> ## Effects of human chorionic gonadotrophin (hCG)
>
> - Luteotrophic effect on corpus luteum that maintains synthesis and secretion of oestrogen and progesterone
> - Stimulates placental progesterone production
> - Possesses thyrotrophic activity
> - May be responsible for nausea and vomiting
> - Stimulates maternal thyroid gland; increases appetite and fat deposition
> - Increases sensitivity to glucose
> - Decreases osmotic threshold for thirst and release of ADH
> - Suppresses maternal lymphocyte response thus preventing rejection of the placenta
> - Promotes myometrial growth
> - Inhibits myometrial contractility
> - Modulates trophoblastic invasion
> - Affects fetal nervous tissue development
> - Affects male sexual differentiation and stimulates fetal testes to produce testosterone
> - Stimulates fetal adrenal glands to increase production of corticosteroids

strate. This diabetogenic effect of pregnancy reduces glucose uptake by maternal cells, thus making more available for fetal use (see below). hPL is also called human chorionic somatomammatrophin.

Relaxin

Relaxin is produced by the corpus luteum, and to a lesser extent by the myometrium and placenta. Levels of relaxin are highest in the first trimester. Relaxin has a role in the softening of elastic ligaments of pelvic bones and has been used clinically to enhance cervical ripening during induction of labour (see Ch. 13). Relaxin acts with progesterone to maintain uterine quiescence; it may also suppress oxytocin release and affect gap junction permeability. The softening and relaxation of the pelvic ligaments allow mobilization and growth of the uterus into the abdomen. Sometimes women experience low-back pain in pregnancy, which is associated with the stretching of these ligaments. Relaxin is also thought to be involved in endometrial differentiation during embryo implantation, wound healing and, possibly, tumour growth and progression (Ivell & Einspanier 2002).

Adrenal and pituitary hormones

The adrenal gland increases in both size and activity during pregnancy. Oestrogen stimulates adrenal cortisol production by inhibiting the metabolism of cortisol and increasing the synthesis of cortisol-binding protein (transcortin). Progesterone increases tissue resistance to cortisol by competing at the receptor level and binding to the cortisol-binding protein; this also results in an increase in cortisol production. Corticotrophin-releasing hormone (CRH) from the hypothalamus affects the release of adrenocorticotrophin (ACTH), melanocyte-stimulating hormone (MSH) and β-endorphin from the anterior pituitary gland. ACTH stimulates the adrenal gland production of cortisol. Cortisol levels increase in response to stress, including increased cardiac output and decreased fasting glucose levels in the second trimester of pregnancy. Both CRH and ACTH are also produced by the placenta as well as by the maternal hypothalamic–pituitary axis; the placental hormones are subject to different feedback control mechanisms and may be important in initiating labour (see Ch. 13).

The increase in circulating levels of cortisol has a positive effect on certain conditions, such as rheumatoid arthritis and eczema. This observation led to the clinical use of exogenous cortisol as a treatment for these conditions. Both progesterone and oestrogen act synergistically to increase aldosterone production. Adrenal synthesis of androgens, oestrogen, progesterone and cholesterol increases in pregnancy.

The pituitary gland enlarges markedly during pregnancy. Much of the increase is due to increased number and activity of cells of the anterior pituitary gland. The gonadotrophs decrease in number as the raised oestrogen concentration inhibits release of FSH and LH, which are barely detectable for most of the pregnancy. However, under the influence of progesterone and oestrogen, the prolactin-secreting cells increase from 10% of the cell population to 50%. Prolactin levels increase progressively through the pregnancy to values 20 times higher than the prepregnant level. Production of ACTH increases, resulting in increased adrenal activity. MSH synthesis also increases so hyperpigmentation may occur (Elling & Powell 1997). Pregnant women frequently observe that they tan more deeply or develop irregular pigmented patches. Towards the second half of pregnancy, oxytocin production from the posterior pituitary increases.

Thyroid hormones

The hypothalamic–pituitary–thyroid axis undergoes marked changes in pregnancy. Oestrogen, hCG and altered hepatic and renal function cause levels of tri-iodothyronine (T_3), thyroxine (T_4) and thyroid-binding globulin (TBG) to change which is important to support the altered metabolism of pregnancy. Oestrogen stimulates hepatic synthesis of TBG by 50–100 times resulting in increased total amounts of T_3 and T_4, although free concentrations remain within normal physiological limits. hCG has mild TSH activity so it stimulates both the production of T_4 and the deiodination of T_4 to T_3 in the peripheral tissues. Pregnancy mimics hyperthyroidism in a number of respects, for instance by increasing body temperature, and stimulating appetite and feelings of fatigue. In 70% of pregnant women, the thyroid gland enlarges because thyroid activity increases and renal iodine loss is increased. Ancient Egyptians used the observation of pregnancy-induced goitre (thyroid gland hypertrophy) as confirmation of pregnancy (Glinoer & Lemone 1992). The thyroid gland hypertrophies as it attempts to increase uptake of iodine for hormone synthesis. Nowadays, with better diets and iodine supplementation of table salt, unless women are at the threshold of iodine deficiency, goitre is rare in pregnancy. Basal metabolic rate increases by 20–25% from the 4th month of pregnancy but much of the increase is related to the increased surface area of the mother and the increased work she has to do maintaining maternal and fetal tissue requirements. Nausea and vomiting have been linked not only to the changes in hCG (see above) but also directly to the rise in free T_4.

The reproductive system

The blood vessels

The vasculature of the uterus undergoes a number of remarkable and unique changes during pregnancy. Uterine blood flow increases: the vessel diameter of the spiral arteries increases and vascular resistance falls (see Ch. 8). These changes accommodate the increased blood flow to the placenta, which is maintained under conditions of low blood pressure. The coursing of blood through the enlarged tortuous arteries produces a uterine 'souffle', which may be heard through a stethoscope or with a sonicaid.

The uterus

The uterus increases in all dimensions and also changes shape (see Chs 2 and 13) during pregnancy. Uterine hyperplasia begins after implantation and is driven by oestrogen and growth factors (it occurs if the embryo is implanted in an extrauterine site) (Blackburn 2003). Early growth results in thickening of the uterine wall. The endometrium thickens into the decidua. The three layers of the myometrium become clearly defined as the uterine muscle undergoes initial hyperplasia (development of new fibres) and subsequent hypertrophy (increase in length and thickness of existing muscle fibres). Later uterine growth is mostly hypertrophy and hyperplasia of the myocytes and remodelling of connective tissue which is driven by distension as the fetus enlarges. The muscle fibres increase in length and width as the timing and speed of the myometrial action potentials change and the muscle cells increase their content of actin and myosin, gap junctions, sarcoplasmic reticulum and mitochondria.

In early pregnancy, the uterine isthmus increases from about 7 mm to 25 mm (Fig. 11.2). From 32 to 34 weeks, the isthmus forms the lower uterine segment (LUS). As effacement commences (at approximately 36 weeks), the external os is incorporated into the LUS (see Ch. 13). The blastocyst usually implants in the fundus (upper part) of the uterus. By 12 weeks, the fetus fills the uterine cavity and the fundus can just be palpated (felt) at the pelvic brim. By 20 weeks the fundus reaches the maternal umbilicus and by 8 months it

reaches the sternum. As the uterus expands during pregnancy, it loses its anteverted and anteflexed configuration and becomes erect, tilting and then rotating to the right under the pressure of the descending colon. The uterus changes from its non-pregnant pear-shape and becomes spherical and then cylindrical.

Uterine quiescence is mediated by progesterone, relaxin, nitric oxide (NO) and prostacyclin (also known as prostaglandin PGI_2). The uterus is never completely quiescent and exhibits low-frequency activity throughout the pregnancy (as it does in the non-pregnant state). Braxton Hicks contractions are painless contractions that are measurable from the first trimester of the pregnancy. These contractions do not dilate the cervix but assist in the circulation of blood to the placenta. The contractions are usually irregular and weak, unsynchronized and multifocal in origin. The contractions of the circular muscles are less than those of the longitudinal ones (Blackburn 2003). The uterine ligaments soften and thicken under the influence of oestrogen, resulting in increased mobility and capacity of the pelvis.

The cervix

The cervix increases in mass and width during the pregnancy. Oestrogen increases the blood supply to the cervix resulting in a lilac coloration and softer tissue texture; the water content of the cervix also changes. The collagen fibre bundles become less tightly bound (see Ch. 13). The cervical mucosa proliferates and the glands become more complex and secrete thickened mucus, which forms a plug or operculum protecting the cervix from ascending infection. The plug is held laterally by projections of thickened mucus in the mouths of the mucus-secreting glands. It

Anatomical internal os

Histological internal os

Isthmus

7mm

Non-pregnant   12 weeks   16 weeks

Fig. 11.2 *The uterine isthmus increases from about 7 mm to 25 mm in the early part of pregnancy. (Reproduced with permission from Miller & Hanretty 1998.)*

is this plug that is released as 'the show' at the onset of labour when the cervix starts to be drawn up to form the lower uterine segment.

The vagina

Blood flow to the vagina increases likewise, resulting in softer vaginal tissue which is more distensible. The lilac coloration of the vagina and cervix was traditionally recognized as being an indicator of pregnancy (described as Jacquemier's sign). The increased blood flow means that the pulsating of the uterine arteries can be felt through the lateral fornices (Osiander's sign). The increased vascularization of the vagina can result in increased sensitivity and sexual arousal. Venous engorgement results in increased vascular transudation, which together with the increased cervical mucus production results in an increased vaginal discharge. The vaginal discharge (leucorrhoea) has a low pH (because of the effect of raised oestrogen levels on the vaginal flora) and is thick and white with an inoffensive odour. Oestrogen also stimulates the vaginal epithelial cell division so the cells acquire a distinctly boat-shaped appearance (which should not be mistaken for carcinoma cells). Early in pregnancy, the hypertrophied corpus luteum, which is about 3–5 cm long, distends from the ovarian surface; this may be palpated in some women or visualized during endoscopic examination in women undergoing egg retrieval for IVF (in vitro fertilization).

The breasts

In early pregnancy, vascularization of the breasts increases. This tends to result in a marbled appearance of the skin owing to the marked dilation of the superficial veins. The breasts, specially the nipple areas, may feel sensitive and tingle because of the engorgement of blood. (Changes to the breast in pregnancy are described in more detail in Ch. 16.)

The signs of pregnancy are summarized in Box 11.2.

The cardiovascular system

The most notable physiological changes occur in the cardiovascular system in preparation for the increased demands of maternal and fetal tissues (Fig. 11.3).

Box 11.2

Signs of pregnancy
- Amenorrhoea
- Softening of vagina and cervix
- Increased blood flow to vagina and cervix causing lilac coloration (Jacquemier's sign)
- Pulsating of uterine arteries (Osiander's sign)
- Tingling and sensitive breasts with dilated superficial veins marbling surface
- Nausea and vomiting, possible changes in taste
- Increased frequency of urination as uterus compresses bladder
- Increased pigmentation of skin
- Bleeding gums
- Tiredness
- Increased appetite and thirst

These changes are caused both indirectly by hormones (oestrogen, progesterone, prostaglandins and other vasoactive substances) and directly by mechanical effects and as a result of the increased load on the system. Heart disease affects less than 1% of pregnancies and causes 10 deaths per million in England and Wales, but symptoms of heart disease (such as breathlessness, palpitations, fainting and oedema) are present in over 90% of pregnant women (de Swiet 1998a). Superimposed on a pre-existing cardiac disease state, pregnancy may be dangerous and even potentially fatal. Measurement of cardiovascular system parameters is technically difficult and notoriously variable. Measurements obviously have to be indirect and are very sensitive to changes such as emotion, exertion and posture. In the research literature, there are many inconsistencies, some of which reflect differences in standardization of conditions (de Swiet 1998a).

Blood volume

Total blood volume increases by 30–50%, more in multiple pregnancies (Brown & Gallery 1994). The rise correlates well with birth weight and, as it begins early in pregnancy, the mechanism of these early changes in the cardiovascular system is thought to be hormonally driven. The increase in blood volume correlates with birth weight. It has been disputed whether the increase in volume (sodium and fluid retention) precedes the increased vascular space ('overfill' hypothesis) or whether the changes are stimulated by

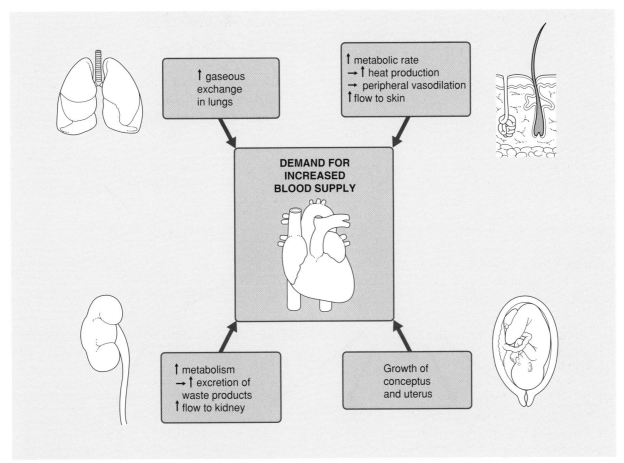

Fig. 11.3 *The changed distribution of blood flow in pregnancy.*

relative hypovolaemia (increased vascular capacity), known as the 'underfill' hypothesis (Schrier 1992). The arguments for the 'underfill' hypothesis are supported by the observation that blood pressure falls before plasma volume expands (Duvekot et al 1993). Often in early pregnancy women feel faint, suggesting that the physiological compensation of the underfill has yet to occur.

Oestrogen stimulates angiogenesis (formation of new blood vessels and vascular beds) and increases the blood flow to the tissues. Oestrogen affects the distribution of collagen in the tunica media of the large vessel walls, increasing venous distensibility. Oestrogen also stimulates endothelium-dependent vasodilatation, by increasing synthesis of NO (a potent vasodilator) and vasodilatory prostaglandins and inhibiting the release of endothelin-I (a vasoconstrictor). Production of both prostacyclin and NO increases in pregnancy (Morris, Eaton & Dekker 1996). These signals affect placental blood flow, particularly remodelling of the spiral arteries (see Ch. 8).

Progesterone relaxes vascular smooth muscle causing vasodilatation and decreased peripheral resistance. Therefore, the circulatory system increases its capacity and is relatively underfilled. Both progesterone and oestrogen increase water retention by affecting the renin–angiotensin system (RAS) and oestrogen increases hepatic angiotensinogen production. This results in a rise in angiotensin II, which increases renal fluid resorption and stimulates the production of aldosterone. All components of the RAS increase in pregnancy, and sensitivity to angiotensin II decreases (so blood pressure does not rise). Renin is produced by the uterus, placenta and fetus, as well as the kidney. Levels of renin are 2–3-fold higher than before pregnancy. These changes in the RAS may mediate the oestrogen-stimulated angiogenesis and increased cell growth and division.

Progesterone stimulates a 10-fold increase in the amount of circulating aldosterone. Progesterone is antagonistic to aldosterone but some progesterone is converted to deoxycorticosterone, which has mild aldosterone-like properties. Progesterone augments its effects on the circulatory volume by resetting the thirst centres in the hypothalamus and increasing thirst. Progesterone also lowers the sodium threshold for the RAS and blocks the vasopressive activity of angiotensin II in pregnancy (Blackburn 2003). The net result of the changes in oestrogen and progesterone is an increase in vascular resistance followed by increased sodium and water retention and expansion of the circulating volume (Fig. 11.4).

Cardiac output

Blood volume and cardiac output increase in parallel (Fig. 11.5). Cardiac output increases by 30–50%, an average increase of 1.5 l/min from 4.5 to 6 l/min. Cardiac output rises quickly in the first trimester and is maintained throughout the pregnancy. The increase in cardiac output is greater in multiple pregnancies. Cardiac output is affected by posture: when the pregnant woman lies supine, her uterus impedes venous

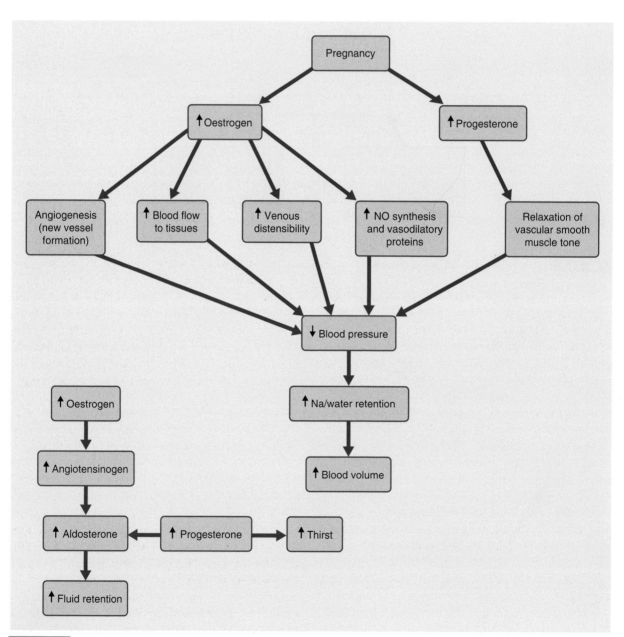

Fig. 11.4 *The likely pathways for blood volume increase in pregnancy.*

A

B

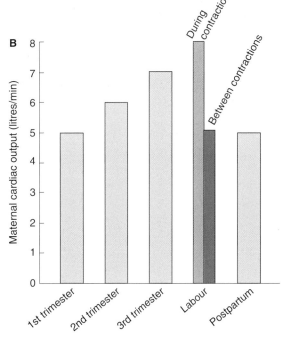

Fig. 11.5 *The parallel increase in A blood volume and B cardiac output during pregnancy. Blood volume is increased up to 40%, thus increasing the load on the heart. (Reproduced with permission from Chamberlain, Dewhurst & Harvey 1991. B after Whitfield CR (ed) 1986 Dewhurst's textbook of obstetrics and gynaecology for postgraduates, 4th edn. Blackwell Scientific, Oxford.)*

return from the inferior vena cava resulting in an apparent decrease in cardiac output. The measured drop in cardiac output in the third trimester, observed by a number of researchers, was most probably the result of measurements being made with the woman lying supine (Mabie et al 1994). In labour, cardiac output increases by about 2.0 l/min.

Cardiac output is the result of two variables: heart rate and stroke volume (see Ch. 1). In pregnancy, both heart rate and stroke volume increase. Heart rate increases soon after implantation, by about 20% (an average of 15 beats more per minute) from about 70 to 85 beats per minute. Stroke volume typically increases by about 10% from 64 ml to 71 ml. Steroid hormones and prolactin may affect the myocardium directly. Oestrogen stimulates an increased accumulation of components of the myocardial cells and increases contractility (Duvekot & Peeters 1998).

Heart

The early changes relating to the heart occur early in the pregnancy and are caused by hormonal changes.

Later, the heart is displaced upwards by elevation of the diaphragm and is rotated forward so the electrocardiogram (ECG) changes and the location of the apex beat is directed forward to the anterior chest wall. The heart increases in size by an average of 70–80 ml (about 12%). This increase is due to increased filling and oestrogen-stimulated cardiac muscle hypertrophy. The remodelling of the heart that occurs in pregnancy in response to increased blood volume and workload is analogous to the ventricular hypertrophy of an athlete's heart in continuous training. The pregnant woman's heart is dilated with increased contractility. Increased blood volume results in an increase in venous return and therefore increased atrial size. The heart sounds change because the mitral valve closes marginally before the closure of the tricuspid valve; thus the first heart sound is louder with an exaggerated split. Many pregnant women (92–95%) develop innocent (non-significant) systolic murmurs in pregnancy. The increased blood flow through the mammary blood vessels may be perceived as a possible heart murmur; this is more common in lactation. The net result of increased contractility, increased venous return, cardiac hypertrophy, decreased peripheral resistance and increased heart rate is increased cardiac output.

Arteriovenous difference

Increased cardiac output exceeds increased oxygen consumption (especially early in pregnancy when cardiac output increases considerably and oxygen consumption is relatively low) so more oxygen is returned to the heart from venous circulation compared with prepregnant values and the arteriovenous (AV) difference is smaller. The AV difference is 34 ml in mid-pregnancy rising towards term but is always less than the non-pregnant values of about 45 ml (de Swiet 1998a). The higher return of oxygen to the heart suggests that the commonly measured decrease in haemoglobin concentration is not physiologically inadequate and the relatively small increase in total haemoglobin (oxygen-carrying capacity) is more than sufficient to compensate for increased oxygen requirements. This supports the argument that the term 'physiological anaemia' is inappropriate (see p. 263). The increased AV difference, especially early in the pregnancy before increased oxygen consumption, means that early fetal development and organogenesis occur in an environment which is adequately oxygenated despite the maternal spiral arteries not connecting with the intervillous spaces in the early part of pregnancy (see Ch. 8).

Blood pressure

Normal pregnancy has relatively little effect on arterial blood pressure. Despite increased cardiac output and increased vascular capacitance, there is relatively little change in systolic pressure in pregnancy. However, diastolic blood pressure is lower in the first two trimesters and returns to prepregnant values in the third trimester. Both the development of new vascular beds and the relaxation of peripheral tone by progesterone result in decreased resistance to flow. This is augmented by a change in the profile of prostaglandins produced. The levels of the prostaglandin PGE_2 and prostacyclin, which stimulate vasodilation, rise early in pregnancy. NO (formerly known as endothelium-derived relaxing factor, EDRF) also appears to play an important vasodilatory role (Palmer et al 1987). The most important stimulator for NO production is shear stress such as that generated from a pulsatile blood flow (Maul et al 2003).

The increased difference between diastolic and systolic blood pressure means that for much of the pregnancy the pulse pressure is increased. Hypotension, particularly in early pregnancy, has been associated with fatigue, headaches and dizziness, which many women experience.

In pregnancy, changes in posture can cause acute haemodynamic changes (Blackburn 2003). Blood pressure in normotensive women is higher when sitting and falls on lying, especially in the supine position. Effects on venous pressure are relatively dramatic compared with the effects on arterial pressure. As there are no valves between the return from the femoral veins to the vena cava and heart, venous pressure in the legs is similar to the pressure in the heart so, if a pregnant woman lies in a supine position, the uterus can compress the aorta and, particularly, the thin-walled vena cava and iliac veins. (The aorta is compressed as well but to a lesser degree because it has a much thicker vessel wall.) Return of blood to the heart can also be impeded by the pressure of the fetal head on the iliac veins and by hydrodynamic obstruction due to outflow of blood from the uterine vessels. Most women experience a drop in blood pressure greater than 10% when they lie down; for some of these women this fall is extreme, reaching up to 50%. The effect of assuming the lithotomy position in labour is to decrease cardiac output significantly (Carbonne et al 1996).

In late pregnancy, most women experience oedema of the lower extremities (see Case study 11.1) owing to the combined effects of progesterone relaxing the vascular tone, the impeding of the venous return by the gravid uterus and gravitational forces. The peripheral circulatory volume is increased by 500–600 ml per limb (de Swiet 1998a). Oedema is further increased in hypertensive women and tends to increase

---

Case study 11.1

It is the height of summer and Kathy, 38 weeks' pregnant, informs her midwife she feels fat and sluggish and cannot cope with the hot weather. Kathy's ankles are visibly swollen.

- Is the midwife right to assume that this is normal?
- What indicators would the midwife be able to use in an assessment to reassure Kathy that all is well?
- What factors may alert the midwife to suspect that all is not well?

with increased maternal age. Fluid drunk by the pregnant woman appears as increased leg volume and the expected diuresis is delayed until she lies down, resulting in increased nocturia. Blood pressure is higher on the side of placental implantation and oedema may also be more marked in the leg on the side of placental implantation (de Swiet 1998a). The effect of increased venous pressure is to increase the incidence and severity of varicose veins of the legs, vulva and haemorrhoids (Fig. 11.6).

The tendency to develop oedema is also affected by the concentration of plasma proteins (see Box 11.3). The increment in plasma volume is not matched by an increase in plasma protein synthesis so there is decreased plasma colloidal pressure. This, together with the increased venous pressure, means there is an

Box 11.3

Oedema and hypertension

The pressures in the right ventricle, pulmonary arteries and pulmonary capillaries do not change but cardiac output increases. The higher pulmonary blood flow therefore has to be absorbed by decreased pulmonary resistance and dilatation of the pulmonary vascular bed so the volume of pulmonary circulation increases to match the increased cardiac output. Conditions where pulmonary resistance is increased or fixed have a poor maternal prognosis such as Eisenmenger's syndrome, which has a 30%–50% mortality rate. Exercise presents an increased demand on the cardiovascular system (see Box 11.4).

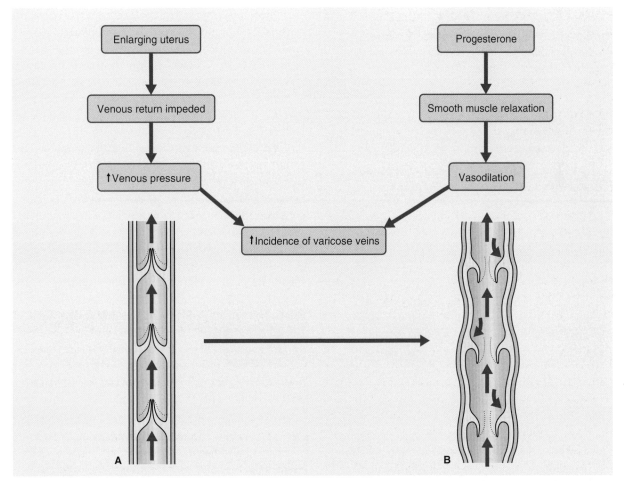

Fig. 11.6 *The effect of increased venous pressure leading to increased incidence of varicose veins of the legs, vulva and haemorrhoids. A Normal vein with normal vascular tone; B varicose vein: the effects of progesterone on muscle tone cause incomplete valve closure, allowing the back-flow of blood.*

increase in fluid loss from the capillaries. There may also be an increase in capillary permeability (Blackburn 2003).

The effects of exercise on the cardiovascular system are summarized in Box 11.4.

Distribution of blood flow

Oestrogen increases blood flow to all tissues but the distribution of flow is affected by posture. Venous tone is affected by progesterone. The increased venous distensibility results in an increased incidence of vari-

---

Box 11.4

Exercise in pregnancy

Exercise affects maternal physiology because there is a hormonal response, weight is redistributed and heat is generated. Many women experience very good physical health especially early in pregnancy. However, the question is whether the adaptive response to exercise compromises fetal oxygenation and well-being. The ability to increase cardiac output in response to exercise progressively declines throughout pregnancy. Theoretically, redistribution of weight could affect the venous return and blood could be preferentially circulated to the skeletal muscles and to the skin for heat dissipation. Studies on animals suggest that uterine blood flow can be decreased substantially before fetal oxygen uptake or temperature regulation is compromised. It has been reported that over a third of the female medal winners in the 1956 Russian Olympic team were pregnant and the cardiovascular changes enhanced for their performance (de Swiet 1998a). In practice, moderate exercise in normal healthy pregnancy is encouraged as maternal and fetal health seem to benefit. However, pregnant women are advised to avoid jumping and jerky movements because of joint instability. Vigorous exercise is not recommended during hot humid weather or if the mother has a fever. It is suggested that heart rate should not exceed 140 beats per minute, strenuous exercise should be done for less than 15 minutes at a time and a pregnant woman should not allow herself to become breathless. A pregnant woman should stop physical exercise if pain, vaginal bleeding or dizziness is experienced or there are known risk factors.

---

cose veins, venous thrombosis and thromboembolism. The uterus is the central target of the increased circulatory flow during pregnancy but distribution of flow to other organ systems, including kidneys, skin, lungs and breasts, increases as well. It is difficult to distinguish between blood flow to the increasing uterine tissue mass and that going specifically to supply the placenta because the uterine vessels are complex and inaccessible. Arteriovenous shunts in the uterine vasculature have been identified; these allow a short circuit of the placental site after delivery of the placenta, rather than being important in increased flow during pregnancy. The increased flow to the uterus is about 500 ml/min more than that to the non-pregnant uterus but changes in uterine flow occur relatively late in pregnancy (de Swiet 1998a).

Blood flow to the kidneys increases by about 400 ml/min from early pregnancy, facilitating elimination of waste products. Vasodilatory prostaglandins are implicated in the peripheral vasodilation, which is particularly evident in the vessels of the breasts, hands and face. Oestrogen and progesterone depress the normal response to angiotensin II and oestrogen abrogates the vasoconstriction mediated by the sympathetic nervous system. Blood flow to the lungs increases, reflecting the increased circulating blood volume and cardiac output. Distribution of blood to the skin is greatly increased (by about 500 ml/min) expediting heat loss. It is common for pregnant women to complain of being hot. Pregnant women usually have warm hands and feet and often complain that midwives' hands are cold. This vasodilatory effect is enhanced in smokers. Blood flow to the hands increases about seven-fold giving a very marked increase in skin temperature. The resulting peripheral vasodilation causes the capillaries to dilate and stimulates angiogenesis, and may give rise to the development of vascular spiders and palmar erythema. The increased flow means there is a decreased tendency to arteriolar spasm, and therefore conditions such as Raynaud's syndrome are abolished.

The increased blood flow to the skin stimulates the growth of nails and hair. The ratio of actively growing hair to resting (prior to falling out) hair is altered from 85:15 to 95:5 (de Swiet 1998a). When this ratio returns to normal in the puerperium, vast amounts of hair can be lost. Mammary blood flow also increases (see Ch. 16). Coronary blood flow probably increases, reflecting the increased workload of the left ventricle, but it is thought that hepatic and cerebral blood flow do not significantly increase (de Swiet 1998a).

In evolutionary terms, heat dissipation from the mucous membranes had been very important in mammals (this is best illustrated by dogs panting to lose heat). The increased flow to the mucous membranes in pregnancy can result in an increased congestion of the mucosa, which is demonstrated by an increased incidence of sinusitis, nosebleeds and snoring in pregnancy. It is suggested that elimination of waste products by the kidneys and heat by the skin is best fulfilled by an increased plasma volume rather than an increase in whole blood, which demonstrates the importance of the apparent physiological anaemia.

Haematological changes

The changes in maternal blood volume and composition increase the efficiency of the transplacental circulation and exchange mechanisms, thus benefiting fetal development. The haematological changes are also part of a maternal adaptive response that protects maternal homeostasis, including the ability to tolerate a sudden blood loss and to cope with placental separation. Thus, even women who have a degree of iron deficiency prior to pregnancy are protected from some decrease in haemoglobin levels at delivery. However, the adaptive responses to pregnancy potentiate the risks of iron-deficiency anaemia, thromboembolism and other clotting problems.

Plasma volume and blood cell mass/number

Pregnancy is a state of hypervolaemia (see p. 256). Blood volume increases in healthy pregnant women by about 1½ litres (30–50%, with a range of individual variation). Plasma volume increases initially rapidly from about 6 weeks' gestation and then the rate of increase becomes slower (Blackburn 2003). The 40–50% increase in plasma volume is not matched by increased red blood cell mass and plasma protein production so there is a haemodilution (an apparent decrease) in haemoglobin and plasma protein concentration. Red blood cell mass increases by about 15–18% in women who do not take iron supplements and by about 25–33% in women supplemented with iron (Blackburn 2003). The differences in plasma volume and red blood cell mass are accentuated by differential timing of the increases. Red blood cell mass begins to expand in the second trimester and the rate peaks in the third trimester. The maternal RAS may be involved; angiotensinogen competes for the erythro-

poietin receptors and may be a precursor of erythropoietin.

The increase in blood volume is higher in multigravidae and women who are obese, have multiple pregnancies or where the pregnancy is prolonged. The increment in plasma volume is positively correlated with birth weight and placental weight; pregnancies resulting in recurrent abortions, stillborn and low-birth-weight babies are associated with an abnormally low increase in plasma volume.

There is no reason for the relationship between plasma volume and blood cell mass, which are controlled by different mechanisms, to be retained throughout the pregnancy. The role of plasma is to fill the vascular space, maintaining the blood pressure, and to dissipate heat. Calculations suggest that the hypervolaemia is adequate to fill the increased vascular space of the pregnant uterus and the enlarged vascular beds of the breasts, muscles, kidneys and skin and to provide a reservoir against the pooling of blood in the lower extremities. It will also decrease the effect of the haemoglobin lost in bleeding at delivery. The decreased viscosity of the blood lessens the resistance to flow and therefore the cardiac effort required to propel the blood. Observation of a 'normal' (prepregnant) or increased haemoglobin level (rather than a lower level seen in healthy pregnancies) may therefore represent an unsatisfactory increase in plasma volume rather than a true increase in haemoglobin concentration. Levels of haemoglobin are at their lowest between 16 and 22 weeks. The assertion that a degree of haemodilution is normal and a requisite adaptation to pregnancy, rather than indicating pathological anaemia, is supported by the increased arteriovenous difference (see above).

Most of the increase in blood cell mass is in the form of red blood cells. An initial depression of erythropoietin levels occurs, but progesterone, prolactin and hPL all stimulate erythropoietin synthesis and so promote red blood cell production; however, red blood cell mass correlates best with hPL levels. These influences result in mild hyperplasia of the bone marrow and an increased reticulocyte count. The function of red blood cells is oxygen transport; therefore red blood cell mass will increase physiologically at high altitude and decrease with prolonged bed rest. In pregnancy, the increment in red blood cells should reflect the need for more oxygen; the estimated increased requirement to supply the increased maternal tissues and conceptus is 15.0–16.5%, which is slightly lower than the measured rise of 18%.

Levels of 2,3-DPG (2,3-diphosphoglycerate) increase from early pregnancy so the oxygen–haemoglobin dissociation curve shifts to the right (see Ch. 1) thus facilitating oxygen unloading at the peripheral tissues. Red blood cells become more spherical, with an increased diameter and thickness, because plasma colloid pressure falls and thus more water crosses the erythrocyte membrane by osmosis.

Iron status

As plasma volume increases, haemoglobin concentration and haematocrit fall, reaching a lowest point at 16–22 weeks (Blackburn 2003). The World Health Organization recommends that haemoglobin concentration should not fall below 11 g/dl at any point in pregnancy; others suggest it should not fall below 10 g/dl. If iron stores can be demonstrated not to be depleted, it would suggest that the decreased haemoglobin concentration is not attributable to iron deficiency. In pregnancy, the most accurate and appropriate method of determining iron status and anaemia is measurement of serum ferritin levels. Serum ferritin, the major iron-storage protein, becomes depleted before clinical indicators reveal anaemia. Serum ferritin is stable, is not affected by recent ingestion of iron and quantitatively reflects iron stores, particularly in the lower range. Serum ferritin levels of less than 50 g/l in early pregnancy indicate a need for iron supplementation and levels above 80 g/l are probably adequate to protect the woman from iron depletion. However, routine iron supplementation in pregnancy, of apparently healthy women with no apparent iron deficiency, results in red blood cells increasing by 30% rather than by 18% in unsupplemented women (Letsky 1998). One method of assessing anaemia in non-pregnant subjects is by observing an increased red blood cell mass in response to increased iron supplementation (Yip & Dallman 1996).

The need for routine iron supplementation in pregnancy is a controversial area (Haram & Nilsen 2001). Letsky (1998) argues strongly that clinical indicators of anaemia are not sensitive enough to demonstrate iron deficiency in practice. Iron depletion causes a reduction in mean blood cell volume (MCV). However, increased erythropoiesis results in a higher proportion of young larger red blood cells, which tends to mask the effect of iron deficiency on cell volume even with established anaemia

Although the amenorrhoea of pregnancy helps to conserve iron stores and absorption of dietary iron increases, the requirement of iron in pregnancy can probably be met only if the woman has good iron stores prior to conception. Letsky argues that, although pregnancy is a physiological state, many women enter pregnancy with insufficient iron stores to supply the high requirements particularly of the third trimester. Active transport of iron across the placenta is maximal in the last 4 weeks of pregnancy. The inadequacy of dietary iron may be related to the move away from the Palaeolithic iron-rich diet that was normal for most of human evolution to a cereal-based one with less meat and fish (Cordain et al 2002). Although most of the body's iron is associated with haemoglobin, iron is also a component of the electron transport chain. Tissue enzyme malfunction occurs in the first stages of iron deficiency before significant anaemia is apparent and supplements can increase perceptions of well-being. Subclinical degrees of iron deficiency may adversely affect maternal exercise tolerance, cerebral function and well-being (Letsky 1998). Offspring of iron-deficient mothers may have reduced iron stores and are at risk of infantile anaemia, which may affect their mental and motor development and have long-term consequences. Maternal iron-deficiency anaemia correlates with high placental fetal weight, suggesting fetal growth is impaired (see Ch. 9). Low birth weight and high placental fetal weight have been associated with hypertension in adult life (Godfrey et al 1991), so iron-deficiency anaemia in pregnancy may have long-lasting and far-reaching effects.

Haemostasis

Pregnancy is a hypercoagulable state. Bleeding time in pregnancy decreases by about 30% because the ratio of clotting and fibrinolytic factors alters. There is an increase in fibrinogen and other clotting factors and a decrease in fibrinolytic substances. The number of platelets decreases slightly towards term but generally remains within the non-pregnant range. This response is variable; there may be increased platelet turnover and low-grade platelet activation (an increased number of aggregated platelets) as the pregnancy progresses, resulting in a larger proportion of younger platelets with increased volume. Low-grade chronic intravascular coagulation in the uteroplacental circulation may be part of the normal physiological response to pregnancy. Platelet count is further decreased in pregnancies with fetal growth retardation, and even in mild pre-eclampsia the lifespan of platelets is reduced.

Synthesis of antithrombin III (the main physiological inhibitor of thrombin and factor Xa) increases in pregnancy in parallel with the increased plasma volume. Levels decrease at delivery (thus increasing the tendency to thrombosis) and increase 1 week postpartum. There is a general increase in clotting factors, particularly in late pregnancy, as demonstrated in Von Willebrand's syndrome (an inherited clotting disorder), which improves with pregnancy. The change in amount of clotting factors seems to be compensatory in preparation for labour. The hypercoagulability is optimal in labour, meeting the demands of placental separation but can increase the risks of thrombosis and disseminated intravascular coagulation. At delivery, total blood loss can be as much as 500 ml. The normal blood flow of 500–800 ml/min is staunched within seconds (aided by myometrial contraction, which decreases blood flow and rapidly closes spiral arteries). A fibrin mesh then rapidly covers the placental site as 5–10% of the total circulating fibrinogen is deposited. Fibrinolytic activity decreases in pregnancy and remains low in labour. It returns to normal within an hour of delivery; the placenta produces inhibitors that block fibrinolysis.

Table 11.1 summarizes the haematological changes in pregnancy.

The respiratory system

Maternal respiratory effort has to be increased in pregnancy to meet the increased metabolic demands of the maternal and fetal tissues. By the end of the pregnancy, 16–20% more oxygen is consumed. The respiratory system is also affected by the expanding uterine volume. In terms of physiological reserve, the stress put on the respiratory system by pregnancy is small compared with the increases that can be measured on exercise (Table 11.2). This contrasts with the much larger proportion of the cardiovascular physiological reserve required in pregnancy. The clinical implication of this is that patients with respiratory disease are much less likely to deteriorate in pregnancy than are those with cardiac disease.

Table 11.1 *Summary of haematological changes in pregnancy*

	Change in pregnancy	Notes
Plasma volume	Increases by about 50% from 2600 ml to 3900 ml	More in second and subsequent pregnancies; correlates with birth weight
Red blood cell mass	Increases by about 18%	Increase is greater with iron supplementation (to 30%)
Neutrophil count	Both cell number and metabolic activity increase	Initial increase occurs early in pregnancy and is similar to the response to other physiological stresses
Plasma proteins	Decrease	Decreased osmotic pressure predisposes to oedema
Clotting factors	Increase	Fibrinolytic factors decrease
Platelet count	Slight fall	Coagulability increases

Table 11.2 *Pregnancy and physiological reserve*

Parameter	Normal	Pregnancy	% increase	Exercise	% increase
Minute volume	7.5 l/min	10.5 l/min	40	80 l/min	1000
Oxygen consumption	220 ml/min	255 ml/min	16		
Cardiac output	4.5 l/min	6 l/min	30	12 l/min	

Anatomy

Early in pregnancy, and therefore not secondary to pressure from the uterus, the diaphragm is displaced upwards by 4 cm (de Swiet 1998b) (Fig. 11.7). The respiratory excursion of the diaphragm increases and there is an increased flaring of the lower ribs (increasing the substernal angle from 68° to 103° by late pregnancy) (Blackburn 2003). This compensatory increase in the diameter of the thorax by about 2 cm (the circumference of the chest increases by about 15 cm) means that the volume of the thoracic cavity is about the same as that before pregnancy. The diaphragm performs the major work of respiration; the breathing is thoracic rather than abdominal. Hormonal influences cause the muscles and cartilage in the thoracic region to relax so the chest broadens. The subsequent decrease in chest wall compliance means the thoracic wall can move further inwards so there is less trapped air and the residual volume decreases. These anatomical changes probably do not completely reverse after the pregnancy (indeed it is said that the increased flaring of the rib cage is beneficial to opera singers after pregnancy).

Progesterone is a respiratory stimulant; it lowers the sensitivity of the peripheral and central chemoreceptors for carbon dioxide (Prabhakar & Peng 2004). This means that respiratory drive is stimulated at lower carbon dioxide levels so pregnant women breathe more deeply. As progesterone increases during the pregnancy, the increased responsiveness to PCO_2 results in an increased tidal volume and therefore minute volume (Table 11.3). So hyperventilation (increased tidal volume) is normal in pregnancy. Oxygen consumption increases but arterial oxygen pressure does not change.

In pregnancy, the respiratory rate is unchanged but minute ventilation increases by 40% because tidal volume increases; this is apparent as early as 7 weeks. This hyperventilation exceeds the increased oxygen consumption. Efficiency of alveolar gas exchange is much more efficient when tidal volume is increased rather than respiratory rate (Fig. 11.8). Alveolar ventilation is further enhanced by the decrease in residual volume. About 150 ml of an inspired breath remains in the upper airways where no gas exchange takes place (this is known as the anatomical dead space). Although the dead space increases by about 60 ml in pregnancy because of dilatation of the smaller bronchioles, the net alveolar ventilation is increased. The increased tidal volume means that the functional residual capacity is reduced, thus an increased volume of fresh air mixes with a much smaller residual volume of air remaining in the lungs. Alveolar ventilation in pregnancy is thus increased by about 70% resulting in increased efficiency of mixing of gases, which facilitates gas exchange because the diffusion gradient is bigger. The increased gradient of carbon dioxide concentrations between maternal and fetal blood aids transfer of carbon dioxide across the placenta and may be particularly important in adverse circumstances. Progesterone increases carbonic anhydrase levels in red blood cells (see Ch. 1) thus further increasing the efficiency of carbon dioxide transfer.

Maternal partial pressures of oxygen increase slightly (from 95–100 mmHg to 101–106 mmHg) and levels of carbon dioxide decrease (from 35–40 mmHg to 26–34 mmHg). The small increase in PO_2 has little effect on haemoglobin saturation. Posture, however, affects alveolar oxygen levels: a supine position in late pregnancy results in a lower alveolar oxygen pressure than when in a sitting position. This change in alveolar oxygenation is probably not significant for the fetus although it may be compensatory at high altitude. Air travel is associated with increased dyspnoea and respiratory rate. The decreased level of carbon dioxide in pregnancy results in a mild respiratory

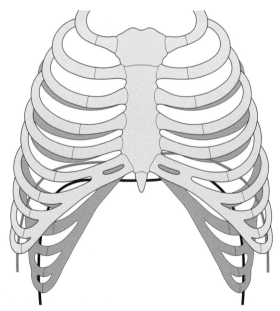

Fig. 11.7 *Displacement of the diaphragm in pregnancy: the ribcage in pregnancy (light) and the non-pregnancy state (dark), showing the increased subcostal angle, the increased transverse diameter and the raised diaphragm in pregnancy.*

Table 11.3 *Lung volumes and capacities*

Parameter	Definition	Normal range	Change in pregnancy
Tidal volume (TV)	Volume of a normal breath at rest	500 ml	Increases by 150–200 ml (25–40%) 75% increase occurs within first trimester
Respiratory rate (RR)	Number of breaths per minute	12 breaths/min	Unchanged/slightly increased to 15 breaths/min
Minute volume (MV)	Total air taken in 1 minute of respiration (= TV × RR)	6000 ml/min 6.5 l/min	Increased by about 40% 10 l/min
Inspiratory reserve volume (IRV)	Volume of air that can be inspired above the resting tidal volume	3100 ml	Unchanged
Expiratory reserve volume (ERV)	Volume of gas that can be expired in addition to the tidal volume	1200 ml	Reduces progressively from early pregnancy to about 1100 ml
Residual volume (RV)	Volume of gas remaining in the lungs after a maximal expiration	1200 ml	Decreases progressively
Total lung capacity (TLC)	Maximum volume of the lungs (= TV + IRV + ERV + dead space)	6000 ml	Unchanged
Vital capacity (VC)	Total volume of gas that can be moved in and out of the lungs (= TLC – residual volume)	4800 ml	Increased 100–200 ml in late pregnancy? (not apparent in obese women)
Inspiratory capacity	Total inspiratory ability of the lungs (= IRC + TV)	2200 ml	Increased about 2500 ml at term
Functional residual capacity (FRC)	Volume of gas remaining in the lungs after a resting breath (= ERV + RV)	2800 ml	Decreases progressively to 2300 ml—increases mixing efficiency
Residual volume (RV)	Volume of gas remaining after a maximal expiration (= FRC – ERV)	2400 ml	
Physiological dead space			Increases by ~ 60 ml
Alveolar ventilation	Difference between TV and volume of physiological dead space		Increased

alkalosis. The change in pH affects levels of circulatory cations such as sodium, potassium and calcium, aiding transfer across the placenta and increasing provision for fetal growth. Metabolic compensation by increased renal excretion of bicarbonate ions occurs. The resulting fall in serum bicarbonate causes maternal pH levels to increase to the upper end of the normal physiological range, from 7.40 to 7.45. Maternal ability to compensate further for metabolic acidosis is

therefore limited, which may create problems in prolonged labour or where there is inadequate tissue perfusion (see Ch. 13).

Progesterone has a local effect on the smooth muscle tone of the airways and the pulmonary blood vessels and decreases airway resistance. Diffusion capacity is the ease with which gases can cross the pulmonary membranes. In early pregnancy, diffusion capacity decreases probably because of the effects of

A

Nonpregnant

Late pregnancy

B

Fig. 11.8 *A Alteration in alveolar gas exchange during pregnancy, and B its mechanisms.*

oestrogen on the composition of the mucopolysaccharides of the capillary walls, which increases diffusion distance (de Swiet 1998b). This effect may last for months after delivery. Increased water retention in the pulmonary tissues also results in a decrease in diffusion capacity. There is an increased closing volume suggesting that the calibre of the small airways is decreased; this may be due to increased lung fluid. The decreased efficiency of pulmonary gas transfer is partially compensated for by progesterone-induced relaxation of bronchiole smooth muscle, which decreases airway resistance. The decreased airway resistance means that air flow is increased. Prostaglandins also affect bronchiole smooth muscle. $PGF_{2\alpha}$, which increases throughout the pregnancy, is a smooth muscle constrictor; PGE_1 and PGE_2, which increase in the third trimester, are smooth muscle dilators. The work of breathing is probably unchanged as the decreased airway resistance compensates for the congestion in the bronchial wall capillaries.

Many pregnant women experience dyspnoea, causing discomfort and anxiety, often early in pregnancy before there are changes in intra-abdominal pressure. This correlates well with PCO_2 and may be due to hyperventilation (de Swiet 1998b). Capillaries in the upper respiratory tract become engorged, which can create difficulties in breathing via the nose and aggravate respiratory infections. Laryngeal changes and oedema of the vocal cords caused by vascular dilation can promote hoarseness and deepening of the voice, and a persistent cough. In severe cases, these changes in laryngeal thickening may cause complications should endotracheal intubation be necessary, for instance in anaesthesia. Forced expiratory volume over 1 second and peak flow rate are not usually affected in pregnancy.

In labour, pain causes an increase in tidal volume and respiratory rate (these effects are abolished by effective epidural anaesthesia). In the second stage, muscle demands result in metabolic acidosis (increased lactate and pyruvate production); this is countered to a degree by the respiratory alkalosis from hyperventilation (Blackburn 2003).

The renal system

During pregnancy, the kidneys increase excretion of waste products in response to the increase in maternal and fetal metabolism, and retention of fluid and electrolytes is altered in response to cardiovascular changes. It is generally accepted that the increased circulating blood volume and haemodilution in pregnancy are achieved by the kidneys increasing their tubular reabsorption rate of sodium. The retention of sodium is stimulated by deoxycorticosterone derived from progesterone. Fluid retention is facilitated by the action of angiotensin II (see above for description of the renin–angiotensin system). Oestrogen increases both angiotensinogen production and renin production. ADH secretion tends to occur at lower plasma osmolality during pregnancy, possibly affected by human chorionic gonadotrophin levels (Blackburn 2003). Likewise, the osmotic threshold for thirst decreases from early pregnancy.

The gross anatomy of the renal system is altered in pregnancy. The kidneys enlarge owing to an increase in renal blood flow and vascular volume. Alterations in both prolactin and prostaglandin levels have effects on renal blood flow (Baylis & Davison 1998). The increased renal blood flow results in an increased glomerular filtration rate (GFR) from early pregnancy. The increased GFR results in more sodium, glucose and amino acids in the filtrate; however, tubular reabsorption also increases so most of the increased sodium load is reabsorbed. The sodium retention results in water accumulation.

The tendency to become insulin-resistant in the latter part of pregnancy results in increased blood glucose. This, together with the increased GFR, results in increased glucose concentration of the filtrate, which can exceed the maximum capacity for glucose reabsorption in the tubules causing some glucose to be present in the urine (glucosuria). This does not necessarily indicate diabetes. Likewise mild proteinuria is common and benign in pregnancy, although with coexisting hypertension it can indicate complications of pre-eclampsia.

There is a cumulative retention of sodium and potassium especially in the last trimester when fetal demands for sodium are high. Urinary excretion of calcium increases but free calcium levels remain stable as dietary absorption of calcium increases (see p. 273). Acid–base balance is also altered in pregnancy (Baylis & Davison 1998). Hydrogen ions fall slightly primarily because of respiratory alkalaemia associated with hyperventilation. Although systemic blood pressure may be reduced, autoregulation (local control of glomerular blood pressure) maintains optimal renal function.

The calyces of the kidneys and the ureters become dilated and lose some of their peristaltic activity in pregnancy. The ureters elongate and become tortuous so they accommodate an increased volume of urine, which is associated with an increased risk of infection. It was generally accepted that this dilation of the ureters was primarily due to the action of progesterone on smooth muscle. However, the ovarian arteries and veins increase in size and compress the ureters, particularly on the right side where the vessels cross over the ureter almost at right-angles, whereas on the left they run approximately parallel to the ureter. This, together with the stress imposed on the ureters by the expanding uterus upon the pelvic brim, explains the extent of these morphological changes.

Bladder function is also affected in pregnancy. Urinary frequency increases early in pregnancy as the growing uterus in the pelvic cavity puts pressure on the bladder. At term, when engagement occurs, the presenting part of the fetus increases stress on the bladder. In the second trimester, the bladder is displaced upwards so urinary frequency is closer to prepregnant levels. Under the effect of progesterone, bladder tone decreases during pregnancy so capacity increases and may be up to a litre by term. The decreased bladder tone and displacement of the ureters by the enlarging uterus can affect competence of the vesicoureteral sphincters (valves created by the normal oblique angle of entry of the ureters into the bladder wall become compromised as the entry of the ureters tends to be perpendicular). The result is possible reflux of urine from the bladder into the ureters, which increases the chance of a urinary infection.

The walls of the bladder become more oedematous and hyperaemic, which increases the vulnerability to infection and trauma. The relatively lax walls of the bladder may also result in incomplete emptying of urine. This urinary stasis increases the risk of a urinary tract infection (UTI) as the urine, which is richer in glucose and amino acids in pregnancy, remains in the bladder allowing the usually harmless number of bacteria in the urine to reach pathological levels. Women with UTI are thought to be at increased risk of premature labour. As the pregnancy progresses the effect of posture on renal function becomes exacerbated. The structural changes of the renal system persist into the puerperium (see Ch. 14) and women who have experienced a UTI during pregnancy are at increased risk of recurrent infection in the puerperium.

Case study 11.2 details an example of a urogenital tract infection.

Case study 11.2

Penny is expecting her second child at 24 weeks' gestation and presents herself at the maternity day assessment unit. Two days previously, Penny noticed her frequency of micturition had dramatically increased. Since then she has felt lower central abdominal pain radiating from the groin round to the right side of her back. The midwife suspects that Penny may have a urinary tract infection (UTI). A provisional diagnosis is made on ward-based urinalysis that indicates the presence of leukocytes and nitrites.

■ What is the significance of these findings and why do they indicate the presence of an infection?

The midwife instructs Penny on how to provide a midstream specimen of urine (MSU) and requests that the duty doctor examine Penny. Penny is prescribed a course of antibiotics with the proviso that this may be changed if the laboratory tests indicate that the antibiotic is inappropriate.

■ How could the midwife describe to Penny the reasons why the UTI has occurred?
■ What else besides taking the antibiotics could the midwife advise Penny to do to (a) help resolve the infection now and (b) avoid further infection in the future?
■ What are the risks and possible consequences if the infection is not treated?

The gastrointestinal system

Maternal nutrition is very important in the outcome of pregnancy but disturbances of gastrointestinal function are the most common cause of complaints in pregnancy (Fig. 11.9). Over 50% of women experience an increased appetite (and consequent increased consumption of food) and even more an increased thirst. hCG affects the hypothalamus decreasing the osmotic threshold for thirst. The changes are most marked in the first half of pregnancy; subsequently they may decline although some persist, albeit to a lesser extent. Surveys have measured an increased intake of food and drink in pregnant women although not all of them are conscious of these changes (Hytten 1991). Changes in maternal appetite do not directly reflect changes in fetal growth or maternal metabolism. Appetite tends to be increased in early pregnancy and may be promoted by several hormones including

Mouth

Oesophagus
Relaxation of lower
oesophageal sphincter
→ regurgitation → heartburn

Gastrointestinal tract
↑ Appetite and thirst
Taste buds change → cravings or
  aversions
Extreme craving = PICA
Excessive salivation (PTYALISM)
  may occur
Gums tend to become swollen and
  bleed easily

Stomach
↓ gastric secretion and
↓ gastric motility
→ slow emptying
→ ↑ pulping of food
May cause nausea

Small intestine
↓ motility
→ ↑ absorption time
  ↑ transit time
(↑ Fe absorption)

Colon
↓ motility
→ ↑ water absorption
May cause constipation
(↑ Na+ absorption)

**Growth of uterus
and conceptus**
→ ↑ appetite and ↑ thirst
In late pregnancy may
↓ capacity for large meals

Haemorrhoids

Fig. 11.9   *Gastrointestinal function in pregnancy.*

leptin. In advanced pregnancy, both appetite and the capacity for food intake decline owing to upward gastric displacement and pressure from the gravid uterus. A pregnant woman can compensate for her limited capacity by increasing the frequency of consumption of small meals and snacks. Oestrogen suppresses appetite but progesterone stimulates it, causing a shift in the central control of energy balance. Decreased plasma glucose and amino acid levels, which are secondary to increased responsiveness to insulin, also stimulate appetite. Cyclical patterns of appetite are also observed during the menstrual cycle. Thirst is increased; progesterone resets the thirst threshold by 10 mOsm so plasma osmolarity falls. Increased angiotensin and prolactin levels are also dipsogenic.

Food cravings and aversions

Changes in food habits can be deliberate, for instance avoiding fried or fatty foods that are considered less healthy. Two-thirds of pregnant women express marked food preferences as cravings or aversions. The commonest cravings are for fruit and highly flavoured foods such as pickles, kippers and cheese. It is suggested that the sensitivity of the taste buds is dulled in pregnancy (Bowen 1992) so highly seasoned foods are more appreciated. Unsatisfied cravings are often thought to explain food-shaped birthmarks (King 2000). Common aversions are to tea and coffee, meat, fried foods and eggs and to caffeinated drinks, alcohol and smoking. Food cravings and aversions need to be assessed as part of a full dietary assessment; they do not necessarily have an adverse effect on dietary quality. Usually cravings cause an increase in energy and calcium intakes and aversions frequently result in decreased intake of alcohol, coffee and animal protein.

Pica, an extreme craving usually for a non-nutritious substance, has been identified for coal, soap, disinfectant, toothpaste, mothballs and ice. Usually pica does not affect either maternal or fetal health. In the southern states of America, there seems to be a social tradition of Black women eating laundry starch, chalk and clay. Sense of smell may be enhanced; pregnant women are especially sensitive to noxious smells such as nicotine and coffee. The timing of the changes in taste and smell appears to reflect secretion of hCG.

Nausea and vomiting in pregnancy

Between 50% and 90% of pregnant women experience nausea and vomiting in pregnancy (NVP), usually in the first trimester although 20% of women experience NVP throughout gestation. It may be the first physical manifestation of pregnancy. NVP is more common in Westernized urban populations and is affected by ethnicity, occupational status and maternal age (Coad et al 2000). The peak of NVP is usually at about 8–12 weeks; symptoms usually resolve by mid-pregnancy. Although about 50% of women suffering from NVP are affected to a greater extent in the morning, some women experience nausea and vomiting in the evening, in a biphasic pattern or throughout the day. It is thought that women who are underweight experience less severe symptoms of NVP compared to women with normal preconceptual weight (Huxley 2000). NVP does not necessarily mean that nutrient intake is decreased. Some women eat more as continual snacking alleviates symptoms and others alter their diet in a way that usually improves dietary quality (Coad et al 2002).

There are several theories about the causes of NVP. Serum hCG peaks in the first trimester but the relationship between NVP and hCG secretion is not clearly established. The effects of progesterone on gastric smooth muscle tone, particularly those on upper gastrointestinal tract motility, the patency of the lower oesophageal sphincter and delayed gastric emptying, suggest a possible role for steroid hormones. NVP is usually conservatively treated with rest and reassurance and advice to consume frequent small meals rich in easily digested carbohydrate and low in fat. Meat and strong smells may aggravate NVP. It has been suggested that NVP is an evolutionary mechanism that protects the embryo by causing pregnant women to physically expel and subsequently avoid foods that might contain teratogenic and abortifacient chemicals (Flaxman & Sherman 2000). An alternative explanation is that NVP has a functional role in stimulating early placental growth by reducing maternal energy intake and suppressing maternal tissue synthesis in early pregnancy so nutrient partitioning favours the developing placenta (Huxley 2000). Although NVP may have a socioeconomic impact and create much misery, it is considered to be favourable prognostic sign and is associated with a positive outcome of pregnancy (Coad et al 2002). Intractable nausea and vomiting causing dehydration, electrolyte imbalances, metabolic disturbances and nutritional deficiencies is known as hyperemesis gravidarum.

Mouth

Gums often become hyperaemic, oedematous and spongy. This is because of the effects of oestrogen on blood flow and connective tissue consistency. Gums therefore bleed more easily and are vulnerable to abrasive food and vigorous tooth brushing. Gingivitis and periodontal disease occur in a large proportion of pregnant women and are more extreme with increased maternal age and parity and where there are pre-existing dental problems. Contrary to folklore belief that a tooth is lost for every baby, there is no evidence of demineralization of dentine resulting from pregnancy as fetal calcium stores are drawn from maternal body stores (skeleton) and not from maternal teeth (Blackburn 2003). However, there is an increase in the number of caries treated during pregnancy. This may be because gum changes result in an increased awareness of dental problems and many women receive free dental care in pregnancy. Saliva becomes more acidic in pregnancy, but the volume produced does not usually change. In rare instances, excessive production of saliva, termed ptyalism or ptyalorrhoea, may occur. It can occur in isolation or in association with hyperemesis gravidarum, where swallowing of saliva induces extreme nausea and vomiting in an affected woman.

Oesophagus

Heartburn, a painful retrosternal burning sensation, is common in pregnancy, affecting 30–70% women. The effects of progesterone on the tone of the lower oesophageal sphincter mean its competence is impaired and regurgitation of gastric acid is more likely. Similar changes occur during the menstrual cycle and in women taking combined oral contraceptive pills. These changes are associated with increased progesterone levels. The risk of a hiatus hernia is increased; the sphincter is displaced and becomes intrathoracic instead of straddling the diaphragm. This usually begins in the second trimester and worsens as the pregnancy progresses. It is due to progesterone-induced relaxation of the lower oesophageal sphincter and a change in pressure gradients across the stomach. The enlarging uterus causes distortion of the stomach and changes the angle of entry of the oesophagus. Because the patency of the pyloric sphincter may also be impaired, both alkaline and acidic secretions may reflux into the oesophagus.

Heartburn is increased with multiple pregnancies, polyhydramnios, obesity and excessive bending over. Alcohol, chocolate and coffee all act directly on the lower oesophageal sphincter, reducing the muscle tone and exacerbating heartburn. Gastric reflux can be limited by advising more frequent intake of smaller meals, the avoidance of seasoned food, and of postural influences such as lying horizontally or bending forwards. Antacid preparations are associated with a number of undesirable side-effects: aluminium salts may cause diarrhoea, magnesium salts are associated with constipation, phosphorus may affect the calcium/phosphorus balance and exacerbate cramp, sodium may affect water balance and long-term use of antacids is associated with malabsorption, particularly of drugs and dietary minerals.

Stomach

Studies on gastric secretion in pregnancy are not conclusive but suggest acid secretion tends to decrease, which may explain why remission of symptoms of a peptic ulcer is not an uncommon event. Secretion of pepsin also falls; this is probably secondary to the decreased acid secretion. Studies have shown that stomach gastric tone and motility markedly decrease in pregnancy. Thus in advanced pregnancy the stomach drapes loosely over the uterine fundus. This tends to delay gastric emptying especially following ingestion of solid foods. The delay of chyme released from the stomach may increase the likelihood of heartburn and nausea and can result in delayed absorption of glucose.

Intestine and colon

Progesterone-induced relaxation of smooth muscle decreases gut tone and motility and thus transit time in the gut increases which may enhance absorption (Blackburn 2003). However, pregnant women may experience bloating and abdominal distension. Duodenal villi hypertrophy and increase in height, which expands absorption capacity. Absorption of several nutrients, such as iron, calcium, glucose, amino acids, water, sodium and chloride is increased (Blackburn 2003); the increased absorption of iron in late pregnancy coincides with raised placental uptake and decreased maternal stores. However, progesterone may inhibit transport mechanisms for other nutrients such as the B group of vitamins.

The relaxation of the smooth muscle in the colon leads to increased water absorption and increases the incidence of constipation (Case study 11.3). The raised levels of angiotensin and aldosterone also increase sodium and water absorption from the colon in pregnancy. As the enlarging uterus compresses the colon, many women experience increased flatulence.

Liver and gall bladder

Progesterone affects the smooth muscle tone of the gall bladder resulting in flaccidity, increased bile

---

Case study 11.3

Josie is 14 weeks pregnant and is suffering from constipation. She is a vegetarian and normally consumes a high-fibre diet.

- What physiological changes may account for her constipation?
- What advice could the midwife give to help alleviate this problem?

volume storage and decreased emptying rate. Water resorption by the epithelium cells of the gall bladder is decreased so the bile is more dilute and contains less cholesterol. There is a tendency to retain bile salts resulting in the formation of cholesterol-based gall-stones in pregnancy. Cholestasis is a condition often observed in late pregnancy where women complain of itchy and irritable skin (though no rash is present) because bile salts are deposited in the skin.

In many species, pregnancy-induced liver enlargement results from increased circulation. In humans, however, morphological changes appear to result from hepatic displacement by the gravid uterus rather than an actual growth increase. Increased glycogen and tri-acylglyceride storage occurs in the hepatic cells. The raised level of oestrogen affects hepatic synthesis of plasma proteins, enzymes and lipids. The most marked changes are the fall in albumin (which is exaggerated by haemodilution), increase in fibrinogen (see above) and increased cholesterol synthesis. Synthesis of many binding proteins involved with placental transport of nutrients increases.

The skin and appearance

A number of changes can be observed in the appearance of a pregnant woman (Box 11.5). The increase in MSH means that there is a progressive increase in skin pigmentation, especially in women with dark hair and complexions. The nipple and the areola darken early in pregnancy. A dark line develops from the navel to pubis; this is the linea nigra showing the embryonic folding and fusion line of the abdomen. Facial chloasma (melasma)—irregular blotchy pigmentation usually in the shape of a butterfly mask ('mask of pregnancy') around the eyes and forehead—is common. Freckles and recent scars may darken and many women tan more deeply in pregnancy. Pigmentation changes may remain after pregnancy in women with darker hair and skin, and chloasma may be exacerbated by exposure to the sun.

The skeleton and joints

Posture and gait change in pregnancy. The weight of the gravid uterus changes the woman's centre of gravity altering the angle of inclination of the pelvic brim to the horizontal plane. The lumbar spine is naturally anteriorly convex, but the combined effects of proges-

---

Box 11.5

Top-to-toe observation of a pregnant woman

- Hair: thicker and glossier
- Face: may have chloasma and/or oedema
- Hands: warm, may develop vascular spiders and palmar erythema
- Skin: warm, well-vascularized, hyperpigmentation (related to MSH production)
- Skin conditions, such as eczema, may improve
- Abdominal wall: pigmentation of linea nigra, lax abdominal muscles, striae gravidarum may be seen (related to cortisol production)
- Pruritus (localized itching usually of abdomen): occurs in about 20% of pregnant women in the third trimester, but earlier in pregnancy it may be a sign of pruritus gravidarum (intrahepatic cholestasis of pregnancy due to raised bile acids), which is associated with premature delivery, fetal distress and perinatal mortality
- Breasts: dilation of superficial veins, pigmentation of nipples and areola
- Legs: oedema may be evident around ankles; varicose veins may develop
- Posture and gait: lordosis, changed centre of gravity (related to effects of hormones on cartilage and connective tissue)

---

terone, relaxin and the weight of the uterus on the intravertebral discs exaggerate this curve. The resulting lordosis of the spine compensates for the shift in the centre of gravity but may result in muscle and ligament strain. By the end of pregnancy, many women adopt a typical posture where they stand and walk with their backs arched and the shoulders held backwards. Lordosis is increased by poor posture generally, obesity, skeletal disorders, tuberculosis and by wearing high-heeled shoes. Oestrogen and relaxin affect the composition of the cartilage and connective tissue of pelvic joints, which soften in preparation for labour. The symphysis pubis and sacroiliac joints become more mobile and flexible so the pelvis becomes wider resulting in a rolling unstable movement and waddling gait when walking. Pregnant women may, therefore, experience muscle and ligament strain and discomfort or pain. The incidence of backache increases particularly after the 5th month. Some women experience severe back pain, often with peak intensity at night.

Occasionally in late pregnancy the symphysis pubis may separate. This condition, described as diastasis, can cause the pregnant woman great discomfort when walking or when her legs are abducted. The lower back is also affected by breast changes, stretching of the round ligament and decreased tone of abdominal muscles. In the third trimester, pressure of the uterus stretching or compressing nerves and blood vessels can result in numbness and tingling of extremities. Leg cramps, especially of the calf and thigh muscles, are common in the second half of pregnancy. They may be related to calcium/phosphorus metabolism and increased neuromuscular irritability. Raised phosphate levels are implicated and reducing dietary intake of milk is often beneficial. About 10% of pregnant women experience restless legs syndrome 10–20 minutes after getting into bed; the cause is unknown (Manconi et al 2004).

Calcium metabolism

There is increased turnover of calcium early in pregnancy. Maternal calcium metabolism changes to facilitate calcium transport to the fetus. The placenta actively transports calcium from the maternal blood. Placental calcium concentrations are higher than maternal levels so the fetus is protected if maternal concentrations fall. Placental efficiency is much greater than the absorptive capability of a fetus's gastrointestinal tract; thus a baby born prematurely with immature gut function cannot absorb calcium efficiently and remains undermineralized. In the last 10 weeks of gestation, the fetus obtains 18 g of calcium and 10 g of phosphorus from the maternal circulation, which is equivalent to 80% of the mother's normal dietary calcium in that period. However, the 28–30 g of calcium accumulated by the fetus represents a very small fraction of the total maternal calcium.

hPL and prolactin stimulate vitamin D synthesis, which increases absorption of calcium. Gastrointestinal absorption of vitamin D increases throughout the pregnancy. hPL increases bone reabsorption of calcium. Oestrogen stimulates parathyroid hormone secretion, which increases calcium absorption, decreases urinary losses and increases release of calcium from bone. Calcitonin secretion is also increased; calcitonin inhibits mineral release from the maternal skeleton but allows the actions of parathyroid hormone on the gut and kidney. Maternal serum calcium levels fall progressively in pregnancy. Levels are related to haemodilution of albumin and increased urinary losses and transport across the placenta. Urinary excretion of calcium decreases after 36 weeks, which augments dietary sources of calcium.

Homeostasis, mediated by maternal hormones, means that the maternal skeleton is conserved. If dietary calcium is adequate, there is no marked change in maternal skeletal mass or bone density. There is no evidence that high parity is associated with increased fractures in later life. Calcium supplements tend to reduce blood pressure by a small amount and may be useful in the treatment of pre-eclampsia (see Ch. 12). Calcium requirements in pregnancy are probably overestimated; clinical deficiency is rarely observed. However, a low vitamin D intake in pregnancy and little exposure to sunlight is associated with osteomalacia, as demonstrated by Asian women in the UK who have lower plasma calcium and an increased incidence of maternal osteomalacia and neonatal rickets.

Vision

The changed hormonal profile of pregnancy influences the maternal nervous system. In the third trimester, mild corneal oedema is common; fluid is retained and the cornea becomes slightly thicker, which affects refraction. Tear composition changes; levels of lysozyme alter and tears often become greasy. This, together with altered corneal sensitivity, may cause blurring or intolerance to contact lenses. Progesterone, relaxin and hCG affect intraocular pressure, which can fall (which will improve glaucoma). Unless they experience problems, it is wise for pregnant women to delay new prescriptions for spectacles. Women with pre-eclampsia and retinal oedema, and those with diabetes, are particularly prone to visual complications.

The nose and larynx

The nasal mucosa becomes hyperaemic and congested in pregnancy, causing nasal stuffiness and obstruction. This seems to be oestrogen-related and may interfere with sleep and sense of smell. It is associated with congestion of the eustachian tubes (often described as blocked ears unrelieved by swallowing), which may cause a transient mild hearing loss. Erythema and oedema of the vocal cords can lead to hoarseness, coughing and vocal changes.

Sleep

Sleep patterns change in pregnancy. An increased desire for sleep and napping in the first trimester has been observed (Brunner et al 1994). It is suggested that progesterone affects neuronal activity in the brain reducing the level of excitatory neurotransmitters (Smith 1991). Oestrogen enhances this effect by increasing the number of receptors for progesterone. The amount of rapid eye movement (REM) sleep increases from 25 weeks, peaking at 33–36 weeks. Stage 4 non-REM sleep (deep sleep) decreases. It is this state that appears important for tissue repair and recovery from fatigue. In the second half of pregnancy,

women tend to sleep less as they frequently are disturbed by nocturia, dyspnoea, heartburn, nasal congestion, muscle aches, stress and anxiety and fetal activity.

Carbohydrate metabolism

Maternal metabolism changes in pregnancy to meet increased maternal needs, including the accumulation of maternal energy stores in readiness for labour and lactation, and to facilitate fetal growth and development (Fig. 11.10). Metabolism in pregnancy must also facilitate both the accumulation of fetal energy

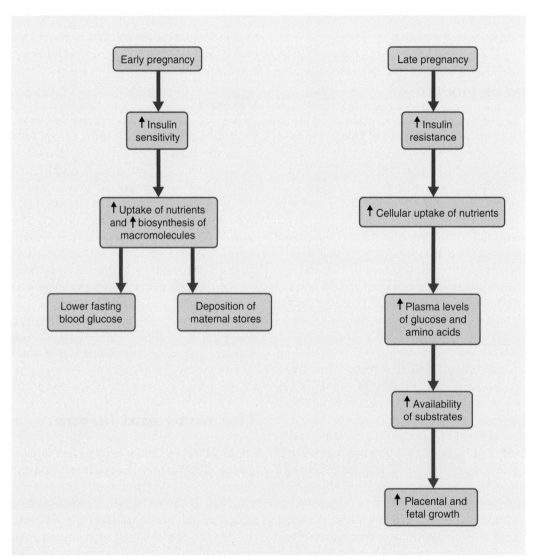

Fig. 11.10   *Changes in maternal carbohydrate handling during pregnancy.*

stores for the transition to extrauterine life (see Ch. 15) and maternal accumulation of fat stores in preparation for labour and lactation. Pregnancy is primarily anabolic: food intake and appetite increase and activity decreases. Pregnancy has been described as a 'state of accelerated starvation' (Frienkel et al 1972) because there is an increased tendency to become ketotic. Pregnancy is a diabetogenic state; women acquire insulin resistance in later pregnancy which appears to represent a temporary excursion into metabolic syndrome.

Early pregnancy

Metabolism in the first trimester is predominantly anabolic with synthesis of new maternal tissues including deposition of maternal fat. It can be considered as a time of preparation for the subsequent high demands of rapid fetal growth; over 90% of fetal growth occurs in the second half of pregnancy (King 2000). Early in the pregnancy, there is an increased response to insulin so fasting blood glucose levels are lower than normal. The tissues exhibit increased sensitivity to insulin so there is increased uptake of nutrients and synthesis of macromolecules by cells which promotes maternal tissue growth. As the pregnancy progresses, most women develop insulin resistance so levels of glucose and amino acids in the blood rise, thus increasing the availability of substrates required by the fetus and placental uptake.

In the first trimester, increased insulin is produced in response to glucose. Early in pregnancy, the raised levels of oestrogen and progesterone orchestrate the changes in metabolism. Oestrogen stimulates pancreatic β-cell growth (hyperplasia and hypertrophy) and therefore insulin secretion. It also enhances glucose utilization in peripheral tissues and increases plasma cortisol. So the net effect is to decrease fasting glucose levels, improve glucose tolerance and increase glycogen storage. Hepatic metabolism of insulin may also be altered. Lowered glucose levels between meals increase the tendency to become ketotic. Placental transfer of amino acids, increased hepatic gluconeogenesis (conversion of amino acids, particularly alanine, to glucose) and raised insulin levels, which stimulate cellular uptake, together result in lowered maternal levels of amino acids. During the first half of pregnancy, the progressive increment in insulin levels, augmented by progesterone and cortisol, stimulates

hepatic lipogenesis (triacylglyceride synthesis and storage) and suppresses lipolysis (fat breakdown). An increase in the numbers of insulin receptors on the adipocytes means there is enhanced removal of triglycerides from circulation. Increased fat storage in early pregnancy results in hypertrophy of adipose cells. During fasting, ketogenesis is increased as the triglycerides are utilized.

Later pregnancy

As the pregnancy progresses, the fetal placental unit grows and levels of placental hormones, which are antagonistic to insulin, increase. Therefore maternal tissues exhibit decreased sensitivity, or resistance, to insulin, which means that insulin is less effective at stimulating glucose uptake. Pregnancy-induced insulin resistance affects adipocytes to a lesser degree. The dominant effect in the second and third trimesters is related to the high levels of hPL, but human placental growth hormone, prolactin, cortisol and progesterone are also involved. Tumour necrosis factor α (TNFα), resistin and leptin may also be involved in the increased insulin resistance that develops in pregnancy. Levels of hPL increase markedly after 20 weeks. hPL is a very potent insulin antagonist with effects similar to those of growth hormone. Raised hPL results in decreased peripheral tissue responses to insulin and therefore increased circulating levels of glucose and amino acids, which are available for transport to the fetus. hPL increases lipolysis and nitrogen retention, decreases urinary potassium excretion and increases calcium excretion.

Progesterone augments insulin secretion, increasing fasting levels, but decreases peripheral insulin effectiveness. Cortisol inhibits glucose uptake and oxidation, increases liver glucose production and possibly augments glucagon secretion. Therefore, in later pregnancy, fasting results in mobilization of maternal triacylglyceride stores leading to a marked increase in levels of maternal fatty acids. This provides an alternative substrate for maternal metabolism so glucose is spared for central nervous system and fetal requirements. As tissue uptake of glucose is suppressed so levels of glucose are raised, which stimulates insulin release from the pancreas. Hyperinsulinaemia is a normal development in the later part of pregnancy; levels of insulin double by the third trimester. The raised level of insulin is important in stimulating protein synthesis. Raised insulin levels counteract the effect of the antagonistic hormones so maternal plasma glucose is maintained at levels similar to prepregnant levels. Insulin sensitivity rebounds after the delivery of the placenta. Women with insulin-dependent diabetes mellitus (IDDM) need to have a marked increase in insulin dose to compensate for the pregnancy-induced resistance to insulin.

In the postabsorptive states between meals, gluconeogenesis and fat mobilization provide substrates for maternal metabolism and placental transfer. Maternal cells metabolize the increased ketones and free fatty acids, thus sparing glucose and amino acids for placental uptake. As blood sugar increases in the pregnancy, it can exceed the transport maxima of the nephrons (i.e. the capacity to reabsorb the glucose from the glomerular filtrate) so some glucose is excreted in the urine. A degree of glucosuria is normal in pregnancy. As renal absorption of glucose is limited (so there are increased losses) and hepatic gluconeogenesis is decreased, hypoglycaemia, hypoalaninaemia and hypoinsulinaemia result.

Gestational diabetes mellitus

Gestational diabetes mellitus is defined as carbohydrate intolerance that begins or was first recognized in pregnancy. It is the extreme end of the spectrum of normal physiological changes in pregnancy. Gestational diabetes mellitus is due to the inability of the maternal pancreas to increase insulin secretion enough to counter the pregnancy-induced insulin resistance. Inability to produce adequate insulin at this stage of pregnancy is probably due to a limitation of the pancreatic β-cells (which may be related to the pregnant woman's own pancreatic development in utero). Inadequate secretion of insulin, and altered carbohydrate metabolism, may become evident again when there is further demand for insulin, as in a subsequent pregnancy or in later life, and is particularly associated with increased body weight (and therefore cell number). Gestational diabetes (or delivery of an infant weighing more then 4.5 kg) is a risk factor both for future pregnancies and for prediabetes and type 2 diabetes mellitus. Infants of diabetic mothers and those with either macrosomia or microsomia also have an increased diabetogenic tendency.

Case study 11.4 is an example of raised glucose levels in pregnancy.

Case study 11.4

Cathy is expecting her fourth baby. At 28 weeks' gestation, a random blood glucose revealed a blood glucose level of 11 mmol/l. Cathy looks well and, as in all her other pregnancies, says she feels exceptionally healthy. Cathy is referred to the consultant clinic for further investigations. Her previous baby was delivered at 37 weeks' gestation weighing 4.960 kg.

■ What is the provisional diagnosis and what investigations will be carried out to confirm this diagnosis?

■ What physiological interactions between the mother and fetus are occurring that could explain this phenomenon?

■ How can the midwife best explain these to Cathy and what advice should she be given?

■ What are the possible consequences for Cathy and her baby if no further investigations are carried out and no treatment advised?

Key points

■ The physiological adaptation to pregnancy is mediated by the increase of steroid hormone secretion. Steroid hormones are initially produced from the corpus luteum under the influence of hCG and subsequently from the placenta.

■ The maternal endocrine system is affected by the increase in steroid hormones so other hormones augment the effects of oestrogen and progesterone. For instance, secretion of MSH and cortisol increases in pregnancy, affecting skin pigmentation and improving some pathological conditions such as eczema.

■ Generally early physiological changes in pregnancy are regulated by hormonal changes, whereas later changes may be due to structural effects of the enlarging uterus.

■ Reproductive system: under the influence of oestrogen, the uterus increases in size and vascularization, and spontaneous uterine contractions are suppressed. The breasts undergo development in preparation for lactation.

■ Cardiovascular system: physiological changes are particularly marked in this system, meeting the increased demands of the maternal and fetal tissues. The vascular system expands as progesterone stimulates vasodilation of the vascular smooth muscle and oestrogen stimulates angiogenesis and increased blood flow. The RAS responds to the underfilled vascular system by increasing sodium and water retention; thus blood volume increases by about 40%. Plasma expansion is greater than blood cell increase leading to overall haemodilution.

- Cardiac output increases early in pregnancy, initially as a result of increased heart rate, which is subsequently followed by increased stroke volume. Myocontractility is increased throughout pregnancy, which stimulates a degree of ventricular hypertrophy.

- Blood pressure decreases in early pregnancy, reaching a minimum in mid-pregnancy, and then returns close to prepregnant values towards term. The effects of posture on blood pressure are marked in pregnancy.

- The dilution of plasma proteins increases the formation of oedema. The ratio of clotting factors changes so bleeding time decreases.

- Respiratory system: excursion of the diaphragm alters as the rib cage flares increasing the efficiency of inspiration. Progesterone affects the sensitivity of the chemoreceptors, which increases respiratory drive. Therefore, hyperventilation is normal in pregnancy and results in lower circulating carbon dioxide levels and higher concentrations of cations, which facilitate exchange across the placenta.

- Gastrointestinal system: progesterone stimulates appetite and thirst and affects the sensitivity of the taste buds. Progesterone also affects the smooth muscle of the gut, which alters motility and transit time. This can result in increased efficiency of absorption but may also cause nausea and constipation. Decreased tone of lower oesophageal sphincter may result in reflux and heartburn.

- Skin: the increase in MSH levels results in increased pigmentation of the nipple and areola, the linea nigra and possibly chloasma. Increased blood flow to the skin, which is important in heat regulation, affects growth of hair and nails and may cause congestion of the mucous membranes.

- Skeleton: posture is affected by changed weight distribution and altered composition of the cartilage and connective tissue resulting in an exaggerated curvature of the spine.

- Metabolism: maternal metabolism is affected by altered thyroid hormone secretion and altered responses to insulin. In the first half of pregnancy, increased sensitivity to insulin favours deposition of maternal fat stores. In the second half of pregnancy, insulin resistance results in raised levels of substrates in the maternal plasma, which favour placental transport and fetal growth. Extremes of insulin resistance result in gestational diabetes mellitus.

Application to practice

Women experience many changes within their bodies and naturally will seek explanations and reassurance from the midwife as the changes occur. The midwife should use her knowledge of the physiological changes to aid her in assessing whether the pregnancy is progressing normally.

Annotated further reading

Blackburn ST 2003 Maternal, fetal, and neonatal physiology: a clinical perspective, 2nd edn. Saunders, Philadelphia
An excellent in-depth description of physiological adaptation to pregnancy and consequent development of the fetus and neonate that draws from physiological research studies. The chapters are clearly organized by physiological systems and link physiological concepts to clinical applications including the assessment and management of low- and high-risk pregnancies.

Bremme KA 2003 Haemostatic changes in pregnancy. Best Practice & Research Clinical Haematology 16:153–168
An in-depth review of the changes in the coagulation and fibrinolytic systems that accompany normal pregnancy

Chamberlain G, Broughton Pipkin F 1998 Clinical physiology in obstetrics, 3rd edn. Blackwell, Oxford
Comprehensively describes the physiological changes in pregnancy and relates recent research findings to practical considerations in the care of pregnant women.

Chamberlain G, Steer P 2001 Turnbull's obstetrics, 3rd edn. Churchill Livingstone, New York
A comprehensive textbook with a medical approach to obstetric principles and practice and the development of clinical protocols.

Creasy RK, Resnik RIJ 2003 Maternal–fetal medicine: principles and practice, 5th edn. Saunders, Philadelphia
Covers all disciplines pertinent to obstetricians including genetics and genetic testing, fetal and placental growth and development, epidemiology, immunology, physiological adaptation to pregnancy as well as clinical applications and medical complications in pregnancy.

Gilbert ES, Harmon JS 2002 Manual of high risk pregnancy and delivery. Mosby, St Louis
This book is an excellent reference for midwives who provide high-risk care in practice and it details many of the pathological problems that can arise during pregnancy and delivery.

References

Baylis C, Davison JM 1998 The urinary system. In: Chamberlain G, Broughton Pipkin F (eds) Clinical physiology in obstetrics, 3rd edn. Blackwell, Oxford, pp 263–307

Blackburn ST 2003 Maternal, fetal, and neonatal physiology: a clinical perspective. 2nd edn. Saunders, Philadelphia

Bowen DJ 1992 Taste and food preference changes across the course of pregnancy. Appetite 19:233–242

Brown MA, Gallery EDM 1994 Volume homeostasis in normal pregnancy and pre-eclampsia: physiology and clinical implications. Baillière's Clinics in Obstetrics and Gynaecology 8:287–310

Brunner DP, Münch M, Biedermann K, Huch R, Huch A, Borbély AA 1994 Changes in sleep and sleep electroencephalogram during pregnancy. Sleep 17(7):576–582

Carbonne B, Benachi A, Léveque ML, Cabrol D, Papiernik E 1996 Maternal position during labor: effects on fetal oxygen saturation measured by pulse oximetry. Obstetrics and Gynecology 88:797–800

Chamberlain G, Dewhurst J, Harvey D 1991 Illustrated textbook of obstetrics. Gower Medical (Mosby), London, p 104

Coad J, Al Rasasi B, Morgan JB 2000 New perspectives on nausea and vomiting in pregnancy. MIDIRS Research Digest 10:451–454

Coad J, Al Rasasi B, Morgan J 2002 Nutrient insult in early pregnancy. Proceedings of the Nutrition Society 61:51–59

Cordain L, Eaton SB, Miller JB, Mann N, Hill K 2002 The paradoxical nature of hunter–gatherer diets: meat-based, yet non-atherogenic. European Journal of Clinical Nutrition 56(Suppl 1):S42–S52

Davison JM, Shiells EA, Philips PR, Lindheimer MD 1990 Influence of humoral and volume factors on altered osmoregulation of normal human pregnancy. American Journal of Physiology 258:F900–F907

de Swiet M 1998a The cardiovascular system. In: Chamberlain G, Broughton Pipkin F (eds) Clinical physiology in obstetrics, 3rd edn. Blackwell, Oxford, pp 33–70

de Swiet M 1998b The respiratory system. In: Chamberlain G, Broughton Pipkin F (eds) Clinical physiology in obstetrics, 3rd edn. Blackwell, Oxford, pp 111–128

Dunlop W 1980 Serial changes in renal haemodynamics during normal human pregnancy. Journal of Obstetrics and Gynaecology 88:1

Duvekot JJ, Peeters LLH 1998 Very early changes in cardiovascular physiology. In: Chamberlain G, Broughton Pipkin F (eds) Clinical physiology in obstetrics, 3rd edn. Blackwell, Oxford, pp 3–32

Duvekot JJ, Cheriex EC, Pieters FA et al 1993 Early pregnancy changes in hemodynamics and volume homeostasis are consecutive adjustments triggered by a primary fall in systemic vascular tone. American Journal of Obstetrics and Gynecology 169(6):1382–1392

Elling SV, Powell FC 1997 Physiological changes in the skin during pregnancy. Clinical Dermatology 15:35–43

Flaxman SM, Sherman PW 2000 Morning sickness: a mechanism for protecting mother and embryo. Quarterly Review of Biology 75:113–148

Frienkel N, Metzger BE, Nitzan M et al 1972 'Accelerated starvation' and mechanisms for the conservation of maternal nitrogen during pregnancy. Israel Journal of Medical Science 8:426

Glinoer D, Lemone M 1992 Goiter and pregnancy: a new insight into an old problem. Thyroid 2:65–70

Godfrey KM, Redman CWG, Barker DJP, Osmond C 1991 The effect of maternal anaemia and iron deficiency on the ratio of fetal weight to placental weight. British Journal of Obstetrics and Gynaecology 98:886–891

Haram K, Nilsen ST, Ulvik RJ 2001 Iron supplementation in pregnancy: evidence and controversies. Acta Obstetrica et Gynecologica Scandinavica 80:683–688

Huxley RR 2000 Nausea and vomiting in early pregnancy: its role in placental development. Obstetrics and Gynecology 95:779–782

Hytten F 1991 The alimentary system. In: Hytten F, Chamberlain G (eds) Clinical physiology in obstetrics, 2nd edn. Blackwell, Oxford, pp 137–149

Iles RK, Chard T 1991 Human chorionic gonadotrophin expression by bladder cancers: biology and clinical potential. Journal of Urology 145(3):481–489

Ivell R, Einspanier A 2002 Relaxin peptides are new global players. Trends in Endocrinology and Metabolism 13:343–348

Johnson MH, Everitt BJ 2000 Essential reproduction, 5th edn. Blackwell, Oxford

King JC 2000 Physiology of pregnancy and nutrient metabolism. American Journal of Clinical Nutrition 71:1218S–1225S

Kornyei JL, Lei ZM, Rao CV 1993 Human myometrial smooth muscle cells are a novel target of direct regulation by human chorionic gonadotrophin. Biology of Reproduction 49:1149–1157

Letsky E 1998 The haematological system. In: Chamberlain G, Broughton Pipkin F (eds) Clinical physiology in obstetrics, 3rd edn. Blackwell, Oxford, pp 71–110

Mabie WC, DiSessa TG, Crocker LG, Sibai BM, Arheart KL 1994 A longitudinal study of cardiac output in normal human pregnancy. American Journal of Obstetrics and Gynecology 170:849–856

Manconi M, Govoni V, De Vito A, Tiberio EN, Cesnik E, Mollica G, Granieri E 2004 Pregnancy as a risk factor for restless legs syndrome. Sleep Medicine 5:305–308

Maul H, Longo M, Saade GR, Garfield RE 2003 Nitric oxide and its role during pregnancy: from ovulation to delivery. Current Pharmaceutical Design 9:359–380

Miller AWF, Hanretty KP 1998 Obstetrics illustrated, 5th edn. Churchill Livingstone, New York, p 34

Morris NH, Eaton BM, Dekker G 1996 Nitric oxide, the endothelium, pregnancy and pre-eclampsia. British Journal of Obstetrics and Gynaecology 103:4–15

Palmer RMJ, Ferrige AG, Moncada S 1987 Nitric oxide release accounts for the biological activity of endothelium-derived relaxing factor. Nature 327:524–526

Picciano MF 2003 Pregnancy and lactation: physiological adjustments, nutritional requirements and the role of dietary supplements. Journal of Nutrition 133:1997S–2002S

Prabhakar NR, Peng YJ 2004 Peripheral chemoreceptors in health and disease. Journal of Applied Physiology 96:359–366

Schrier RW 1992 A unifying hypothesis of body fluid volume regulation. Journal of the Royal College of Physicians of London 26:295–306

Smith SS 1991 Progesterone administration attenuates excitatory amino acid responses of cerebellar Purkinje cells. Neuroscience 42:309–320

Sweet B, Tiran D 1996 Mayes midwifery, 12th edn. Baillière Tindall, London, p 131

Yip R, Dallman PR 1996 Iron. In: Ziegler EE, Filer LJ (eds) Present knowledge in nutrition, 7th edn. ILSI, Washington DC, pp 277–292

12 Maternal nutrition and health

Learning objectives

■ To review nutritional requirements and explain the role of the main nutrient groups in human health.

■ To identify how and why nutrient requirements might change during pregnancy.

■ To describe how the fetus adapts to low nutrient levels.

■ To relate undernutrition to outcome of pregnancy.

■ To discuss other factors that may affect weight gain in pregnancy and birth weight.

Introduction

It is common for pregnancy to affect a woman's sense of well-being. Some aspects of health may be affected positively and others negatively. The role of nutrition, both before and after pregnancy, is important for the health of both the mother and fetus. Pregnant women are often receptive to advice and may make changes to their diet which may persist (Anderson 2001). Maternal stressors, including perceived stress, chronic and acute stresses related to life events, work-related stress and pregnancy-related anxiety, as well as nutritional stress, are associated with adverse outcomes of pregnancy such as low birth weight (LBW), prematurity and intrauterine growth retardation (IUGR) (Hobel & Culhane 2003). Although stress, of all types, is a risk for preterm birth and premature labour, not all stressed women deliver prematurely suggesting that pregnant women (or their fetuses) have differing vulnerability to the effects of stress.

Chapter case study

Both Zara and James follow a vegetarian diet and try to lead a healthy lifestyle. At her first visit to the midwife, Zara was calculated as having a body mass index (BMI) of 24, which the midwife calculated from what Zara reported as her non-pregnant weight. During the pregnancy, Zara's baby appeared to be growing as expected and her midwife has measured Zara's uterine growth in centimetres using the symphysis pubis as the reference point; as expected, the fundal height has increased by 1 cm per week of pregnancy.

At 34 weeks' gestation, Zara is concerned that she only seems to have gained 9 pounds over her non-pregnant weight unlike her sister who has put on over 20 pounds and has been told by her midwife that her baby is a little bit on the small side. What factors could explain the differences in weight gain between Zara and her sister? What are the benefits of calculating the BMI of pregnant mothers and why is it preferable to calculate the BMI using the non-pregnant values if they are available? Does Zara's smaller weight gain give any cause for concern? What other reasons could explain why Zara's sister appears to have gained a lot more weight than Zara has?

Overview of nutrition

Growth, development and optimal health rely on good nutrition and an adequate quality and quantity of nutrients for the cells. However, diet is influenced by many factors including wealth, religion, culture, and geographical and social factors. The insoluble macro-molecules of food must be digested into soluble and absorbable subunits (see Ch. 1). The major components of the diet, or macronutrients, are carbohydrates, proteins and fats. Essential micronutrients are vitamins and minerals. Water is also an essential part of the diet.

Carbohydrates

Carbohydrates are the major energy source in the majority of human diets, but the amount and type of carbohydrate consumed varies amongst different population groups. With increased affluence in the Western world, there is a tendency to increase the proportion of fat in the diet at the expense of carbohydrate. There are two major types of carbohydrate: polysaccharides (or complex carbohydrates) and simple sugars (monosaccharides and disaccharides).

Monosaccharides, such as glucose, fructose and galactose, are not usually consumed in high quantities although they do occur in fruit. The major source of carbohydrate in the diet is starch from plant sources, plus some glycogen from animal liver and muscle. Dietary disaccharides include sucrose (table sugar), lactose (in milk) and maltose, which occurs in malt, beer and some sprouting seeds. Most starchy foods are high in carbohydrate and low in fat. With increasing affluence, added sugars tend to contribute more to the carbohydrate content at the expense of polysaccharides; soft drinks and sweet snacks may constitute a significant part of the carbohydrate intake.

Carbohydrates have differing effects on blood glucose levels and carbohydrate-rich foods can be compared using glycaemic index (GI) ranking. GI values for different foods are calculated by comparing their effect on blood glucose with the effects of a reference food (usually glucose or white bread). Carbohydrates with high GI are digested quickly and absorbed faster so the blood glucose response is fast. Carbohydrates that break down slowly, and result in a slow and sustained release of glucose into the circulation, have a low GI. Low GI foods prolong carbohydrate absorption, attenuate insulin secretion, increase the translocation of the insulin-responsive glucose transporter (GLUT4) to the cell membrane; they also result in more colonic fermentation of carbohydrate and beneficial short-chain fatty acid production (Brand-Miller 2003). High GI foods provide a rapid rise in blood sugar levels and are recommended for post-exercise energy recovery, whereas low GI foods release energy slowly and steadily and are appropriate for diabetics, dieters and endurance athletes.

Many carbohydrate-rich foods contain indigestible non-starch polysaccharides (NSP or 'dietary fibre'). Dietary fibre is indigestible carbohydrate. Insoluble fibre promotes the formation of bulkier and softer faecal stools. Soluble fibre slows absorption of glucose and reduces blood cholesterol levels; it is associated with decreased incidence of gut diseases. Foods rich in complex carbohydrates include cereal grains, starchy vegetables, legumes, seeds and wholegrain cereals, all of which contain reasonable proportions (3–15%) of NSP. Most other vegetables, and most fruits, contain small amounts of both starch and NSP and variable amounts of sugars. Most foods that are not highly processed, with the exception of honey and dried fruits, do not contain much sugar, whereas most processed foods contain added sugars, usually sucrose.

Proteins

Proteins are made up of 20 types of amino acids linked together by peptide bonds. Indispensable or essential amino acids are those that cannot be synthesized from other amino acids and, therefore, are required in the diet (Table 12.1). There are conditions, in which requirement is high or there is limited ability to interconvert amino acids, that result in an amino acid that can usually be synthesized from an indispensable

Table 12.1 *Amino acids*

Essential amino acids	Conditionally essential amino acids	Non-essential amino acids
Lysine	Cysteine	Alanine
Threonine	Tyrosine	Glutamic acid
Histidine	Arginine	Aspartic acid
Isoleucine	Citrulline*	Glycine
Leucine	Taurine*	Serine
Methionine	Carnitine	Proline
Phenylalanine		Glutamine
Tryptophan		Asparagine
Valine		

*Conditionally essential or essential only at certain ages or in certain conditions.

amino acid being required in the diet. These amino acids are described as being conditionally indispensable, for instance premature babies with immature enzyme function or under conditions of stress may require amino acids that they will be able to synthesize when they are older.

Protein quality depends on the proportion of dietary protein that is absorbed across the gut (digestibility) and the ratio of the essential amino acids in the protein. A protein that is absorbed completely and utilized completely because the indispensable amino acids are in the optimum proportion for synthesis of new proteins is described as a high-quality protein, with a net protein utilization (NPU) value of 1.0 or 100%. Human milk and whole egg have an NPU of 1.0, whereas the overall protein availability in the Western diet is typically 0.7. The NPU of diets dependent on poor-quality proteins, such as those based on cassava (made from tapioca root), can be as low as 0.5.

In the absence of alternative sources of energy, protein can be metabolized as an energy source. Excess protein in the diet will also be used as a metabolic fuel. An adult is usually in nitrogen balance: protein intake is equal to protein breakdown so nitrogen in the diet is equal to excreted levels of nitrogen. Under conditions of growth and protein synthesis, there is a net accumulation of protein, and hence nitrogen, which is described as a state of positive nitrogen balance. States of growth, including pregnancy, result in positive nitrogen balance. Negative nitrogen balance usually indicates tissue breakdown or nutrient deficiency resulting in energy generation from protein sources. Illness and trauma cause negative nitrogen balance, although it also occurs with reduced activity and decreasing muscle mass and during uterine involution (see Ch. 13).

Fat

Fat is used for energy requirements. There is also a requirement for essential long-chain fatty acids, which cannot be synthesized by the body. These are the precursors of prostaglandins and leukotrienes. Fat also provides the vehicle for absorption of fat-soluble vitamins. Most fat is present in the diet as triglycerides; a triglyceride is a glycerol molecule with three fatty acids (Fig. 12.1). There is a range of fatty acids of different chain length and degree of saturation, which is related to the number of double bonds in the fatty acid molecule. Saturated fatty acids have no double bonds, monounsaturated fatty acids have one double bond and polyunsaturated fatty acids have two or more double bonds. The body handles fatty acids differently depending on their length and the degree of saturation (Fig. 12.1C). Fats in foods are formed of triglycerides containing a combination of different fatty acids, but are described by the predominant type. For instance, olive oil is particularly rich in monounsaturated fatty acids (with single double bonds).

Saturated fats are likely to be solid at room temperature and are usually of animal origin, although coconut and palm oils and cocoa butter are saturated. Saturated fats become rancid very slowly so they store well. Unsaturated fats are usually liquid at room temperature and mostly of plant origin. The C=C double bond is not very stable so it oxidizes easily and the fat becomes rancid. In food processing, unsaturated vegetable oils are hydrogenated (have hydrogen atoms added to saturate the C=C bonds), which makes the fat harder and extends the shelf-life and flavour stability. Unsaturated fatty acids from vegetable and most animal sources adopt a cis configuration, although ruminants produce some trans fatty acids which are thus found in low concentrations in milk and meat from ruminant animals. Positional isomerism, where the fatty acid has the same length and number and position of double bonds, but the atoms lie in different positions, is described as a trans configuration (Fig. 12.2). Hydrogenation and heating can convert the cis bonds to the trans isomer. Many cellular processes depend on the fluidity of the membrane lipids which depends on the properties of fatty acid chains. Saturated fatty acids are more ordered and rigid. The double bonds of unsaturated fatty acids produce bends in the fatty acid which means that the fatty acids of the membrane pack less tightly together, thus conferring a greater degree of fluidity and flexibility to the cell membrane. Trans fatty acids are straighter and are more like saturated fatty acids in conformation even though they have double bonds. Cholesterol also inserts into the cell membrane bilayer and affects fluidity.

Diets high in saturated fat are associated with an increased incidence of atherosclerosis (damage to arterial blood vessels, causing hardening and plaque formation) and an increase in low-density lipoprotein (LDL) cholesterol levels which is a marker for heart disease. Diets higher in polyunsaturated fat are associated with increased high-density lipoprotein (HDL) cholesterol levels and an increased HDL:LDL ratio

A

Palmitic acid (saturated)

Stearic acid (saturated)

Oleic acid (mono-unsaturated)

Triacylglycerol (triglyceride)

B

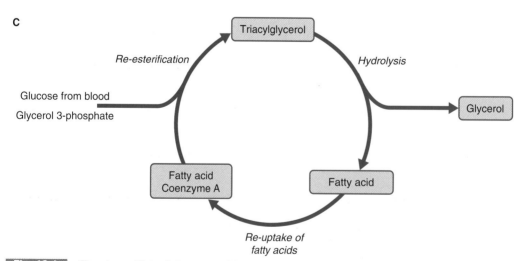

Fatty acid (palmitic acid)

Glycerol

C

Triacylglycerol

Re-esterification

Hydrolysis

Glucose from blood
Glycerol 3-phosphate

Glycerol

Fatty acid
Coenzyme A

Fatty acid

Re-uptake of
fatty acids

Fig. 12.1 *Structure of fats: A A saturated fatty acid; B a triglyceride; C the fatty acid cycle.*

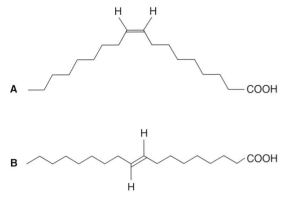

A

B

Fig. 12.2 *A Cis and B trans isomerism of fatty acids.*

which is at the omega position 3 of the chain). The body can further elongate and desaturate (lengthen and add more double bonds to) these essential fatty acids. However, there are two things to note. First, the fetus has limited ability to elongate and desaturate fatty acids so it is dependent on placental supply for both long-chain polyunsaturated fatty acids (LC-PUFA) and the indispensable fatty acids. Second, the enzymes involved in the pathways of elongation and desaturation of the indispensable fatty acids into their longer chain metabolites are competitive. This means that the ratio of ω-6 fatty acids to ω-3 fatty acids is important for optimal development.

which is associated with more favourable cardio-vascular health. Trans fatty acids are implicated in increased risk of myocardial infarction and other cardiovascular problems.

There are two polyunsaturated fatty acids that are indispensable ('essential') in the diet as they cannot be synthesized by the body. These are linoleic acid (18:2, ω-6; chain length of 18 carbons and two double bonds, the first of which is at the omega position 6 of the chain) and α-linoleic acid (18:3, ω-3; chain length of 18 carbons and three double bonds, the first of

Vitamins

Vitamins are organic substances required in small amounts for metabolism, growth and maintenance; they are not synthesized by the body (either at all or in adequate amounts) and so are essential nutrients. Vitamins do not provide sources of energy but act as regulators of metabolic processes. They can be divided into water-soluble (Table 12.2) and fat-soluble vitamins (Table 12.3). The fat-soluble vitamins are more stable than water-soluble vitamins and are stored in

Table 12.2 *Water-soluble vitamins*

Vitamin	Role	Source
Thiamin (B_1)	Carbohydrate metabolism	Pork, wheat germ, yeast
Riboflavin (B_2)	Protein metabolism	Offal, milk, grains, legumes, eggs, vegetables
Niacin (B_3)	Production of energy from glucose; synthesis of fatty acids	Meat, nuts, legumes
Pyridoxine (B_6)	Synthesis and catabolism of amino acids; synthesis of antibodies and neurotransmitters	Pork, offal, grains, legumes, potatoes, bananas
Cyanocobalamine (B_{12})	Reactions preceding use of folic acid in DNA synthesis	Animal and dairy products, eggs, yeast
Folate	Formation of DNA	Liver, green leafy vegetables, kidney beans, oranges, melon
Pantothenic acid	Metabolism; synthesis of acetylcholine	Liver, egg yolk, milk, dried and spouting beans
Biotin	Synthesis of fatty acids, amino acids and purines (required for DNA and RNA)	Offal, egg yolk, tomatoes
C	Collagen formation, tissue formation and integrity, antioxidant, iron absorption	Citrus fruit, tomatoes, other fruit and vegetables

Table 12.3 *Fat-soluble vitamins*

Vitamin	Role	Source
A	Visual perception (rhodopsin synthesis); growth of epithelial tissue and bones, antioxidant	Liver, kidney, egg yolk
D	Hormone involved in bone mineralization and calcium homeostasis	Synthesized in skin, fish oils
E	Tissue growth + integrity of cell membranes; antioxidant	Vegetable oils, grains, milk, eggs, fish, meat
K	Synthesis of blood-clotting factors; bone metabolism	Gut flora, liver, green leafy vegetables

the body, so when taken in excess they are more likely to cause toxicity than water-soluble vitamins. As B vitamins function as coenzymes in energy metabolism, requirement for B vitamins increases in parallel with increased energy consumption. Vitamins A, C and E function as antioxidants protecting cells from free-radical damage.

Minerals

Minerals regulate body function and are essential to good health. They are inorganic and become part of the body structure (Table 12.4). Excessive intake of minerals can be toxic or lead to illness indirectly because of the competitive nature of mineral absorption in the body. For example, excess iron can lead to zinc deficiency and excess zinc can lead to copper deficiency.

Preconceptual nutritional status

The sensitivity of the hypothalamus to environmental influences, such as nutrient availability, was probably of immense importance in promoting pregnancy in seasons when the fetus and infant had optimal chances of survival. Weight loss affects cyclical ovarian function in women. Anorexia nervosa disrupts the hypothalamic–pituitary–ovarian axis (see Ch. 4) and may cause amenorrhoea. Amenorrhoea related to inadequate nutrient intake is often reported in ballet dancers, competitive runners and other athletes (Frisch 1990). It not only affects the ovulatory cycle but also can result in low levels of oestrogens, which reduce bone density and predispose to osteoporosis. It has been suggested that the menarche depended on women reaching a 'critical weight' (Frisch & McArthur 1974). However, low body weight is not always asso-

ciated with amenorrhoea (Franks & Robinson 1996). Conversely, dieting, high energy expenditure, nutrient restriction or erratic eating patterns (such as crash dieting and binging) can suppress normal reproductive cycles in women even if their weight stays within a normal range (Coad 2003).

A minimal level of nutrient intake and fuel metabolism seem to be required to maintain reproductive functions, particularly the pulse generating secretion of gonadotrophin-releasing hormone (GnRH; see Ch. 4). Fluctuations in body fat can also disturb the transport and metabolism of the steroid hormones, which are fat-soluble. Nutrient deficiency may itself suppress appetite. Studies in animals suggest optimal pregnancy outcome may depend on long-term nutritional status rather than a period of 'flushing' or short-term good-quality diet (Wynn & Wynn 1991). Although restricted nutrient intake can suppress reproductive function, excess energy intake may also be disruptive. Obesity also affects conception rate. Polycystic ovary syndrome (PCOS), which is often associated with anovulation (see Ch. 6), disrupts glucose–insulin homeostasis. The symptoms and effects of PCOS on reproduction are more severe with increased body weight. In PCOS, increased obesity disrupts normal production of steroid hormones and affects carbohydrate handling. Disruption of ovulation is associated with insulin resistance and hyperinsulinaemia (Franks & Robinson 1996).

A woman's weight, particularly if it is related to her height, indicates her nutritional status to some degree. Weight loss and nutrient fluctuation caused by self-imposed dieting, affecting reproductive function, may be the cause of infertility in a large proportion of the women seeking fertility treatment. It has been suggested that nearly 80% of women attending infertility clinics can be classified as underweight (Wynn & Wynn 1991). Maternal nutritional status can be assessed by calculation of body mass index (BMI;

Table 12.4 *Minerals*

Mineral	Function	Dietary source
Sodium (Na)	Extracellular ion essential for the generation of action potentials; required in the active transport of small molecules into the cell	Table salt (NaCl)
Potassium (K)	Intracellular ion essential for the generation of action potentials; utilized by the cell to maintain ion concentration gradients	Meat, milk, fruits, vegetables
Calcium (Ca)	Bone and teeth structural component; essential for blood clotting, muscle contraction and nerve impulse conduction	Dairy products, fortified flour, cereals, green vegetables
Chlorine (Cl)	Cation in body fluids; gastric acid excretions	Salt (NaCl)
Phosphorus (P)	Structural component of bones and teeth; essential for formation of ATP for energy storage	Meat, dairy products cereals, bread
Magnesium (Mg)	Required by some enzyme activities; present in cells, body fluids and bone	Vegetables, milk, cereals, bread
Iron (Fe)	Transfer of oxygen in haemoglobin molecule; oxidation processes; electron transfer chain	Meat, vegetables, flour
Zinc	Enzyme activity; growth and development of the immune system; spermatogenesis; tissue growth	Oysters, steak, crab meat, red meat, milk-products
Iodide	Thyroid hormones	Seafood, sea salt
Copper	Constituent of enzymes; energy production and release	Legumes, grains, nuts and seeds, offal
Manganese	Synthesis of urea; conversion of pyruvate in TCA cycle	Plant products
Fluoride	Essential to reduce decay in bone and tooth tissues	Fluoridated drinking water
Chromium	Carbohydrate and lipid metabolism	Unrefined foods, brewers yeast, whole grains and nuts
Selenium	Antioxidant; catalyst for the production of thyroid hormone	Liver, shellfish, fish meat

Box 12.1). BMI is correlated to fat mass (and health prognosis) but there are limitations to its use; BMI tends to overestimate fat mass in individuals who are active and have a high muscle mass. There are also racial differences in the correlation between BMI and fat mass; individuals from African and Polynesian races have less fat per BMI class compared with individuals from Caucasian races, whereas individuals from Asian races tend to have more fat. A BMI of about 24 kg/m^2 is thought to be optimal for women planning pregnancy. A BMI of less than 20 kg/m^2 is not associated with good fertility or pregnancy outcome. A BMI of greater than 30 kg/m^2 in a prepregnant woman is considered a considerable risk factor in the obstetric management of the pregnancy.

Maternal protein intake affects gonadotrophin secretion and ovulatory maturation (Wynn & Wynn 1991). Diets with abnormally high protein content and also those with very low protein content affect the menstrual cycle and fertility. It is possible that high-protein diets may cause one of the coenzymes involved in protein metabolism to become limiting. It is also suggested that low levels of B vitamins depress pituitary hormone secretion. Both embryonic development, especially early in gestation, and follicular development involve a rapid rate of protein synthesis and cell division, which are associated with a high energy and nutrient requirement. Preconceptual nutrient deficiency may retard development of the follicle and corpus luteum, affecting subsequent embryonic

The body mass index

Body mass index (BMI) is used to indicate nutritional status and risk factors associated with obesity. It is a ratio of weight (measured in kilograms) against height (measured in metres squared).

Calculation:

$$BMI = \frac{weight}{height^2} \left\{ \frac{kg}{m^2} \right\}$$

Interpretation:

Grade	BMI*	Definition
–	<20	Underweight
0	20–24.9	Desirable weight
I	25–29.9	Overweight
II	30–39.9	Mild obesity
III	40	Severe obesity

*Normal: 19.8–26.0

A healthy shape is considered to be that usually associated with a BMI of 20–25 kg/m². Waist circumference and waist to height ratios are also used as indicators of healthy shape. A waist circumference of less than 80 cm is considered healthy in women and less than 94 cm in adult men, with waist circumferences above 88 cm and 102 cm, respectively, indicating risk. A waist:height ratio of less than 0.5 is also considered healthy with a ratio greater than 0.6 indicating risk to health.

growth, even if the level of deficiency is not adequate to cause infertility. Excess intakes of some nutrients may increase mutation rate. Nutrient deficiency also affects male fertility, by altering DNA synthesis and rates of cell division. Selenium availability may be an important factor in male fertility.

Whether the mother enters pregnancy with high nutritional stores may affect the outcome of the pregnancy. Placental size in humans appears to be governed by genetic growth potential, anoxia and nutrient availability. In sheep, a period of poor nutrition early in gestation increases placental size, presumably as an adaptive mechanism to increase nutrient extraction (McCrabb et al 1992). Provided this nutrient restriction is transient and the sheep are then returned to richer pasture, the increase in placental size is associated with an increase in lamb birth weight. In humans, an increased placental:fetal weight ratio is associated

with poorer outcome and long-term health prognosis (Barker 1998). However, larger babies have larger placentas but in proportion to their birth weight. Morning sickness may produce a period of poor nutrition in early pregnancy, which could stimulate placental growth (Coad et al 2002). Provided the woman entered pregnancy with good nutrient stores and the effects on nutrient consumption were limited, nausea in pregnancy could promote placental enlargement and positively affect the fetal growth trajectory. An adequate interpregnancy interval may be important to allow replenishment of maternal stores, especially of vitamins such as folate.

Case study 12.1 looks at an example of nutritional status in pregnancy.

Non-nutritional factors affecting reproductive function

Food can provide nutrition but it is also the source of a number of maternal infections (Box 12.2). Pregnant women are advised to be particularly careful about food hygiene. Although nutrient intake and weight gain are associated with clear effects on birth weight, a number of other factors have been shown to affect fetal size and growth potential (Box 12.3).

Age affects cell proliferation and gamete formation. Some diseases accelerate premature ageing of the germ cells. These include diabetes, parental gene mutation, multiple sclerosis, ulcerative colitis and Crohn's disease (Wynn & Wynn 1991). Smoking, drugs, alcohol and radiation all affect cell division; indeed, smoking is probably the most important single factor influencing incidence of LBW babies in developed countries (Chiriboga 2003). Viruses are mutagenic and have long been associated with abnormal fetal development. Sexually transmitted diseases (STDs) can cause pelvic inflammatory disease, which may affect fertility and pregnancy outcome. Diseases caused by larger organisms, such as syphilis and gonorrhoea, are

Fiona informs the midwife at the booking appointment that she has a healthy balanced diet.

■ How can the midwife assess that this is an accurate statement?

relatively easy to diagnose and treat. However, STDs caused by smaller microorganisms, such as chlamydia, papilloma, HIV, herpes and mycoplasmas, are difficult to eradicate. STD prevalence is associated with increased mobility of the population.

Nutritional requirements in pregnancy

Energy requirements

The nutritional costs of pregnancy can be calculated by estimating the cost of the new maternal tissues (particularly maternal fat deposition) and the tissues of the conceptus (fetus, placenta, membranes and other tissues)—the 'capital gains'—and the metabolic costs of maintaining these growing tissues—the 'running costs' (Campbell-Brown & Hytten 1998). Tissue accrued accounts for about 185 MJ (50 000 kcal), and increased metabolism accounts for about 150 MJ (36 000 kcal), bringing the total specific cost of pregnancy to about 335 MJ (80 000 kcal) (Fig. 12.3). As more studies about nutritional requirements during pregnancy are performed, the recommended daily allowances of energy and other nutrients have progressively decreased. However, recommended allowances are intended to be a standard against which the nutritional status of a population, rather than that of an individual person, can be assessed.

Energy requirements during the pregnancy are highest in the middle (from 10–30 weeks) when maternal fat stores are being assimilated. During the last 10 weeks of the pregnancy, the rapid growth of the fetus has a high energy requirement but the rate of maternal fat storage is decreased (and often maternal intake is limited). In effect, the increased nutritional requirements of the pregnancy are spread fairly evenly over the later three-quarters of the pregnancy. The daily increase in energy requirement is calculated to be about 1.2 MJ (300 kcal) over the final three-quarters of pregnancy (Campbell-Brown & Hytten 1998). This is calculated from the total cost of the pregnancy, estimated to be 335 MJ (80 000 kcal) divided by 270 days of pregnancy. The actual energy consumed in pregnancy by women 'eating to appetite' (with free access to food) is about 0.8 MJ (200 kcal) extra per day, less than the theoretical expected cost of the pregnancy. Many women, including those in developing countries and the poorer parts of affluent countries, successfully reproduce supported by energy intakes far below the recommended level.

Some of the additional energy requirements of pregnancy can be met by increased efficiency of maternal metabolism (decreased metabolic rate or diet-induced thermogenesis) and decreased energy expenditure (Durnin 1987). The additional requirements are a relatively small proportion (about 25%)

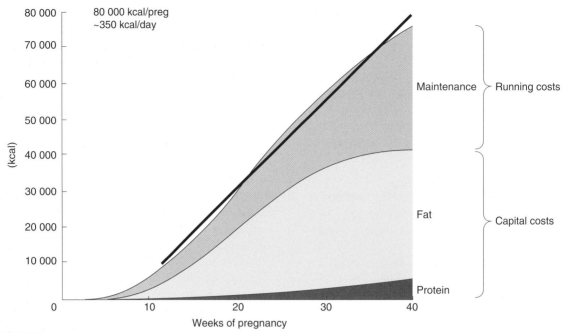

Fig. 12.3 *The cumulative energy costs of pregnancy. (Reproduced with permission from Hytten 1991.)*

of the average total energy requirements for a non-pregnant woman. Thus decreased activity can make up a considerable proportion of the extra requirement. Decreased energy expenditure in the second and third trimesters of pregnancy has been observed in the Five Country Study of pregnant women (Lawrence et al 1987), which compared women living in Scotland, Holland, the Gambia, the Philippines and Thailand. Leisure activities and the rate at which heavy work was done decreased. Women who have a long history of poor nutrition, for instance those in subsistence farming communities, seem to be able to adapt more to sparing nutrients and economizing to support the cost of the pregnancy. This may be because these women are more physically active and so can decrease their energy expenditure by a greater degree.

Dieting or energy restriction is not appropriate for pregnant women; it is unlikely to be beneficial and may harm the fetus. Historically, women at risk of developing pre-eclampsia and obese women were recommended to limit their energy intake and weight gain. However, energy restriction has no effect on the development of pre-eclampsia; excessive weight gain is the result, not the cause, of the underlying clinical pathology. In obese women, energy restriction is associated with lower infant birth weight (Merialdi et al 2003). Inadequate energy intake, particularly in the first trimester, is associated with an increased incidence of LBW infants and congenital abnormalities

(Carmichael et al 2003). Excessive weight loss and fat mobilization in pregnancy can produce metabolites that can create metabolic stress and are detrimental to fetal development. Maternal health and later lactational capability may be compromised by dietary restriction in pregnancy.

Protein requirements

Protein requirements increase in pregnancy, to support maternal tissue synthesis and fetal growth. Metabolic adaptations enhancing the efficiency of protein synthesis are evident from early pregnancy onwards (Duggleby & Jackson 2002). Low-protein diets are associated with an adverse outcome of pregnancy but low-protein intakes are unlikely in affluent developed countries. Protein requirements for the growth of maternal tissues and the growth of the conceptus can be calculated. The increased protein synthesis, and therefore increased dietary requirement, in late pregnancy is about 6 g/day. In Britain and other developed countries, where the average net protein utilization (NPU) value is 0.7, this is equivalent to about 8–9 g of additional dietary protein being required to maintain nitrogen balance.

During the pregnancy, there is a fall in blood protein levels from about 70 g/l to 60 g/l. Much of this fall is due to decreased plasma albumin concentration resulting from haemodilution. Albumin functions as a non-specific carrier of lipophilic substances such as some drugs, hormones, free fatty acids, unconjugated bilirubin and some ions. It has an important role in maintaining the plasma osmotic pressure. The fall in plasma colloid osmotic pressure increases movement of water out of the blood vessels (see Ch. 1), thus increasing lower limb oedema and affecting glomerular filtration rate (GFR). Plasma globulins increase in pregnancy.

Plasma levels of most amino acids fall in pregnancy. The most marked falls are observed in glucogenic amino acids, which can be used to form glucose, then those involved in the urea cycle and then the ketogenic branched-chain amino acids. Amino acids are actively transported across the placenta. The transfer of amino acids across the placenta is only just adequate for fetal protein synthesis so any factor adversely affecting amino acid transport mechanisms has the potential to limit growth. Imbalances in maternal amino acid concentration will be reflected by placental uptake. For instance, women with phenylketonuria (PKU) are advised to resume a low-phenylalanine diet (and take tyrosine supplements) prior to conception as high levels of phenylalanine can harm the fetus, even if the fetus does not have PKU. High phenylalanine levels in pregnancy are associated with fetal IUGR, congenital heart disease, microcephaly and mental retardation. The amino acid methionine is involved in folate metabolism; women who have higher dietary intakes of methionine seem to be at lower risk of delivering a baby with a neural tube defect (NTD) (Shoob et al 2001). Good sources of methionine tend to be foods such as animal proteins that are rich in other amino acids and total protein, iron, zinc and calcium.

The optimum birth weight in humans can be considered to be within the range of birth weights associated with the lowest incidence of perinatal mortality and morbidity, in the range 3500–4500 g (Wynn & Wynn 1991). Mothers of babies in the optimal birth-weight range tend to eat more protein than women who give birth to babies with lower birth weight. Maternal intakes of B vitamins and some minerals, particularly magnesium, have been found to correlate well with birth weight (Wynn & Wynn 1991). The main regulator of fetal growth seems to be availability of nutrients, which can affect growth directly by changing the availability of substrates required for growth, or indirectly by altering hormonal control of growth.

The normal protein intake of women in most developed countries, who regularly consume foods such as lean meat and poultry, fish, reduced-fat milk products, wholegrains and legumes as part of a balanced and varied diet, appears to be sufficient to provide the additional requirements of pregnancy. Vegetarian and vegan women must ensure a range of wholegrains and legumes are consumed daily to provide adequate protein. The US Institute of Medicine (2002) recommends an additional 25 g of protein per day for pregnancy in addition to the recommended daily intake (RDI) of 46 g of protein per day (0.80 g/kg/day), a total RDI of 71 g of protein per day for pregnant women (or 1.1 g/kg/day). Women with twin pregnancies are recommended to consume an additional 50 g of protein per day together with an appropriate energy increment to optimize efficient utilization of the protein (Institute of Medicine 2002). Women with very low energy intakes may be at risk of inadequate protein intake. The use of formulated protein supplements, powders or high-protein formulated beverages should be discouraged because clinical studies suggest they may be potentially harmful to the fetus (Kramer & Kakuma 2003). Some popular weight-restriction diets have promoted high protein intake. However, the fetus has limited ability to detoxify ammonia and excrete urea, particularly during the vulnerable periods of organogenesis in the first trimester. In experimental animals, high protein intakes and apparent high levels of ammonia have been associated with increased rates of congenital abnormalities.

Fat requirements

In pregnancy, plasma lipids alter markedly. Levels of free fatty acids, triacylglycerides, cholesterol, lipoproteins and phospholipids transiently fall early in pregnancy and then rise (Butte 2000). The changes in handling of lipids are orchestrated by hormonal changes and are associated with changed insulin resistance during the pregnancy (Robinson et al 1992). The initial low maternal levels of fatty acids reflect maternal fat storage, which is highest early in pregnancy when maternal maintenance costs of pregnancy and fetal growth are relatively low (Campbell-Brown & Hytten 1998). This appears to anticipate requirements later in pregnancy. In the later stages of pregnancy, when fetal requirements are maximal, maternal nutrient intake could be restricted by lack of availability of food or by restricted capacity for eating and gastrointestinal disturbances. Maternal fat stores, which are 3.5 kg on average, can subsidize a considerable part of the pregnancy. Oxidation of 3.5 kg of fat could theoretically produce 132 MJ (30 000 kcal).

During early gestation the fetus depends on placental transfer for fatty acid requirements (Herrera & Amusquivar 2000). Lipids are transported across the placenta as lipoprotein complexes, classified by their density (Fig. 12.4). Triglyceride levels increase throughout gestation. Placental uptake of triglycerides occurs in the form of very-low-density lipoproteins (VLDL). Placental lipase may hydrolyse VLDL, releasing the products for energy metabolism by the fetus (Robinson et al 1992). The rising level of maternal fatty acids in the third trimester probably reflects mobilization of maternal fat stores. In later gestation, maternal fatty acids are predominantly used for maternal metabolism and ketone body synthesis. The more mature fetus can synthesis fatty acids de novo, using ketone bodies as fuels and lipogenic substrates.

LCPUFA requirements of pregnant women are particularly high, especially in the third trimester when fetal brain and nervous tissue growth is maximal; about half of brain lipids are LCPUFA. Arachidonic acid (20:4, ω-6) is essential for neonatal growth and is the precursor for eicosanoids, prostaglandins and leukotrienes, and docosahexaenoic acid (DHA; 22:6, ω-3) has a key role in fetal brain development and visual function. Therefore, fetal demand for indispensable fatty acids (linoleic acid, 18:2, ω-6; and α-linoleic acid, 18:3, ω-3) must be met from either maternal intake or be released from maternal adipose tissue. The placenta transports the indispensable fatty acids and their preformed long-chain derivatives, arachidonic acid and DHA from the maternal circulation to the fetus. Low maternal intake of these indispensable fatty acids is correlated with reduced neonatal growth (Herrera 2002).

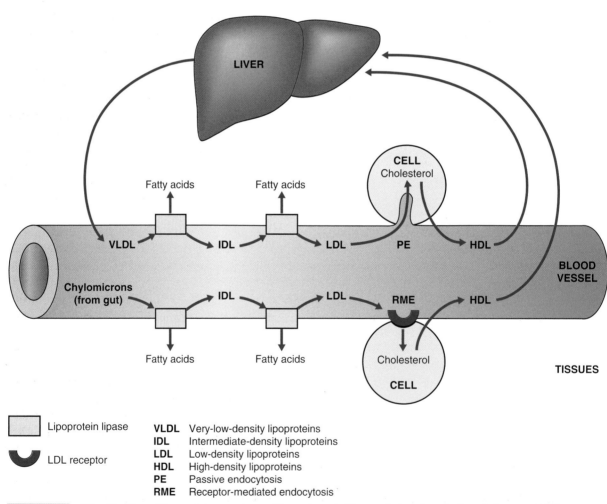

Lipoprotein lipase

LDL receptor

VLDL Very-low-density lipoproteins
IDL Intermediate-density lipoproteins
LDL Low-density lipoproteins
HDL High-density lipoproteins
PE Passive endocytosis
RME Receptor-mediated endocytosis

Fig. 12.4   *Classification of lipoprotein complexes. (Reproduced with permission from Saffrey & Stewart 1997.)*

Consumption of fish, and therefore DHA, in pregnancy is associated with a reduced incidence of preterm delivery and LBW (Olsen & Secher 2002), probably because ω-3 fatty acids from marine sources inhibit ω-6-derived eicosanoids involved in cervical ripening and the initiation of parturition. Women who eat more marine foods also seem less likely to develop pregnancy-induced hypertension (Al et al 2000). These positive effects of fish consumption on gestational duration and fetal development have generated much interest in requirements of LCPUFA for optimal outcome of pregnancy. However, it is not clear that supplementation with LCPUFA or fish oil might be beneficial as excess intake of LCPUFA can potentially increase the risk of oxidative damage (Herrera 2002). The higher the content of PUFAs in the diet, the more likely damaging free radicals will be formed which are potentially toxic and can reduce antioxidant capacity.

Western diets are relatively rich in ω-6 fatty acids but poor in ω-3 fatty acids and intake of preformed DHA is low, so the supply of DHA to the fetus may be compromised. The ratio of ω-6 fatty acids to ω-3 fatty acids is estimated to be significantly higher than it was in the Neolithic era when the big brain of modern man evolved. Obese women with insulin resistance and thin women with little body fat are likely to be even more dependent on dietary DHA. Eating fish in pregnancy would increase DHA intake but much of the advice about fish liver oils containing vitamin A and not consuming an excess of fish in case of heavy metal contamination of fish has led pregnant women to avoid fish totally in pregnancy rather than increase their intake because they are pregnant.

A high fat intake is not recommended in pregnancy as there is an association between increased fat intake and the development of glucose abnormalities (Saldana et al 2004). Ketonaemia appears to have a negative effect on fetal development and later intellectual performance (Rizzo et al 1991). High-fat, low-carbohydrate diets are not optimal for pregnancy; it is suggested that a diet <30% fat and >50% carbohydrate reduces the risk of glucose intolerance and gestational diabetes.

Carbohydrate requirements

Adequate carbohydrate intake is important in pregnancy to ensure adequate glucose for maternal brain metabolism and transfer to the fetus. Metabolism of carbohydrates and lipids alters, under hormonal influ-
ence, throughout pregnancy to ensure that the fetus receives a continuous supply of nutrients despite maternal intake being intermittent (Butte 2000). Maternal glucose concentration is maintained at a significantly higher level in later pregnancy by increased hepatic glucose production in order to meet the increasing requirements of the placenta and fetus. The developing fetus utilizes glucose as its primary energy-producing substrate but it can also metabolize maternally derived ketoacids.

Maternal pre-existing diabetes (type 1 or type 2, but not gestational diabetes which develops later in pregnancy), high sucrose intake or prepregnancy obesity are all associated with an increased risk of NTD (Shaw et al 2003). This is probably because the embryo does not have pancreatic function when the neural tube is developing and closing so it is unable to regulate excess of glucose at this time; high glucose levels lead to oxidative stress and embryonic depletion of inositol which can also affect neural tube development (Baker et al 1990). The developing embryo may also be vulnerable to the effects of maternal hypoglycaemia following hyperglycaemia. Thus, good control of glucose metabolism in early pregnancy, which is more is likely to be achieved by a diet higher in foods with low GI, lowers the risk of congenital abnormalities. Gestational diabetes, because it becomes evident in the second half of pregnancy after embryonic development is completed, is not associated with an increased risk of congenital abnormalities but a high carbohydrate (low fat) diet with plentiful low GI foods is associated with a decrease in newborn macrosomia (Romon et al 2001).

Adequate dietary fibre is particularly important in pregnancy because the high progesterone levels affect smooth muscle tone and result in a decreased rate of gastrointestinal transit. This has advantages for nutrient absorption as gut contents are in contact with sites of absorption for longer times but water is also absorbed to a greater extent, which often results in constipation. Recommending that pregnant women increase their intake of complex carbohydrates, such as wholemeal or wholegrain breads, cereals, legumes, fruit and vegetables, would provide carbohydrate with good sources of fibre. Promoting foods high in fibre will help to address problems of constipation as well as generally increasing carbohydrate intake. The other advantage of this is that many foods with higher fibre content also have a lower GI, which is particularly important for women who have, or are risk of developing, diabetes. Increasing intake of complex carbohydrate also has the positive outcome of displacing intakes of fat and added sugars.

Vitamins and minerals

It is thought that a range of micronutrient deficiencies might contribute to congenital malformations and the failure of human embryos to implant or survive (Keen et al 2003). However, supplementation needs to be evaluated carefully as nutrient–nutrient interactions can be detrimental and some micronutrients are toxic in excess. Thus, both micronutrient deficiency and excess are associated with adverse pregnancy outcome. Levels of fat-soluble vitamins increase during pregnancy and levels of water-soluble vitamins fall. However, levels of vitamin A fall but levels of carotenoids rise. Fat-soluble vitamins cross the placenta more readily than water-soluble vitamins and their transport increases with gestational length; decreased levels of maternal plasma levels may be due to haemodilution rather than to increased uptake by maternal and fetal tissue. Thus, lower circulating levels of nutrients in pregnancy cannot be simply interpreted as indicating a deficiency. It is suggested that hormonal resetting of homeostatic mechanisms favours transfer of nutrients to the fetus (Campbell-Brown & Hytten 1998). Low levels of nutrients in maternal plasma may limit maternal cell uptake while optimizing placental uptake. The placenta can extract nutrients from maternal plasma and transfer them to the fetus, maintaining transport against a concentration gradient. Thus, fetal concentration of vitamins may be 5–10 times the level in maternal blood. The 'pump' mechanisms of the placenta appear to be specific for vitamins; most minerals are not transported by similar mechanisms.

A good-quality maternal diet is probably able to provide the increased vitamin and mineral requirements of the pregnancy, particularly if energy intake is increased from a source of high-nutrient-density food. However, a poor-quality diet may adversely affect both fetal growth and the establishment of adequate stores for neonatal growth. Micronutrient requirements increase slightly in pregnancy but, unless the woman is at the threshold of a deficiency, most women consuming a varied and balanced diet should have adequate reserve. The possible exceptions to this generalization are iron and calcium nutritional status which should be assessed early in antenatal care. Periconceptual folate requirements are higher than can

usually be provided by the diet. Vitamin A potentially presents some challenges in pregnancy, as both deficiency and excess are teratogenic. Certain subgroups within the population are at increased risk of vitamin D deficiency, such as Asian women.

Folate and folic acid

'Folate' is a generic term applied to dietary sources of related compounds that have the same biological activity in the body. Dietary folates are vulnerable to being broken down during food preparation. Folic acid is a synthetic form which is more bioavailable and more stable. Folate deficiency in early pregnancy is teratogenic and is associated with an increased incidence of NTDs; it can also cause megaloblastic anaemia of pregnancy, cervical dysplasia and atherosclerosis (Stover 2004). There is a well-established protective effect of folic acid supplements that significantly reduce the incidence of NTDs.

Folate is involved in single-carbon transfer reactions in the metabolism of nucleic and amino acids, and hence the synthesis of DNA, RNA and proteins. Requirements for folate increase in pregnancy because the number of single-carbon transfer reactions increases, for instance for nucleotide synthesis and cell division. Blood folate levels fall in pregnancy, reflecting the high rate of DNA synthesis and cell division. Any factor that reduces DNA, RNA and protein synthesis increases the risk of congenital malformations, which are usually associated with a reduced cell number rather than a reduced cell size.

There is considerable interaction between folate and other vitamins, such as choline and vitamins B_6 and B_{12}, which also have a role in single-carbon methyl donation and, thus, recycling homocysteine to methionine. Deficiency of any of these vitamins can contribute to hyperhomocysteinaemia. Raised levels of homocysteine in pregnancy are associated with complications and adverse outcomes of pregnancy such as an increased risk of pre-eclampsia, NTDs and other congenital abnormalities, LBW and preterm delivery, placental abruption and spontaneous pregnancy loss (Holmes 2003).

NTDs are the most common congenital abnormality resulting from failure of the neural tube to close effectively between 22 and 27 days postconception, which is usually before women realize they are pregnant. Increased intake of folic acid periconceptually overcomes unidentified abnormalities in folate utilization (Boddie et al 2000) which are related to mutations of genes expressing enzymes in the folate metabolic pathways of genetically predisposed women. The incidence of NTD is 1.6 per 10 000 livebirths in England and 3.1 per 10 000 in Wales; NTDs are a clinical reason for offering termination of pregnancy so the actual incidence of pregnancies affected by NTDs is higher than the livebirth rate suggests.

Folic acid supplements, of 400 µg/day, are recommended for all pregnant women or women who might become pregnant. It is recommended that women who are at higher risk for pregnancy affected by NTD (because they have previously had an NTD-affected pregnancy, have a family history of NTD, have insulin-dependent diabetes, or are taking anticonvulsants known to affect folate metabolism) take a high-dose folic acid supplement (those who have already had one conception affected by a NTD should consume 4 mg folic acid per day to reduce the risk of recurrence). Although pregnant women seem aware of campaigns recommending increased folic acid consumption, many seem reluctant to take it (Health Education Authority 1996). Possibly advice to supplement the diet with folic acid may appear to conflict with the usual health advice to avoid unnecessary drugs in pregnancy. Renaming folic acid as 'vitamin B$_9$' as is done in some parts of Europe might alter the perception of folic acid as a drug.

The levels of folic acid that are associated with reduced incidence of NTD are significantly higher than those that could be easily achieved from the diet. It is difficult to increase levels of folate-rich food to the level recommended (Cuskelly, McNulty & Scott 1996). Increased consumption of folate to reduce the risk of NTD is 4 weeks before and after conception, which presents difficulties in many developed countries like the UK because about half of all pregnancies are unplanned.

The argument for supplementing a staple food, such as bread or flour, with folic acid (Wald & Bower 1995) has been strengthened by the other advantages of increasing folate consumption. Folate is important in maintaining optimal levels of homocysteine; hyperhomocysteinaemia (accumulation of circulating homocysteine) is associated with cardiovascular disease, stroke, depression, Alzheimer's disease and some types of cancer. However, folic acid supplementation can mask the symptoms of pernicious anaemia due to low vitamin B$_{12}$ intake which can delay the diagnosis of deficiency, increasing the risk of permanent neurological damage. Some drugs are folate antagonists and so increase the risk of NTDs (Pimental 2000). These include anti-epileptic drugs (such as carbamazepine and valproate), retinoids (used to treat acne) and some anti-tumour agents. Women who are pregnant with more than one fetus, breastfeeding women nursing more than one infant and those women with a high alcohol intake or are on chronic anticonvulsant or methotrexate therapy have increased requirement for folate.

Case study 12.2 looks at the issue of folic acid supplementation.

Calcium

Calcium requirements increase mostly in the third trimester when the fetal skeleton develops rapidly, incorporating a total of about 30 g of calcium. However, this is a tiny proportion of the calcium deposited in the maternal skeleton, which can act as a reservoir if dietary calcium is low. However, if the mother's own skeleton is still growing, as in adolescent pregnancy, there may be competition between the maternal and fetal skeletons for calcium. Young girls who become pregnant within 2 years of starting to menstruate are most at risk.

Vitamin D concentrations rise in pregnancy, resulting in increased intestinal calcium absorption, and calcium retention is increased; this occurs in advance of mineralization of the fetal skeleton. Calcium supplementation has been used therapeutically during pregnancy to prevent hypertensive disorders and related problems. Calcium is one of the main nutrients which need to be considered in the antenatal assessment; it is not uncommon for women of reproductive age to have an intake that is below the recommended intake.

Case study 12.2

Jane seeks preconceptual nutritional counselling. She has had a previous miscarriage and is keen to improve the quality of her diet. Jane expresses concern about taking drugs in pregnancy, including folic acid, and is adamant that the human race could not have evolved requiring nutrients that could not be provided by a healthy diet.

- How might a midwife summarize the characteristics of a balanced diet?
- What rich sources of folate could be identified and how might consumption be increased?
- Is the connection between a previous miscarriage and diet valid?
- How could Jane's fears about folic acid supplementation be addressed?

Pregnant adolescents are particularly at risk of inadequate intake of calcium as are women of all ages who do not consume dairy products. Pregnant women should be encouraged to consume at least three servings of calcium-rich foods a day. Although dietary sources of calcium are preferable, it may be necessary for women who avoid dairy produce and other calcium-rich foods to be prescribed a calcium supplement. Women who are prescribed both iron and calcium supplements should avoid taking them at the same time of day to maximize absorption of both.

Iron

The requirements for additional iron in pregnancy remain controversial (see Ch. 11). First-trimester iron requirements are lower than for non-pregnant women due to menstrual savings but requirements are markedly higher by the third trimester (Hallberg 2001). It is estimated that about 600 mg of iron are required for the fetus and placenta and blood lost at parturition (Campbell-Brown & Hytten 1998). The expansion of maternal red blood cell mass accounts for about 290 mg of iron (Letsky 1998), but this expansion probably accommodates for the blood lost at parturition. Amenorrhoea of pregnancy saves about 120 mg of iron, which is not lost in menstruation and iron absorption increases.

Iron depletion (low iron stores) or deficiency (anaemia) appears to be common in pregnant women and the consequences are significant for both mother and fetus. Maternal anaemia increases risk of morbidity and mortality, and is associated with risk of heart failure, haemorrhage and infection. The risks of fetal death, perinatal mortality, preterm delivery and lower birth weight are also increased (Scholl & Reilly 2000). Maternal iron deficiency affects cognition, behaviour, motor development and activity of offspring (Allen 1997), probably irreversibly. Infants of iron-deficient mothers are more likely to have low iron stores and be susceptible to iron deficiency themselves. Maternal iron deficiency affects the mother's physical work capacity and interaction with the infant.

There are two pathways of iron absorption; haem and non-haem iron absorption (Fig. 12.5). Haem iron from meat is highly bioavailable and affected to a negligible degree by other components of the diet. However, most dietary iron is non-haem iron, absorption of which varies with other dietary constituents, particularly those which influence the reduction of the insoluble ferric iron to soluble ferrous iron. Vitamin C and other organic acids significantly enhance dietary

Fig. 12.5 *Pathways of iron absorption. Haem iron from meat, poultry and fish is absorbed efficiently via the haem transporter, whereas absorption of non-haem iron is affected by other dietary components. For instance, vitamin C enhances the conversion of Fe^{3+} (ferric iron) to the more soluble Fe^{2+} (ferrous iron) which is better absorbed. Some dietary components, such as phytate and polyphenols, bind to the iron and make it less available. Non-haem iron is transported across the gut wall via the divalent metal transporter (DMT). Zinc and copper can compete for transport by DMT and therefore inhibit iron absorption.*

absorption of non-haem iron, as does the presence of meat, fish or poultry, though the mechanism is not clear. Inhibitors of non-haem absorption bind iron and render it less available; these include phytate (in legumes, grains and rice), polyphenols (in tea and coffee, grains, oregano and red wine) and vegetable proteins such as those in soybeans. Calcium inhibits absorption of both haem and non-haem iron with a dose-related effect. Non-haem iron is transported across the gut by the same divalent metal transporter which also transports other metals such as zinc and copper; this means that supplementation with one metal can affect the absorption of the others. The bioavailability of iron from meat is significantly higher than from plant-based foods, and the meat and other animal proteins enhance non-haem iron absorption, so individuals who consume omnivorous diets absorb more iron than do vegans or vegetarians.

Risk factors for iron deficiency in pregnancy include depleted iron stores prior to pregnancy (usually related to menstrual loss), not eating meat, chronic use of non-steroidal anti-inflammatory drugs (NSAIDs) such as aspirin (resulting in gastrointestinal lesions), low intake of factors which increase iron absorption (particularly vitamin C) and high intake of factors which decrease absorption. Iron deficiency is more likely with low socioeconomic status, poorer educational attainment and multiple gestation; adolescent women and those with a short interpregnancy interval are also at increased risk of iron deficiency. Use of oral contraceptives prior to pregnancy tends to result in a favourable iron status because menstrual loss is limited.

Pregnant women who are at risk of iron deficiency are usually prescribed iron supplements. Some women experience gastrointestinal effects in response to supplementary iron. Absorption of iron is best in the absence of other food (empty stomach) but may be associated with more side-effects. Low-dose supplements are associated with fewer side-effects and ferrous gluconate appears to be less irritating. However, iron is potentially toxic in excess; concerns focus on iron overload causing the generation of free radicals which can cause cellular damage. Thus, iron supplementation should be prescribed on the basis of biological criteria rather than being administered routinely.

Haemochromatosis is the most common genetic disorder affecting Caucasian populations (Heath & Fairweather-Tait 2003); it is a recessively inherited disease resulting in iron overload. The clinical effects of haemochromatosis, due to deposition of iron in the liver, heart and pancreas, are not usually manifest or of concern in women of childbearing age as menstrual losses help to maintain iron balance. However, routine assessment of blood parameters such as transferrin saturation in pregnant women could help to identify those women who might be at risk in later life.

To meet the additional requirements of pregnancy, women need to markedly increase their intake of iron-rich foods and the dietary factors that promote iron absorption. Nutritional assessment and dietary advice for pregnant women should take into consideration both sources of iron and the intake of factors affecting non-haem iron absorption. Timing of consumption of foods can influence nutrient–nutrient interaction. For instance, drinking fruit juice (high vitamin C content) with a good iron source will favour absorption, and drinking tea, which has a high tannin level, should be avoided with iron sources. Vegetarian and vegan women may find it difficult to meet their iron requirements solely from food sources; they should consume grains, vegetables and legumes, and have vitamin C-rich foods or drinks (raw fruits, fruit juice or vegetables) with meals. As adolescents have a higher iron requirement, this group is particularly vulnerable in being able to achieve an adequate iron intake particularly in the latter part of pregnancy and especially if they avoid meat. Supplementation may be necessary for those with low iron stores and/or low dietary iron intakes, but supplementation must always be given in conjunction with appropriate dietary advice, and under supervision from a health professional. There are concerns about excessive intake of supplementary iron and its potential effects on free radical generation; also, the implications of iron supplementation on zinc and copper status need to be considered.

Zinc

Zinc is involved in cell proliferation, protein synthesis, protection from oxidative damage, apoptosis, hormone binding (by means of zinc fingers) and transcription, and is thus likely to affect embryonic and fetal development (Keen et al 2003). Zinc deficiency in pregnancy is teratogenic; it is associated with increased risk of congenital abnormality (including NTDs) and other complications of pregnancy and delivery, growth retardation, retarded neurobehavioural and immunological development and premature delivery (Velie et al 1999). Iron supplementation can decrease zinc absorption, and zinc in excess may induce a secondary copper deficiency, as there is competition for the divalent metal transporters. Bioavailability of zinc in foods is particularly affected by high phytate content in foods such as cereal grains, legumes and nuts.

Selenium

Selenium forms part of the enzyme glutathione peroxidase, which metabolizes hydrogen peroxide formed from polyunsaturated fatty acids. Selenium is incorporated into proteins to make selenoproteins, some of which function as antioxidant enzymes preventing cellular damage from free radicals (natural by-products of oxygen metabolism). Other selenoproteins are involved in thyroid hormone metabolism (Thomson 2004). The requirement for selenium is uncertain; a relatively low intake of selenium is required to prevent Keshan disease, a cardiomyopathy, but higher intakes of selenium may be protective against cancer and cardiovascular disease, by protecting against free radical damage. Pregnant women have increased selenium requirements to allow for growth of the embryo and increased selenoprotein synthesis and tissue accumulation. The placenta actively transports selenium to the fetus (Hytten & Leitch 1971), but it is not known whether maternal absorption of selenium increases in pregnancy. Requirements for selenium are increased with increased oxidative stress such as that caused by smoking and intense exercise. The main sources of selenium are fish and seafood, meat and poultry, eggs, dairy produce and bread.

Magnesium

Magnesium status has been implicated in the incidence of preterm labour (via uterine hyperirritability), pregnancy-induced hypertension, fetal growth retardation, cerebral palsy and mental retardation (Institute of Medicine 1997). Studies of women from poor socioeconomic backgrounds, who have a higher risk of poor pregnancy outcome, have observed low intakes of magnesium (Doyle et al 1989). Some intervention studies have found that magnesium supplementation increases birth weight (Merialdi et al 2003). Magnesium forms part of the chlorophyll molecule so green vegetables such as spinach are rich in magnesium; other sources include nuts, seeds, wholegrains, wheat bran, wheat germ and breakfast cereals, dairy products, dried fruit and hard water. Women who consume a wide variety of foods including plenty of fruit and vegetables are unlikely to be deficient in magnesium.

Iodine

Iodine is a component of the thyroid hormones thyroxine (T_4) and its active form 3,3',5-tri-iodothyronine (T_3), which are important in growth and development and in energy production. Pregnant women have increased requirements for iodine as the fetus has a high growth rate. The fetal brain is very vulnerable to maternal hypothyroidism; iodine deficiency is the major cause of preventable mental retardation worldwide. In pregnancy, severe iodine deficiency is associated with LBW and preterm delivery, congenital abnormalities, increased pregnancy loss, stillbirth, increased perinatal and infant mortality, psychomotor, speech and hearing defects, dwarfism, spastic diplegia, cretinism and mental retardation (Zimmermann & Delange 2004). Mild-to-moderate iodine deficiency during pregnancy adversely affects both maternal and infant thyroid function and has implications for the mental development of the infant. Marginal iodine deficiency in pregnancy may be associated with impaired development but small effects on mental development such as IQ score reduced by a few points are difficult to assess, particularly as it is difficult to measure dietary iodine intake. Although iodized tablesalt is mandatory in the UK, some individuals are consuming less salt for well-founded health reasons and there is reduced use of iodophors in the dairy industry. It has been proposed that pregnant women and women planning pregnancy should take an iodine-containing supplement of about 150 µg/day (Zimmermann 2004); however, iodine preparations often have stability issues and problems with quality control.

Vitamin A

Vitamin A (retinal) status in pregnancy is positively correlated with outcome of pregnancy in terms of infant size and gestational length. It is involved in vision, reproduction, gene expression, embryological development, growth, immune function, integrity of the epithelium and bone remodelling. Both deficiency and excess of vitamin A in pregnancy cause fetal abnormalities. Low vitamin A status in pregnancy is associated with increased maternal mortality, decreased birth weight and increased risk of congenital abnormalities (Ramakrishnan et al 1999). A high vitamin A intake is also associated with teratogenicity; this occurs in the first trimester and causes birth defects deriving from cranial neural crest cells such as craniofacial deformations (cleft lip and palate) and abnormalities of the central nervous system (not NTDs), heart and thymus.

Changes in animal husbandry, and increased use of growth-promoting agents and vitamin supplements given to animals, may make the livers of farmed animals considerably richer in vitamin A than they used to be. Birth defects in humans have been associated with the use of vitamin A analogues for treatment of acne. Women taking medications for the treatment of dermatological problems such as acne should check whether the medication contains large doses of vitamin A and, if so, discontinue its use prior to and during pregnancy. With some acne preparations, it is recommended that conception be avoided for a year after stopping treatment. Preformed vitamin A (retinal) is only available from animal-derived foods. Pro-vitamin A from carotenoids in coloured fruit and vegetables is not efficiently converted into retinal so pregnant women who avoid dairy products and meat need to consume at least five servings of fruit and vegetables per day and to select rich sources of carotenoids. No adverse effects of carotenoids from normal dietary levels of intake have been reported.

Vitamin D

Vitamin D maintains serum calcium and phosphorus concentrations within the range that optimizes bone health, by affecting the absorption of these minerals from the small intestine, their mobilization from bone and calcium resorption by the kidney. Vitamin D is synthesized in the skin; dietary requirements depend on exposure to sunlight. In pregnancy, vitamin D requirements increase substantially. Vitamin D deficiency is associated with decreased fetal growth via the effect on maternal calcium homeostasis (Brunvand et al 1996).

Dietary vitamin D is required for those individuals whose skin is not adequately exposed to sunlight (Hollis & Wagner 2004). Women who are regularly exposed to sunlight are much less dependent on dietary sources of vitamin D. Risk factors for low vitamin D are low socioeconomic status, being covered or otherwise restricting access to ultraviolet light, and having a low educational level. Synthesis of vitamin D is affected by the season of the year and the amount of UV light. Less vitamin D is synthesized in the skin of dark-skinned people as melanin absorbs ultraviolet light. Being housebound or not exposing the face, hands and body to sunlight for cultural or religious reasons will limit vitamin D synthesis. Pregnant women who do not receive regular exposure to sunlight (estimated to be about 30–40 minutes of exposure of face and arms) are recommended to have a supplement of 5.0 µg (or 200 IU) of vitamin D per day (Institute of Medicine 1997). It is prudent to recommend that exposure to sunlight is in the morning or late afternoon to reduce the risk of sunburn and excessive exposure to harmful UVR. (It is not known to what extent the use of sunscreen affects vitamin D synthesis but it is important to encourage pregnant women to routinely use sunscreen.)

Vitamin K

Vitamin K is a coenzyme used in the synthesis of a number of proteins involved in bone metabolism and the blood coagulation cascade. Use of drugs that interfere with metabolism of vitamin K, such as warfarin, can increase the risk of fetal intraventricular haemorrhage, cerebral microbleedings, microencephaly and mental retardation. Anti-epileptic treatments can inhibit placental transport of vitamin K affecting fetal synthesis of clotting factors and increasing risk of haemorrhage. For this reason, it is recommended that pregnant women with epilepsy take a vitamin K supplement in the month before delivery and during labour. In addition, microbial synthesis of vitamin K may be compromised by the use of broad-spectrum antibiotic therapy (particularly if it is required for a prolonged period).

Vitamin B_{12}

Vitamin B_{12} is a coenzyme involved in homocysteine-to-methionine conversion and for the reaction that converts L-methylmalonyl-coenzyme A to succinyl-CoA. Vitamin B_{12} is involved in maternal and fetal erythropoiesis so requirements are increased particularly in the first two trimesters. Deficiency of vitamin B_{12} increases the risk of neurological abnormalities in the fetus. Absorption of vitamin B_{12} may increase in pregnancy; the fetus is dependent on maternal dietary intake (Allen 2002). The placenta concentrates vitamin B_{12} and then transfers it to the fetus down a concentration gradient so fetal levels of vitamin B_{12} are about double maternal levels. The placenta preferentially transports newly absorbed vitamin B_{12} rather than that from maternal liver stores, so transfer to the fetus may be compromised even though the mother shows no overt signs of deficiency.

Plants do not synthesize vitamin B_{12} so strict vegetarians and those people who consume low amounts of animal products are more likely to be deficient. Plant foods exposed to vitamin B_{12}-producing bacteria, or contaminated with soil, insects or other substances containing B_{12} or foods fortified with vitamin B_{12} are the only dietary sources for strict vegetarians. Fetal levels of vitamin B_{12} may be compromised even if the mother has only recently become a vegetarian. Pregnant women who are strict vegetarians need to take vitamin B_{12} supplements or eat foods that have been fortified with vitamin B_{12}, and continue doing so while they are breastfeeding. Infants are less tolerant to vitamin B_{12} deficiency than adults; breastfed infants may develop severe megaloblastic anaemia and neurological damage, even if their vitamin B_{12}-deficient mothers are not showing clinical signs of deficiency. The first symptoms of infant vitamin B_{12} deficiency are drowsiness, repetitive vomiting, swallowing problems, severe constipation and tremor (particularly involving tongue, face, pharynx and legs). Progression to unconsciousness, coma and, ultimately, death can be swift.

Vitamin C

Vitamin C is a water-soluble antioxidant and a cofactor for enzymes involved in the synthesis of collagen, neurotransmitters and carnitine. It is involved in the recycling of vitamin E and also enhances absorption of non-haem iron. Haemodilution in pregnancy results in plasma vitamin C concentration falling. Pregnant women have increased vitamin C requirements to ensure adequate transfer to the fetus and maternal needs are met. The placenta transports ascorbate from the maternal circulation, oxidizes it and transfers it to the fetus (Choi & Rose 1989). Vitamin C deficiency is associated with premature rupture of the placental membranes (Siega-Riz et al 2003), preterm delivery (Ramakrishnan et al 1999) and infection (Casanueva et al 1993). Intervention studies have shown reduced incidence of pre-eclampsia in at-risk women supplemented with vitamin C and vitamin E (Chappell et al 2002). Additional vitamin C is recommended for pregnant women exposed to increased oxidative stress; these include smokers and women who use recreational drugs or consume significant qualities of alcohol or regularly take aspirin (Cogswell et al 2003).

Undernutrition in pregnancy

In experimental animals, maternal undernutrition in pregnancy usually leads to decreased birth weight. Maternal weight gain in human pregnancy is positively associated with birth weight and developmental outcome. However, in nutritional assessment it is important to determine prepregnancy weight from objective data and to assess the level of oedema. Women who are underweight have an increased risk of pregnancy loss and small babies that have increased morbidity and mortality. It is difficult to dissociate the effects of a poor diet in pregnancy from other variables. Women who consume a poor diet in pregnancy are likely to have consumed a poor diet before pregnancy and more likely to have had a poorer diet during their own growth and development. Many of them are shorter than average and a poor diet is associated with an increased incidence of smoking. Maternal shortness is also associated with a poorer social background, young maternal age and less formal education.

Diet quality

Although most nutritional studies have focused on energy requirements and consumption in pregnancy, the quality of the diet as well as the quantity may be important. In Britain, nutrient-deficiency diseases are rare but the quality of the diet varies markedly (see below). Mothers of LBW babies have not only low energy intakes but also diets of low nutrient density. Even in affluent countries, many women have daily intakes of B vitamins below the recommended level. Lifestyle changes, such as car ownership and less-active work patterns, mean energy requirements fall. However, nutrient requirements may not fall in parallel; indeed pollution and smoking increase requirements of certain nutrients. This means that, although energy consumption needs to fall to match reduced energy expenditure, the density of nutrients within the diet may need to increase to ensure that requirements are met.

Supplementation

Nutrient supplementation studies of the diet in pregnancy have produced inconsistent and inconclusive results. High-density protein supplementation depresses birth weight (Rush 1989). Lower concentrations of protein have disappointingly small effects. Some of the studies are probably methodologically flawed and supplements may be used as alternatives rather than increasing nutrient consumption, or the target group may not consume them. Supplementation in the second and third trimesters of pregnancy may be too late to have an effect on birth weight; however, it may benefit maternal health and work potential and improve breast-feeding efficiency. Earlier supplementation may have a greater effect because nutrient support of early follicular development and maternal nutrient stores prior to conception may programme the fetal growth trajectory.

Fetal adaptation to undernutrition

Subjected to inadequate substrate levels of either nutrients or oxygen, the fetus adapts by changing its metabolic activity in order to survive in utero and to optimize chances of surviving after birth in a nutritionally poor environment. Slowing of growth and reducing energy expenditure are part of this adaptation. Growth accounts for a large proportion of energy expenditure. Adapting to a lower growth trajectory means that nutrient requirement decreases and available nutrient levels may then be adequate. The placenta, which has a high nutrient and oxygen requirement itself, may also adapt. Although a number of adult-onset diseases are associated with impaired fetal nutrition (Fig. 12.6), they tend not to affect reproductive ability as they cause pathological problems late in life. Animal studies have demonstrated that marginal malnourishment for many generations requires optimal nutrition for several generations before normal size and behaviour are expressed (Stewart et al 1980). This intergenerational effect may be one of the reasons why dietary supplementation in pregnancy has such a small effect on outcome.

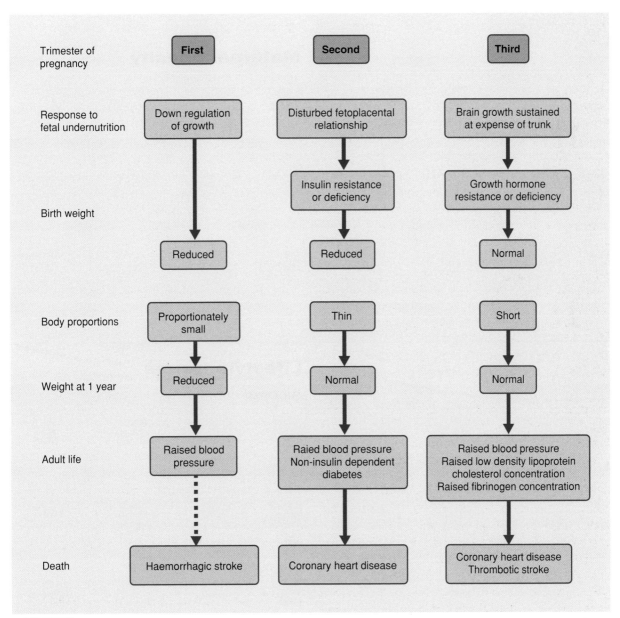

Fig. 12.6 *Association of adult-onset diseases and impaired fetal nutrition. (Reproduced with permission from Barker 1995.)*

Malnutrition

Interesting results come from studies looking at the effect of nutrient deprivation on previously well-nourished women. The Dutch Hunger Winter, from September 1944 to May 1945, was due to the Nazi blockade of food supplies exacerbated by very severe winter weather conditions. The severe nutritional deficiency affected fertility and birth weights and the birth rate fell dramatically, by about 50%, 9 months later (Lumley 1992, Stein & Susser 1975a). This was due both to effects on ovulation and an increased incidence of pregnancy failure. Congenital malformation rate increased among babies conceived during the famine and in the following 4 months, which demonstrates the importance of good preconceptual nutrition. However, many women were already pregnant at the time of the food shortage. If the women were deprived of energy in the second half of their pregnancy, the birth weight of their babies was reduced by 350 g on average. These babies were thin but of normal length. They appeared to develop and grow normally. However, in adulthood the male babies who had been exposed to deficiency late in development had lower rates of obesity compared with those who had experienced restricted nutrient levels early in development (Ravelli et al 1976). Young women who had been exposed to nutrient deficiency early in gestation, but not later, had normal birth weights themselves. However, their babies were smaller than expected (Stein & Susser 1975b). Adults of lower birth weight have increased risk of developing type 2 diabetes mellitus, heart disease, hypertension, obstructive lung disease, hypercholesterolaemia and renal disease (Godfrey & Barker 2000). However, results from the longer, more severe, Leningrad siege do not show any association between intrauterine malnutrition and glucose intolerance and coronary heart disease in adulthood (Stanner et al 1997).

Transient nutrient deficiency may alter fetal growth patterns without affecting final birth weight very much (Harding & Johnson 1995). Birth weight is a crude outcome measure of optimal gestational growth and development. Suboptimal maternal body composition and nutrient intake can have a long-term effect on the offspring without necessarily affecting size at birth (Godfrey 2001). Birth weight does not differentiate between the more subtle effects of nutrition on body composition and development of specific tissues and organs. It may not identify growth restriction; a similar birth weight can be attained with different growth trajectories. For instance, if an infant does not reach its potential birth weight but is born above 2500 g, it will not be classified as being of LBW even though its growth is not optimal. Nutrient deprivation before pregnancy or early in gestation affects brain growth and development in animals, which suggests that 'programming' of later brain growth is determined by nutrient availability before the demand for nutrients occurs. Lung growth is affected by later nutritional deficiency; lung weight and composition, muscle function, defence mechanisms and surfactant production are all susceptible to nutritional insult in late pregnancy.

Maternal obesity

Maternal obesity is associated with larger babies, macrosomia and increased perinatal mortality. Large-for-gestational-age babies are not longer in length but have increased deposition of adipose tissue. Routine antenatal care is more difficult in obese women, and labour is more likely to be prolonged and unsuccessful. Obese women tend to have increased problems during delivery; operative delivery is more complicated and there is increased risk in the puerperium (Fraser & Chan 2003). Maternal obesity is also associated with an increased incidence of congenital malformations (Prentice & Goldberg 1996), particularly NTD. In obese women, folic acid seems to lose its protective effect.

Lifestyle issues

Alcohol

Alcohol readily crosses the placenta so maternal alcohol levels determine alcohol levels in fetal blood and may affect embryonic development, fetal brain function and later behaviour. Exposure of the fetus to alcohol can cause long-term behavioural and developmental problems. Whether there is a 'safe' limit of alcohol exposure is uncertain; other dietary factors and genetics also play a role in the effects of alcohol. Therefore, it is prudent to advise all pregnant women to avoid alcohol completely if possible. Also, total abstinence is often found easier to adhere to.

Fetal alcohol syndrome, the most easily recognizable outcome of fetal alcohol exposure, is characterized by intrauterine and postnatal growth retardation, characteristic unusual facial features and adverse effects on brain function leading to mental retardation and/or behavioural disturbances. It occurs if the fetus is exposed to regular heavy alcohol intake or to very high alcohol concentrations at critical periods in development. However, fetuses exposed to lower amounts of alcohol may also be affected with fetal alcohol spectrum disorder which results in a range of symptoms that can be more difficult to diagnose definitively. These symptoms include attention deficit hyperactivity disorder (ADHD), inability to foresee consequences and learn from previous experience, inappropriate or immature behaviour, lack of organization, learning difficulties, poor abstract thinking, poor adaptability, poor impulse control, poor judgement and communication problems (Koren et al 2003). Infants exposed to alcohol in utero may demonstrate withdrawal symptoms after birth such as hyperactivity, excessive crying, irritability, weak sucking, disturbed sleep, tremors and seizures.

It can be difficult to reassure women who have had a small amount to drink before realizing that they were pregnant and still maintain advocacy for abstinence (Koren et al 2003).

Smoking

Although some women stop or reduce smoking when they become pregnant, a significant proportion continue to smoke throughout pregnancy. Smoking (and environmental or second-hand tobacco smoke) is associated with increased early spontaneous abortion and placental complications such as premature placental abruption, sudden infant death syndrome, decreased birth weight and preterm delivery (Lambers & Clark 1996). Both nicotine and carbon monoxide are vasoconstrictors and may affect blood flow to placental and fetal tissues. Nicotine can increase maternal blood pressure and heart rate which may compromise uterine blood flow. Carbon monoxide binds to haemoglobin forming carboxyhaemoglobin which can cause fetal hypoxia and is implicated in sudden infant death syndrome (Haustein 1999). Cigarette smoke also contains lead, cadmium and thiocyanate all of which are potentially hazardous to the fetus. Cigarette smoke is a source of free radicals and oxidative stress. Smoking is also thought to affect absorption of micronutrients and to increase nutrient utilization (Cogswell et al 2003). Thus, smoking increases maternal micronutrient requirements but may also decrease the appetite and food consumption. Smokers are more likely to consume alcohol and other substances which interact with nutrient metabolism and are less likely to take nutrient supplements. Many women who smoke in pregnancy or who quit smoking during pregnancy and resume in the postpartum period are influenced by weight concerns (Levine & Marcus 2004).

Caffeine

Caffeine is a mild stimulant present in beverages, such as coffee, tea and cola, chocolate and medications such as cold remedies, allergy preparations, headache medications, diuretics and stimulants. High doses of caffeine in pregnancy have been associated with increased risk of fertility problems, congenital abnormalities, pregnancy loss, growth retardation and behavioural problems; however, the usual range of caffeine intake is below the threshold which is thought to have adverse reproductive effects (Christian & Brent 2001). It is recommended that pregnant women limit their caffeine consumption to 300 mg/day. The caffeine content of tea and coffee ranges markedly but 300 mg caffeine is roughly equivalent to four cups of instant coffee, three average cups of brewed coffee, six average cups of tea, eight cans of regular cola drinks, four cans of 'energy' drinks and 400 g of plain chocolate (caffeine in milk chocolate is about half that in plain chocolate).

Drug use, medication, herbs and 'smart' drinks

Most medications prescribed to pregnant or breast-feeding women will have been evaluated for safety and the maternal benefit weighed against the risk of the drug being transported across the placenta and affecting the fetus. No drug is without side-effects (Shehata & Nelson-Piercy 2000) and anxiety about birth defects is a major parental concern. Anti-anxiety drugs, antidepressants, and neuroleptic drugs may affect neurotransmitter function of the developing central nervous system. Many recreational drugs such as amphetamines, heroin, marijuana and hallucinogens are harmful in pregnancy. It is important that pregnant women discuss their condition with health practitioners including pharmacists.

Many women use herbs and herbal teas during pregnancy. A number of herbs have pharmacological actions and the safety and effectiveness of others are not known; there are also concerns about quality control and contamination. Some herbs are known to be unsuitable in pregnancy; for instance, raspberry leaf tea can stimulate contractions and is used to induce labour. Other herbs that should be avoided in pregnancy include cohosh, pennyroyal, mugwort, Ma Huang or ephedra. Pregnant women are recommended to choose herbal teas made with ingredients that are a normal part of their diet such as mint, blackcurrant or orange extracts and avoid unfamiliar substances. Herbal teas should preferably be purchased from reputable sources.

Carbonated drinks are not harmful for pregnant and breastfeeding women per se; carbonation itself does not present problems. Carbonated drinks are usually not nutrient-dense and may contribute only sugars; they may displace drinks which could provide more nutrients. Other ingredients in 'smart' drinks (also known as 'new age', 'designer' or 'energy' drinks) may be of concern. High levels of caffeine are commonly added to energy drinks. Guarana, a Brazilian berry extract, is a stimulant related to caffeine. Ginseng is not recommended for pregnant women. Many of the smart drinks also contain higher levels of amino acids and vitamins than are considered optimal for pregnant women.

Exercise

Pregnant women who exercise have reduced fat gain, more rapid weight loss after pregnancy, improved mood and improved sleep patterns (Kramer 2002). It is suggested that labour progresses faster and more effectively in women who exercise, reducing the need for induction, pain relief and operative delivery (Brown 2002, Lumbers 2002). However, all women tend to decrease their activity as pregnancy progresses. Physiological adaptations to exercise during pregnancy protect the fetus, maintain placental and fetal tissue perfusion and oxygenation and facilitate nutrient delivery (Clapp III 2000). Exercise begun in early pregnancy enhances placental development and fetal growth, whereas initiating significant exercise programmes later in pregnancy may reduce fetoplacental growth (Clapp III et al 2000). Women should therefore be encouraged to begin or continue low-volume exercise throughout pregnancy but decrease exercise towards the end of gestation to optimize outcome.

The aim should be to maintain a good fitness level during pregnancy rather than to reach peak fitness or train for competitive events. Moderate aerobic and strength-conditioning exercises (such as swimming, yoga, stretching, biking and walking) as part of a healthy lifestyle are considered safe and beneficial (Jarski & Trippett 1990). Activities which minimize the risk of loss of balance and fetal trauma are recommended (Davies et al 2003), whereas activities that result in respiratory stress (hyperventilation) or hyperthermia should be avoided. Certain activities such as contact sports and walking or running on rocky or unstable ground should be avoided (as joint laxity and centre of gravity are affected by pregnancy). In late pregnancy, exercises that involve lying on the back are best avoided as the weight of the uterus can impede venous return to the heart and may cause postural hypotension (see Ch. 11). Women are advised to seek advice before starting an exercise programme in pregnancy. Pregnant women with certain conditions such as a history of bleeding or preterm labour, placenta praevia (where the placenta is low in the uterus), anaemia, pre-eclampsia or hypertension, and medical conditions which limit cardiovascular reserve may be advised to avoid exercise programmes. Pregnant women taking part in physical activity should wear appropriate footwear, take frequent breaks and avoid exercising in extremely hot weather.

There are differences in physiological responses in pregnant women who are acclimatized to high altitude (live at high altitude) and pregnant visitors to high altitude (Niermeyer 1999). Fetal oxygenation does not seem to be affected by air travel but exercise at high altitude may be associated with pregnancy complications such as dehydration, bleeding and preterm labour.

Work and stress

Strenuous work can potentially influence micronutrient status and outcome of pregnancy. Women in employment may be at risk of compromised diets because they have less time for shopping and cooking. Peak energy expenditure, length of time spent standing (which has been shown to affect patterns of meals consumed) and type of activity (for instance, lifting may result in greater intra-abdominal pressure) may be more significant. Particular occupations, long and/or irregular working hours and shift work have been implicated in being associated with a poorer outcome of pregnancy (Shaw 2003).

Key points

■ The diet before pregnancy, as well as that consumed during pregnancy, can affect the nutrient status of the woman.

■ The increased energy requirements of pregnancy can be met by a combination of increasing intake, decreasing activity and changing metabolism.

■ A good-quality, nutrient-dense diet can supply the additional protein, vitamin and mineral requirements of pregnancy.

■ Energy restriction and obesity affect reproductive function: both fertility and fetal growth.

■ Pregnancy-induced hormonal changes, including insulin resistance, affect transfer of nutrients to the placenta and fetus.

■ Adaptation to poor nutrition in pregnancy results in changes in growth in utero and birth weight and may be linked to disease in adult life.

Application to practice

Advice on nutrition in pregnancy is important before and during pregnancy, and also for subsequent pregnancies.

Women who have a poor history of nutrition are at risk and the midwife needs to be aware of this to aid in the detection of problems associated with poor dietary intake.

Annotated further reading

Barker DJP 1992 Fetal and infant origins of adult disease. BMJ Books, London
Describes the research underlying the fetal origins of adult disease (the Barker Hypothesis) in a compilation of the 31 key papers in this area.

Edelman CL, Mandle CL 1998 Health promotion throughout the lifespan, 4th edn. Times Mirror-Mosby, St Louis
Provides a focus upon health promotion including lifestyle and health choices in preconceptual, antenatal and the postnatal periods as well as health needs throughout the lifespan.

Morgan JB, Dickerson JWT 2002 Nutrition in early life. Wiley, Chichester
This book focuses on good nutrition for and during pregnancy, in low-birth-weight infants, and during infancy; it has a strong public health emphasis and provides a useful scientific basis and applications to practice.

Shanklin DR 2000 Maternal nutrition and child health. 2nd edn, Charles C Thomas
Reviews scientific studies linking maternal and early nutrition to later health of the offspring.

Worthington-Roberts B, Rodwell-Williams S 1996 Nutrition in pregnancy and lactation, 6th edn. Times Mirror-Mosby, St Louis
A comprehensive textbook about nutritional needs before and during pregnancy and during lactation. Includes practical information on assessing nutritional risk and counselling and supporting breastfeeding mothers.

References

Al MDM, van Houwelingen AC, Hornstra G 2000 Long-chain polyunsaturated fatty acids, pregnancy, and pregnancy outcome. American Journal of Clinical Nutrition 71:285S–291S

Allen LH 1997 Pregnancy and iron deficiency: unresolved issues. Nutrition Reviews 55:91–101

Allen LH 2002 Impact of vitamin B-12 deficiency during lactation on maternal and infant health. Advances in Experimental Medicine and Biology 503:57–67

Anderson AS 2001 Pregnancy as a time for dietary change? Proceedings of the Nutrition Society 60:497–504

Barker DJP 1995 Fetal origins of coronary heart disease. British Medical Journal 311:171–174

Baker L, Piddington R, Goldman A, Egler J, Moehring J 1990 Myo-inositol and prostaglandins reverse the glucose inhibition of neural tube fusion in cultured mouse embryos. Diabetologia 33:593–596

Barker DJP 1998 Mothers, babies and health in later life. Churchill Livingstone, New York

Boddie AM, Dedlow ER, Nackashi JA, Opalko FJ, Kauwell GP, Gregory JF III, Bailey LB 2000 Folate absorption in women with a history of neural tube defect-affected pregnancy. American Journal of Clinical Nutrition 72:154–158

Bottiglieri T 1996 Folate, vitamin B$_{12}$ and neuropsychiatric disorders. Nutrition Reviews 54:382–390

Brand-Miller JC 2003 Glycemic load and chronic disease. Nutrition Reviews 61:S49–S55

Brown W 2002 The benefits of physical activity during pregnancy. Journal of Science and Medicine in Sport 5:37–45

Brunvand L, Quigstad E, Urdal P, Haug E 1996 Vitamin D deficiency and fetal growth. Early Human Development 45:27–33

Butte NF 2000 Carbohydrate and lipid metabolism in pregnancy: normal compared with gestational diabetes mellitus. American Journal of Clinical Nutrition 71:1256S–1261S

Campbell-Brown M, Hytten FE 1998 Nutrition. In: Chamberlain G, Broughton Pipkin F (eds) Clinical physiology in obstetrics, 3rd edn. Blackwell, Oxford, pp 165–191

Carmichael SL, Shaw GM, Schaffer DM, Laurent C, Selvin S 2003 Dieting behaviors and risk of neural tube defects. American Journal of Epidemiology 158:1127–1131

Casanueva E, Polo E, Tejero E, Meza C 1993 Premature rupture of amniotic membranes as functional assessment of vitamin C status during pregnancy. Annals of the New York Academy of Sciences 678:369–370

Chappell LC, Seed PT, Kelly FJ, Briley A, Hunt BJ, Charnock-Jones D, Mallet A, Poston L 2002 Vitamin C and E supplementation in women at risk of preeclampsia is associated with changes in indices of oxidative stress and placental function. American Journal of Obstetrics and Gynecology 187:777–784

Chiriboga CA 2003 Fetal alcohol and drug effects. Neurologist 9:267–279

Choi JL, Rose RC 1989 Transport and metabolism of ascorbic acid in human placenta. American Journal of Physiology 257: C110–C113

Christian MS, Brent RL 2001 Teratogen update: evaluation of the reproductive and developmental risks of caffeine. Teratology 64:51–78

Clapp JF III 2000 Exercise during pregnancy. A clinical update. Clinics in Sports Medicine 19:273–286

Clapp JF III, Kim H, Burciu B, Lopez B 2000 Beginning regular exercise in early pregnancy: effect on fetoplacental growth. American Journal of Obstetrics and Gynecology 183:1484–1488

Coad J 2003 Pre- and periconceptual nutrition. In: Morgan JB, Dickerson JWT (eds) Nutrition in early life. Wiley, Chichester, pp 39–71

Coad J, Al Rasasi B, Morgan J 2002 Nutrient insult in early pregnancy. Proceedings of the Nutrition Society 61:51–59

Cogswell ME, Weisberg P, Spong C 2003 Cigarette smoking, alcohol use and adverse pregnancy outcomes: implications for micronutrient supplementation. Journal of Nutrition 133: 1722S–1731S

Cuskelly GJ, McNulty H, Scott JM 1996 Effect of increasing dietary folate on red-cell folate: implications for the prevention of neural tube defects. Lancet 347:657–659

Davies GA, Wolfe LA, Mottola MF, MacKinnon C, Arsenault MY, Bartellas E et al 2003 Exercise in pregnancy and the postpartum period. Journal of Obstetrics and Gynaecology of Canada 25:516–529

Doyle W, Crawford MA, Wynn AW 1989 Maternal magnesium intake and pregnancy outcome. Magnesium Research 2:205–210

Duggleby SL, Jackson AA 2002 Protein, amino acid and nitrogen metabolism during pregnancy: how might the mother meet the needs of her fetus? Current Opinion in Clinical Nutrition & Metabolic Care 5:503–509

Durnin DVGA 1987 Energy requirements of pregnancy: an integration of the longitudinal data from the five country study. Lancet ii:1131

Franks S, Robinson S 1996 Nutrition, metabolism and reproduction. In: Hill SG, Kitchener HC, Neilson JP (eds) Scientific essentials of reproductive medicine. Saunders, Philadelphia, pp 242–249

Fraser LB, Chan KL 2003 Problems of obesity in obstetric care. Current Obstetrics & Gynaecology 13:239–243

Frisch RE 1990 The right weight, body fat, menarche and ovulation. Baillière's Clinics in Obstetrics and Gynaecology 4:3

Frisch RE, McArthur JW 1974 Menstrual cycles: fatness as a determinant of minimum weight necessary for their maintenance or onset. Science 185:949–951

Godfrey KM 2001 The 'gold standard' for optimal fetal growth and development. Journal of Pediatric Endocrinology and Metabolism 14(Suppl 6):1507–1513

Godfrey KM, Barker DJP 2000 Fetal nutrition and adult disease. American Journal of Clinical Nutrition 71:1344S–1352S

Hallberg L 2001 Perspectives on nutritional iron deficiency. Annual Review of Nutrition 21:1–21

Harding JE, Johnson BM 1995 Nutrition and fetal growth. Reproduction, Fertility and Development 7:539–547

Haustein KO 1999 Cigarette smoking, nicotine and pregnancy. International Journal of Clinical Pharmacology and Therapeutics 37:417–427

Health Education Authority 1996 Awareness, attitudes and behaviour towards folic acid amongst women: a report by the HEA. HEA, London

Heath AL, Fairweather-Tait SJ 2003 Health implications of iron overload: the role of diet and genotype. Nutrition Reviews 61:45–62

Herrera E 2002 Lipid metabolism in pregnancy and its consequences in the fetus and newborn. Endocrine 19:43–55

Herrera E, Amusquivar E 2000 Lipid metabolism in the fetus and the newborn. Diabetes/Metabolism Research and Reviews 16:202–210

Hobel C, Culhane J 2003 Role of psychosocial and nutritional stress on poor pregnancy outcome. Journal of Nutrition 133: 1709S–1717S

Hollis BW, Wagner CL 2004 Assessment of dietary vitamin D requirements during pregnancy and lactation. American Journal of Clinical Nutrition 79:717–726

Holmes VA 2003 Changes in haemostasis during normal pregnancy: does homocysteine play a role in maintaining homeostasis? Proceedings of the Nutrition Society 62:479–493

Hytten FE 1991 Nutrition. In: Hytten F, Chamberlain G (eds) Clinical physiology in obstetrics, 2nd edn. Blackwell, Oxford, p 153

Hytten FE, Leitch I 1971 The physiology of human pregnancy. Blackwell Scientific Publications, Oxford

Illingworth PJ, Jung RT, Howie PJ, Isles TE 1987 Reduction in postprandial energy expenditure in pregnancy. British Medical Journal 294:1573–1576

Institute of Medicine 1997 Dietary reference intakes for calcium, phosphorus, magnesium, vitamin d and fluoride. Standing Committee on the Scientific Evaluation of Dietary Reference Intakes, Food and Nutrition Board, Institute of Medicine. The National Academy of Sciences

Institute of Medicine 2002 Dietary reference values for energy, carbohydrates, fiber, fat, protein and amino acids (macronutrients). Standing Committee on the Scientific Evaluation of Dietary Reference Intakes, Food and Nutrition Board, Institute of Medicine. The National Academy of Sciences

Jarski RW, Trippett DL 1990 The risks and benefits of exercise during pregnancy. Journal of Family Practice 30:185–189

Jennings E 1995 Folic acid as a cancer-preventing agent. Medical Hypotheses 45:297–303

Keen CL, Clegg MS, Hanna LA, Lanoue L, Rogers JM, Daston GP, Oteiza P, Uriu-Adams JY 2003 The plausibility of micronutrient deficiencies being a significant contributing factor to the occurrence of pregnancy complications. Journal of Nutrition 133:1597S–1605S

Koren G, Nulman I, Chudley AE 2003 Fetal alcohol spectrum disorder. Canadian Medical Association Journal 169:1181–1185

Kramer MS 2002 Aerobic exercise for women during pregnancy. Cochrane Database Systematic Reviews CD000180

Kramer MS, Kakuma R 2003 Energy and protein intake in pregnancy. Cochrane Database Systematic Reviews CD000032

Lambers DS, Clark KE 1996 The maternal and fetal physiologic effects of nicotine. Seminars in Perinatology 20:115–126

Lawrence M, Lawrence F, Coward WA, Cole TJ, Whitehead RG 1987 The energy requirements of pregnancy in the Gambia. Lancet ii:1072

Letsky E 1998 The haematological system. In: Chamberlain G, Broughton Pipkin F (eds) Clinical physiology in obstetrics, 3rd edn. Blackwell, Oxford, pp 71–110

Levine MD, Marcus MD 2004 Do changes in mood and concerns about weight relate to smoking relapse in the postpartum period? Archives of Women's Mental Health 7:155–166

Lumbers ER 2002 Exercise in pregnancy: physiological basis of exercise prescription for the pregnant woman. Journal of Science and Medicine in Sport 5:20–31

Lumley LH 1992 Decreased birthweights in infants after maternal in utero exposure to the Dutch famine of 1944–45. Paediatric and Perinatal Epidemiology 6:240

McCrabb GJ, Egan AR, Hosking BJ 1992 Maternal undernutrition during mid-pregnancy in sheep: variable effects on placental growth. Journal of Agricultural Science 1189:127–132

Merialdi M, Carroli G, Villar J, Abalos E, Gülmezoglu AM, Kulier R, de Onis M 2003 Nutritional interventions during pregnancy for the prevention or treatment of impaired fetal growth: an overview of randomized controlled trials. Journal of Nutrition 133:1626S–1631S

Naismith DJ, Morgan BL 1976 The biphasic nature of protein metabolism during pregnancy in the rat. British Journal of Nutrition 36(3):563–566

Niermeyer S 1999 The pregnant altitude visitor. Advances in Experimental Medicine and Biology 474:65–77

Olsen SF, Secher NJ 2002 Low consumption of seafood in early pregnancy as a risk factor for preterm delivery: prospective cohort study. BMJ 324:447

Pimentel J 2000 Current issues on epileptic women. Current Pharmaceutical Design 6:865–872

Prentice A, Goldberg G 1996 Maternal obesity increases congenital malformations. Nutrition Reviews 54:146–152

Ramakrishnan U, Manjrekar R, Rivera J, Gonzáles-Cossío T, Martorell R 1999 Micronutrients and pregnancy outcome: a review of the literature. Nutrition Research 19:103–159

Ravelli GP, Stein ZA, Susser MW 1976 Obesity in young men after famine exposure in utero and early infancy. New England Journal of Medicine 295:349

Rizzo T, Metzger BE, Burns WJ, Burns K 1991 Correlations between antepartum maternal metabolism and child intelligence. New England Journal of Medicine 325:911–916

Robinson S, Viita J, Learner J et al 1992 Insulin insensitivity is associated with a decrease in postprandial thermogenesis in normal pregnancy. Diabetic Medicine 10:139–145

Romon M, Nuttens MC, Vambergue A, Verier-Mine O, Biausque S, Lemaire C, Fontaine P, Salomez JL, Beuscart R 2001 Higher carbohydrate intake is associated with decreased incidence of newborn macrosomia in women with gestational diabetes. Journal of the American Dietetic Association 101:897–902

Rosa FW, Wilk AL, Kelsey FO 1986 Teratogen update: vitamin A congeners. Teratology 33(3):355–364

Rush D 1989 Effects of changes in protein and calorie intake during pregnancy on the growth of the human fetus. In: Chalmers I, Enkin M, Kierse MJNC (eds) Effective care in pregnancy and childbirth, Vol 1. Oxford University Press, Oxford, pp 255–280

Saffrey J, Stewart M (eds) 1997 Maintaining the whole. SK 220 Human biology and health, Book 3. Open University Press, Milton Keynes

Saldana TM, Siega-Riz AM, Adair LS 2004 Effect of macronutrient intake on the development of glucose intolerance during pregnancy. American Journal of Clinical Nutrition 79:479–486

Scholl TO, Reilly T 2000 Anemia, iron and pregnancy outcome. Journal of Nutrition 130:443S–4437S

Scott J, Kirke P, Molloy A, Daly L, Weir D 1994 The role of folate in the prevention of neural tube defects. Proceedings of the Nutrition Society 53:631

Shaw GM 2003 Strenuous work, nutrition and adverse pregnancy outcomes: a brief review. Journal of Nutrition 133:1718S–1721S

Shaw GM, Quach T, Nelson V, Carmichael SL, Schaffer DM, Selvin S, Yang W 2003 Neural tube defects associated with maternal periconceptional dietary intake of simple sugars and glycemic index. American Journal of Clinical Nutrition 78:972–978

Shehata HA, Nelson-Piercy C 2000 Drugs to avoid in pregnancy. Current Obstetrics & Gynaecology 10:44–52

Shoob HD, Sargent RG, Thompson SJ, Best RG, Drane JW, Tocharoen A 2001 Dietary methionine is involved in the etiology of neural tube defect-affected pregnancies in humans. Journal of Nutrition 131:2653–2658

Siega-Riz AM, Promislow JH, Savitz DA, Thorp JM Jr, McDonald T 2003 Vitamin C intake and the risk of preterm delivery. American Journal of Obstetrics and Gynecology 189:519–525

Stanner SA, Bulmer K, Andres C et al 1997 Does malnutrition in utero determine diabetes and coronary heart disease in adulthood? Results from the Leningrad siege study, a cross sectional study. British Medical Journal 315:1342–1349

Stein Z, Susser M 1975a Fertility, fecundity, famine: food rations in the Dutch famine 1944/5 have a causal relation to fertility and probably to fecundity. Human Biology 47:131

Stein Z, Susser M 1975b The Dutch famine 1944–45 and the reproductive process. 1. Effects on six indices at birth. Paediatric Research 9:70

Stewart RJC, Sheppard H, Preece R, Waterlow JC 1980 The effect of rehabilitation at different stages of development in rats marginally malnourished for ten to twelve generations. British Journal of Nutrition 43:403–412

Stover PJ 2004 Physiology of folate and vitamin B12 in health and disease. Nutrition Reviews 62:S3–S12

Thomson CD 2004 Selenium and iodine intakes and status in New Zealand and Australia. British Journal of Nutrition 91:661–672

Velie EM, Block G, Shaw GM, Samuels SJ, Schaffer DM, Kulldorff M 1999 Maternal supplemental and dietary zinc intake and the occurrence of neural tube defects in California. American Journal of Epidemiology 150:605–616

Wald NJ, Bower C 1995 Folic acid and the prevention of neural tube defects. British Medical Journal 310:1019–1020

Ward M, McNulty H, McPartlin J, Strain JJ, Weir DC, Scott JM 1997 Plasma homocysteine, a risk factor for cardiovascular disease, is lowered by physiological doses of folic acid. Quarterly Journal of Medicine 90(8):519–524

Wynn M, Wynn A 1991 The case for preconception care of men and women. AB Academic, Bicester

Zimmermann MB 2004 Assessing iodine status and monitoring progress of iodized salt programs. Journal of Nutrition 134(7):1673–1677

Zimmermann M, Delange F 2004 Iodine supplementation of pregnant women in Europe: a review and recommendations. European Journal of Clinical Nutrition 58:979–984

13 Physiology of parturition

Learning objectives

- To describe uterine changes in pregnancy and its preparation for labour.
- To discuss theories of the initiation and timing of parturition in humans.
- To relate factors thought to be involved with initiation of labour to methods for inducing labour, possible causes and treatment of preterm labour.
- To describe the effects of labour on maternal and fetal physiology.
- To outline the physiology of pain in relation to childbirth and the rationale for choice of pain relief.

Introduction

The success of pregnancy and, ultimately, the survival of the species, depends on the baby being born healthy and mature enough to survive. In pregnancy and labour, the uterus has to fulfil two very different functions. It has to grow but remain quiescent during the pregnancy to allow fetal development and then, at the appropriate time, commence the powerful and coordinated contractions which result in the delivery of the infant. However, parturition also requires the maturation of the fetal systems essential for extrauterine survival. The mother also needs to be physiologically prepared for lactation. Therefore, the maturation of the fetus and the onset of labour need to be synchronized. Asynchrony leads to preterm birth.

Most human infants are capable of surviving at delivery and are born at term (defined as between the end of the 37th week and 42 weeks of pregnancy). Preterm birth occurs in about 8–10% of pregnancies (Challis et al 2000). The incidence of preterm birth has not fallen over the last 50 years. In fact, modern practices such as women giving birth at a later age and fertility treatment (and subsequent multiple gestation) have increased the incidence of preterm birth. Low socioeconomic status, bacterial vaginosis, smoking and a history of preterm delivery and abortion are all risk factors for preterm birth (Friese 2003).

Preterm babies account for 85% of the early neonatal deaths that are not associated with a lethal deformity (López Bernal et al 1993). The shorter the gestation, the poorer the prognosis is. Even though very low-birth-weight babies (i.e. those born below 1000 g) may now survive, it is generally at the expense of high morbidity rates and much emotional stress for their parents, as well as a high financial burden on neonatal intensive care units. There are also long-term health and education costs associated with physical and mental handicap and neurodevelopmental complications. It can be argued that one of the principal objectives of obstetrics is to reduce preterm labour. There are three categories of causes of preterm birth: iatrogenic, where complications of pregnancy enforce obstetric intervention and the deliberate induction of premature delivery (10–30% of cases); premature rupture of fetal membranes, which may be associated with infection (30–40% of cases); and idiopathic preterm labour (40–50% of cases) (Challis et al 2001).

The factors controlling the transition from one state to the other are not well understood but are very important both in determining the possible causes of preterm labour and in understanding how to induce labour successfully without eliciting fetal distress. The control of the onset of human (and primate) parturition remains elusive. There are marked differences between human and other mammalian species in the cascade of factors leading to parturition. Humans have a very high rate of premature delivery (about 5–10%) compared with other species. For most domestic and laboratory animals the duration of gestation is remarkably constant; for example, there is less than 1% variation in sheep (Jenkin & Young 2004). Theoretically, the length of gestation does not matter to the mother. The crucial aspect is that the baby can survive at delivery. It seems likely, therefore, that the fetus controls the length of gestation. Certainly in animals there is proven fetal involvement in the timing of labour but it is difficult to obtain such evidence in humans.

In other species, it seems that the same signal controls fetal maturation and triggers the onset of labour so parturition is synchronized. In humans, the two pathways seem to be separable (Fig. 13.1). The human fetus appears to undergo lung maturation 4–6 weeks before labour, unlike other species in which the signals initiating labour also stimulate fetal organ maturity. It is not clear why the events leading to parturition should be so complex in the human; however, it seems likely that a variable length of gestation is advantageous. The complexity of control of parturition in humans might allow a transfer of control from mother to fetus. Thus, in early pregnancy, it may be physiologically expedient for the mother to terminate the pregnancy if it is harmful for her long-term health to continue. Continuing with a pregnancy that is unlikely to be completed, for example because maternal nutrient intake is insufficient, prevents needless maternal investment. Later in gestation, once the fetus is mature enough to survive, fetal control of parturition would allow the fetus to remain in the uterus if the environment was favourable. The fetus could respond to stress by switching from cell division and growth to accelerated maturation and earlier initiation of parturition. This would suggest that intrauterine growth restriction is part of an adaptive response to fetal stress which increases survival as long as the stressor is not too early or too severe. It is not surprising, therefore, that many of the signals involved in parturition are also involved in physiological stress responses.

Midwifery management of women in labour is often interventionist. This chapter covers the physiology of parturition; for information about clinical management, readers are referred to midwifery texts in the list of further reading.

Chapter case study

While working in Africa, Zara had been able to assist several of her African friends during childbirth, all of which had occurred at home and attended by mostly female relatives who had informed Zara that they would only call the local midwife if they felt things were going wrong. All her friends had had uncomplicated deliveries and Zara felt quite privileged to have witnessed childbirth in such a different way to how it is presented within most modern Western societies.

Zara is keen to have a waterbirth at home and wants to avoid all forms of pain relief. She also wants her sister and some of her close friends who are also heavily pregnant to be present if possible. As Zara has had all her antenatal care from her midwife, she particularly wants her midwife to care for her in labour, especially as her midwife has extensive experience of waterbirth. What factors do you think will be a positive influence on enabling Zara to have a normal birth?

Stages of labour

From a clinical point of view, labour is often divided into three stages (Fig. 13.2). However, physiologically there is no abrupt transition between stages. The events leading to the onset of labour are gradually and inconspicuously initiated earlier in the pregnancy, and the three stages overlap. The first stage is that of progressive cervical dilatation, timed from the onset of regular coordinated contractions accompanied by progressive effacement (thinning) and dilatation of the cervix. The end of this stage is marked by the full dilatation of the cervix as the uterine contractions pull the entire tissue of the cervix upwards until it becomes incorporated into the lower uterine segment, continuous with the uterine walls. This stage lasts an average of 12–14 hours in primigravidae, but tends to be shorter in multigravidae. The second stage is fetal expulsion, from full cervical dilatation until the delivery of the baby. The contractions are strong and aided by the respiratory muscles. The second stage may take

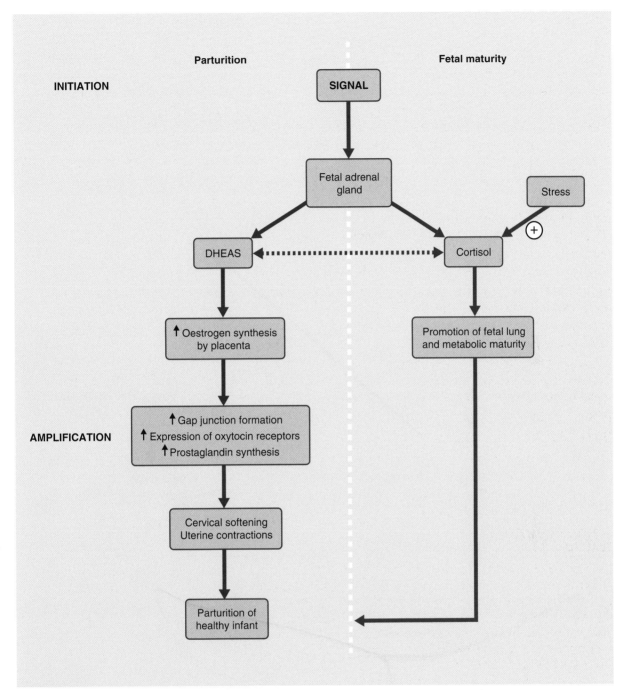

Fig. 13.1 *The two distinct pathways controlling parturition and fetal development in the human.*

over an hour in primigravidae and as little as a few minutes in multigravidae. The third stage of labour involves separation and complete expulsion of the placenta and membranes, and control of bleeding from the uteroplacental circulation. The return to the prepregnant state is described as the puerperium (see Ch. 14).

From a physiological point of view, it is useful to think of labour being related to phases of uterine myometrial activity. For most of pregnancy, the uterus is relatively quiescent predominantly under the influence of progesterone (the literal meaning of progesterone is 'pro-gestation', i.e. promoting and sustaining pregnancy). In late pregnancy, the uterus changes from

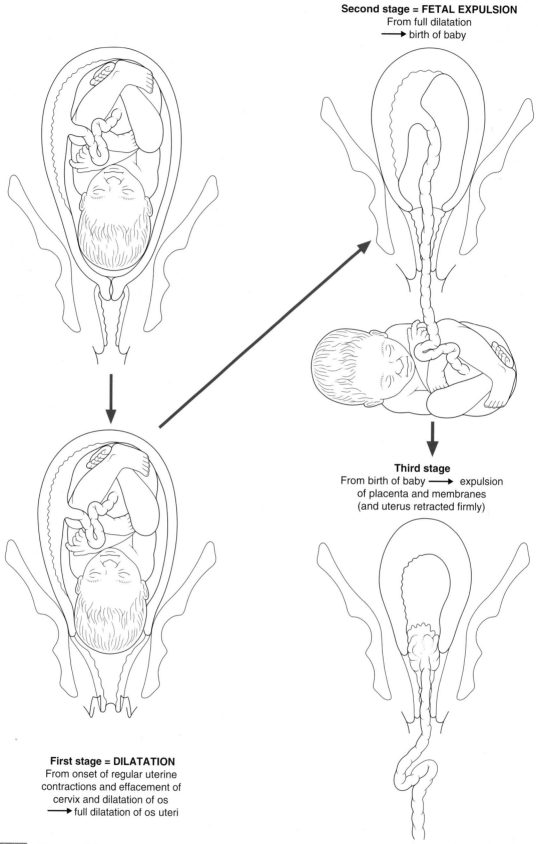

Second stage = FETAL EXPULSION
From full dilatation
⟶ birth of baby

Third stage
From birth of baby ⟶ expulsion
of placenta and membranes
(and uterus retracted firmly)

First stage = DILATATION
From onset of regular uterine
contractions and effacement of
cervix and dilatation of os
⟶ full dilatation of os uteri

Fig. 13.2   *Stages of labour.*

being quiescent (having a low level of muscle activity) to being activated. This transition to activation is the initiation of labour; labour results from activation and then stimulation of the myometrium. Activation is stimulated by mechanical stretch of the uterus together with changes in signalling via endocrine pathways, resulting from an increased activity of the fetal hypothalamic–pituitary–adrenal (HPA) axis. The activated uterus is spontaneously excitable and responsive to uterotonins; it develops coordinated, effective and strong contractions. The activation of the uterus is the start of a positive feedback loop whereby the initial signals become further amplified and the uterus becomes fully stimulated allowing progression of the first and second stages of labour. The uterus is able to perform a remarkable mechanical effort to expel its contents—the baby, placenta and associated membranes and fluids—through the birth canal (Fig. 13.3).

The uterus at term

Uterine growth in pregnancy

The uterine muscle undergoes exceptional growth throughout pregnancy to accommodate the growing fetus. The prepregnant weight of the uterus is about 50 g in a nulliparous woman and about 60–70 g in a multiparous woman with a capacity of about 10 ml. During pregnancy, uterine size increases 20-fold, to about 800–1200 g and a capacity of about 5 litres. Initially, the uterus grows by hyperplasia (increasing cell number). This is under the influence of oestrogen and, unlike later growth, occurs regardless of the site of implantation. By the 4th month, the uterine wall has thickened from 10 mm to 25 mm. Subsequent growth is due to hypertrophy stimulated by uterine distension. The uterine wall thins and the smooth muscle cells increase markedly in length (from 50 µm

Fig. 13.3 *Expulsion through the birth canal.*

to 500 μm long and from 5 μm to 15 μm wide) as they accumulate contractile proteins. The increased size is accompanied by a change in uterine shape from a sphere to a cylinder. By term, the organization of the myometrial cells allows coordinated, strong and effective contractions to develop. The uterine muscle is innervated by adrenergic, cholinergic and peptidergic fibres, which are more abundant in the cervix and uterine tubes. The uterus also has many sensory nerves. By the third trimester, the uterine wall is thin, about 5–10 mm by term; the fetus movements are visible and the fetus can be palpated through the uterine wall (Blackburn 2003). The uterus almost reaches the liver and displaces the stomach and intestine. The blood vessels in the non-pregnant uterus are extremely tortuous and coiled (see Ch. 2); this allows them to adapt to the increased requirements of the expanding uterine tissue. Uterine blood flow increases in pregnancy as the blood vessel diameter increases and resistance to flow decreases.

tent. The lower segment forms at about weeks 28–30 of pregnancy. Caesarean sections late in gestation are usually via the lower segment of the uterus (lower-segment caesarean section, LSCS), whereas the incision in an emergency 'classic' caesarean section earlier in pregnancy usually is on the midline of the uterus and is likely to dictate the method of delivery in future deliveries. Contractile strength is related to the proportion of smooth muscle (Petersen et al 1991). Therefore, the upper part of the uterus contracts strongly and the lower segment, which has a diminishing proportion of muscle, contracts weakly and passively (see Fig. 13.10, p. 332).

The uterine muscle forms three distinct anatomical layers, which are more evident with the hypertrophy of the uterus that occurs in pregnancy (Fig. 13.4). The innermost layer has muscle mostly in a longitudinal orientation. The outermost layer has longitudinal and circular fibres. The middle layer of uterine muscle has spiralling fibres and is particularly well vascularized.

Uterine muscle organization

The uterus is predominantly comprised bundles each of 10–50 myometrial (smooth muscle) cells separated by connective tissue, formed of collagen and elastin. The distribution of the smooth muscle varies throughout the length of the uterus. The smooth muscle density is highest in the fundus of the uterus (an approximate ratio of smooth muscle fibres:connective tissue of 90:10) and gradually declines until the cervix where the ratio is 20:80. The isthmus, which forms the lower segment of the uterus, has a lower smooth muscle con-

The myometrium

The myometrium is formed of myometrial cells embedded in a collagen matrix. The cytoplasm of these myometrial cells is packed with long random bundles of actin and myosin. Compared with skeletal muscles, the concentration of actin is higher and the myosin has longer filaments, which increases the maximum shortening of the contractile cells. Myosin is both a structural protein and an Mg-ATPase, an enzyme that can hydrolyse ATP and utilize the energy for movement. When ATP is hydrolysed (broken

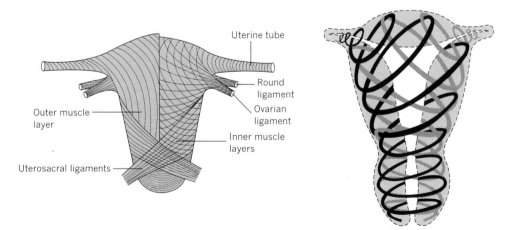

Fig. 13.4 *Uterine muscle layers: A the inner and outer muscle layers; B spiral organization of central smooth muscle fibres. (Reproduced with permission from Sweet & Tiran 1996.)*

down), actin and myosin cross-bridges form so actin and myosin slide past each other, shortening the cell so that the muscle contracts (Fig. 13.5). Myosin is made up of two heavy chains forming the ATPase and two light chains, which bind calcium and undergo phosphorylation. Phosphorylation is the incorporation of a phosphate group catalysed by a kinase, in this case myosin light-chain kinase (MLCK) which effectively activates the protein. Factors that negatively affect myometrial contractility may be important in maintaining uterine quiescence through pregnancy; those that increase contractility may be important in facilitating the progression of labour.

The role of calcium

Muscle contraction is triggered by a rise in the intracellular concentration of calcium ions. Electrical activity, calcium ion influx and development of myometrial tension are precisely synchronized (López Bernal 2003). Calcium ions bind to the calcium-binding protein calmodulin (CAM) which regulates the activity of many of the intracellular enzymes generating a cascade of reactions leading to binding of actin and myosin (Wray et al 2003). Binding of calcium to CAM forms a Ca–CAM complex which activates MLCK. MLCK is inhibited when calcium levels are low. The activated MLCK undergoes a conformational change which exposes the catalytic site so the MLCK can be phosphorylated and will interact with actin, initiating contractions. Removal of calcium results in dephosphorylation of myosin by myosin dephosphorylase and causes muscle relaxation. Smooth muscle contraction can therefore be increased either by activating MLCK or by inhibiting myosin phosphatase.

Calcium enters the myometrial cell from the extracellular fluid or is released from intracellular binding sites and organelles including the sarcoplasmic reticulum of the myometrial cells. Calcium released from the sarcoplasmic reticulum can prime contractions that need to be sustained by calcium influx. Voltage-operated calcium channels regulate contractility by allowing calcium entry. Calcium-activated potassium channels set the threshold of activation of the cell membrane. There is a good correlation between intracellular calcium concentration and the muscular force developed with ionized calcium (Ca^{2+}) concentration increasing from approximately 100 nm to 500 nm during contraction. Uterotonins (substances that stimulate myometrial contractility), such as prostaglandins and oxytocin, increase calcium influx and decrease calcium storage, therefore increasing intracellular calcium concentrations and MLCK phosphorylation and increasing myometrial activity. Agents that inhibit myometrial activity, such as progesterone, β-mimetics, relaxin and prostacyclin, decrease intracellular calcium by promoting calcium uptake into the intracellular stores such as the sarcoplasmic reticulum so free calcium levels decrease and the uterine muscle relaxes. Calcium channel blockers, such as nifedipine, prevent calcium entry into the cells promoting relaxation of the uterus.

The control of myometrial contractions

Intracellular calcium levels (and myometrial activity) are controlled by various receptors on the myometrial cell surface. Most hormones that affect myometrial contractility bind to receptor sites that are coupled to one of two G-proteins: G_αs or G_αq (see Ch. 3) (Bernal et al 1995). The G-proteins act as transducers between the receptor and the effector regulating the cellular response by coupling the receptor to one or other signal-generating enzymes within the cell. These enzymes, in turn, generate an amplifying cascade of second messengers. The G-proteins allow the myometrial tissue to respond to a large number of agonists with a limited number of effects, either relaxation or contraction (Fig. 13.6). One of the G-protein pathways (G_αq) is linked to the inositol phosphate pathway. Binding of agonists

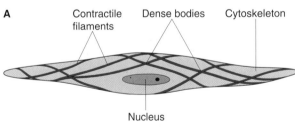

A   Contractile filaments   Dense bodies   Cytoskeleton

Nucleus

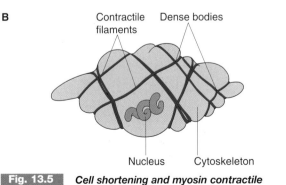

B   Contractile filaments   Dense bodies

Nucleus   Cytoskeleton

Fig. 13.5 *Cell shortening and myosin contractile elements in myometrial muscle contraction: A relaxed; B contracted.*

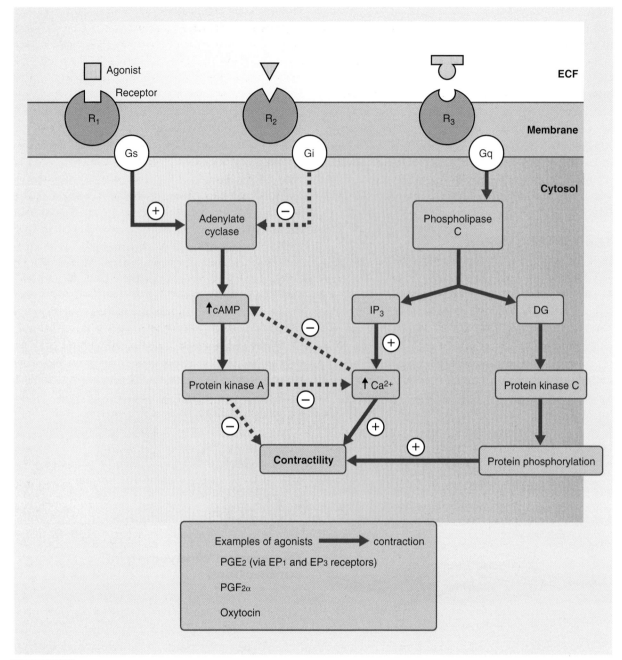

Fig. 13.6 *The regulation of muscle contraction by G-proteins.*

(uterotonins) to receptors coupled to this G-protein activates phospholipase C (PLC), generating inositol triphosphate and diacylglycerol. Inositol trisphosphate stimulates the release of calcium ions from the sarcoplasmic reticulum and diacylglycerol activates the enzymes protein kinase C and phospholipase A. The latter releases arachidonic acid from membrane phospholipids; arachidonic acid is the precursor of prostaglandins. The result is a rise in intracellular calcium and therefore smooth muscle contraction. The other G-protein pathway ($G_\alpha s$) activates adenylate cyclase, an enzyme that generates cyclic adenosine monophosphate (cAMP) and inhibits release of calcium. Agonists that stimulate this pathway, such as β-adrenergic receptor agonists and prostacyclin, will cause increased calcium binding and dephosphorylation of myosin (so MLCK cannot bind Ca–CAM) and thus uterine relaxation.

Gap junctions

The onset of regular uterine contractions is gradual. As pregnancy progresses, the resting potential of the myometrial cells falls so that action potentials are generated with greater ease. Initially spontaneous uterine contractility is inhibited but becomes significant by mid-gestation. At about 20–24 weeks, hardening of the uterus can be felt as muscle contractions start. Initially, uterine activity is mostly of low amplitude and high frequency, with peak activity at night. This circadian rhythm stops at about 3 weeks before delivery, and may be mediated by cortisol (Germain et al 1993). At first, small groups of myometrial cells contract together causing small fluctuations in intrauterine pressure. As pregnancy progresses, adjacent cells begin to contract synchronously so the contractions become more coordinated. This increased coordination results from cell–cell coupling and is due to the formation of intercellular gap junctions.

Gap junctions are formed from bundles of proteins, called connexins, that align forming pore-like sym-metrical channels protruding through adjacent cells, so allowing contact and communication. Gap junctions exist in other tissues that act together in a coordinated fashion, such as cardiac muscle and pancreatic islets. In the open state, gap junctions allow rapid transmission of signals such as electrical stimuli and second messengers such as calcium and inositol trisphosphate (Fig. 13.7). This means that depolarization and smooth muscle contraction in one cell are quickly communicated to adjacent cells so there is a spread of excitement and a synchrony of contractions.

The number of gap junctions increases during gestation to about 1000 per myometrial cell. Physiological regulation of connexins and formation of gap junctions is by prostaglandins and steroid hormones; oestrogen and some prostaglandins increase and progesterone and nitric oxide suppress gap junction formation (Garfield et al 1988). Gap junction density can be determined by measuring electrical resistance of tissue. The resistance of human myometrium at term is about half of that in the non-pregnant uterus and much

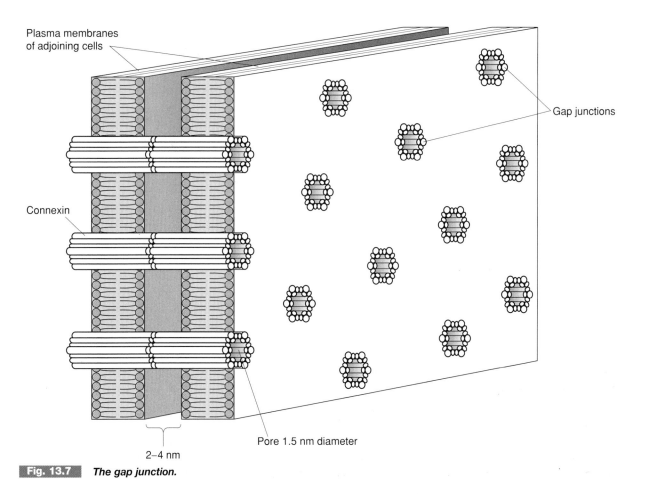

Fig. 13.7 *The gap junction.*

Plasma membranes of adjoining cells

Gap junctions

Connexin

Pore 1.5 nm diameter

2–4 nm

less than that in other smooth muscle (for instance bladder and stomach), which indicates that the cells of the pregnant myometrium are very well coupled. Gap junction formation increases prior to spontaneous labour, resulting in synchronization and coordination of high-amplitude high-frequency myometrial contractions so increased intrauterine pressure is generated (Neulen & Breckwoldt 1994). Suppression of gap junctions may be important at the time of implantation and in early pregnancy (Grummer & Winterhager 1998).

Uterine contractions and quiescence

The uterus exhibits spontaneous contractility. A biopsy specimen of uterine tissue, placed in a physiological solution, will contract involuntarily every 2–5 minutes without stimulation. During the menstrual cycle, three patterns of uterine contractility have been described (de Ziegler et al 2001). At the beginning of the cycle (menstruation), all layers of the myometrium contract exerting antegrade (from fundus to cervix) expulsive forces; these contractions may be associated with painful cramps (dysmenorrhoea). During the receptive window, in the late follicular phase, uterine contractility involves only the inner layers of the myometrium and is gentle and not perceived by women; this facilitates retrograde (cervix to fundus) transport of sperm towards the uterine tubes where fertilization usually takes place (see Ch. 7). As progesterone levels rise after ovulation, the uterus reaches a stage of quiescence. In pregnancy, progesterone continues to increase and to suppress the rhythmic activity of the uterus. Other inhibitors of uterine contractions early in pregnancy include relaxin, prostacyclin and nitric oxide, all of which increase intracellular cAMP and/or decrease intracellular calcium levels. It is also suggested that human chorionic gonadotrophin (hCG) inhibits myometrial contractility (Slattery et al 2001).

However, the uterus is never completely quiescent. From about 7 weeks, the contractions, or 'contractures', are irregular, not synchronized and focal in origin; they have a very high frequency and a very low intensity (Wray 1993). From mid-gestation, the contractions increase gradually in intensity and frequency until about 6 weeks before term when their intensity increases more markedly. The early Braxton Hicks contractions can be perceived but, although strong, they are not normally painful as the cervix remains closed. In labour, the contractions become synchronized, regular and more intense with increased duration.

The cervix

The consistency of the cervix changes in pregnancy to become softer in preparation for labour. Connective tissue changes affect the whole uterus but are more evident in the cervix. The uterine contractions imposed on the softened cervix result in it changing shape. During the pregnancy, the role of the cervix is to act as a closure for the uterus containing its contents and protecting them from ascending infection. Prior to the delivery of the baby, the cervix loses its structural rigidity and is pulled by the uterine contractions so it changes from being a tubular closure to becoming a wide-funnelled canal with very thin edges that is continuous with the rest of the uterine structure. In primigravida women, this shape change occurs in two distinct stages.

The first stage of cervical change is effacement, where the cylindrical shape is transformed into a funnel, but the internal sphincter, or os, is still patent and closed. The longitudinal muscle fibres of the cervix shorten. The differential localization of the fibres means that the outer margins of the cervix develop more tension so maximum uptake of the cervix occurs at the lower end and the external os and softer cervical tissue move upwards into the lower uterine segment (Gee & Olah 1993). During vaginal examination, a midwife might feel an 'effacement ridge' of the cervical tissue undergoing effacement (Fig. 13.8).

The second stage is dilatation (opening of the internal os); the uterus and vagina form one continuous 'sleeve' opening for the exit of the fetus. In multiparous women, the transition from one stage to the other is far less abrupt so effacement and dilatation occur simultaneously. Dilatation is due to the retraction or shortening of the upper part of the uterus, rather than pressure from the descending presenting fetal part. Therefore, if there is no effective presenting part, as in a transverse lie, cervical dilatation still occurs. The dramatic changes in the cervix result from a combination of structural changes in the tissue and forces exerted by the uterine contractions.

The cervix is predominantly composed of fibrous connective tissue plus some smooth muscle and fibroblasts together with blood vessels, epithelium and mucus-secreting glands. There are two elements

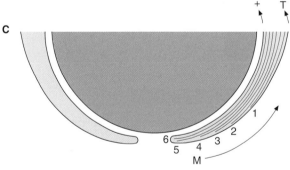

Fig. 13.8   *The differential movement of tissue planes at the time of cervical effacement and early dilatation. M direction of movement of collagen bundles; T, + differential tension across the myometrium. (Reproduced with permission from Sweet & Tiran 1996.)*

nantly composed of proteoglycans, which coat the collagen fibres and modify their physical properties, determining the water content of the tissue. Hormones that promote cervical softening affect the composition of the ground substance. Prior to the onset of labour, the composition of the proteoglycans changes so that dermatan sulphate decreases and hyaluronic acid increases. Dermatan sulphate binds collagen fibrils tightly, whereas hyaluronic acid has a lesser affinity for collagen and attracts water. Although the proteoglycans are a minor constituent of the cervix, they have an amazing ability to bind water: 1 g of hyaluronic acid can bind about 1 litre of water (Uldbjerg & Malstrom 1991). The increased level of hyaluronic acid may act as a signal to activate resident macrophages and neutrophils to secrete interleukins. Interleukins increase prostaglandin activity and neutrophil migration and degranulation (releasing collagenase and elastase). Two other glycoproteins are also involved in cervical changes. Decorin binds and immobilizes the collagen fibres thus stabilizing the structure of the extracellular matrix in early pregnancy. Concentrations of decorin fall in late gestation. Fibronectin binds dermatan sulphate and collagen, protecting collagen from collagenase and stabilizing the extracellular matrix. Hyaluronic acid weakens the interaction of collagen with fibronectin.

The mechanical strength of the ground substance changes as the water content increases and the number of cross-links between elements of the connective tissue diminishes. The collagen increases in solubility and becomes disorganized and weakened (like a fraying rope) so it is more vulnerable to enzymatic digestion. Collagen is resistant to most proteases except collagenase from fibroblasts and neutrophil elastase. Amounts of neutrophil elastase in the cervix significantly increase at term. The association between intrauterine infection and premature labour may be linked to neutrophil infiltration and activation. The effects of oestrogen on cervical ripening are suggested to be mediated by insulin-like growth factor I (IGF-I) (Stjernholm et al 1996). Collagenolysis is a complex balance between availability of free collagenase and the inhibitory proteins. Connective tissue in the body of the uterus also changes at term altering uterine compliance. The level of elastin increases throughout the pregnancy. It provides the elastic recoil that coordinates the contraction–retraction cycle and is important in the return of the uterus to its normal shape after delivery.

to cervical softening: increased vascularity and water content, and structural changes in the connective tissue. At term, 90% of the weight of the cervix is water. Connective tissue is formed of collagen fibres and elastin held together by an extracellular matrix, or ground substance. The ground substance is predomi-

Although the cervix has relatively little smooth muscle tissue, it may have an important functional role as a sphincter. The cervix constricts with uterine contractions in early labour (Olah 1994). It is suggested that this coordinated muscular activity is important in the maintenance of cervical integrity during Braxton Hicks contractions before labour (Steer & Johnson 1998).

Assessment of cervical effacement

In practice, the cervix can be assessed by using a simple scoring system, the Bishop's score (Table 13.1). This is particularly useful prior to induction of labour and for monitoring the changes in the cervix as the induction progresses.

If the cervix is soft, effaced and has started to dilate, induction may be implemented by artificial rupture of the membranes, which augments endogenous prostaglandin production. If the cervix is less favourable, prostaglandin E_2 (PGE_2) is administered into the posterior fornix of the vagina to facilitate effacement. However, PGE_2 should be used with caution in multiparous women because they have a greater sensitivity to it.

The cause of these structural changes in the cervix is not clear. It is thought to be hormonally controlled. Relaxin has been shown to be important in cervical ripening in rodents and has been used clinically to promote cervical ripening in humans. However, the levels of endogenous relaxin in pregnant women seem to be highest at the beginning of the second trimester. Oestrogen affects the synthesis of connective tissue components in vitro but has limited success when used pharmacologically as an induction method. PGE_2 causes cervical softening or 'ripening' and is produced naturally by both the cervix and the fetal membranes.

PGE_2 appears to act by increasing collagenolytic activity rather than by changing the composition of the ground substance, which probably precedes prostaglandin use in successful induction of labour. Following delivery, glycoproteins that bind strongly to collagen are re-formed so the rigidity of the cervix is re-established; however, it never completely regains its original form (see Ch. 14). Damage to the cervix may have long-term consequences (Box 13.1).

Initiation of parturition

Animal models of parturition

Parturition in sheep has been studied in detail. Based on the assumption that mammals are likely to share similar physiological mechanisms for the onset of labour, clinical procedures derived from understanding the mechanisms of parturition in sheep were developed, both for inducing labour and for inhibiting preterm labour in humans. Initiation of labour in sheep is driven by the maturation of the fetal brain; the effect is that progesterone falls resulting in increased uterine activity. Expression of pro-opiomelanocortin, the precursor of adrenocorticotrophic hormone (ACTH), progressively increases in the pituitary from mid-gestation as the fetal brain matures (Challis et al 2000). Regulation of secretion of pituitary ACTH in the fetal lamb is by antidiuretic hormone (ADH, also known as vasopressin) and corticotrophin-releasing hormone (CRH). Thus, the first indicator of impend-

Table 13.1 *Bishop's score*

Bishop's score	0	1	2
Station of presenting part	−3	−2	−1
Position of cervix	Posterior	Mid	Anterior
Consistency	Firm	Soft	Very soft
Length	3–4 cm	1–2 cm	< 1 cm
Dilation of cervix	0	1–2 cm	>2 cm
Total =	(Bishop's score)		

Box 13.1

Clinical issues relating to the cervix

Longitudinal fibres allow full dilatation of the cervix to be achieved without the pressure of a presenting part, for instance in the case of a transverse lie. Artificial dilatation of an unprepared cervix may damage the collagen fibres. This can result in the cervix failing to remain intact during subsequent pregnancies, resulting in habitual spontaneous abortion, usually in mid-trimester. Preoperative preparation to avoid this involves the administration of a prostaglandin derivative, which induces cervical softening and aids artificial dilatation of the cervix. This method is used prior to procedures involving exploration of the uterine cavity such as termination of pregnancy, evacuation of retained products of conception, surgical ablation of the endometrium and investigation of infertility.

ing labour in sheep is a sharp rise in fetal cortisol levels due to mature secretion of ACTH from the pituitary gland and increased adrenal sensitivity to ACTH. Removal or abnormal development of the fetal lamb pituitary gland prevents the onset of labour. Infusion of ACTH, cortisone or dexamethasone (a cortisol analogue, frequently used as an anti-inflammatory drug) into the sheep fetus induces labour. Fetal stress such as hypoxia and undernutrition can stimulate preterm birth in sheep (Warnes et al 1998) by increasing fetal HPA maturation.

The effects of raised cortisol levels are both to promote fetal organ maturity and to initiate labour. Cortisol induces 17α-hydroxylase activity in the placenta that promotes the conversion of C21 steroids to C18 steroids. Thus 17α-hydroxylase converts progesterone to oestrogen so that the progesterone:oestrogen ratio alters in favour of oestrogen. This increases prostaglandin ($PGF_{2\alpha}$) synthesis by the placenta and myometrium. The alteration in oestrogen and progesterone levels can be measured prior to the onset of labour. Exogenous oestrogen induces labour and infusion of progesterone inhibits labour in the sheep. Increasing oestrogen or decreasing progesterone levels stimulates the synthesis of $PGF_{2\alpha}$. Prostaglandins increase myometrial sensitivity to oxytocin. $PGF_{2\alpha}$ is important in cervical softening and increases uterine contractility. A positive feedback mechanism, known as the Ferguson reflex, amplifies the signals. The pressure of the fetal presenting part on the cervix activates a neurohumoral reflex whereby afferent nerves from the cervix impinge on the hypothalamus and increase oxytocin release from the posterior pituitary gland. Oxytocin stimulates uterine contractions and causes further release of $PGF_{2\alpha}$ from the uterus. However, initiation of labour in the human is different in a number of respects from that in the sheep. (Note that pregnancy in some species, such as goats, rabbits and rodents, depends on progesterone secretion from the corpus luteum. Luteolysis, mediated by $PGF_{2\alpha}$, causes a fall in progesterone and initiation of parturition in these species.)

Initiation of parturition in humans

The mean length of human gestation is 39.6 weeks and the majority of births occur between 38 and 42 weeks (Steer & Johnson 1998). Such a wide range of gestation times in normal pregnancy suggests the timing mechanism is not precise, possibly because it is affected by a number of factors including external influences. The fetus seems to maintain the pregnancy actively. Labour invariably ensues after fetal death has occurred, although it might be delayed by a few weeks (and therefore be pre-empted by mechanical removal of the products of conception). Labour occurs sooner if placental damage has occurred. The critical events permitting extrauterine survival are adequate maturation of the fetal lung and nervous system. The fetal brain may monitor this maturation and control the timing mechanism. Mothers of fetuses with brain abnormalities still progress into labour spontaneously but with a much wider range of gestation (see below). This suggests the fetal brain affects the precise timing of labour in humans, rather than controlling the exact length of gestation.

Hormonal changes at parturition in humans

The role of the fetal pituitary–adrenal axis

In sheep, maturation of the fetal HPA initiates parturition. Human fetal malformations such as anencephaly (no cerebrum), malformed pituitary glands or hypoplasia of the adrenal glands are associated with an increased range of gestation length (both longer and shorter) but women still undergo spontaneous labour (Steer & Johnson 1998). In sheep, similar fetal malformations, either accidental or deliberate, result in significantly prolonged gestation which adversely affects the fetus (Challis et al 2001). This implies that the fetal–adrenal axis has a supportive rather than a direct role in parturition, acting to fine tune the gestational length in humans, rather than functioning as the 'on–off switch' for the initiation of labour, as seen in sheep.

Cortisol

It is evident that the human fetal anterior pituitary gland undergoes maturational changes in the last weeks of gestation as the profile of hormonal release changes. However, there are no defined changes measurable in the maternal circulation prior to the onset of labour. The raised cortisol levels in the cord blood of infants who had experienced a spontaneous delivery rather than an induced one, or delivery by caesarean section, are maternally derived and are secondary to maternal pain. Labour itself, whether spontaneous or induced, causes stress and therefore an increased production of cortisol, which can cross the placenta. It is possible to differentiate between cortisol of maternal origin and cortisol of fetal origin by comparing the levels in umbilical cord arterial blood with those in the cord vein. Blood in the vein flows from the placenta to the fetus so if cortisol levels are higher in the vein than in the arteries this suggests the source of cortisol is maternal.

Exogenous corticosteroids (such as dexamethasone and betamethasone) given to a pregnant woman at 24–34 weeks to promote fetal lung maturity (see Ch. 15) do not initiate parturition, although oestrogen and cortisol levels fall. Pharmacological doses of glucocorticoids introduced into the amniotic fluid increase uterine activity and induce labour; however, this effect is not observed with physiological doses. Most researchers have not been able to measure an increase in cortisol prior to the onset of labour, nor an effect on placental hormone production. Therefore, it now seems unlikely that cortisol is important in initiating labour in humans, although it has a vital role in the maturation of fetal lungs and other organs. Several factors may affect physiological responses to cortisol; these include corticosteroid-binding protein (CBP) and the relative concentration of free cortisol, metabolism of cortisol to inactive cortisone by 11β-hydroxysteroid dehydrogenase and modification of corticosteroid receptor expression.

Progesterone:oestrogen ratio

In the sheep, fetal cortisol affects steroidogenesis so progesterone levels fall and oestrogen levels increase. This is a result of increased expression and activity of placental 17α-hydroxylase (see above). Across almost all species, the fall in plasma progesterone concentration is a common endocrine event leading to parturition. However, progesterone levels do not fall prior to labour in humans. In humans, the placenta does not express inducible 17α-hydroxylase activity and therefore cannot convert progesterone to oestrogen. However, increases in free oestriol levels have been observed in saliva of women before the onset of labour, both preterm and at term (Goodwin 1999).

High progesterone levels inhibit myometrial activity during implantation and favour uterine quiescence throughout the pregnancy. This suppression of myometrial activity is essential to the maintenance of pregnancy, although parturition begins without a measurable decrease in maternal peripheral progesterone levels. Large doses of progesterone are relatively unsuccessful in inhibiting preterm labour in humans. However, mifepristone, an anti-progestin also known as RU-486, blocks the effect of progesterone and can induce labour (Thong & Baird 1992).

It is possible that there could be local changes in progesterone concentration, not reflected in peripheral blood, that may affect myometrial activity. As the uterus enlarges during the pregnancy, the part of the uterine wall distal to the site of implantation, and therefore furthest away from the major source of progesterone production, may re-establish uterine contractions and trigger the onset of labour (Challis et al 2000). Measurement of absolute progesterone levels may therefore be misleading as the biological effects will be altered by receptor density, levels of binding proteins or postreceptor changes. The fetal membranes can both metabolize progesterone and produce cortisol. Cortisol is antagonistic to progesterone and can increase the synthesis of CRH (Karalis et al 1996). Fetal membranes, therefore, offer a mechanism for local control of progesterone concentration. Alternative mechanisms have been suggested for the apparent lack of progesterone withdrawal prior to human parturition. These include sequestration of progesterone, another progesterone-like steroid being involved as a natural antagonist or local inactivation of progesterone, for instance progesterone is converted into an inactive metabolite that competes for receptor sites (Challis et al 2000). It has also been suggested that in humans there is a regionalization of uterine activity and high progesterone levels are important in promoting relaxation of the lower uterine segment while contractions in the fundal area facilitate the descent of the fetus (Challis et al 2000). Changes in progesterone receptor expression could potentially act as a functional progesterone block and thus control myometrial progesterone responsiveness (Mesiano 2004). The altered progesterone receptor profile is postulated to affect oestrogen effects (and hence oxytocin responses) via expression of oestrogen receptors. The human progesterone receptor exists in two isoforms, PR-A and PR-B, and the ratio of the two forms changes during gestation thus affecting the response of the uterine tissue and the ability of progesterone to suppress myometrial activity (Astle et al 2003).

Human placental production of oestrogen increases throughout labour and the rate seems to increase in the latter part of gestation. In sheep, increased oestrogen causes increased contraction-associated proteins (CAPs) and up-regulation of prostaglandin synthase and consequent increased synthesis of PGE_2, promoting a positive feedback of myometrial contractility.

However, spontaneous labour in humans can occur in the absence of measurable changes in oestrogen concentration. Exogenous oestrogen infusion in humans causes a transient increase in uterine activity and decreases the oxytocin threshold of the uterus but does not induce premature delivery or fetal membrane changes (Challis et al 2000).

Synthesis of placental oestrogen depends on fetal cooperation in the provision of the precursors, and could thus potentially provide an opportunity for the human fetus to manipulate the progesterone:oestrogen ratio and uterine activity. The fetal adrenal gland in humans and higher primates has three zones: the outer adult zone produces mostly aldosterone, the unique fetal zone produces dehydroepiandrosterone sulphate (DHEAS) and the transitional zone produces mostly cortisol. This large fetal zone of the adrenal gland disappears in the neonatal period and may be regulated by hCG levels. DHEAS is the fetal adrenal C19 steroid precursor for placental oestradiol-17α and oestrone synthesis, which are implicated as having a role in labour. DHEAS is converted to oestrogens by placental sulphatase, aromatase and other enzymes (see Ch. 3). Production of DHEAS is controlled by ACTH from the anterior pituitary, which is itself regulated by hypothalamic CRH. CRH of placental origin can also stimulate production of DHEAS from the fetal zone (see below). However, women who have placental sulphatase or aromatase deficiencies and produce very little placental oestrogen can have normal pregnancy and labour (López Bernal 2003). Thus, the changing ratio of oestrogen to progesterone may facilitate effective uterine contractions but is probably not critical for the induction of labour (Steer & Johnson 1998).

Corticotrophin-releasing hormone

Placental CRH seems to have an important role in the initiation of parturition in higher primates and humans. CRH is synthesized by the placenta and reaches the maternal circulation (Riley & Challis 1991). Levels steadily increase from mid-term until about 35 weeks when levels sharply rise and are usually particularly high in pregnancies ending with premature labour (Wolfe et al 1990). CRH activity is attenuated by CRH-binding protein (CRH-BP), which is synthesized by the liver, placenta and brain so most CRH is in the bound (inactive) form during pregnancy. However, towards term, when levels of CRH increase, levels of CRH-BP simultaneously fall so circulating levels of physiologically active, free CRH markedly increase. CRH establishes positive feedback loops, increasing prostaglandin production and fetal glucocorticoid levels (Petraglia et al 1995), both of which further increase placental synthesis of CRH. Fetal stresses such as hypoxia and hypoglycaemia result in increased CRH concentrations. CRH is a vasodilator in the placental vascular bed (Clifton et al 1994) so increased CRH should result in increased blood flow and abrogation of the fetal insult. However, if the insult persists, then CRH would increase ACTH secretion and increase DHEAS production thus increasing oestrogen synthesis which leads to myometrial activation. Thus, CRH appears to be a mechanism by which a compromised fetus can precipitate labour when intrauterine life becomes unfavourable.

It has been suggested that the ratio of placental CRH and CRH-BP acts as a placental 'clock' which controls gestational length and allows a distressed fetus to 'wind-on' the clock to initiate premature labour. CRH receptors can couple to different G-proteins in different tissues and at different times (Karteris et al 1998). So for most of pregnancy, CRH is coupled to the G-protein (G_αs) involved in increasing cAMP levels. It therefore has a 'protective' role and promotes myometrial quiescence via the generation of cAMP and cGMP, and up-regulation of nitric oxide synthase expression. Near term, CRH couples to the other G-protein pathway (G_αq) as well so it activates PLC and mobilizes calcium thus promoting increased myometrial contractility and labour (Hillhouse & Grammatopoulos 2003). Myometrial contractility is also enhanced by up-regulation of oxytocin receptor expression and cross-talk between the oxytocin and CRH receptors.

Loss of uterine quiescence

It is argued that an alternative pathway for initiation of parturition is the switching off of mechanisms that cause relaxation (see above) (López Bernal 2003). Cyclic nucleotides (cAMP, etc.) promote myometrial relaxation and β_2-adrenergeric agonists are effective tocolytic agents (see Table 13.2). The enzyme adenylyl cyclase catalyses the production of cAMP from ATP. Coupling of receptors to adenylyl cyclase may be responsible for uterine quiescence. As progesterone inhibits activity of the phosphodiesterase which breaks down cAMP, thus terminating its action, progesterone sustains the effect of cAMP and promotes uterine relaxation during pregnancy.

Table 13.2 *Intervention in labour*

Drug/treatment	Effect	Notes
Treatment of preterm labour (tocolytic agents)		
Indomethacin	Inhibits prostaglandin synthesis	Adverse effects on fetal renal function, associated with oligohydramnios
β-Adrenergic agonists ('β-agonists'), e.g. ritodrine, terbutaline, fenoterol	Inhibit uterine contractions	Effects often short-lived; unpleasant side-effects (cardiovascular and metabolic)
Magnesium sulphate	Inhibits myometrial contractility	Limited usefulness as a tocolytic agent but useful as cerebroprotective agent
Atosiban	Oxytocin antagonist	Clinical trials taking place; potentially useful as oxytocin receptors have limited distribution
Prostaglandin synthase inhibitors, e.g. indomethacin	Inhibit preterm contractions	Serious neonatal complications in infants born <30 weeks
Calcium-channel blockers, e.g. nifedipine	Decrease intracellular calcium, cause uterine relaxation	May affect placental and uterine blood flow; cardiovascular side-effects
Alcohol		Risk of aspiration, intoxication, depression and incontinence
Treatment of post-term labour (methods of induction)		
Oxytocin	Used to augment labour; oxytocin has little effect on unripe cervix	Production of endogenous oxytocin can be increased by nipple stimulation
PGF_2 agonists, e.g. dinoprostone, Cervidil, Prepidil	Cervical ripening, induction of labour	Effects depend on expression of receptors
Misoprostol (Cytotec)	Synthetic PGE_1 analogue; used to reduce acid in the stomach	Can cause the uterus to contract; nausea and diarrhoea
Mifepristone (RU-486; Mifegyne)	Antiprogestin	Primarily used to induce first trimester abortion

Signal amplification

Once parturition has been initiated and the myometrium is activated, there is a positive fast-forward stimulation of myometrial activity. This signal amplification is mediated by prolabour factors, known as contraction-associated proteins (CAPs) or utero-tonins. These include prostaglandins and prostanoid receptors, oxytocin and oxytocin receptors, gap junctions and ion channels. It has not been easy to discriminate between those hormones and signals that initiate labour and those that amplify the triggering signals.

Prostaglandins

Prostaglandins (PGs) of the 2-series are known to be important in the fast-forward signal amplification and progression of labour; they promote myometrial contractions, cervical dilatation and membrane rupture. Prostaglandins are present in the circulation in low concentrations and are cleared in the pulmonary circulation so they are difficult to measure as they have paracrine activity and a short half-life. Prostaglandins can be formed as a consequence of tissue trauma (including labour itself and any manipulative or tactile stimuli). In late pregnancy, prostaglandin synthesis is readily stimulated by minor local stimuli, such as coitus, vaginal examination, sweeping the membranes or amniotomy, which are associated with inducing labour. Exogenous prostaglandins can be used therapeutically to ripen the cervix and to induce uterine contractions and labour. Mid-trimester abortion can be induced by procedures, such as intra-amniotic injection of hypertonic saline, that result in the increased synthesis and release of prostaglandins. Increasing DHEAS or oestrogen concentration and decreasing progesterone concentration increase production of prostaglandins (Challis et al 2000). An increase is myometrial expression of prostaglandins receptors, particularly the receptor of $PGF_{2\alpha}$ is implicated in the causes of some preterm labour (Olson et al 2003).

Prostaglandins are synthesized in the fetal membranes, decidua, myometrium and cervix; levels fall abruptly following placental separation. The rate-limiting step of prostaglandin production may be important in initiating labour. Activity of phospholipase A_2 (PLA_2) may regulate the level of arachidonic acid, which is the precursor of prostaglandins (see Ch. 3). Increased oestrogen (or decreased progesterone) stimulates the release of PLA_2 from decidual lysozymes and therefore increases free arachidonic acid and subsequent prostaglandin synthesis. Arachidonic acid can also be produced indirectly via phospholipase C activity. Alternatively, the activity of cyclo-oxygenase (COX) may be rate-limiting (Aitken, Rice & Brennecke 1990).

The two most important prostaglandins in labour appear to be $PGF_{2\alpha}$ and PGE_2. At term, concentrations of PGE_2 and $PGF_{2\alpha}$ are higher in the decidua and myometrium (but these tissues are subject to tissue trauma so some authors believe raised prostaglandin levels are caused by increased uterine activity). PGE_2 is involved in cervical ripening and is metabolized by the myometrium to produce $PGF_{2\alpha}$. However, women with extrauterine pregnancies go into labour at term and experience painful uterine contractions even though there are no fetal membranes in contact with the uterus.

Maintenance of human pregnancy may depend on the synthesis of PGE_2 being inhibited and this inhibition of prostaglandin synthase being attenuated at the onset of labour. Prostaglandin concentrations in the pregnant uterus are very low (about 200 times lower than at any stage in the menstrual cycle), but increase sharply in the maternal circulation from 36 weeks' gestation probably in response to the increasing level of CRH (Hertelendy & Zakar 2004). Arachidonic acid, the precursor, is plentiful but synthesis of prostaglandins is inhibited, even if the pregnancy is extrauterine. Progesterone or the fetus may directly or indirectly moderate synthesis or metabolism of prostaglandins. Endogenous inhibitors of prostaglandin synthesis have been identified in maternal plasma; levels fall towards the end of gestation.

Inhibitors of prostaglandin synthase, such as aspirin and indomethacin, are used therapeutically to treat preterm labour. Prostaglandin synthase activity is up-regulated by cortisol (and dexamethasone), oestradiol, CRH and the inflammatory cytokines interleukin 1β (IL-1β) and tumour necrosis factor α (TNFα) (Bowen et al 2002).

Low doses of prostaglandins, particularly $PGF_{2\alpha}$, increase myometrial responsiveness to prostaglandins and oxytocin possibly by increasing the formation of gap junctions. In vitro, PGE_2 has a biphasic effect, stimulating at nanomolar concentrations and inhibiting at micromolar concentrations. It also has a dual action: when its effects are mediated by the EP_1 and EP_3 receptors, PGE_2 increases intracellular calcium concentration, but the EP_2 receptor is coupled to adenylate cyclase so PGE_2 acting at this receptor decreases intracellular calcium and favours relaxation. Variations in regional prostaglandin synthesis may occur (Wilmsatt et al 1995).

Prostacyclin (PGI_2) is synthesized in the myometrium and cervix. It promotes myometrial quiescence. It has an important role in maintaining uterine blood flow in labour; it causes vasodilation of smooth muscle and inhibits platelet aggregation, potentially inhibiting thromboembolic complications. Myometrial relaxation between uterine contractions in labour prevents occlusion of the uterine vessels and hypoxia which could lead to uterine dystocia (Hertelendy & Zakar 2004). Placental thromboxane (TxA_2) has opposing effects to PGI_2 and is important in the closure of the fetal ductus arteriosus and haemostasis after delivery. In pre-eclampsia, levels of prostacyclin are low and levels of thromboxane are high. This is the rationale for aspirin treatment of pre-eclampsia. Aspirin-like drugs are inhibitors of the COX enzyme responsible for prostaglandin synthase and restore thromboxane levels in pre-eclampsia. Trials using aspirin caused a slight prolongation of gestation and diminution of uterine contractions, but also increased the risk of premature closure of the ductus arteriosus and postnatal bleeding problems in the mother.

Prostaglandins are metabolized by the enzyme prostaglandin dehydrogenase (PGDH) which is located in the fetal membranes. Deficiency of PGDH is associated with preterm labour. Expression of PGDH is up-regulated by progesterone and IL-10 and suppressed by cortisol (and dexamethasone), oestradiol, CRH, IL-1β and TNFα. Parturition is, therefore, essentially an inflammatory process. The association between infection and preterm labour is thought to be due to the release of phospholipases from bacterial organisms (Romero et al 2003), which cause an increase in arachidonic acid release and so prostaglandin synthesis. Decidual macrophages respond to bacterial products by releasing pro-inflammatory cytokines. Bacterial endotoxins, such as lipopolysaccharide, can either increase prostaglandin release directly or further stimulate release of cytokines which then increase prostaglandin synthesis. Lipopolysaccharide also contributes to premature rupture of the membranes.

Prostaglandins also have an important role in the establishment of a neonatal circulatory pattern (see Ch. 15). Respiratory distress syndrome is associated with high levels of $PGF_{2\alpha}$ in the infant's circulation, and patent ductus arteriosus with high PGE_2 levels. PGE_2 can prevent the ductus from closing and inhibitors of prostaglandin synthesis can promote closure of the ductus. There is indirect evidence (i.e. fetal breathing movements stop) that PGE_2 increases in the fetal circulation 48–72 hours before the onset of labour (Thorburn 1992). It is possible that this is mirrored by a local increase in PGE_2 concentration in uterine tissue, which initiates labour.

Oxytocin

Oxytocin is a peptide synthesized by the hypothalamus and released from the posterior pituitary gland (see Ch. 3). A synthetic form is used extensively for induction and augmentation of human labour and endogenous production can be stimulated, for instance by nipple stimulation, with a favourable outcome. However, it is not certain whether oxytocin is important in the initiation of labour. As oxytocin receptors are generally localized to the uterus, mammary glands and pituitary, oxytocin antagonists and agonists have few systemic effects. Maternal oxytocin levels are very low and do not change very much before labour. Maternal pituitary production of oxytocin dramatically increases in the first stage of labour. However, focusing on circulating levels of oxytocin may be misleading. The concentration of oxytocin receptors in the myometrium and decidua rise dramatically (by 100–200 times) during late pregnancy so the sensitivity of the uterus increases (Fuchs et al 1984). This means the uterus can be stimulated by low concentrations of maternal oxytocin levels that previously had no effect. Therapeutic doses adequate to augment labour are very variable, which probably reflects individual differences in receptor number. The

pattern of oxytocin release changes at the onset of labour, with an increased frequency of pulses (Fuchs et al 1991). It may be important that maternal oxytocin levels stay low during the pregnancy so the sensitivity of the uterus to oxytocin is maintained. Oxytocin antagonists, such as antosiban, have been used to inhibit uterine contractility in preterm labour (see Table 13.2) but not always effectively.

Exposure of decidual cells to oxytocin increases the release of prostaglandins. Vaginal examination in late pregnancy stimulates the Ferguson reflex so oxytocin is released from the posterior pituitary, which stimulates uterine prostaglandin production. Earlier in pregnancy, this response does not occur, presumably because there are inadequate oxytocin receptors. Women who go into preterm labour seem to have an increased expression of oxytocin receptors and higher myometrial sensitivity to oxytocin. Failed induction of labour is associated with a reduced number of oxytocin receptors. Therefore the initiation of labour depends on mechanisms that induce the expression of oxytocin receptors in the myometrium rather affect the oxytocin level itself. Both oestrogen and prostaglandins increase uterine responsiveness to oxytocin.

Oxytocin is also synthesized by the decidua and may act locally (Miller, Chibbar & Mitchell 1993). The fetal posterior pituitary produces both oxytocin and ADH (vasopressin). Exogenous oxytocin can cause uterine contractions in sheep and anencephalic humans (Honnebier et al 1974); however, the physiological relevance of this is not clear as maternal oxytocin secretion does not rise until labour has been initiated. In spontaneous labour, fetal secretion of oxytocin is high and transferred across the placenta at levels comparable to those used to induce uterine activity (Husslein 1985). The increment in oxytocin levels is greater in the umbilical arteries than in the umbilical vein and is much higher than maternal levels, suggesting it is synthesized by the fetus and transferred across the placenta. Initiation and maintenance of human labour may therefore be influenced by fetal oxytocin production. ADH (vasopressin) is produced at even higher concentrations than oxytocin and may regulate prostaglandin production.

Relaxin

Relaxin is a polypeptide hormone produced by the corpus luteum, and decidua and placenta in pregnancy, which promotes tissue remodelling during reproduction (Bani 1997). It has been found to inhibit myometrial contractility and promote vasodilation, via nitric oxide synthesis, until late pregnancy. It also appears to promote cervical ripening at parturition. Concentrations of relaxin appear to be highest in the first trimester and then fall. A very early fall is associated with preterm labour. Histologically, the number of cells staining positively for relaxin are much less after spontaneous delivery compared with caesarean section. Relaxin may inhibit PGE_2 production during pregnancy but favours its production in labour. It may act synergistically with progesterone during the pregnancy, maintaining uterine quiescence and inhibiting oxytocin release.

The maternal endocrine system

Ovaries are not necessary for the initiation of labour. Hypophysectomized women (who have no pituitary glands) and women with diabetes insipidus (a posterior pituitary defect) go into labour at term. However, the posterior pituitary stores oxytocin, which is synthesized in the hypothalamus. In the absence of a functional pituitary gland, oxytocin is probably secreted directly by the hypothalamus. Adrenalectomized women on corticosteroid maintenance therapy go into labour spontaneously but women with Addison's disease tend to have prolonged pregnancy.

The maternal nervous system

There is a higher density of adrenergic and cholinergic innervation towards the cervix. The non-pregnant uterus contracts in response to both adrenaline and noradrenaline but, at term, noradrenaline increases uterine contractions and adrenaline causes relaxation. α-Receptor antagonists, such as phentolamine, decrease uterine activity and inhibit the response to noradrenaline so adrenergic drugs are used to suppress contractions in preterm labour; β-receptor antagonists, such as propranolol, increase uterine activity. Catecholamines both stimulate and inhibit uterine activity, acting via the α_2-receptors and β_2-receptors respectively. The α_1-receptors increase intracellular calcium concentrations and promote contractile activity. However, labour occurs normally in paraplegic women (who have no nervous input to the uterus), suggesting that the onset and progress of labour is under hormonal, rather than nervous, control. Neural control appears to modulate uterine activity but is subordinate to hormonal control.

Stretch

In a normal pregnancy, growth of the uterus keeps pace with the growth of its contents and the limit of stretchability is probably not reached. In fact, mechanical stretching of the uterine wall by the growing fetus induces smooth muscle hypertrophy and increases its tensile strength. However, overstretching, for instance with multiple pregnancy and polyhydramnios, is associated with a shorter gestation period. The probable mechanism is that stretching of the muscle fibres increases their excitability and that mechanical stress can increase responsiveness to uterotonins.

The timing of parturition

In some mammalian species there is a clear seasonal influence on ovulation and delivery. There are obvious advantages to ensuring the young are born at the optimal time of year when there is a plentiful food supply and less threat from predators. In these species, the length of the daylight period mediated by melatonin production appears to play an important role. The human fetus possibly has the potential to survive birth as early as the 24th week of gestation. Most babies are delivered after the 37th week of gestation. However, there is a range of gestational periods producing healthy babies capable of survival. It is suggested that this variation in apparently normal gestation could allow changing environmental conditions to influence the precise timing. One suggestion is that the time of the lunar month could affect the timing after 37 weeks. Other suggestions are that gestational length may be linked to the length of the individual woman's ovarian cycle or may have a familial pattern. Women with longer menstrual cycles may have a lower level of oestrogen, which could affect the initiation of parturition (see above).

Mammals tend to labour most effectively during the period of the day in which they normally rest. They usually seek isolation and privacy and protection from terrestrial predators. Nocturnal species tend to give birth during the day and diurnal species tend to give birth at night (Rosenberg & Trevathan 2002). This timing may be because the effect of the parasympathetic nervous system is then dominant; labour is inhibited by sympathetic stimulation. Both the start of labour and the actual time of delivery occur more frequently at night and in the early hours of the morning (Honnebier & Nathanielsz 1994). Circadian rhythms occur in several variables including pregnancy-associated hormones and prelabour myometrial activity. Uterine activity and oxytocin levels are higher at night until about 3 weeks before delivery. The maternal circadian system probably entrains fetal cooperation. Circadian rhythms do not occur in sheep (Apostolakis et al 1993).

The evolutionary context of human labour

Humans have large and complex brains and are the only living mammal that habitually walks on two legs. They have a complicated mechanism of labour and routinely seek assistance when they give birth. The development of bipedal locomotion has resulted in a changed pelvic structure and physiology. One suggestion is that eye contact in sexual intercourse has led to the vagina forming a right-angle with the brim of the pelvis and uterus, presenting a laborious passageway in childbirth (Stewart 1984). The relatively straight cylindrical pelvis of our forebears has evolved into a tilted conical birth canal. Pelvic size has decreased to enhance adaptation to the upright posture and swift movement.

It is thought that the upright stance of human ancestors led to thickening and lengthening of the pelvic bones and the forward curvature of the sacrum (Stewart 1984); this stance imposes extra pressure on the pregnant cervix. Humans have a particularly high concentration of cervical collagen compared with other species. Unlike most other animals, where the cervix remains firmly closed until just before delivery, there is usually some degree of cervical softening relatively early in human pregnancy (Fig. 13.9); partial dilatation of the cervix occurs much earlier in gestation (Leppert 1995). Because there is such a wide variation in the cervical changes among pregnant women, cervical assessment in isolation of other signs is an unreliable indicator of the imminence of labour. Towards the end of the first stage of labour, the changing shape of the cervix means that its tissue becomes integrated with the rest of the uterus (Fig. 13.8) (see below).

The evolution of the human brain resulted in cephalization, the marked enlargement of head size in relation to overall body mass (Stewart 1984). This creates the potential problem of obstructed labour, which occurs at a much higher rate in humans compared to other animals. The fetus has to negotiate rather than simply pass through the pelvic cavity. It seems that humans have adapted by the fetus completing in utero development at a relatively early stage, and being born at a much smaller proportion of the adult weight. Cephalization has resulted in secondary altriciality, the infant being born at an immature and helpless state of development. Human infants are born with a smaller proportion of adult brain size than other primates. This has significant implications for parental behaviour and social relationships as well as placing a higher emphasis on the importance of nutrition in

 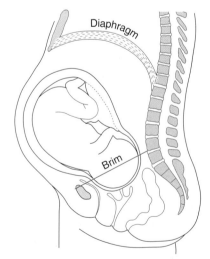

Fig. 13.9   *A Prior to lightening: the fundus is in close proximity to the diaphragm and the lower uterine segment is still firm so the fetal head remains high. B After lightening (2–3 weeks before the onset of labour): the lower uterine segment has softened and dilated so the fetal head descends and the fundus sinks below the diaphragm, easing breathing. (Reproduced with permission from Bennett & Brown 1999.)*

providing for development of the nervous system in the postnatal year.

Humans are not the only animals that have difficulty in childbirth (Rosenberg & Trevathan 2002). The smaller bodied primates, such as monkeys and gibbons, have similar cephalopelvic constraints; the neonate at birth has a head size that is close to the size of its mother's birth canal. Monkeys usually deliver in a squatting position away from other members of the social group, who may observe from a distance. The mother monkey may wipe mucus from the infant's mouth and nose and guide the infant, who is usually dexterous with developed motor skills, out of the birth canal towards the nipples (Rosenberg & Trevathan 2002). Because of mechanical differences in the birth process, however, the human fetus has to rotate within the pelvic cavity and is usually born in an occipito-anterior position (head facing away from the maternal pubic bones, in the opposite direction from the mother). In this position, it is difficult for the mother to reach to clear a breathing passage or remove the umbilical cord from the infant's neck. Thus, human mothers actively seek assistance in childbirth and birth is a social rather than a solitary occurrence.

Whereas most primates squat during delivery, unless women are used to squatting, the semi-upright positions of kneeling and sitting are thought to be optimal (Rosenberg & Trevathan 2002). The upright position (standing, squatting or sitting) results in a shortened second stage of labour and more favourable maternal and infant outcomes. Being upright allows maternal effort to be aided by gravity. The presenting part bears the force of the neonate. The occiput has well developed cranial plates and is best able to withstand the stress (Rosenberg & Trevathan 2002).

It is suggested that the physiological control of birth is mediated by hormones that are derived from archaic brain structures such as the hypothalamus and pituitary gland (Odent 2001) and that labour is facilitated by an environment that promotes these primitive pathways. The neocortex, on the other hand, is thought to inhibit the primitive pathways. The neocortex responds to bright light and to language. Thus, it is suggested that bright lights, feelings of being observed (and use of cameras and monitoring equipment) and use of language which stimulate neocortical activity might interfere with the primitive physiological processes and impede the progress of labour. Maternal levels of catecholamines peak towards the end of labour which increases maternal awareness and alertness as the baby is born. This is suggested to be an evolutionary advantage, promoting maternal behaviour and protectionism, even aggressiveness (Odent 2001).

The first stage of labour

Uterine contractions in labour

If softening of the cervix has taken place, the coordinated uterine contractions exert a steady pull thus stretching the cervix. This effacement of the cervix often takes place before the contractions become completely regular so it may occur a week or so before labour. As the cervix effaces, the presenting part of the fetus, usually the head, descends into the cavity of the pelvis. The fetal position alters so that it fits well; this is described as engagement.

Contractions are involuntary and will therefore occur in an unconscious woman. However, they can be temporarily abolished by emotional disturbances (including moving from home to hospital and by a change in staff shifts). The frequency and strength of the contractions can be increased by enemas, prostaglandins and oxytocin preparations, and by stretching of the cervix or pelvic floor by the presenting part. Contractions are regular and intermittent. The intermittent nature is important as it allows recovery of both the uterus and the labouring woman and a resumed oxygen supply to the fetus.

Contractions begin to feel painful once the cervix starts to dilate. Backache often precedes cervical dilation. The pain is due to ischaemia in the muscle during the contraction because the uterine blood vessels are compressed. Similar pain occurs for the same reason in spasmodic dysmenorrhoea. Uterine pain is analogous to myocardial pain in angina when blood flow in the coronary arteries supplying the cardiac muscle is restricted. Baseline tone in labour is about 10–12 mmHg (Blackburn 2003). An increase in intrauterine pressure of about 10–20 mmHg can be palpated abdominally and perceived by the women at 15–20 mmHg. Pain is often perceived when the pressure rises above 25 mmHg. Pressures may rise to 50 mmHg in the first stage and to 75–100 mmHg in the second stage. Weak contractions have a shorter duration with longer intervals between each contraction. The sensation of pain is related not just to the strength of contraction and the interval between each contraction but also to the well-being of the mother. An anxious or tired woman experiences pain at lower uterine pressure intensity (see below). Maternal position and use of analgesics may influence the strength and timing of contractions.

Contraction waves

The uterus is also analogous to the heart in another respect in that it appears to exhibit pacemaker activity, although specific pacemaker cells have not been localized. Specific areas that depolarize more rapidly have not been identified, although it was believed that they were each side of the fundus, near the uterotubal junctions or cornuae. All myometrial cells have spontaneous pacemaker activity. The contractions tend to originate from cells near the fundus and spread as a wave, as the electrical activity moves through the gap junctions of the muscle fibres (Fig. 13.10). The waves are strongest at the fundus, which has the highest density of muscle fibres, and take about 15–30 seconds to

travel down the length of the uterus (Blackburn 2003). There is a polarity of wave contraction with rhythmic coordination between the upper segment, which contracts for longer and retracts, and the lower segment, which contracts slightly later, to a less extent and dilates. This is described as fundal dominance; it is similar to the peristaltic waves generated by smooth muscle in other viscera. If the wave pattern is abnormal, for instance if the lower part contracts first or more strongly, the waves become erratic and uncoordinated and labour does not progress efficiently. This is described as 'incoordinate uterine activity'.

The uterus relaxes between contractions, which is important for oxygenation of the fetus and myometrium. The upper part of the uterus does not relax fully between contractions but retracts instead. This means that the muscle fibres do not return fully

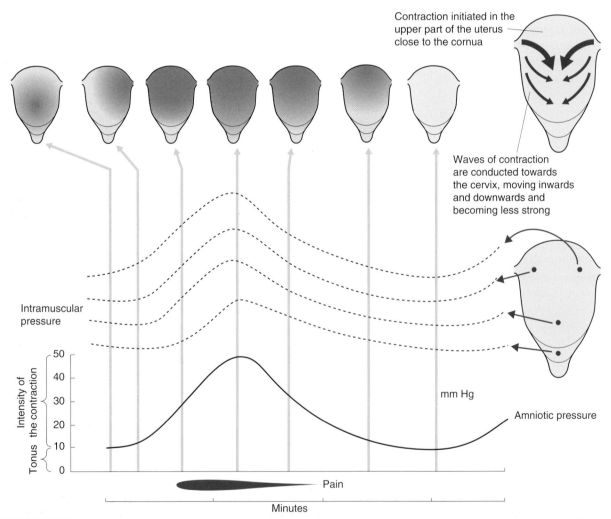

Fig. 13.10   *Contraction and retraction of uterine muscle cells. (Reproduced with permission from Sweet & Tiran 1996.)*

to the original length but progressively and gradually get a little bit shorter and thicker with each contraction (Fig. 13.11). This means that the less active lower segment is pulled up towards the shortening upper part of the uterus. (If the uterine muscle relaxed completely following each contraction, the uterus would remain the same size and labour would not progress.) The weakest points are the os and cervix which are effaced and dilated, enlarging the opening of the uterus.

Formation of hindwaters and forewaters

As the lower segment stretches and the cervix starts to efface and change its position, the chorion becomes detached from the uterine wall. The operculum tends to become dislodged from the receding cervical canal. The loss of this mucus closure, which may be blood-streaked, is described as 'the show' and indicates dilatation is progressing. The membranes are extruded through the opening cervix by the pressure of the amniotic fluid (Fig. 13.12). The head of the fetus tends to act as a ball-valve separating the amniotic fluid pushing through the cervix (forewaters) from the remainder of the fluid (hindwaters). The forewaters transmit the pressure generated from the waves of contraction, spreading the force evenly over the cervix, which aids its further effacement and dilatation. The hindwaters help to cushion the fetus from the contraction pressures. As the fundus presses on the upper aspect of the fetus (usually breech) during contractions, the pressure is transmitted through the fetal body to the lower segment and cervix (this is known as the fetal axis pressure). As uterine contractions progress, the pressure of the fluid in the forewaters rises and the membranes tend to rupture.

Membrane rupture

The fetal membranes rupture when the contractions cause the presenting part to distend them. There is a loss of lubricant between the chorion and amnion leading to increased shear force and cell rupture

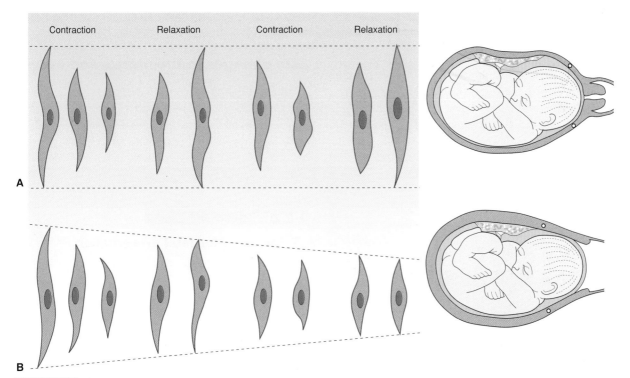

Fig. 13.11   *Uterine muscle contraction. Rather than the uterine myometrial cells relaxing fully (as in A), during labour the myometrial cells in the upper segment of the uterus retract getting progressively shorter (as in B). The lower uterine segment and the cervix dilate in response to the forces of contraction generated by the shortening upper segment thus the fetus is expelled.*

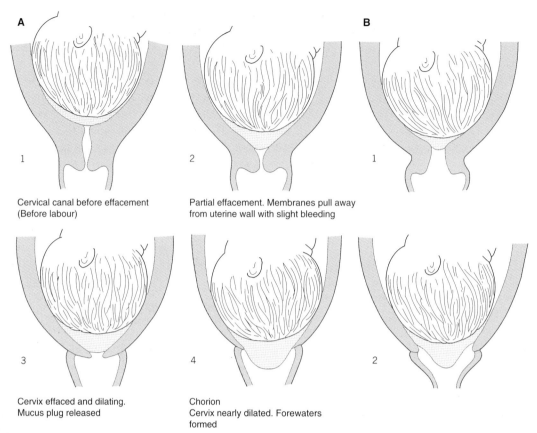

A

1 Cervical canal before effacement
(Before labour)

2 Partial effacement. Membranes pull away
from uterine wall with slight bleeding

3 Cervix effaced and dilating.
Mucus plug released

4 Chorion
Cervix nearly dilated. Forewaters
formed

B

1

2

Fig. 13.12 *Effacement and dilatation of the cervix. A. in a primigravidae; b. occuring simultaneously in a multigravidae. (Reproduced with permission from Sweet and Tiran 1996.)*

(Blackburn 2003). In 5–10% of pregnancies, premature rupture of the membranes (PROM) occurs spontaneously before the onset of uterine contractions as the earliest sign of labour (Duff 1996); about 60% of these are classified as term gestation. Spontaneous rupture of the membranes before 37 weeks' gestation often culminates in premature labour and delivery. Early rupture of the membranes as the first event in the course of labour is a cause for concern as it may indicate an ill-fitting presentation or high head at term in a primigravida, polyhydramnios or chorioamnionitis (a local infection which may be due to chlamydia or streptococcus).

Rupture of the amniotic membrane is associated with collagen degradation in the membrane (Hampson et al 1997). Usually coordinated contractions and dilatation of the cervix follow rupture of the membranes but if there is a delay the fetus is at risk from ascending infections so clinical intervention may be necessary if labour has not followed within 24 hours. There is controversy about artificial rupture of membranes and the effect it has on speeding up labour; it is thought that labour may progress more abruptly and painfully (Barrett et al 1992).

Size changes in the uterus and cervix

As the size of the upper segment of the uterus gradually diminishes because of the repeated cycles of contraction and retraction, the fetus is pushed into the lower segment so its presenting part (Box 13.2) exerts pressure on the obstructing maternal tissues. This results in increased oxytocin release from the posterior pituitary

Box 13.2

Terms used for fetal presentation

■ Attitude: relationship between fetal head and limbs and fetal trunk
■ Lie: relationship of fetus to long axis of uterus
■ Presentation: part of fetus presenting in lower aspect of uterus
■ Presenting part: part of presentation immediately inside internal os
■ Position: relationship of presentation, or presenting part, to maternal pelvis
■ Denominator: part of presenting part marking position

gland, which increases uterine activity by positive feedback mechanisms (see Ch. 1). Later in labour, when the baby has been born and the placenta has been expelled, retraction aids the uterine walls to come together so the cavity is obliterated as the uterine walls lie in apposition. A physiological retraction ring forms at the junction between the thick retracted segment of the upper segment and the thin distended wall of the lower segment. Under normal conditions, this ring is not visibly evident or palpable by abdominal examination. A pathological visible 'Bandl's ring' is the consequence of failure to recognize and manage obstructed labour appropriately and is a sign of imminent uterine rupture.

The rate of cervical dilatation is not constant; initially the cervix dilates slowly, but early changes are reinforced by positive feedback mechanisms and the rate accelerates. The latent phase of the first stage is slower and can take up to 12 hours (Box 13.3, Fig. 13.13). It is during this stage, when dilatation to 3–4 cm is achieved, that the cervix positively contracts in response to oxytocin (Olah et al 1993). This probably facilitates effacement. After a transition stage of about 15 minutes when the cervix does not contract, the cervix then dilates in response to myometrial contractions during the faster active phase.

Case study 13.1 is an example of the first stage of labour.

Table 13.2 details the possible types of intervention in labour.

The second stage of labour

By the end of the first stage of labour, the lower uterine segment, the cervix, the pelvic floor and the vulval outlet form one continuous dilated birth canal. The forces required to expel the fetus are both from the uterine muscle activity and from the secondary muscles of the abdomen and diaphragm, which augment the contractions of the uterus. The forces generated by the uterus can be described as the primary power and the complementary force from the voluntary movement of the respiratory muscles as the secondary power. By this stage, the uterus is markedly retracted and undergoing a pattern of strong, regular and repetitive contractions. The mother is compelled involuntarily to bear down or push. As she inspires before pushing, the diaphragm is lowered and the abdominal muscles contract, augmenting the contractile forces of the uterus. Bearing down by the mother helps to overcome the resistance of the soft tissues of the vagina and the pelvic floor. The fetal attitude (see Box 13.2) extends as it is directed through the birth canal, which aids the efficiency of the uterine contractions. The pain experienced in the second stage of labour is often less as cervical dilatation is complete and the woman is aware that progress is more rapid.

As the fetal head passes through the pelvis, the pressure on the sacral nerves may be associated with cramp in the legs and pain from the trauma to the tissue. The fetus distends the vagina and displaces the pelvic floor. The anterior part of the pelvic floor is drawn up causing the urethra to elongate and become compressed. The bladder is therefore repositioned within the protective environs of the abdomen. Posteriorly, the pelvic floor is stretched forward in relation to the presenting part and the rectum is compressed, which may lead to defecation. The perineum is flattened and lengthened by the fetus.

During a contraction, the presenting part (usually the fetal head) advances forward. In the interval between contractions, the presenting part recedes slightly but, as the uterine muscle retracts with each contraction, progression in the forward direction is maintained. This progression has been likened to taking two steps forward and one step back. When the widest part of the fetal head (the biparietal diameter) distends the vulva, the stretching is at its maximum, hence pain may be severe if not managed effectively with analgesia. This is described as 'crowning' of the head. The severity of the pain may cause a labouring woman to gasp and inhale sharply. The momentary break in the bearing-down movement has an important role in protecting the perineum from too much trauma, which can cause tearing of the tissue. The birth is usually accomplished with the next contraction following 'crowning'. A gush of amniotic fluid

---

Box 13.3

Progression of labour

The medical model of care in labour has defined an acceptable rate of progress in labour. Failure of labour to progress at this rate is described as abnormal and used as the rationale for medical intervention. Progress in labour is assessed through the use of a partogram. Cervical dilatation at the rate of 1 cm/h is accepted as normal. Progression of cervical dilatation can be graphically plotted and compared with predefined lines of progress referred to as Studd curves (Studd & Duiagnan 1972). Intervention is usually recommended if the rate of progress falls below 2 cm of the expected progress.

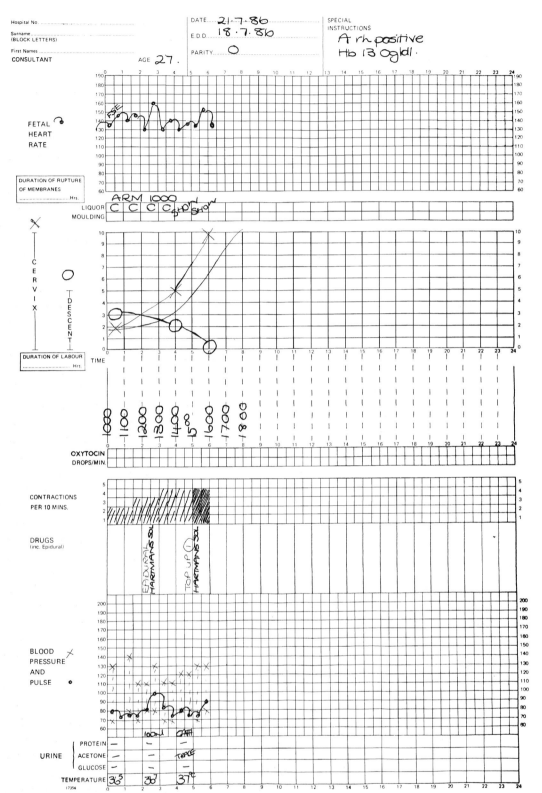

Fig. 13.13   *The partogram is a complete visual record of measurements made during labour and delivery. (Reproduced with permission from Symonds & Symonds 1997.)*

escapes. The fetus undergoes a pattern of passive corkscrew movements as it follows the shape and curvature of the pelvis (curvature of Carus). The gutter shape of the pelvic floor facilitates the rotation of the presenting part enabling the widest diameters of the pelvis to accommodate the largest dimensions of the fetal head and shoulders (Fig. 13.14).

Influences of pelvic and pelvic floor morphology and parturition

The passage of the fetus through the pelvis is described in practice as the mechanism of labour. Engagement describes the descent of the presenting part into the true pelvic cavity; the term relates to the widest transverse diameter of the fetal skull having negotiated the pelvic brim or inlet. If the baby has a cephalic (head-first) presentation, this is described in terms of number of fifths palpable (Fig. 13.15). Verification of the degree of engagement can be achieved through vaginal examination. With a cephalic presentation, the level of the biparietal prominences is judged in relation to the pelvic brim and the pelvic outlet at the level of the ischial spines. Engagement may occur long before the onset of labour, or may occur during, or even late on in, labour (more common in multiparous women). In a primigravida, engagement usually occurs at about 36 weeks' gestation in response to effacement of the cervix. Engagement does not indicate cavity and outlet measurements.

The third stage of labour

During the third stage, the placenta separates from the wall of the uterus and is expelled. Before separation, the placental extracellular matrix is thought to be weakened by proteases including matrix metalloproteinases (Salamonsen 2003). The uterus retracts markedly and bleeding from the placental wound site is constrained. Following the safe delivery of a healthy baby, the third stage of labour still presents a number of potential hazards. Should part of the placenta be retained, control of bleeding is impaired and a life-threatening postpartum haemorrhage could ensue. Immediately after delivery, the uterus markedly decreases in size. The pattern of contractions is interrupted for a minute or so, until contractions resume at a slow rate. As the uterus retracts, the placental site is greatly diminished. The placenta is not elastic, thus it tends to wrinkle and buckle and be sheared off the elastic uterine wall (like a paper label coming away from a deflating balloon). It is at this stage that some fetal blood from the placental circulation can enter the maternal circulation, potentially causing problems if there is Rhesus incompatibility (see Ch. 10). The marked retraction of the uterus impedes the venous drainage of the maternal intervillous spaces. Separation usually begins in the centre of the placenta and the extravasculated blood forms a haematoma or retroplacental clot between the placenta and decidua aiding its separation as the clot adds to the placental weight peeling the membranes from the uterine wall. As the uterus retracts, its progressively shortening muscle fibres tighten around the maternal vessels, forming 'living ligatures', which impede blood flow. This restricts the flow of maternal blood to the uterus and placental wound site, preventing excessive blood loss.

It is the commencement of spontaneous or stimulated uterine contractions following the completion of the second stage of labour that causes the placenta to separate from the uterine wall. The weight of the placenta completes the detachment of the membranes, which peel off and are expelled (Fig. 13.16). The site of placental implantation determines the speed of separation and the method of placental expulsion. The fetal membranes are expelled with the maternal or fetal surface prominent. The Schultze method of expulsion whereby the fetal side presents is most common and is

Fig. 13.14 *Rotation of the presenting part: A delivery of the head; B restitution; C external rotation. (Reproduced with permission from Bennett & Brown 1999.)*

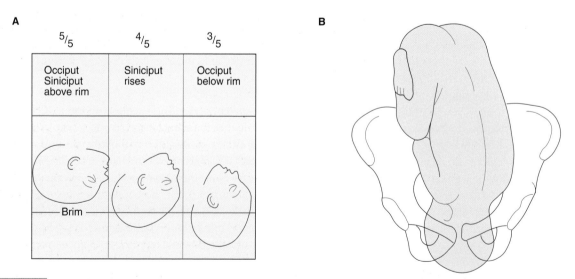

Fig. 13.15 *A Flexion and descent of the presenting part into the pelvic cavity; B engagement of the head. (A reproduced with permission from Bennett & Brown 1999; B reproduced with permission from Sweet & Tiran 1996.)*

A   B   C

D   E

Fig. 13.16 *The mechanism of placental separation and expulsion: A uterine wall partially retracted but not sufficiently to cause placental separation; B further contraction and retraction thicken uterine wall, reduce placental site and aid placental separation; C complete separation and formation of retroplacental clot (note: the thin lower segment has collapsed like a concertina following the birth of the baby); D Schultze method of expulsion; E Matthews-Duncan method of expulsion.*

associated with a fundal site implantation and the Matthews-Duncan expulsion (whereby the placenta slips out sideways like a button through a button-hole) is more likely with a lateral implantation. In some cultures, the placenta has important significance and women keep it for ritual ceremonies.

Active management

The third stage of labour can be physiologically managed, taking about 20–30 minutes to complete, but active management is widely practised by midwives, shortening the time of placental delivery to a few minutes. Active management involves the injection of an anti-tocolytic agent such as Syntometrine (see below) at the birth of the anterior shoulder or shortly after the delivery of the baby and delivering the placenta and membranes by controlled cord traction (CCT; also known as the Brandt–Andrews manoeuvre). The sheared-off placenta is extracted rather than expelled if active management of the third stage of labour is implemented. The use of CCT is subject to some discussion and is not practised in all countries.

The placenta should be separated and the uterus should be well contracted before CCT to ensure that it does not cause uterine inversion. The woman may be asked to bear down to assist expulsion of the placenta.

Syntometrine is a combination of oxytocin and ergometrine which is used to prevent postpartum haemorrhage. Oxytocin acts within 2–3 minutes following intramuscular injection, by causing intermittent contractions. These effectively continue the retraction process behind the placental site, thus encouraging separation and early expulsion. Ergometrine becomes effective about 5–7 minutes after administration. By this time, aided by CCT, the placenta has been expelled. The midwife applies cord traction by gripping the umbilical cord with one hand and applying a downward traction (Fig. 13.17). The other hand is placed on the lower abdomen, applying pressure to avoid inversion of the uterus. Ergometrine produces a sustained uterine contraction, which promotes the haemostatic action of the living ligatures. It is essential, therefore, to deliver the placenta before ergometrine stimulates closure of the cervix.

Physiological management of the third stage of labour involves no routine use of anti-tocolytic drugs, not clamping the umbilical cord until pulsations cease, no uterine manipulation or controlled cord traction, and delivery of the placenta and membranes solely by maternal effort within 1 hour of birth.

Fig. 13.17 *Controlled cord traction (Brandt–Andrews method). (Reproduced with permission from Bennett & Brown 1999.)*

The effects of labour on maternal physiology

Cardiovascular system

The stress of labour prepares the woman for the inevitable blood loss at delivery and limitation of bleeding after placental separation. Dehydration and muscle activity increase the haemoglobin concentration. Erythropoiesis and white blood cell number also increase as part of the normal response to stress. Concentrations of clotting factors increase, clotting times shorten and fibrinolytic activity is decreased on completion of the third stage of labour. The placenta and decidua are very rich sources of thromboplastin which can activate coagulation (see Ch. 1). About 5–10% of the total body fibrin is deposited as a haemostatic endometrial mesh over the placental wound site (Blackburn 2003). This hypercoagulable state is further developed in the puerperium (see Ch. 14).

The cardiovascular system is affected by pain, anxiety, apprehension, position and anaesthesia, as well as by the muscular activity of the uterus itself and the dramatic increase in catecholamine production during labour. Uterine contractions progressively increase cardiac output as venous return and circulating volume are increased. Each contraction can contribute 300–500 ml of blood to the circulation (Sullivan & Ramanathan 1985), which significantly increases cardiac output and blood pressure. In the supine position, stroke volume and cardiac output tend to be lower and heart rate raised.

Catecholamines affect vascular tone and increase blood pressure; this effect is reduced with anaesthetics. Pain and anxiety result in tachycardia (increased heart rate) and affect blood pressure. During a contraction, systolic blood pressure increases by at least 35 mmHg and diastolic blood pressure may increase between 25 and 65 mmHg (Blackburn 2003). The increment in blood pressure precedes each contraction and falls to baseline between contractions. The greatest haemodynamic changes occur in women delivering their baby vaginally, which is an important consideration for women who have cardiac disease.

The respiratory system

Labour affects the respiratory system as the muscular work increases metabolic rate and oxygen consumption. Respiratory rate and depth of respiration increase. Anxiety, drugs and use of a gas mask mouthpiece can all affect respiratory rate. There is a tendency for a labouring woman to hyperventilate. Hyperventilation is a natural response to pain. Contractions occurring at high frequency can affect oxygenation causing muscular hypoxia and acidosis. Hypoxia can increase the amount of pain experienced.

The increased ventilation causes a progressive and marked decrease in partial pressure of carbon dioxide (to about 25 mmHg) particularly if the contractions are painful. In early labour, hyperventilation can cause respiratory alkalosis and increased blood pH. This can result in the woman experiencing dizziness and tingling of her fingers and toes, and possibly developing muscle spasms. At extremely low P_aCO_2, blood flow can be affected and the oxygen–haemoglobin dissociation curve (see Ch. 1) shifts to the left so release of oxygen is impaired. The remedy of breath counting to slow respiratory rate, especially if the woman counts them with her partner or a midwife who deliberately slows down counting, can prevent or correct hyperventilatory effects.

By the end of the first stage, maternal acidosis due to isometric muscle contractions is likely and is compensated for, to a degree, by the respiratory alkalosis. The muscle contractions reduce blood flow to the uterine muscle, which becomes hypoxic and undergoes anaerobic metabolism. Flow to the intervillous space also decreases so fetal levels of carbon dioxide increase and the fetus tends to become acidotic. During bearing down, when the mother's accessory respiratory muscles are involved, mild respiratory acidosis is likely. In the second stage of labour lactate levels increase, thus pH falls. This metabolic acidosis is not compensated for.

The renin–angiotensin system

Labour and delivery affect the renin–angiotensin system of both fetus and mother. Levels of renin and angiotensinogen increase, which is important in maintaining blood flow, but can also affect handling and excretion of drugs. Glomerular filtration rate, renal blood flow and sodium excretion are also affected by raised catecholamine levels or general anaesthetic. Oxytocin has structural similarities with ADH and has inherent antidiuretic properties, therefore fluid retention is increased in labour. Women in labour can be at risk of iatrogenic water intoxication due to loss of electrolytes, use of oxytocin, or intravenous fluid administration.

Metabolic rate

Maternal glucose consumption markedly increases in labour to provide energy required by the uterus and skeletal muscles. Glucose and triacylglycerides are used as energy sources. Oxytocin has some insulin-like properties. An increased body temperature during labour may indicate dehydration or infection. It is common for women to experience a transient postpartum chill about 15 minutes after the birth of the baby or delivery of the placenta. In the following 24 hours, postpartum women frequently have a slightly raised temperature secondary to dehydration.

Nutrition in labour

Food and drink consumption in labour is controversial. There are two conflicting arguments. The first is that a woman in labour might possibly require a general anaesthetic and therefore should be treated as a preoperative patient at risk of gastric aspiration (Parsons 2003). Pulmonary aspiration of gastric acid (Mendelson's syndrome) or particulate food matter, although rare, is a major cause of morbidity and mortality for women in labour. The risks of gastric aspiration are thought to be greatly reduced if oral intake is limited (Rowe 1997). Pregnant women have a slower gastric emptying rate (see Ch. 11), which is further delayed by labour (Carp et al 1992), and decreased tone of the lower oesophageal sphincter but it is not known whether this delayed gastric emptying predisposes to gastric aspiration.

The opposing view is that a more liberal policy is more beneficial and that women are being needlessly deprived of food (Baker 1996, Ludka & Roberts 1993, Sharp 1997, Parsons 2004). It is argued that general anaesthesia is relatively rare now and that techniques have improved, which make aspiration of gastric contents unlikely. It is argued that prolonged fasting could have detrimental psychological and physiological effects, including increased anxiety and stress.

Pregnant women are predisposed to ketosis, particularly in labour. Pregnancy is a ketotic state and fasting in pregnancy is invariably associated with ketonuria (Scheepers et al 2001). It is estimated that a woman in labour has an energy requirement of 700–1100 kcal/h. When glycogen stores are exhausted, adipose tissue is mobilized. Fatty acid oxidation increases ketosis, an excess of ketone bodies in the plasma, which are excreted into the urine. Lipolysis provides fatty acid substrates for maternal energy needs and spares glucose for the fetus. The critical question is whether ketosis is detrimental to the progress of labour. Ketones can increase acidity, cause excessive renal excretion of sodium and cross the placenta to the fetus. Although the length of labour is correlated with the degree of ketosis, it is not clear whether longer labour results in increased ketosis or whether ketosis prolongs labour.

It is suggested that fasting in labour can increase the need for medical intervention. Allowing women to eat in labour reduces the plasma level of ketones, which may aid the progress of labour (Scutton et al 1996). Ketonuria can be treated by administration of intravenous dextrose but this is associated with fluid and electrolyte imbalance. A number of women experience nausea and vomiting in labour. But, in practice, more maternity units are cautiously adopting a liberal policy offering a non-particulate diet while using antacids and H_2-antagonists to reduce gastric pH and decrease volume of gastric contents, thus minimizing the risk of aspiration and lung damage.

The effects of labour on the fetus

Labour has profound effects on the fetus and is important in aiding the adaptation to extrauterine life (see Ch. 15). Understanding the effects of labour on the fetus is important in differentiating between normal healthy responses and diagnosing fetal distress.

Behaviour of the fetus during pregnancy

The use of ultrasound led to the observation that, after 36 weeks, the fetus exhibits a number of clearly definable behavioural states, which are analogous to the neonatal states (see Ch. 15). These states have characteristic patterns of fetal heart rate (FHR), fetal breathing movements (FBM), eye movements, voiding and mouthing movements (Table 13.3). The patterns of fetal behaviour change with gestational age and are assumed to reflect the activity of the fetal central nervous system and can potentially be used to recognize a compromised fetus (Nijhuis 2003). The movements evidently demonstrate fetal ability to respond to external stimuli. Many factors such as time of day, meals,

Table 13.3 *Fetal behavioural states*

State 1F (1 fetal); quiet sleep	Fetal quiescence with brief gross startles; high-voltage electrocortical activity; no eye movement; FHR accelerations; minimal heart rate variability; isolated fetal heart rate
State 2F (2 fetal); active sleep	Paradoxical/irregular sleep; frequent and periodic stretches; retroflexion and movements of extremities; low-voltage electrocortical activity; continuous eye movements; increased FHR variability with frequent accelerations
State 3F (3 fetal); quiet awake	Absence of gross movements; continuous rapid eye movements; stable, but widely oscillating FHR, no accelerations
State 4F (4 fetal); active awake	Vigorous and continual movements; rapid eye movement; unstable heart rate—large, long accelerations and tachycardia

smoking, etc. affect fetal behaviour. Most of the movements that are discernible in the third trimester can be tracked back to the first trimester. Both the movements and the periods of quiescence between them are important.

FBM can be detected from the end of the first trimester (Nijhuis 2003). FBM are more regular in state 1F than in state 2F, they occur more frequently in state 2F and are present but irregular in states 3F and 4F. It has been suggested that FBM are more likely to be state-dependent when maternal glucose levels are lower (Mulder et al 1994). There is a postprandial increase in FBM and smoking diminishes them. Fetal voiding movements are inhibited in state 1F but occur at the transition to state 2F. Sucking and swallowing can be seen from the end of the first trimester. Regular or rhythmic mouthing movements are most often observed in state 1F, when they occur in bursts of 10–20 minutes, whereas powerful sucking movements can be seen in state 3F. Both regular mouthing and sucking can entrain fetal heart rate patterns which can bewilder clinical interpretation.

States 1F and 2F account for about 90% of fetal life in late gestation. FHR patterns during these four behavioural states may mimic fetal distress. The fetal behavioural states and the transitions between them can be observed throughout labour. States 1F and 2F predominate as they do before labour. It is thought that diminished FHR variability and absent accelerations in a healthy term fetus probably represent fetal sleep rather than fetal distress. In the deep sleep state 1F, FHR pattern is usually unaffected even by strong uterine contractions. A period of low fetal heart variability (FHV) or tachycardia may indicate that fetal oxygenation is being compromised. In the second stage of labour, the length of the behavioural cycles decreases; this is related to the gamut of sensory stimuli and head compression incurred during this stage of labour.

FBM increase in frequency and in length of episode as gestation progresses. By the third trimester, FBM occur for 30% of the time and are closely associated with behavioural state, especially active sleep (2F). A few days before the onset of labour, FBM are depressed, probably because increased levels of prostaglandin, especially PGE_2, inhibit the fetal respiratory centre. During the latent stage of labour, FBM occur for about 10% of the time but almost cease in the active stage. In preterm labour, the decrease in FBM is less acute. FBM may be affected by changes in oxygenation and pH. FBM require energy so the fetus decreases FBM in response to hypoxia as an adaptive response to conserve oxygen. The hypoxia-induced decrease in FBM is more marked near term possibly because the responses to hypoxia have become more sensitive as the respiratory centre becomes more mature.

Although hypoxia normally decreases FBM, deeper, sustained inspiration or gasping is stimulated synergistically by raised carbon dioxide levels in the presence of hypoxia. In perinatal aspiration, this gasping can cause meconium inspiration. Paradoxically, maternal hyperventilation decreases FBM. Hypoglycaemia and central nervous system depressants, such as ethanol, barbiturates and diazepam, decrease FBM. Theophylline increases FBM and is used to treat postnatal apnoea in premature infants. Prostaglandin inhibitors, such as indomethacin, stimulate FBM but have to be used with caution because of their effects on fetal vascular function.

Changes in fetal behaviour over the course of pregnancy are summarized in Box 13.4.

Changes during labour

The stress of labour causes a reflex increase in maternal catecholamine levels well above those seen in non-pregnant women or pregnant women before labour.

Box 13.4

Changes in fetal behaviour during pregnancy

First trimester
- Specific sequence of movements
- Continual activity
- Coordinated and graceful quality

Second trimester
- Body movements diminish
- Breathing movements increase
- Quiescence increases
- Rest–activity cycles develop

Third trimester
- Clear fetal behavioural states
- Specific combination of variables
- Stable with state transitions
- Breathing is state-dependent

The physiological stress and hypoxia associated with the pain and anxiety increase adrenaline secretion. The physiological work of labour, which is highest in the second stage of labour, increases noradrenaline release. Placental metabolism of maternal catecholamines reduces the transfer to the fetus. However, maternal catecholamines can affect placental blood flow and affect the fetus in labour. Animal studies show that adrenaline is associated with vasoconstriction and a reduction in uterine blood flow. As the rise in adrenaline level is associated with maternal stress in labour, there is a clear advantage to limiting maternal psychological distress and pain.

Normal labour and delivery are associated with increased physiological stress resulting in raised cord levels of catecholamines in the neonate (Gluckman et al 1999). This increase in fetal catecholamines may be a response to fetal compression, mild acidosis and other stimuli experienced during the birth. It is suggested that this is an adaptive response that facilitates extrauterine adaptation. The increased catecholamines stimulate breathing, increase fluid absorption from the lungs, stimulate surfactant release, enhance irritability, and play a role in metabolism by mobilizing glucose and fatty acids (Gluckman et al 1999).

Fetal tissues are metabolically active; heat dissipation is via the placenta to the mother. Cord exclusion in animals results in an increase in fetal temperature. It seems likely that uterine contractions affecting uterine blood flow will impair heat transfer, particularly in active labour. At delivery, there is a transition from a heat-producing fetus to a neonate dependent on heat generation. In utero, PGE_2 and adenosine derived from the placenta may have a role in suppressing the activity of brown adipose tissue and therefore minimizing heat production by the fetus. Occlusion of the umbilical cord is the signal to increase heat generation. Non-shivering thermogenesis by brown adipose tissue is under the control of noradrenaline (see Ch. 1) released during labour.

A healthy term fetus has good energy stores and a normal base excess so it can tolerate temporary reductions in uterine perfusion in labour. There is a marked increase in fetal glycogen storage in the last month of gestation. The fetus also has the enzymes required for glycogenolysis. However, under normal uterine conditions, placental transfer of maternal glucose means that the fetal glucose pool is of maternal origin. Until labour, the fetus still depends on maternal sources of glucose. The changes in catecholamine secretion boost neonatal metabolism.

The placenta also provides the route of oxygen transfer and carbon dioxide removal. Maternal hyperventilation in labour increases carbon dioxide diffusion across the placenta, therefore increasing respiratory alkalosis (increasing pH). However, respiratory depression caused by oversedation or magnesium sulphate could have the opposite effect. In the presence of a reduced oxygen supply, anaerobic metabolism will cause metabolic acidosis. Lactate diffusion across the placenta is slow and the fetal kidney is not efficient at clearing organic acids. It seems likely that the respiratory alkalosis related to maternal hyperventilation compensates for at least some of the metabolic acidosis, owing to anaerobic glycolysis, thus restoring fetal pH to a normal range. Normal labour nevertheless will cause a gradual decrease in fetal pH, oxygen and bicarbonate ions and a corresponding rise in partial pressure of carbon dioxide.

Uterine blood flow is largely determined by maternal blood pressure, cardiac output and uterine muscular tone. Labour compromises uterine blood flow. The maternal spiral arteries, which perfuse the intervillous spaces, are occluded and venous drainage of the spaces is obstructed during uterine contractions. Doppler measurements show that blood flow through the uterine arteries is gradually reduced during a contraction and gradually returns when the uterus relaxes. Most animal models demonstrate that the placenta has an anatomical redundancy; over 70% of the placental capillary bed must be occluded before impedance to gas exchange rises significantly. If placental reserve is reduced, uterine contractions may have a significant effect on fetal hypoxia and acidosis. Even with a healthy placenta and normal uterine blood flow, contractions with excessive strength of frequency can cause fetal hypoxia and bradycardia. Maternal conditions may exacerbate this by reducing uterine perfusion; supine posture can reduce venous return, therefore cardiac output and regional anaesthesia can cause vasodilation so decreasing maternal cardiac output.

Labour promotes the clearance of fetal lung fluid. Transient tachypnoea, caused by residual lung fluid, is more common in babies born by elective caesarean section than in those experiencing a vaginal delivery. Chest compression mechanically expels a small volume of fluid. Late in gestation, the pulmonary epithelial cells actively secrete chloride ions, which creates a gradient maintaining adequate lung volume in utero. Before birth the lung epithelial cells change from being predominantly chloride-secreting to being sodium-absorbing, which draws fluid into the interstitial spaces. The sodium-pumping activity is increased in spontaneous labour; this may be related to the catecholamine surge.

A mature sucking pattern is evident from 36 weeks of gestation. Although fetal swallowing can be observed as early as 11 weeks' gestation, near-term discrete episodes of swallowing occur, probably triggered by 'thirst', gastric emptying or changed composition of amniotic fluid (Boyle 1992). This swallowing may be important for gut development and maturation. In labour there is some evidence that swallowing increases. Meconium passage is rare until about 38 weeks when the control of intestinal peristalsis is more mature. Early meconium passage is associated with listeriosis. Meconium-stained amniotic fluid occurs in about a third of pregnancies beyond 42 weeks. Hypoxia induces vasoconstriction of the fetal gut, hyperperistalsis and anal sphincter relaxation, so passage of meconium has been associated with fetal distress (Houlihan & Knuppel 1994). However, it has been argued that meconium-stained fluid could reflect normal maturity of the fetal gut function (Katz & Bowes 1992). Less than 2% of babies born with meconium-stained fluid go on to develop severe meconium aspiration syndrome. It has been suggested that the primary cause of this syndrome is pulmonary epithelial damage or airway obstruction, which results in ineffectual clearance of meconium. The residual meconium can interfere with surfactant dispersal and increase the severity of the respiratory problems.

The fetal skull and fetal presentation

The dimensions of the fetal head correlate well with those of the maternal pelvis. Examination of the shape of the baby's head soon after delivery shows how it passed through the pelvis (Fig. 13.18). The bones of the fetal skull are relatively mobile and mould under compression during labour. The sutures and fontanelles (Fig. 13.19) allow the skull bones to overlap partially so the dimensions of the presenting part can be reduced by about 0.5–1 cm. Diameters that are not compressed elongate to compensate for those that are reduced. If the pressure generated against the cervix impedes the circulation in the scalp then oedema may occur forming a caput or swelling. The area of the caput and the degree of moulding indicate the degree of head compression endured in labour. The caput is usually absorbed within a few days of delivery and requires no treatment. If the head is compressed in an abnormal diameter, or if the moulding is too excessive or rapid, the dura mater forming the falx cerebri may be pulled from the tentorium cerebellum resulting in rupture of the venous sinuses and intercranial haemorrhage (Fig. 13.20).

The position of the fetus (see Box 13.2, p. 334, for an explanation of terms) is determined on abdominal examination in later pregnancy and early labour (Fig. 13.21). The midwife can gently palpate the pregnant woman's abdomen to determine how the fetus is lying and how the presenting part of the fetus relates to the pelvis. The degree of engagement of the fetal head into the brim of the pelvis can also be ascertained. Auscultation of the fetal heart confirms the initial findings. The lie of the fetus describes the relative position of the long axis of the fetus to the long axis of the uterus. Usually the lie is longitudinal, rather than oblique or transverse, particularly in the last weeks of pregnancy. The attitude is the degree of flexion of the fetus. In the fully flexed attitude, the fit of the fetus in the uterus is comfortable. The presentation describes the presenting part of the fetus. Cephalic presentation occurs in most pregnancies. The fetal position is described by the relationship of the denominator (the presenting part) to areas of the maternal pelvis. The pelvic areas are: left and right, anterior, lateral or posterior areas. The occiput (the bone at the back of the fetal skull) is the denominator of a cephalic position so the fetus could, for instance, be described to be in a right occipito-anterior position. Anterior positions are more common because the fetal spine is against the mother's abdominal wall. Occipito-posterior positions tend to result in the fetus assuming a deflexed attitude, which can result in less-effective contraction, prolonged labour, uneven cervical dilatation, increased risk of trauma to the perineum and unfavourable compression of the fetal head.

Pain in labour

Many women experience severe pain in labour. Pain is a complex and personal phenomenon. Although it is easier to understand the neurophysiological aspects of tissue damage, the experience of pain is always subjective and is related to psychological state and past experience. Pain can be defined as a sensation (sensory and emotional experience) usually evoked by tissue damage or inflammation that stimulates the activity of specific receptors transmitting information to pain centres in the brain. Although pain can often be considered to be part of a protective mechanism (a rapid warning system) against tissue damage, there are some exceptions. For instance, pain associated with radiation (as in sunburn) or tumour growth tends to occur well after the tissue damage has occurred so it does not function as a warning. Chronic pain associated with degenerative diseases, such as arthritis, also cannot be regarded as a protective reflex. In labour, some aspects of pain experienced can be protective, such as the pain due to stretching of the soft tissue as the baby's head is crowned, which causes the woman to gasp.

The perception of pain depends on a number of physiological factors. The location and intensity of the stimuli affect the quality and severity of the perceived pain; generally, the higher the intensity of the stimuli, the greater is the pain experienced. However, psychological and cultural factors are important in the perception of pain (Box 13.5). Mood and personality type are important; generally, anxious or tired people are less able to tolerate pain but emotional arousal limits pain perception. In certain primitive cultures, the father has the 'labour pains' and the mother quietly gives birth.

Pain receptors

Pain or nociceptive receptors respond to stimuli that cause tissue damage. They are specific, responding

Suboccipitobregmatic 9.5 cm
vertex presentation

Occipito-anterior position

Occipitofrontal 11.5 cm persistent
occipitoposterior position

Persistent occipito-posterior position

Submentobregmatic 9.5 cm
face presentation

Face presentation

Mentovertical 13.5 cm
brow presentation

Brow presentation

Fig. 13.18   *The relationship between the shape of the baby's head and the moulding of the fetal skull.*

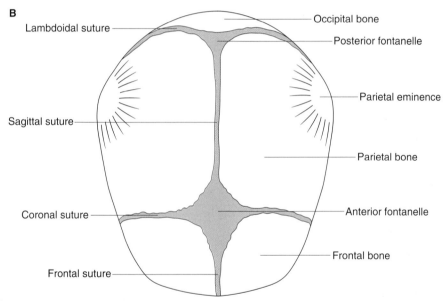

Fig. 13.19 *Sutures and fontanelles of the fetal skull.*

to chemical mediators of tissue damage, such as plasmakinins, acetylcholine, histamine and substance P. Pain receptors are distributed unevenly with a higher density in skin, dental pulp, some internal organs, periosteum, meninges, arterial walls and joint surfaces. Pain receptors are free nerve endings that form part of small afferent myelinated Aδ fibres and larger (but unmyelinated) C fibres (Table 13.4). There is controversy over the pain being caused by overstimulation of other receptor types such as those that respond to temperature and pressure (Box 13.6).

Pain transmission

Transmission of pain depends on the type of fibre in which the nerve ending triggers the impulse. In general the speed of transmission is faster in larger fibres and those that are myelinated (see Ch. 1). Sharp stabbing sensations are thought to be conducted by Aδ fibres and dull aching or burning pain by the slower unmyelinated C fibres. Myelinated fibres are more sensitive to ischaemia. Small unmyelinated fibres are more susceptible to local anaesthetics such as procaine, which is effective at blocking aching pain.

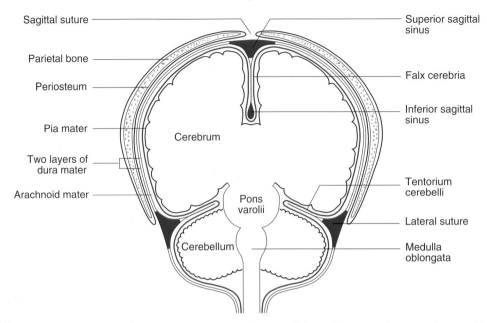

Fig. 13.20 *Coronal section through the fetal head to show intracranial membranes and venous sinuses. (Reproduced with permission from Bennett & Brown 1999.)*

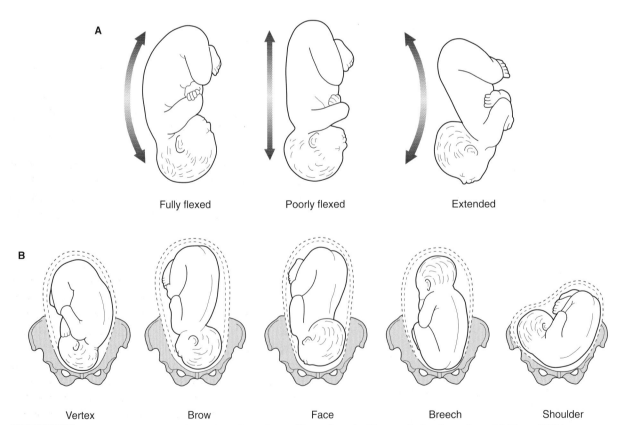

Fig. 13.21   *A Attitude and B presentation of the fetus. (Reproduced with permission from Sweet & Tiran 1996.)*

Factors affecting pain perception

- Anatomy
- Physiology
- Psychology
- Sociology
- Culture
- Cognition
- Learning

Pain receptors

Large

- Aα (Ia and Ib) (myelinated): position proprioception, touch, pressure, vibration
- Aβ (II) (myelinated): fine discriminative touch, pressure, vibration
- Aγ (myelinated): burning sensation

Small

- Aδ (III) (myelinated): well-localizable sharp pain, temperature
- C (IV) (unmyelinated): dull aching pain, temperature

The nerve fibres enter the spinal cord and terminate in the grey matter of the dorsal horn (Fig. 13.22). Aδ fibres have a relatively direct route of transmission, synapsing with neurons in the dorsal horn to the brain stem and via the spinothalamic tract to the thalamus and cerebral cortex. Therefore the pain is perceived as sharp and is easy to localize. The unmyelinated C fibres synapse in the grey matter of the spinal cord as well but are routed through the spinoreticular tract and reticular formation to the thalamus and cortex. Within the reticular formation, a number of physiological processes take place, stimulating the nervous system and affecting electrical activity in the brain, wakefulness and attention. The state of excitement that is generated means the pain is difficult to localize and produces unpleasant symptoms. The limbic system (which includes the hypothalamus and the amygdala) at the base of the brain is stimulated, which affects emotional responses such as fear, anger, pleas-

ure and satisfaction. The thalamus integrates the sensation of pain and relays the information that tissue damage has occurred. The somatosensory cortex discriminates and identifies the precise position of the tissue damage and the parietal cortex is involved in interpreting the information and relating the learned meaningfulness to past experience. The main excitatory neurotransmitter in pain perception is glutamate.

The gate control theory

There is a relationship between the pain receptors and the touch receptors at the level of the spinal cord. The pain gate control theory, proposed by Melzack & Wall in 1965, suggests that interneurons in the substantia gelatinosa of the dorsal horn of the spinal cord can regulate the conduction of the ascending afferent nerve (Fig. 13.23). So input from the large-diameter myelinated fibres from the touch receptors can inhibit the impulses on the smaller-diameter fibres from the pain receptors, acting as a gate. This means that touch, like massage, can inhibit transmission from the pain receptor unless activity along the smaller fibres markedly increases. Descending fibres from the brain can also modify transmission of pain signals, thus 'opening' or 'closing' the gate. This explains the relationship between psychological factors and pain perception. If a labouring woman is feeling relaxed and confident, the descending inhibition is high so less pain is perceived. If she becomes tired or anxious, the descending inhibition is reduced. Transcutaneous electrical nerve stimulation (TENS) acts both to stimulate the large-diameter touch afferent nerves and possibly to stimulate powerful descending inhibitory pathways.

Table 13.4 *Fast and slow pain receptors*

Fast pain	Slow pain
Bright, sharp, localized sensation	Dull, intense, diffuse unpleasant feeling
Aδ	C fibres
2–5 μm diameter	0.4–1.2 μm diameter
Myelinated	Non-myelinated
Conduct at 12–30 m/s	Conduct at 0.5–2 m/s
Terminate on neurons in laminars I and V	Terminate on neurons in laminars I and II
Spinothalamic tract	Spinorecticular tract
Somatic pain	Visceral pain

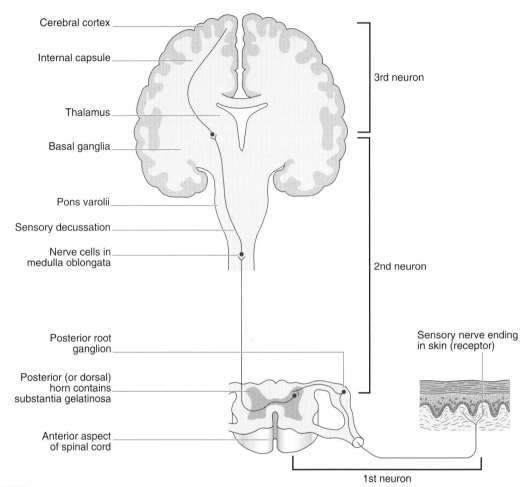

Cerebral cortex

Internal capsule

3rd neuron

Thalamus

Basal ganglia

Pons varolii

Sensory decussation

Nerve cells in
medulla oblongata

2nd neuron

Posterior root
ganglion

Sensory nerve ending
in skin (receptor)

Posterior (or dorsal)
horn contains
substantia gelatinosa

Anterior aspect
of spinal cord

1st neuron

Fig. 13.22 *Pathways of pain transmission. (Reproduced with permission from Bennett & Brown 1999.)*

Pain from muscle contractions

Both visceral pain from the uterus and somatic pain from trauma to the soft tissues of the birth canal are experienced in labour. Visceral pain tends to predominate in the first stage of labour when the uterus is contracting and the cervix is stretching and dilating. Rhythmic muscle contraction in the presence of an adequate blood flow does not usually cause pain. In labour, uterine contractions compress blood vessels and reduce flow; the ischaemic pain persists until the flow is restored. It is hypothesized that a chemical mediator reaches critical levels when flow is limited and stimulates the pain receptors. When flow is restored, the chemical mediator is diluted or metabolized. This is similar to exertion causing myocardial ischaemia and angina pain, which is relieved by rest and decreased myocardial oxygen requirements. Initially, pain is transmitted by the afferent fibres entering the spinal cord at T11 and T12, spreading to T10 and L1.

Referred pain

In referred pain, damage from one part of the body is experienced as though it had occurred in another part of the body. The pain fibres from the damaged area enter the spinal cord at the same level as the afferent nerves from the referred area. Usually the pain is referred to another tissue or structure that developed from the same embryonic structure or dermatome in which the pain originates. So, for instance, development of the diaphragm begins in the neck but, as the lungs develop, the diaphragm and the phrenic nerve migrate towards the abdomen. The afferent fibres in the phrenic nerve enter the spinal cord with the afferent fibres from the tip of the shoulder. Irritation of the diaphragm is therefore referred as a pain in the shoulder. However, previous experience is important in referred pain. Pain from the abdominal viscera including the uterus is usually referred to the midline. But in patients who have experienced abdominal surgery,

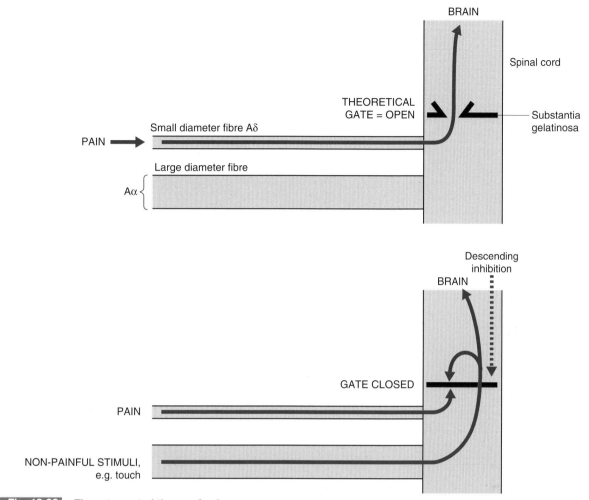

BRAIN

Spinal cord

THEORETICAL
GATE = OPEN

Small diameter fibre Aδ

Substantia
gelatinosa

PAIN

Large diameter fibre

Aα

Descending
inhibition

BRAIN

GATE CLOSED

PAIN

NON-PAINFUL STIMULI,
e.g. touch

Fig. 13.23 *The gate control theory of pain.*

such as a caesarean section, the pain is referred to the scar site. Pain during this stage arising from the uterus and cervix may be referred. A labouring woman may experience pain over her abdominal wall, between the naval and pubic bone, radiating down her thighs and in the lumbar and sacral regions.

Somatic pain

Somatic pain caused by the presenting part impinging on the birth canal, vulva and perineum tends to occur in the transition and in second stage of labour. Pain is transmitted by the pudendal nerves S2, S3 and S4. The conscious sensation of pain is accompanied by a number of physiological responses including increased ventilation and cardiac output, inhibition of gastrointestinal function, increased oxygen demand and

metabolic rate and increased catecholamine release. The increased catecholamine release may detrimentally affect placental perfusion and uterine contractions. Non-pharmacological methods of pain relief, such as imagery, relaxation techniques and provision of information about the progress of labour, probably decrease anxiety and stress and responses mediated by the sympathetic nervous system.

Endogenous opiates

The endogenous opiates are of particular interest in pain perceived in labour. These include β-endorphin, enkephalins and dynorphin, which are analgesic peptides. They bind to the presynaptic receptors on the neuron membrane and block pain transmission. Enkephalins comprise two short peptide chains (consisting of five amino acids) that are very unstable and have a half-life of less than a minute. Enkephalins are fragments of β-endorphin, which is more stable and also binds to opiate receptors; β-endorphin is a fragment of the pituitary hormone β-lipotrophin. β-Lipotrophin and ACTH are both derived from the same precursor.

Endogenous opiates inhibit prostaglandin synthesis. Prostaglandins are possible chemical mediators of pain. They also inhibit actions of a number of other pain transmitters. β-Endorphin levels increase throughout pregnancy, peaking at delivery, and may be further stimulated by the stress of labour. It is suggested that it is this high level of endogenous opiates that allows women to tolerate surprisingly high levels of pain during delivery; this phenomenon is known as 'pregnancy-induced analgesia'. Acupuncture may increase enkephalin activity. Placebo responses where pain relief occurs as a result of expectation of pain relief rather than because of being given an analgesic may be due to release of endogenous opiates and genuine analgesia.

Pain relief

Pain relief in labour needs to work rapidly and effectively relieve the pain without slowing down the course of labour. It needs to be safe for the mother and fetus and not adversely affect the neonate. There is no ideal analgesic (Table 13.5); all have some side-effects but pain also can adversely affect the fetus. Maternal analgesia can alter the balance of factors promoting uterine contraction and can potentially result in increased effects of oxytocin, promoting tetanic uterine contractions, decreasing oxygen delivery and causing transient fetal bradycardia (Eberle & Norris 1996). There are three main mechanisms of pain relief blocking the pain receptors, the propagation of the action potential or the perception of pain within the central nervous system (CNS). Mild analgesics block at the pain receptor level. The sensitivity of the pain receptors is increased by prostaglandins. Drugs which inhibit prostaglandin synthesis, such as aspirin, decrease levels of prostaglandins both at the receptor and where prostaglandins are involved in pain transmission higher in the pathway.

Local anaesthetics

Local anaesthetics prevent the propagation of action potentials by blocking the sodium channels. They are particularly effective in blocking pain carried by the C fibres, possibly because unmyelinated fibres allow easier penetration. For instance, lignocaine (lidocaine) injected into the perineum is effective at blocking the pain of episiotomy.

Centrally acting opiates

Centrally acting opiates or narcotics, such as morphine and pethidine, block nerve transmission in the brain and spinal cord and decrease pain perception. There are also opiate-binding sites in the substantia gelatinosa of the dorsal horn of the spinal cord, which affect the release of neurotransmitters. Opiates increase the activity of the descending inhibitory pathways from the brain stem and act on the limbic system to elevate mood. Opiates have other physiological effects such as depressing the medullary respiratory centre, causing nausea and vomiting, sedating and affecting the heart rate.

Position in labour

Certain positions have advantages in optimizing uterine efficiency or increasing maternal comfort

---

Table 13.5 *Types of analgesics*

Pain relief	Example	Mechanism	Disadvantages/advantages
Opioids	Pethidine	Depression of CNS	Nausea, vomiting, sedation; potentiate effect of epidural
Paracervical block	Spinal	Action potentials blocked from nerves	Risk of fetal injection; could provide surgical anaesthesia
Epidural	Bolus, intermittent or continuous infusion	Inhibition of neurotransmission across synapses	Maternal hypotension, motor blockade

(Blackburn 2003). The lithotomy position and lying supine are probably advantageous only to those assisting at the delivery, unless medical intervention/delivery is required. Fetal monitoring and a number of procedures can usually be adapted to a variety of maternal positions. There seems to be no physiological advantage in lying supine. Fetal alignment, pelvic diameter and efficiency of contractions are not optimal. Contractions are more frequent but less intense so labour is prolonged and drug use seems to be increased. Many women appear to choose a supine position because they are presented with a bed and have no alternative option.

A lateral recumbent position reduces obstructive pressure on maternal blood vessels so venous return and cardiac output are optimal for uterine perfusion and fetal oxygenation. Uterine contractions are more intense but less frequent and have increased efficiency. In an upright position, the abdominal wall relaxes and the effect of gravity will augment the effect of the fetal head pressing on the cervix and the subsequent feedback to the myometrial activity. Both frequency and intensity of contractions are increased so uterine activity is enhanced and labour tends to be shorter. Squatting increases maternal pelvic diameter, enhances engagement and the descent of the fetal head.

During bearing down, in the second stage of labour, directed pushing with a Valsalva manoeuvre against a closed glottis increases sympathetic discharge and catecholamine release. Minimal straining with an open glottis has fewer negative effects on maternal blood pressure, maternal and fetal oxygenation levels and is associated with reduced need for episiotomy.

Key points

- Parturition in humans is poorly understood; animal studies offer limited insight into the process owing to the evolution of species-specific differences.

- Parturition is a continuous process: the defining of the various stages of labour enables clinical judgement of progress and thus intervention under the biomedical model of care.

- The fundal region of the uterus has the highest density of smooth muscle so it is responsible for the strong expelling contractions of the uterus during labour.

- Human cervical structure is complex owing to the upright stance causing an increased gravitational force as the contents of the uterus increase in mass. Structural changes within the cervix have to occur before dilatation can be achieved by uterine contractions.

- Coordinated effective contractions are facilitated by the development of gap junctions between the myometrial cells.

- The first stage of labour is measured from the onset of strong and regular effective contractions to full effacement and dilation of the cervix.

- The second stage of labour is characterized by strong expulsive contractions, aided by respiratory muscle involvement, until the fetus is delivered.

- The passage of the fetus through the pelvis is described as the mechanism of labour and is achieved through the contractions forcing the presenting part to rotate against the muscle tone, structural resistance and shape of the pelvic floor.

- The third stage of labour covers the delivery of the placenta and fetal membranes and staunching of maternal blood loss.

- Maternal blood loss immediately following separation of the placenta is limited by the myometrial fibres contracting, thus occluding the uterine vessels.

- The onset of labour is poorly understood; a fetal signal probably alters the ratio of progesterone and oestrogen and other factors, such as prostaglandin secretion and oxytocin receptor expression, are involved in the amplification of the signal.

- The evolution of bipedal locomotion and increasing cephalization have influenced parturition in humans so the presenting part has to negotiate, by rotational manoeuvres, rather than just pass through the pelvic girdle.

- The process of labour induces many changes within the fetus in preparation for extrauterine existence, which are mediated by increasing hypoxia and catecholamine production.

- Pain in labour has a complex aetiology; there are visceral and somatic components further complicated by psychological and social factors.

Midwives need to understand the physiological interactions and external factors that can affect human parturition in order to underpin intrapartum care.

The development of observational skills allows the midwife not only to interpret how a woman may be coping with labour, but also to determine how the labour is progressing from observing behaviour and physical responses of the labouring woman. By ignoring, not noticing or misunderstanding certain physical cues, the midwife may inadvertently provide suboptimal support.

Intervention in labour must be justified and decisions surrounding this must be underpinned to maximize maternal and fetal well-being. Knowledge of the effects of intervention upon fetal and maternal physiology is essential so that the midwife can judge the effectiveness and quickly identify possible adverse outcomes of such interventions.

Annotated further reading

Abitbol MM 1996 Birth and human evolution: anatomical and obstetric mechanics in primates. Greenwood Press
This book describes the evolutionary development of the mechanisms of birth in monkeys and primates including humans.

Blackburn ST 2003 Maternal, fetal and neonatal physiology: a clinical perspective, 2nd edn. Saunders, Philadelphia
An excellent in-depth description of physiological adaptation to pregnancy and consequent development of the fetus and neonate that draws from physiological research studies. The chapters are clearly organized by physiological systems and link physiological concepts to clinical applications including the assessment and management of low- and high-risk pregnancies.

Gee H, Glynn M 1997 The physiology and clinical management of labour. In: Henderson C, Jones K (eds) Essential midwifery. Mosby, St Louis, pp 171–202
This chapter provides a useful overview to midwifery management of labour in relation to the physiological processes and their progression.

Greer IA 1995 The physiology and biochemistry of labour. In: Chamberlain G (Ed) Turnbull's obstetrics, 2nd edn. Churchill Livingstone, New York, pp 551–567

An in-depth exploration of the factors that may contribute to the onset and regulation of human parturition including interventions to inhibit preterm labour and induce labour at term.

Kean L, Baker P, Edelstone (eds) (2000) Best practice in labour ward management.
This book provides guidance on the clinical management of complications associated with labour.

Kierse MJN C 2003 The history of tocolysis. British Journal of Obstetrics and Gynaecology 110:94–97
A brief historical review which evaluates different types of drugs used to prevent premature delivery.

Liggins GC 1994 Mechanism of the onset of labour: the New Zealand perspective. Australian and New Zealand Journal of Obstetrics and Gynaecology 34:338–342
A comprehensive and thoughtful review of the factors involved in the onset of parturition by one of the pioneers of the field.

López Bernal A 1996 Parturition. In: Hillier SG, Kitchener HC, Neilson JP (eds) Scientific essentials of reproductive medicine. Saunders, Philadelphia, pp 364–375
A good summary of factors that influence parturition in the human, their likely mechanisms and how these can be combined to create a model of physiological control of labour.

Mander R 1997 The control of labour pain. In: Henderson C, Jones K (eds) Essential midwifery. Mosby, St Louis, pp 203–218
Looks at pain pathways, management of pain and the interventions used at delivery to achieve pain relief.

Steer PJ, Johnson MR 1998 The genital system. In: Chamberlain G, Broughton Pipkin F (eds) Clinical physiology in obstetrics, 3rd edn. Blackwell, Oxford, pp 308–355
A comprehensive chapter describing the anatomy and physiology of the uterus and cervix. It includes changes in pregnancy and prior to labour, interaction of the placenta and uterus, factors influencing the onset of labour, and the involution of the uterus.

Tribe RM 2001 Regulation of human myometrial contractility during pregnancy and labour: are calcium homeostatic pathways important? Experimental Physiology 86(2): 247–254
A review about the contribution of calcium in the regulation of myometrial activity in the context of developing strategies to treat and manage preterm and dysfunctional preterm labour.

References

Aitken MA, Rice GE, Brennecke SP 1990 Gestational tissue phospholipase A_2 messenger RNA content and the onset of spontaneous labour in the human. Reproduction Fertility and Development 2:575–580

Apostolakis EM, Rice KE, Longo LD, Seron-Ferre M, Yellon SM 1993 Time of day of birth and absence of endocrine and uterine contractile activity rhythms in sheep. American Journal of Physiology 264:E534–E540

Astle S, Slater DM, Thornton S 2003 The involvement of progesterone in the onset of human labour. European Journal of Obstetrics Gynecology and Reproductive Biology 108(2):177–181

Baker C 1996 Nutrition and hydration in labour. British Journal of Midwifery 4:568–572

Bani D 1997 Relaxin: a pleiotropic hormone. General Pharmacology 28:13–22

Barret JFR, Savage J, Phillips K, Liford RJ 1992 Randomised trial of amniotomy in labour versus the intention to leave membranes intact until the second stage. British Journal of Obstetrics and Gynaecology 99:5

Bennett VR, Brown LK 1999 Myles' textbook for midwives, 13th edn. Churchill Livingstone, Edinburgh, pp 393, 396, 431, 451, 468, 473, 509, 993

Bernal AL, Europe-Finner GN, Phaneuf S, Watson SP 1995 Preterm labour: a pharmacological challenge. Trends in Pharmacological Science 16:129–133

Blackburn ST 2003 Maternal, fetal, and neonatal physiology: a clinical perspective, 2nd edn. Saunders, Philadelphia

Bowen JM, Chamley L, Keelan JA, Mitchell MD 2002 Cytokines of the placenta and extra-placental membranes: roles and regulation during human pregnancy and parturition. Placenta 23(4):257–273

Boyle JT 1992 Motility of the upper gastrointestinal tract in the fetus and neonate. In: Polin RA, Fox WW (eds) Fetal and neonatal physiology, Vol 2. Saunders, Philadelphia, pp 1028–1032

Carp H, Jayaram A, Stoll M 1992 Ultrasound examination of the stomach contents of parturients. Anesthesia and Analgesia 74:683–687

Challis JRG, Matthews SG, Gibb W, Lye SJ 2000 Endocrine and paracrine regulation of birth at term and preterm. Endocrine Reviews 21:514–550

Challis JR, Lye SJ, Gibb W, Whittle W, Patel F, Alfaidy N 2001 Understanding preterm labor. Ann. N. Y. Acad. Sci. 943:225–34

Chamberlain G, Dewhurst J, Harvey D 1991 Illustrated textbook of obstetrics. Gower Medical (Mosby), London, p 115

Clifton VL, Read MA, Leitch IM, Boura AL, Robinson PJ, Smith R 1994 Corticotropin-releasing hormone-induced vasodilatation in the human fetal placental circulation. Journal of Clinical Endocrinology and Metabolism 79(2):666–669

De Ziegler D, Bulletti C, Fanchin R, Epiney M, Brioschi PA 2001 Contractility of the nonpregnant uterus: the follicular phase. Ann. N. Y. Acad. Sci. 943:172–84

Duff P 1996 Premature rupture of the membranes in term patients. Seminars in Perinatology 20:401–408

Eberle RL, Norris MC 1996 Labor analgesia: a risk-benefit analysis. Drug Safety 14:239–251

Friese K 2003 The role of infection in preterm labour. British Journal of Obstetrics and Gynaecology 110(Suppl 20):52–54

Fuchs AR, Fuchs F, Husslein P, Soloff MS 1984 Oxytocin receptors in the human uterus during pregnancy and parturition. American Journal of Obstetrics and Gynecology 150:734–741

Fuchs AR, Romero R, Keefe D, Parra M, Oyarzun E, Behnke E 1991 Oxytocin secretion and human parturition: pulse frequency and duration increase during spontaneous labour in women. American Journal of Obstetrics and Gynecology 165:1515–1522

Garfield RE, Blennerhassett MG, Miller SM 1988 Control of myometrial contractility: role and regulation of gap junctions. Oxford Review of Reproductive Biology 10:436–490

Gee H, Olah KS 1993 Failure to progress in labour. Progress in Obstetrics and Gynaecology 10:159–181

Germain AM, Valenzuela GJ, Ivankovic M, Ducsay CA, Gabella C, Seron-Ferre M 1993 Relationship of circadian rhythms of uterine activity with term and preterm delivery. American Journal of Obstetrics and Gynecology 168:1271–1277

Goodwin TM 1999 A role for estriol in human labor, term and preterm. American Journal of Obstetrics and Gynecology 180(1 Pt 3):S208–S213

Gluckman PD, Sizonenko SV, Bassett NS 1999 The transition from fetus to neonate: an endocrine perspective. Acta Paediatrica Supplement 88(428):7–11

Grummer R, Winterhager E 1998 Regulation of gap junction connexins in the endometrium during early pregnancy. Cell and Tissue Research 293(2):189–194

Hampson V, Lui D, Billett E, Kirk S 1997 Amniotic membrane collagen content and type distribution in women with preterm premature rupture of the membranes in pregnancy. British Journal of Obstetrics and Gynaecology 104:1087–1091

Hertelendy F, Zakar T 2004 Prostaglandins and the myometrium and cervix. Prostaglandins Leukotrienes and Essential Fatty Acids 70(2):207–222

Hillhouse EW, Grammatopoulos DK 2002 Role of stress peptides during human pregnancy and labour. Reproduction 124(3):323–329

Honnebier MBOM, Nathanielsz PW 1994 Primate parturition and the role of the maternal circadian system. European Journal of Obstetrics, Gynecology and Reproductive Biology 55:193–203

Honnebier WJ, Jobsis AC, Swaab DF 1974 The effect of hypophysial hormones and human chorionic gonadotrophin (HCG) on the anencephalic fetal adrenal cortex and on parturition in the human. Journal of Obstetrics and Gynaecology of the British Commonwealth 81(6):423–438

Houlihan CM, Knuppel RA 1994 Meconium-stained amniotic fluid: current controversies. Journal of Reproductive Medicine 39(11):888–898

Husslein P 1985 Pregnancy and plasma oxytocin levels. Journal of Perinatal Medicine 13:314–315

Jenkin G, Young IR 2004 Mechanisms responsible for parturition; the use of experimental models. Animal Reproduction Science 82–83:567–581

Kanayama N, Terao T 1991 The relationship between granulocyte elastase-like activity of cervical mucus and cervical maturation. Acta Obstetrica et Gynecologica Scandinavica 70:29

Karalis K, Goodwin G, Majzoub J A 1996 Cortisol blockade of progesterone: a possible mechanism involved in the initiation of labour. Nature Medicine 2:556–560

Katz V, Bowes WA 1992 Meconium aspiration syndrome: reflections on a murky subject. American Journal of Obstetrics and Gynecology 166(1 Pt 1):171–183

Karteris E, Grammatopoulos D, Dai Y, Olah KB, Ghobara TB, Easton A, Hillhouse EW 1998 The human placenta and fetal membranes express the corticotropin-releasing hormone receptor 1alpha (CRH-1alpha) and the CRH-C variant receptor. Journal of Clinical Endocrinology and Metabolism 83(4):1376–1379

Leppert PC 1995 Anatomy and physiology of cervical ripening. Clinical Obstetric Gynecology 38(2):267–279

López Bernal A 2003 Mechanisms of labour: biochemical aspects. British Journal of Obstetrics and Gynaecology 110(Suppl 20):39–45

López Bernal A, Watson SP, Phaneuf S, Europe-Finner GN 1993 Biochemistry and physiology of preterm labour and delivery. Baillière's Clinics in Obstetrics and Gynaecology 7:523–552

Ludka LM, Roberts CC 1993 Eating and drinking in labour. Journal of Nurse-Midwifery 38:199–207

Melzack R, Wall PD 1965 Pain mechanisms: a new theory. Science 150(699):971–979

Mesiano S 2004 Myometrial progesterone responsiveness and the control of human parturition. Journal of the Society for Gynecologic Investigation 11(4):193–202

Miller FD, Chibbar R, Mitchell BF 1993 Synthesis of oxytocin in amnion, chorion and decidua: a potential paracrine role for oxytocin in the onset of human parturition. Regulatory Peptides 45:247

Mulder EJH, Boersma M, Meeuse M, Van der Wal M, Van De Weerd E, Visser GHA 1994 Patterns of breathing movements in the near-term fetus: relationship to behavioural states. Early Human Development 36:127–135

Neulen J, Breckwoldt M 1994 Placental progesterone, prostaglandins and mechanisms leading to initiation of parturition in the human. Experimental and Clinical Endocrinology 102(3):195–202

Nijhuis JG 2003 Fetal behavior. Neurobiology of Aging 24(Suppl 1):S41–S46

Odent M 2001 New reasons and new ways to study birth physiology. International Journal of Gynecology & Obstetrics 75:S39–S45

Olah KS 1994 Changes in cervical electromyographic activity and their correlation with cervical response to myometrial activity during labour. European Journal of Obstetrics, Gynecology and Reproductive Biology 3:157–150

Olah KS, Gee H, Brown JS 1993 Cervical contractions: the response of the cervix to oxytocic stimulation in the latent phase of labour. British Journal of Obstetrics and Gynaecology 100:635–640

Olson DM, Zaragoza DB, Shallow MC, Cook JL, Mitchell BF, Grigsby P, Hirst J 2003 Myometrial activation and preterm labour: evidence supporting a role for the prostaglandin F receptor: a review. Placenta 24(Suppl A):S47–S54

Parsons M 2003 Midwifery dilemma: to fast or feed the labouring woman. Part 1: The case for restricting oral intake in labour. Australian Journal of Midwifery 16(4):7–13

Parsons M 2004 Midwifery dilemma: to fast or feed the labouring woman. Part 2: The case supporting oral intake in labour. Australian Journal of Midwifery 17(1):5–9

Petersen LK, Oxlund H, Uldberg N, Forman A 1991 In vitro analysis of muscular contractile ability and passive biomechanical properties of uterine cervical samples from non-pregnant women. Obstetrics and Gynecology 77:772–776

Petraglia F, Benedetto C, Florio P et al 1995 Effect of corticotropin-releasing factor-binding protein on prostaglandin release from cultured maternal decidua and on contractile activity of human myometrium in-vitro. Journal of Clinical Endocrinology and Metabolism 80:3073–3076

Riley SC, Challis JRG 1991 Corticotropin-releasing hormone production by the placenta and fetal membranes. Placenta 12:105–119

Romero R, Chaiworapongsa T, Espinoza J 2003 Micronutrients and intrauterine infection, preterm birth and the fetal inflammatory response syndrome. Journal of Nutrition 133(5 Suppl 2):1668S–1673S

Rosenberg K, Trevathan W 2002 Birth, obstetrics and human evolution. British Journal of Obstetrics and Gynaecology 109(11):1199–1206

Rowe TF 1997 Acute gastric aspiration: prevention and treatment. Seminars in Perinatology 21:313–319

Salamonsen LA 2003 Tissue injury and repair in the female human reproductive tract. Reproduction 125(3):301–311

Scheepers HC, de Jong PA, Essed GG, Kanhai HH 2001 Fetal and maternal energy metabolism during labor in relation to the available caloric sustrate. Journal of Perinatal Medicine 29(6):457–464

Scutton M, Lowy C, O'Sullivan G 1996 Eating in labour: an assessment of the risks and benefits. International Journal of Obstetric Anesthesia 5:214–215

Sharp DA 1997 Restriction of oral intake for women in labour. British Journal of Midwifery 5:408–412

Slattery MM, Brennan C, O'Leary MJ, Morrison JJ 2001 Human chorionic gonadotrophin inhibition of pregnant human myometrial contractility. British Journal of Obstetrics and Gynaecology 108(7):704–708

Steer PJ, Johnson MR 1998 The genital system. In: Chamberlain G, Broughton Pipkin F (eds) Clinical physiology in obstetrics, 3rd edn. Blackwell, Oxford, pp 308–355

Stewart DB 1984 The pelvis as a passageway I. Evolution and adaptations. British Journal of Obstetrics and Gynaecology 91:611–617

Stjernholm Y, Sahlin L, Akerberg S et al 1996 Cervical ripening in humans: potential roles of estrogen, progesterone and insulin-like growth factor-I. American Journal of Obstetrics and Gynecology 174:1065–1071

Studd J, Duiagnan N 1972 Graphic records in labour. British Medical Journal 4(837):4

Sullivan JM, Ramanathan KB 1985 Management of medical problems in pregnancy: severe cardiac disease. New England Journal of Medicine 313:304–309

Sweet B, Tiran D 1996 Mayes' midwifery, 12th edn. Baillière Tindall, London pp 31, 224, 225, 340, 358, 993

Symonds EM, Symonds IM 1997 Essential obstetrics and gynaecology, 3rd edn. Churchill Livingstone, Edinburgh, p 134

Thong KJ, Baird DT 1992 Induction of abortion with mifepristone and misoprostol in early pregnancy. British Journal of Obstetrics and Gynaecology 99:1004–1007

Thorburn GD 1992 The placenta, PGE2 and parturition. Early Human Development 29:63–73

Uldbjerg N, Malstrom A 1991 The role of proteoglycans in cervical dilatation. Seminars in Perinatology 15:127–132

Warnes KE, Morris MJ, Symonds ME et al 1998 Effects of increasing gestation, cortisol and maternal undernutrition on hypothalamic neuropeptide Y expression in the sheep fetus. Journal of Neuroendocrinology 10:51–57

Wilmsatt J, Myers DA, Myers TR, Nathanielsz PW 1995 Prostaglandin synthase activity of fetal sheep cotyledons at 122 days of gestation and term-expression of prostaglandin synthetic capacity in fetal cotyledonary tissue near labor is location-dependent. Biology of Reproduction 52:737–744

Wolfe CDA, Petruckevitch A, Quartero R et al 1990 The rate of rise of corticotropin releasing-factor and endogenous digoxin-like immunoreactivity in normal and abnormal pregnancy. British Journal of Obstetrics and Gynaecology 97:832–837

Wray S 1993 Uterine contraction and physiological mechanisms of modulation. American Journal of Physiology 264:C1–C18

Wray S, Jones K, Kupittayanant S, Li Y, Matthew A, Monir-Bishty E, Noble K, Pierce SJ, Quenby S, Shmygol AV 2003 Calcium signaling and uterine contractility. Journal of the Society for Gynecologic Investigation 10(5):252–264

14 The puerperium

L e a r n i n g   o b j e c t i v e s

- To describe the physiological processes that achieve haemostasis in the early puerperium.
- To discuss the timing of the physiological changes in the puerperium.
- To understand the aetiology of the common problems experienced within the puerperium.
- To recognize signs of pathological conditions associated with the puerperium.

Introduction

The puerperium has been traditionally defined as the 6-week period immediately following the birth of a baby and represents the period of time in which maternal physiology, particularly the reproductive system, returns to a near prepregnant state. It probably originates from the tradition of 'churching' or the 'lying-in period,' which was a religious ceremony where women were accepted back into the church after a period of 40 days during which they were considered unclean. The time after childbirth is imbued with social, cultural and religious significance and, in many cultures, the puerperal woman is given special treatment. Two important landmarks are often observed: the cessation of lochial discharge (women often being considered 'unclean' when lochia is present) and the shrivelling and loss of the remnants of the umbilical cord from the infant. With the rise of medical dominance, the end of the puerperium was marked by the postnatal examination of the woman by a doctor. This has structured the traditional descriptions of the puerperium as a period of maternal recovery, underpinned by the medicalization of pregnancy. It is the midwife's responsibility to maintain a careful watch on the physiological changes in the puerperium and to recognize early signs of pathological conditions.

The puerperium is sometimes considered to be the 'Cinderella' of midwifery and obstetrics as the excitement of the birth is over and after delivery the effects of pregnancy on maternal physiology receive little emphasis. There is not very much research into the timing or mechanisms of the changes in the puerperium. However, the puerperal woman can be very vulnerable to physiological stress, which can become pathological. The midwife's role is to observe and monitor the early changes and to be able to differentiate between those which are normal and abnormal.

A woman adapts to pregnancy progressively over a period of months, but after childbirth she suddenly no longer needs the physiological changes. During the puerperium, there is a marked decrease in the levels of oestrogen and progesterone within the maternal system. Although the placenta is the main source of progesterone in pregnancy, the corpus luteum continues to produce progesterone for several days into the puerperal period. The fall in concentrations of steroid hormones facilitates the initiation of lactation (see Ch. 16) and allows the physiological systems to return to their prepregnant state. In reality, the puerperium should be described as a transitional phase. It begins at the birth of a child and it ends with the return of fertility. Women do not return to the same physiological and anatomical state, however. The puerperium also, within a social context, represents many transitions for the parents, child and other members of the family. Many of the physiological changes within the puerperium, such as the establishment of parenting skills, lactation and feeding, are modified by the past and present social interactions of the individuals within the new family situation.

Chapter case study

Zak was born 2 days after his expected date of delivery and was the first son born to his proud parents, Zara and James. Zak was delivered at around 04:30 hours and Zara had laboured in a birthing pool attended by her named midwife. As labour had progressed quickly without complications, the midwife followed Zara's request for no active management in the third stage of labour. The midwife was unable to accurately estimate Zara's blood loss due to the waterbirth. Once out of the bath, the midwife assessed Zara's perineal trauma, which appeared to be a first-degree tear that was not bleeding and did not require suturing. How can the midwife effectively assess Zara's well-being following the delivery, given that she has been unable to estimate Zara's total blood loss? What factors that have occurred during Zak's delivery will optimize Zara's transition to parenthood?

Physiological and structural changes

Involution of the uterus

Clinical observation and management of the puerperium is essentially based on the return of the uterus to its 'normal' size. The puerperium begins as soon as the placenta and membranes are expelled from the uterus together with a substantial proportion of the endometrium. Oxytocin released from the posterior pituitary gland induces strong intermittent myometrial contractions, and as the uterine cavity is empty the whole uterus contracts down fully and the uterine walls become realigned in apposition to each other. The myometrial spiral fibres that occlude the uterine blood vessels (see Ch. 13) restrict the blood supply to the placental site (Fig. 14.1). Uterine vascular resistance increases soon after delivery (Tekay & Jouppila 1993).

About an hour after delivery, the myometrium relaxes slightly but further active bleeding is prevented by the activation of the blood-clotting mechanisms, which are altered greatly during pregnancy to facilitate a swift clotting response. Haemostasis is achieved in three ways:

- ischaemia
- pressure: apposition of the uterine walls forming the T-shaped cavity
- clotting mechanisms.

The midwife has the responsibility to inspect the placenta and membranes to assess that they are complete and that no tissue remains within the uterine cavity. Retained products impede the contraction of the uterus and may be the source of abnormal bleeding and cause secondary postpartum haemorrhage (secondary PPH) as they become the focus of infection. Retained products are often spontaneously voided usually associated with the passing of a blood clot, which facilitates the cleansing of the uterine cavity.

Immediately after delivery the uterus weighs about 900–1000 g and the fundus is palpable about 11–12 cm above the symphysis pubis (Howie 1995). The placental site is raw and exposed. Initially, the uterus is continuous with the vagina with the cervix draping from the body of the uterus. Uterine involution is rapid so 50% of the total mass of the tissue is lost within a week (Howie 1995). This physiological destruction of most of the uterine tissue is unique in adult life and the mechanisms are not clearly understood. It is suggested that 90% of uterine protein is degraded in the first 10 days of the puerperium (Hytten 1995). There are rapid and marked changes in collagen and elastin content (Stone & Franzblau 1995), and water and protein are lost. Involution results from a withdrawal of placental hormones and is thought to be mediated by hydrolytic and proteolytic enzymes released from myometrial cells, endothelial cells of blood vessels and macrophages. Cytoplasmic organelles are autodigested, and intracellular cytoplasm and extracellular collagen are reduced (Howie 1995). The breakdown of protein from the myometrial cells releases the amino acid components into the circulation and thence into the urine; thus a puerperal woman is in a state of negative nitrogen balance (see Ch. 12). The myometrial cells are thought to reduce in size (Fig. 14.2) rather than being destroyed and replaced, although there may be an 'overshoot' in uterine involution with rebuilding to the resting non-pregnant state. The uterus ultimately returns almost to its prepregnant size (Fig. 14.3), although the proportion of fibrous tissue present in the uterus is progressively increased with successive pregnancies.

Initially the cervix is soft, bruised and lacerated following a vaginal delivery (particularly so in primiparae and with premature labour). The cervix rapidly re-forms and closes; by the end of the first puerperal week it will admit one finger. However, the cervix never returns to its original state and always shows evidence of parturition. The external os re-forms with a slit rather than the nulliparous dimple (Fig. 14.4).

A

B

Muscle fibre

Blood vessel

Muscle fibre

Blood vessel

Fig. 14.1 *A Myometrial spiral fibres around uterine blood vessels; B occlusion of blood supply to the placental site. (Reproduced with permission from Sweet & Tiran 1996.)*

The uterus involutes quite quickly, initially at about 1 cm/day; thus by the 10th day it should no longer be palpable above the symphysis pubis. Involution is slower in women who have undergone lower-segment caesarean section (LSCS), but it can be judged by a detectable decrease in fundal height. Subinvolution (a slow rate of uterine involution) may indicate retained products of conception and/or a secondary infection, which is usually found in conjunction with continued lochia rubra that may have an offensive odour. The uterus should be well contracted, hard and central; if it is higher than the umbilicus and soft on palpation (often described as 'boggy') then this may also indicate the presence of infection. The endometrial cavity is a potential space in non-pregnant women but gas is commonly detected in the endometrial cavity puerperally (Hytten 1995).

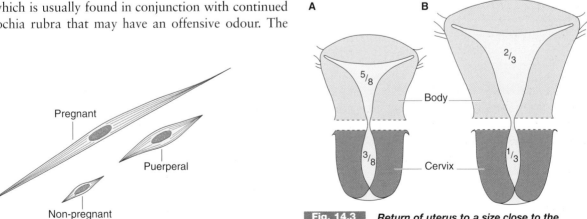

Pregnant

Puerperal

Non-pregnant

Fig. 14.2 *Reduction in size of myometrial cells. (Reproduced with permission from Miller & Hanretty 1998.)*

A

B

$5/8$

$2/3$

Body

$3/8$

$1/3$

Cervix

Fig. 14.3 *Return of uterus to a size close to the prepregnant dimensions: A nulliparous uterus; B parous uterus. (Reproduced with permission from Miller & Hanretty 1998.)*

A
B

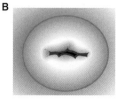

Fig. 14.4 *Re-formation of the external os:*
A nulliparous cervix; B parous cervix.
(Reproduced with permission from Miller &
Hanretty 1998.)

The initiation of breastfeeding and the infant suckling in the early puerperium augments stimulation of oxytocin release. The oxytocin stimulates further contraction of the myometrium and so uterine evacuation. Involution of the uterus in breastfeeding mothers is more efficient. 'After-pains' associated with lactation are often experienced, particularly by multiparous women who often complain of increased vaginal loss while feeding. Initially oral analgesia such as paracetamol may be offered but the intensity of the pain usually subsides after about 24 hours because expression of myometrial oxytocin receptors is reduced as a result of oestrogen withdrawal.

The superficial layer of the decidua becomes necrotic and is shed in the lochia in the first few days of the puerperium. The epithelium rapidly regenerates, re-forming an intact layer over most of the surface within 7–10 days of delivery. The placental site takes 3 weeks or longer to recover. The endometrium regenerates from the basal layers and grows in from the margins of the placental wound site and from glandular remnants within it (Howie 1995).

Soft tissue damage and repair

It is not uncommon for soft tissue damage to occur during the delivery of a baby. Trauma to the female genital tract is described as follows:

- *Superficial*—this usually describes grazes to the skin where the epidermis has split owing to pressure of distension. These require no treatment; however, they often cause discomfort through stinging because of the disruption of the many nerve endings found within the superficial layer of the tissue. Voiding of urine can also be uncomfortable as the urine comes in contact with the grazes.
- *First degree*—this describes a tear in the skin and underlying superficial tissues (not including the muscle). Often the wound will heal spontaneously as the skin edges are usually in apposition. Ragged tears may result in the formation of excess scar tissue.
- *Second degree*—when a tear involves perineal muscle damage it is described as being second degree. Usually these wounds are sutured to aid healing.
- *Episiotomy*—this is a surgical incision to enlarge the introitus to facilitate the delivery of the baby. It falls into the same category as the second-degree tear.
- *Third degree*—here the muscle of the anal sphincter is involved. Obstetric repair is essential so that the sphincter activity of the muscle is restored thus avoiding complications of faecal incontinence at a later time.
- *Fourth degree*—when the tear is extensive the anal sphincter may become completely divided and the tear continues through the rectal mucosa. Specialist surgical repair is required to ensure the resumption of normal anal function.

Repair to the perineum involves the clinician suturing the perineum. There is a wide variety of suture materials and techniques for repair; however, suturing aims to achieve the following:

- *Haemostasis*—this is to ensure that any active bleeding points are ligated to minimize blood loss and the postnatal complication of a haematoma (formation of a blood clot within the wound) which can be extremely painful.
- *Alignment*—this is to bring the tissues back into alignment to optimize healing and to achieve a near pre-tear condition. If wounds are left gaping, alignment may not occur and as healing is by granulation this can result in the formation of scar tissue. This can result in a rigid misshapen perineum, which can cause dyspareunia (pain on intercourse).

The majority of perineal traumas can be described as being deep wounds as the tissue trauma involves layers below the epidermis and the dermis. Wound healing occurs in three phases: inflammation, tissue formation and tissue remodelling (see also Box 14.1). Some features of wound healing are common to all tissues; others are specific to the tissue involved. For instance, granulation tissue does not develop in the endometrium and the wounds do not heal with scarring. In this respect, there are similarities with fetal wounds which also heal without scarring suggesting

Box 14.1

The stages of wound healing

0–3 days
- Blood clot forms, reinforced with fibrin fibres
- Acute inflammatory response occurs: polymorphs and macrophages migrate to site; high-protein exudate leads to local oedema

1 week later
- Eschar dries out, hardens and eventually becomes detached
- Wound contracts
- Mitotic activity occurs in epidermal cells, which migrate over living tissue
- New blood capillaries form from endothelial buds, bringing nutrients to healing tissue
- New connective tissue, formed by fibroblasts, supports capillary loops

6 months later
- Surface depression may still be visible at wound site; scar tissue becomes paler
- Epithelialization is complete
- Connective tissue is reorganized, less vascular and stronger

that the process of endometrial remodelling is more a developmental mechanism than merely repair.

1. First is the inflammatory response; inflammation is a normal reaction to tissue trauma. Perineal inflammation can initially cause great discomfort for women in the very early postnatal period. An analgesic such as diclofenac sodium is useful as it acts as an anti-inflammatory agent (though it should be used with caution if the woman is asthmatic). Paracetamol and codeine-based products can also be used but codeine can cause or exacerbate bowel constipation so appropriate advice is required. However, a degree of inflammation is vital to ensure tissue healing, so analgesics should be used only when the response is severe and perineal pain restricts normal activity. The inflammation acts to isolate the damaged tissues, reducing the spread of infection. White blood cells, such as neutrophils and macrophages, invade the tissue owing to the increased vasodilatation in the surrounding blood vessels. These cells ingest any invading bacteria and break down any necrotic tissue within the wound.

2. The migratory phase involves the infiltration of the wound by mesenchymal cells that form fibroblasts, initially creating a scab over the open wound site. Following this, blood vessels grow into the wound and the wound is gradually filled from the bottom up by new tissue growth called granulation tissue.

3. There then follows a proliferative phase where epithelial cells grow under the scab. It concludes with the maturation of the new cells and the shedding of the scab.

Lochia

The initial vaginal loss is termed the lochia rubra and consists of blood that has collected within the reproductive tract together with autolytic products of degenerated necrotic decidua from the placental site and any trophoblastic remains. The outward flow of blood lost at delivery and the subsequent discharge of lochia are important in removal of potential sources of ascending infection and, thus, protection of the placental wound site. The alkalinity of the lochia is also important in protecting the vulnerable site. Lochia is the normal discharge in the puerperium; it has a characteristic sweetish smell unless there is an infection.

Lochia may be described by its visual appearance (Box 14.2); normally, the lochia lightens progressively in both volume and colour. However, at about day 7 after delivery, the fibrinous mesh deposited over the

Box 14.2

Lochia

- Lochia rubra (red)
  - decidua and frank blood loss from placental site
  - initially sterile then uterus begins to be colonized by vaginal flora
  - red colour persists for about 3 days

- Lochia serosa (pink/brown)
  - contains leukocytes, mucus, vaginal epithelial cells, necrotic decidua, non-pathological bacteria
  - may be blood stained for 3–4 weeks
  - characteristic sweetish odour

- Lochia alba (yellow–white)
  - mostly serous fluid and leukocytes
  - plus some cervical mucus and microorganisms

placental site may be shed as part of the normal healing process so the vaginal loss may be transiently heavier and flushed with fresh blood. By day 10, the lochia is normally scant and pink in colour although discharge of lochia may persist for up to 6 weeks. Prolonged duration of lochia discharge suggests the placental wound site is not completely epithelialized or that the woman has some retained debris which is still disintegrating (Hytten 1995). The duration of lochia discharge tends to be longer with the first pregnancy and is also related to birth weight.

Heavy discharge of lochia with an offensive odour, maternal pyrexia and/or a feeling of general malaise can all indicate possible intrauterine infection. If the lochia remains abnormally heavy and further bleeding occurs, dilatation and curettage (D&C) to empty the uterine cavity may be necessary. The procedure is also termed evacuation of retained products of conception (ERPC). The cervix is dilated and the retained products are scraped from the decidua. This procedure is not without complications, however. Excessive scraping can damage or remove the entire endometrium. If the basal layer of the endometrium is removed (see Ch. 2) then proliferation during the menstrual cycle fails to occur, affecting fertility; this is termed Asherman's syndrome.

Blood loss

Excessive blood loss, i.e. more than 500 ml or any amount that jeopardizes the well-being of the mother, at and within 24 hours of delivery is termed a primary postpartum haemorrhage, or primary PPH. It is usually caused by failure of the myometrium to contract completely, or failure of the blood-clotting mechanisms, or both (see Ch. 13); PPH may be very serious (Box 14.3, Case study 14.1).

The risk of primary PPH is lower 24–72 hours following delivery, but until involution of the uterus is complete there is a risk of a secondary PPH if there is an infection within the uterine cavity. The bleeding is usually due to the fibrinolytic action of bacteria such as haemolytic streptococcus. These bacteria are usually anaerobes (able to thrive in the absence of oxygen) and so specific antibiotic treatment with antibiotics such as metronidazole (Flagyl) may be required.

Hormonal changes

In late pregnancy, most of the steroid hormones are derived from the placenta, although the corpus luteum

---

Box 14.3

Disseminated intravascular coagulation

Disseminated intravascular coagulation (DIC) is a condition caused by abnormal activation of the clotting mechanisms. The blood-clotting factors are induced on a wide basis resulting in fibrin deposits being produced that line the major part of the vascular bed. Once this has occurred, bleeding continues owing to the absence of clotting factors, which were exhausted during the DIC phase and the activation of fibrinolysis. Liver dysfunction occurs in pre-eclampsia and may be associated with DIC and microangiopathic haemolysis (erythrocyte breakdown in small blood vessels). The acronym HELLP refers to *H*aemolysis, *E*levated *L*iver enzymes and *L*ow *P*latelet counts.

DIC is an extremely severe condition. Although such a life-threatening case would normally be managed by intensive care staff rather than by the midwifery unit, it is important that midwives are able to recognize the symptoms and implications of DIC.

---

and ovary continue to contribute some progesterone. Levels of progesterone and oestrogen fall to non-pregnant levels within 72 hours of delivery. The placental protein hormones have a longer half-life so plasma levels fall more slowly. During pregnancy, production of the gonadotrophins is suppressed. Follicle-stimulating hormone (FSH) levels are restored to prepregnant concentrations within 3 weeks of delivery, but restoration of luteinizing hormone (LH) secretion takes longer, depending on the duration of lactation. Levels of oxytocin and prolactin also depend on lactational performance.

Case study 14.1

Lucy is a 35-year-old primigravida who is delivered by emergency LSCS at 30 weeks' gestation owing to fulminating pre-eclampsia. Following delivery, the blood loss per vaginum is noted to be quite brisk and a Syntocinon (oxytocin) infusion is commenced in an attempt to control the bleeding. On investigation it is discovered that Lucy's platelet count is extremely low and that the clotting time for her blood is greatly prolonged. A provisional diagnosis of DIC secondary to HELLP syndrome is made.

The haematological system and cardiovascular changes

The blood lost at delivery, accepted to be about 300–500 ml normally, is adequately compensated for by the increase in blood volume acquired during pregnancy (see Ch. 11). Women can lose about 1000 ml of their predelivery blood volume before postnatal haemoglobin concentration is compromised (Letsky 1998) (Case study 14.2). Erythropoiesis is stimulated before and after delivery (Richter, Huch & Huch 1995). Diuresis further decreases plasma volume in the first days, although as interstitial fluid is mobilized subsequently the plasma volume tends to increase transiently causing haemodilution of both haemoglobin and plasma proteins, such as clotting factors. It is this variability in blood lost at delivery and restoration of normal water balance that may result in raised concentrations of clotting factor and hypercoagulability. The tendency to coagulate is also affected by the loss of placental and fetal factors affecting clotting and water regulation (Blackburn 2003).

Haemoglobin levels return to normal prepregnant levels within 4–6 weeks and white blood cell numbers fall to normal within a week of delivery (Blackburn 2003). Platelet number increases in the first few days following delivery, thereafter falling gradually to prepregnant levels. Fibrinolytic activity is maximal for about 48 hours after delivery in response to the removal of the placenta, which produces fibrinolytic inhibitors (Lanir et al 2003). Clotting factors, which peaked in labour, gradually decrease. The net result is that the hypercoagulable state of pregnancy is increased in the early puerperium and then slowly returns to a prepregnant state over a few weeks.

In previous eras, wealthy women were advised to rest in bed after childbirth and received indulgent cosseting (Hytten 1995). However, trials of early ambulation led to early mobility being highly recommended as it facilitates rapid disposal of oedema and optimizes cardiovascular health. Mobilization is essential to optimize venous return and avoid stasis within the vascular bed, in order to minimize the risk of deep vein thrombosis (DVT) formation (see p. 369). Women who are unable to mobilize owing to obstetric complications, such as an LSCS, are given prophylactic treatment as the risks of DVT and complications are much increased. Women are advised to report any discomfort or swelling in the lower legs as this may indicate DVT formation; the risks of DVT progressively diminish.

The cardiovascular system is rendered transiently unstable by delivery owing to the blood loss and the ensuing compensatory mechanisms. During the brief period of instability of fluid balance in the first week after delivery, many women experience headaches. Initially there is a marked increase in cardiac output as the uteroplacental flow is returned to the venous system and the gravid uterus no longer impedes the vena cava blood flow. This is augmented by the mobilization of extracellular fluid. Although pregnant women are normally able to tolerate normal blood lost at delivery, those women who had decreased vascular expansion during pregnancy, such as those with preeclampsia (see Ch. 11), may be less able to tolerate blood loss. Vaginal delivery is associated with a higher haemoglobin concentration than operative deliveries because vaginal delivery tends to have less blood loss and to promote diuresis more markedly (Blackburn 2003).

Parameters of the cardiovascular system return towards prepregnant values but remain significantly different. Resolution of ventricular hypertrophy is slow. Vascular remodelling of pregnancy persists for at least a year after delivery and is enhanced by second and subsequent pregnancies (Clapp & Capeless 1997). Because circulating blood volume and cardiac output fall early in the puerperium and the hypertrophied ventricle is slowly remodelled, the stroke volume remains relatively high. This means that heart rate falls in the puerperium, as the stroke volume contributes proportionately more to the decreased cardiac output. Thus it is normal for puerperal women to exhibit bradycardia (a reduced pulse rate of about 60–70 beats per minute). A raised pulse may indicate severe anaemia, venous thrombosis or infection (see below).

Case study 14.2

Prior to delivery Megan had a haemoglobin (Hb) concentration of 10.1 g/dl. At delivery, her blood loss is estimated at around 1000 ml. The midwife is quite concerned over this although Megan was asymptomatic. Prior to discharge on day 3, Megan's Hb concentration is rechecked and is estimated at being 9.8 g/dl.

- How can you account for the Megan's Hb concentration being relatively stable despite her suffering a postpartum haemorrhage?
- What advice/treatment would you give to Megan following her discharge?

Respiratory system

The decreased progesterone concentration following delivery of the placenta restores prepregnant sensitivity to carbon dioxide concentration so partial pressures of carbon dioxide return to prepregnant levels. The diaphragm can increase its excursion distance once the gravid uterus no longer impedes it so full ventilation of the basal lobes of the lung is possible. Chest wall compliance, tidal volume and respiratory rate return to normal within 1–3 weeks.

Urinary system

It is important that bladder function is assessed in the early postnatal period. The trauma experienced by the bladder during delivery usually results in oedema and hyperaemia of the bladder, which has reduced muscle tone in pregnancy. Effects on the bladder are increased by prolonged labour, use of forceps, analgesia and anaesthetic procedures and pressure of the descending presenting part during delivery. The resulting transient loss of bladder sensation, which may result in overdistension and incomplete emptying, can last from days to weeks. Bladder changes are associated with increased risk of urinary tract infections in the puerperium. Trauma to the sphincter of the bladder increases the frequency of stress incontinence, which is marked by urine leakage occurring with coughing, laughing, sudden movement or exercise.

If bladder function is impaired, an indwelling catheter may be inserted to enable the damaged tissue to recover; however, catheterization itself increases the risk of a urinary tract infection (UTI). If the uterus can be palpated high up or is displaced over to one side following the woman voiding urine, this indicates that there is retention of urine as the full bladder displaces the uterus. This is compounded by the increased diuresis that occurs in the postnatal period due to the reduction of the increased plasma volume acquired during pregnancy. It is normal for women to have frequency of micturition as long as they are voiding large amounts of urine each time. Frequency involving just small amounts of urine being voided may indicate a degree of urinary retention.

Pain associated with micturition may indicate a UTI. Dilation of the ureters, overdistension of the bladder and instrumental or operative deliveries all increase the risk of infection. By day 10, full bladder function should be observed and assessed; there should be no evidence of unprovoked urinary incontinence.

Parameters of the renal system, such as renal plasma flow, glomerular filtration rate and plasma creatinine, are back to normal non-pregnant levels by the 6-week check. Urinary excretion of mineral and vitamins is normal within the first week after delivery. Plasma renin and angiotensin levels adjust to the loss of fetal hormones affecting their control so levels fall and then increase before returning back to normal (Blackburn 2003). This fluctuation in hormone levels affecting water retention, together with the redistribution of body fluid, results in rapid and sustained natriuresis and diuresis, which is particularly marked between the 2nd and 5th day after delivery. Fluid and electrolyte balance is normal with 21 days after delivery. Oxytocin, which has antidiuretic hormone (ADH)-like activity, falls after delivery, augmenting diuresis. The voiding volume increases and many women experience night sweats in the puerperium, which also increase fluid loss. Pregnancy-induced changes in the urinary system may persist for several months. Although the dilated smooth muscle of the urinary tract appears normal within a week of delivery, it remains potentially distensible. The kidneys return to their prepregnant size within 6 months of pregnancy.

Gastrointestinal system and defecation

During labour, gastric motility is reduced, particularly in association with pain, fear and narcotic drugs. The reduced tone of the lower oesophageal sphincter, reduced gastric motility and increased gastric acidity result in delayed gastric emptying. The tone and pressure of the lower oesophageal sphincter are normal by 6 weeks after delivery. However, in the early puerperium, the reduced gastrointestinal muscle tone and motility and the relaxed abdomen can increase gas distension and constipation immediately after delivery.

The first bowel movements usually occur within 2 or 3 days following delivery. This may become complicated by the presence of haemorrhoids, which are associated with evacuation problems. Haemorrhoids are common during late pregnancy because of the effects of progesterone on vascular smooth muscle tone. Usually haemorrhoids resolve quickly after birth and cause only minor discomfort in the postnatal period. Sometimes, particularly if they are severe, owing to displacement by the passage of the present-ing part through the birth canal, they can become traumatized and localized thrombosis can occur. This can be further complicated if constipation develops and the woman, because of perineal trauma, resists opening her bowels. Problems with constipation are increased by intestinal atony, lax abdominal muscula-ture, irregular food intake and dehydration in labour. By day 10, the woman should have achieved normal bowel function. Faecal incontinence may indicate anal sphincter damage or inadequate repair.

Fig. 14.5 *Carunculae myrtiformes. (Reproduced with permission from Miller & Hanretty 1998.)*

Weight change

Although weight is lost at delivery of the products of conception, many women experience a weight gain in the first couple of days following delivery. This is due to a combination of increased adrenocorticotrophin (ACTH), ADH and stress, all of which increase sodium and water retention. Women who have a higher blood loss at delivery tend to gain slightly more weight during the early days of the puerperium as water is retained for compensatory expansion of their blood volume. Weight usually starts to fall from the 4th day after delivery as diuresis increases. Weight is lost steadily, usually over a period of several months. Postpartum weight retention is affected by changes in lifestyle during and after pregnancy rather than by pregnancy itself (Ohlin & Rossner 1994). Weight loss tends to be greater with lower parity, maternal age and lower prepregnant weight. Lactation and maternal nutrition affect the rate of weight loss (see Ch. 16).

Other structural changes

Immediately after delivery, the vagina is smooth, soft and oedematous. The elasticity of the tissue returns within a few days. As the vagina is extremely well vas-cularized, episiotomies and tears usually heal well. The rugae of the vagina re-form in the third week but are less prominent than prior to pregnancy. The labia regress to a less prominent and fleshy state than in nul-liparous women. The fall in oestrogen at delivery results in the vaginal epithelium becoming thinner and many women experience problems with vaginal lubrication immediately after delivery. Tags of the hymen remain and are renamed carunculae myrtiformes (Fig. 14.5).

Pelvic floor muscle strength and neuromuscular control are impaired to a greater extent in women who deliver vaginally and experience more mechanical trauma, particularly in the first week of the puer-perium (Peschers et al 1997); however, for most women, muscular tone and strength are normal within 2 months. Weakened circumvaginal muscles are asso-ciated with perineal outcome, episiotomy, length of second stage of labour, the weight of the baby and pushing techniques (Cosner et al 1991). Problems associated with a lax ineffective pelvic floor such as uterine prolapse, urinary incontinence and prolapse of the rectum are more likely as parity increases. Pelvic floor exercises help to restore the muscle tone and function of the pelvic floor; specialist advice from an obstetric physiotherapist may be required for persist-ent problems with incontinence.

The abdominal wall may remain soft and flabby for several weeks. Severe stretching, for instance in a mul-tiple pregnancy or with polyhydramnios, can result in permanently lax muscles. The softened pelvic joints and ligaments slowly return to normal over a period of a few months. Relaxation of pelvic joints may cause backache in the puerperium. The striae gravidarum become paler over a period of several months but fade rather than completely disappear.

Pregnancy-induced changes in the skin sponta-neously regress or fade. Hair loss may be marked fol-lowing delivery and initial regrowth may be initially less abundant. Corneal sensitivity and pressure return to normal within 2 months of delivery. Nasal conges-tion and effects on the ear and larynx are restored to prepregnant status within a few days of delivery.

Body temperature

In the first 24 hours following delivery, body temper-ature may increase slightly (to 38°C) in response to the stress of labour, particularly dehydration. This temperature fluctuation is normally transient; a persistent raised temperature may indicate infection (see below).

Sleep

The puerperium is associated with disrupted sleep patterns, particularly immediately after delivery (Swain et al 1997). The first 3 days can be extremely difficult for the mother compounded by fatigue accumulated during labour and being unable to rest comfortably due to perineal pain (see Case study 14.3). Postpartum perineal pain correlates well with the duration of the second stage of labour (Thranov et al 1990). Euphoria, urinary, breast and perineal discomfort and infant disturbances can all lead to reduced sleep, which may affect memory and psychomotor tasks. Theoretically, sleep patterns are close to normal within 2 or 3 weeks of delivery but breastfeeding mothers obviously have more disrupted sleep (Quillin 1997).

Psychological state

Usually by day 10 the mother and baby have established a feeding cycle. Although fatigue is common and normal, the mother should be developing strategies to cope with this, such as daytime sleeps. The mother should be independently caring for herself and the baby and interacting fully with members of her family and other people. Offspring provide their mothers with stimuli that elicit behavioural responses and emotional reactions;

comparative studies suggest that these nurturing responses are evolutionarily conserved (Stern 1997).

Many women experience a lack of libido (sex drive) during the first few months following delivery. This may be complicated by trauma to the reproductive tract during delivery. Sexual desire, expression and satisfaction may be reduced after delivery. Sexual activity may be affected by fatigue, altered body image, marital adjustment, dyspareunia, lactation, traditional taboos, vaginal bleeding or discharge, insufficient lubrication or fear of waking the baby.

Return to fertility

In pregnancy, ovarian function is suppressed by the high level of placental steroids. Women who do not breastfeed begin to menstruate, on average, about 55–60 days after delivery and to ovulate at about 40–50 days after delivery (Wang & Fraser 1994), whereas lactation can delay ovulation to 30–40 weeks after delivery and menstruation to 8–15 months, depending on the duration and extent of breastfeeding. Although ovarian activity is almost invariably suspended, there have been reported cases of women who conceive within 2 weeks of giving birth (Hytten 1995). The return to fertility exhibits similar hormonal profiles as puberty with a circadian pattern of LH secretion. A proportion of women become pregnant during lactational amenorrhoea but the degree of suppression of fertility depends on infant-feeding patterns and perhaps on maternal nutrition. Lactational effects on fertility are reduced as the spaces between the feeds increase and as the baby receives supplementary feeding. Where the number of sucking episodes is 10–20 per day, as is normal in many developing countries, resumption of ovarian activity is unlikely. With 5–6 feeds per day, the duration of feeds is important in suppressing ovulation. However, lactational amenorrhoea appears to reduce the likelihood of conception for a few months (Lewis et al 1991), although it is probably more successful in achieving birth spacing.

Many women purposely choose to limit the number of children they wish to have. There are many economical and social issues that impinge on this; however, it is important to recognize that there are some women for whom certain (or all) methods of contraception are not acceptable on cultural and religious grounds. The return of fertility is very difficult to assess as factors such as breastfeeding, cultural and religious practice, genetic variation and disease may

---

Case study 14.3

Sandra is a first-time mother who delivered a healthy male infant 3 days ago. She went home on the day of the birth as she appeared to be coping well with breastfeeding and caring for her infant. The community midwife visits at lunchtime on the 3rd day to find a very distressed mother, partner and infant. They have had no sleep and the baby has been very fractious and wakeful.

- What are the possible physiological causes that have contributed to this situation?
- What would reassure the midwife that everything was normal and what support, help and advice could the midwife give to the family during this difficult period?

all compound the identification of return of the fertility cycle. It is important to emphasize that ovulation precedes menstruation so amenorrhoea does not guarantee the absence of fertility.

The role of the midwife

In the UK, most women are discharged from midwifery care by day 10; however, the midwife may visit up to day 28 in the postnatal period if required. Once the midwife is satisfied that the physiological transition is progressing normally then the discharge can be completed. The health visitor and general practitioner (GP) continue care of the mother and baby. The responsibilities of the midwife in the puerperium and at discharge include giving advice to women on a number of issues including infant-feeding, parentcraft, pelvic floor exercises, contraception and sources of psychological support.

Complications of the puerperium

Thromboembolic disorders

The increase in potential clot formation can have a physiological disadvantage both in pregnancy and following delivery because thrombi (blood clots) can form within the venous system. During the third trimester, the pregnant woman develops a state of hypercoagulation, such that her blood is more likely to clot than it would in the non-pregnant state and the effects of progesterone on venous muscle tone increase stasis of flow. The risk of thromboembolic disorders in pregnancy is about six times higher than previously, and increases further in the puerperium. This is enhanced by a decrease in fibrinolytic activity (the breakdown of fibrin forming a blood clot) and raised concentration of clotting factors. This tendency of the blood to clot more readily imparts a physiological advantage to the woman to prevent excess blood loss during and immediately after delivery of the placenta and membranes. Haemoconcentration of the blood from physiological diuresis following delivery augments the increase in clotting factors.

Thrombophlebitis

Thrombophlebitis is inflammation due to the formation of a thrombus (clot) in a superficial vein. The commonest site of thrombus formation is in the saphenous vein supplying the calf of the leg. Symptoms include a tender reddened area over the thrombosed vein and possibly a small increase in pulse and temperature. Motility and elevating the legs at rest reduce the risk of thrombus formation; compression stockings may be helpful. Thrombophlebitis is unlikely to progress to pulmonary embolism.

Deep vein thrombosis

DVT is less common but carries the risk of a clot dislodging, which can cause pulmonary embolism. Hypercoagulability is increased with increased maternal age, parity, dehydration following delivery and delivery by caesarean section. Risk factors include immobility, pelvic or leg trauma, obesity, pre-eclampsia, caesarean section, instrument-assisted delivery, haemorrhage, multiparity, varicose veins, a previous history of a thromboembolic event and hereditary or acquired thrombophilias (Colman-Brochu 2004). It has been observed clinically that there is an increased risk of DVT in the left leg, especially after a caesarean section, because blood flow velocity is reduced to a greater extent (Macklon & Greer 1997). DVT may cause no symptoms or the woman may experience pain and swelling over the affected area and occasionally pyrexia. There may be marked differences in calf size or, in extreme cases, circulation to the leg below the thrombosis may be affected so the leg appears cold and white and possibly oedematous. DVT is confirmed by Doppler ultrasound or impedance plethysmography.

Pulmonary embolism

Pulmonary embolism (PE) is an obstetric emergency that may follow DVT or occur without warning. PE is a condition that contributes towards maternal mortality associated with pregnancy. If a thrombus (a fragment of the blood clot) breaks away and enters the venous system, it is then carried in the venous system to the right side of the heart and the pulmonary circulation. As the pulmonary arteries reduce in size, the thrombus may occlude arterial vessels within the lungs, causing major damage. Symptoms are sudden collapse, acute severe chest pain, dyspnoea, cyanosis, haemoptysis and shock. A woman with a PE will require intensive treatment and care. A PE is more common in the postnatal period compared to the antepartum period. This may be due to the physiological reversal of haemodilution happening much faster (usually by day 3) than the physiological reversal of increased clotting factors which may take up to 6 weeks to return to prepregnancy values.

Women assessed to be at increased risk of thrombus formation are treated with prophylactic anticoagulants, such as heparin and synthetic analogues such as enoxaparin. DVT is usually treated with heparin and, if required, long-term anticoagulation therapy with drugs such as warfarin is commenced. Warfarin use in pregnancy is contraindicated as it is transported across the placenta; but postnatal women who choose to breastfeed can have warfarin treatment as it not secreted in significant levels in the breast milk.

Risk of infection

In the puerperium, the woman is at increased risk of infection, particularly that associated with the genital tract, urinary system, breast and any site of thrombophlebitis. The placental wound site, lacerations and incisions of the perineum and the lax urinary system are especially vulnerable. The lochia provides ideal culture conditions for microorganisms. Other predisposing factors include anaemia, fatigue, malnutrition, traumatic delivery and the presence of retained tissue in the uterus. Both maternal and neonatal infection (see Ch. 15) may be caused by endogenous or exogenous organisms (Box 14.4).

Symptoms of infection include pyrexia (up to 40°C), tachycardia (up to 140 beats per minute), subinvolution of the uterus, headache, malaise, lower abdominal pain and heavy offensive-smelling lochia. Infection in the acute phase can inhibit lactation. When choosing antibiotics to treat infection in the puerperium one needs to take into consideration whether the woman is breastfeeding and the potential effect of the transfer of the drug into breastmilk.

Box 14.4

Examples of microorganisms causing puerperal infection

Endogenous
- *Escherichia coli*
- *Clostridium perfringens*
- *Streptococcus faecalis*
- *Pseudomonas aeruginosa*

Exogenous
- β-Haemolytic streptococci
- *Staphylococcus aureus*

Breast discomfort and after-pains

The establishment of lactation is covered in detail in Chapter 16; however, it is worth mentioning here two common problems that can occur during this period in relation to breastfeeding.

- If the baby has been incorrectly positioned, often because it is fractious or hungry and wanting to feed constantly, the nipple may become sore, cracked and bleed as a consequence. A break in the integrity of the nipple skin increases the risk of mastitis (localized and ascending infection usually caused by *Staphylococcus aureus*). Women experiencing early feeding problems need a lot of help and support. The baby needs to 'fix' or 'latch on' properly in order to provide adequate nipple stimulation to establish the feeding cycle.
- Sometimes the breasts become engorged or extended. Initially this may be a venous cause due to the increased vascularization of the breast. However, when milk production increases (described as the milk 'coming in'), the breast may initially be overproductive. The breasts may overfill with milk causing them to become distended and hardened, which may be uncomfortable or painful. The baby may need help achieving an appropriate position; however, once the feeding cycle is established the demand/supply balance is achieved and the breast engorgement problems will resolve.

Pharmacological effects

The majority of deliveries within the UK have the third stage actively managed as opposed to passive or physiological management where the women delivers the placenta naturally (see Ch. 13). However, the administration of an anti-tocolytic (or 'uterotonic') drug such as Syntometrine (which contains ergometrine and oxytocin) may cause side-effects following completion of the third stage; for example:

- nausea and vomiting
- transient rise in blood pressure
- palpitations and tachycardia
- chest pain
- headache.

Also during the early puerperium, women may suffer side-effects from pharmacological methods of pain relief administered during labour. Pethidine may induce drowsiness, fatigue and nausea within the mother and reduce the suckling instinct of the infant, thus interfering with feeding. The effects of an epidural anaesthetic may take several hours to wear off, which affects maternal mobility and the ability to void urine.

Psychological problems

Women in the postpartum period have increased vulnerability to affective disorders which are classified on the basis of severity, such as postpartum 'blues', postpartum depression and postpartum psychosis. It is estimated that as many as 80% of women may experience some fluctuations in mood, mostly transient emotional disorders at about day 3 described as 'the blues' (Steiner 1998). 10–20% of puerperal women develop true depressive illness, which may have a later onset (or referral) and delayed recovery. A few women (0.1–0.2%) develop severe prolonged psychotic illness following childbirth. Although many of these cases may be recognized in the early postnatal period, some become evident much later. Certain symptoms are recognized to be important in the diagnosis of postnatal depression (Box 14.5). These figures mean that postnatal depression is the most common disorder of the puerperium.

The aetiology of these depressive disorders is not fully understood. Immediately after delivery, the infant may feed often and this may be increased at night adding to maternal fatigue. Initially the mother's fatigue is overcome by intense feelings of relief and excitement at the birth of her baby. By day 3, however, the woman may become emotional, tearful and tired and need a lot of support and comfort during this period. This low ebb of hormonal withdrawal is physiologically marked by the commencement of full lactogenesis following the

initial production of small volumes of colostrum (see Ch. 16). The 'blues' coincide with lactation, breast engorgement, perineal pain and wound discomfort.

As the withdrawal of steroid hormones has been postulated to have a role in the aetiology of postnatal depression, clinical trials have investigated whether either progesterone or oestrogen supplementation might be of prophylactic or therapeutic value in postnatal depression. Some uncontrolled studies (e.g. Dalton 1980) reported the benefit of progesterone in preventing postnatal depression. However, use of synthetic progesterone is positively associated with depression in the postnatal period and should be used with caution (Karuppaswamy & Vlies 2003).

Oestrogen has also been associated with psychological well-being (Brace & McCauley 1997); sudden changes in oestrogen levels such as those experienced in the puerperium may result in effects on neurotransmitter release. Oestrogen therapy may be of modest value in severe postnatal depression but more research is needed.

Other authors suggest that levels of cortisol or β-endorphin have a stronger association with postnatal depression (Harris et al 1996). The hypothalamic–pituitary–adrenal (HPA) axis is very active in the third trimester as placental corticotrophin-releasing hormone (CRH) production increases and CRH-binding protein (CRH-BP) levels fall. Suppression of hypothalamic CRH secretion is implicated in the aetiology of postnatal depression (Magiakou et al 1996). The relationship between breastfeeding and postnatal depression is controversial. However, hormones involved in lactation affect cortisol levels (Amico et al 1994). Lactation may also predispose the breastfeeding mother to depression by isolating her and increasing levels of fatigue. Women who develop postnatal depression make a good recovery with the right treatment and support. Exercise programmes have been found to decrease anxiety and depression in the puerperium significantly (Koltyn & Schultes 1997). The recurrence of postnatal depression is high, which allows identification of women at increased risk. It has been suggested that women who have a low intake of fish (and omega-3 fatty acids) are more likely to suffer from postnatal depression (Hibbeln 2002). Certainly the high docosahexaenoic acid (DHA) requirements of the fetus and for breastmilk may deplete women. There is no evidence that dietary treatment of postnatal depression is successful.

Case study 14.4 describes an example of a hormonal complication of the puerperium.

Box 14.5

Classic signs of postnatal depression

- Depressed mood
- Sleep disturbance not related to discomfort and infant wakening
- Unable to cope—guilt
- Thoughts of harming self or baby
- Rejection of baby
- Altered libido
- Anxiety

Case study 14.4

At delivery Lucy suffered a large haemorrhage that was difficult to control; she finally underwent a hysterectomy following a total blood loss of over 4 litres. Her recovery was uneventful but within 6 months she was diagnosed as suffering from Sheehan's syndrome—necrosis of the pituitary gland.

- What would her symptoms be?
- What endocrine function would be disrupted as a result of this condition?

Application to practice

In comparison to pregnancy, when the changes induced by endocrine effects are at a relatively slow pace, the reversal of this in the puerperium is much more dramatic. These rapid changes occur at the same time as another endocrine-induced change resulting in the initiation of lactation.

Fatigue from labour, perineal pain from trauma and the demands of a newborn infant can also complicate the situation.

The midwife needs to use her knowledge of the puerperium to support women through this often difficult period of adaptation.

Annotated further reading

Abbott H, Bick D, McArthur C 1997 Health after birth. In: Henderson C, Jones K (eds) Essential midwifery. Mosby, St Louis
Describes the postnatal period and the care required for the mother and baby from a health perspective.

Hytten F 1995 The clinical physiology of the puerperium. Farrand Press
This comprehensive reference text covers the postnatal adjustments of each physiological system referring to sociology and cultural history as well as the clinical implications.

Greer IA 2003 Prevention of venous thromboembolism in pregnancy. Best Practice & Research Clinical Haematology 16(2):261–278
A recent review about pulmonary thromboembolism, the major cause of maternal death in developed countries, which discusses risk factors and clinical management.

Hussein J, Fortney JA 2004 Puerperal sepsis and maternal mortality: what role can new technologies play? International Journal of Gynecology & Obstetrics 85(Suppl 1):S52–S61
A practical review of infection-control protocols and evidence-based procedures such as use of prophylactic antibiotics for caesarean section or preterm rupture of membranes, hand rubs, needle-disposal systems, and rapid microbiological diagnostic tests in sepsis management.

Kennedy KI 2002 Efficacy and effectiveness of LAM. Advances in Experimental Medicine and Biology 503: 207–216
A review covering issues surrounding the efficacy and effectiveness of the lactational amenorrhoea method of

Key points

- Maternal physiology and anatomy adapt rapidly to the withdrawal of steroid hormones, following the delivery of the placenta. These dramatic physiological changes increase the risk of infection, haemorrhage and psychological and emotional changes.

- The uterus rapidly involutes after delivery; normal involution can be monitored by assessment of fundal height and characteristics of the lochia.

- After delivery, there is a dramatic and rapid decrease in circulating blood volume followed by a return to normal cardiovascular parameters. As stroke volume initially remains high, bradycardia is usual, particularly in the first 2 weeks.

- The postpartum physiological changes allow the woman to tolerate considerable blood loss at delivery, but alteration in clotting factor concentration and venous stasis predispose the woman to thromboembolic disorders; the risk is enhanced by immobility and sepsis.

- Marked diuresis is normal in the puerperium but overdistension, or decreased sensitivity, of the bladder can predispose the woman to urinary problems.

- Ovulation occurs before menstruation and is delayed by breastfeeding; lactational amenorrhoea is useful in birth spacing rather than being a reliable method of contraception.

contraception (LAM) and discussed in the context of existing information from industrialized countries.

Royal College of Obstetricians and Gynaecologists 2004 Thromboprophylaxis during pregnancy, labour and after vaginal delivery. Guideline 37. RCOG, London
Clinical guidance and management for the prevention of venous thromboembolism.

Sibai BM 2004 Diagnosis, controversies, and management of the syndrome of haemolysis, elevated liver enzymes, and low platelet count. Obstetrics and Gynecology 103 (5 Pt 1): 981–991
A review of observational studies and randomized trials for the HELLP syndrome, together with recommendations for diagnosis, identification of risk factors and treatment of women with this syndrome.

Varner MW 1998 Medical conditions of the puerperium. Clinics in Perinatology 25:403–416
This article reviews the physiological and emotional changes that occur during the puerperium and the clinical management of common problems such as infection and haemorrhage.

References

Amico JA, Johnston JM, Vagnucci AH 1994 Suckling-induced attenuation of plasma cortisol concentrations in postpartum lactating women. Endocrinology Research 20:79–87

Blackburn ST 2003 Maternal, fetal, and neonatal physiology: a clinical perspective, 2nd edn. Saunders, Philadelphia

Brace M, McCauley E 1997 Oestrogens and psychological well-being. Annals of Medicine 29:283–290

Clapp JF, Capeless E 1997 Cardiovascular function before, during, and after the first and subsequent pregnancies. American Journal of Cardiology 80:1469–1473

Colman-Brochu S 2004 Deep vein thrombosis in pregnancy. MCN: American Journal of Maternal Child Nursing 29(3):186–192

Cosner KR, Dougherty MC, Bishop KR 1991 Dynamic characteristics of the circumvaginal muscles during pregnancy and the postpartum. Journal of Nurse-Midwifery 36:221–225

Dalton K 1980 Depression after childbirth. OUP, Oxford

Harris B, Lovett L, Smith J, Read G, Walker R, Newcombe R 1996 Cardiff puerperal mood and hormone study III: postnatal depression at 5 to 6 weeks postpartum, and its hormonal correlates across the peripartum period. British Journal of Psychology 168:739–744

Hibbeln JR 2002 Seafood consumption, the DHA content of mothers' milk and prevalence rates of postpartum depression: a cross-national, ecological analysis. Journal of Affective Disorders 69(1–3):15–29

Howie PW 1995 The physiology of the puerperium and lactation. In: Chamberlain G (ed) Turnbull's obstetrics, 2nd edn. Churchill Livingstone, New York

Hytten F 1995 The clinical physiology of the puerperium. Farand Press

Karuppaswamy J, Vlies R 2003 The benefit of oestrogens and progestogens in postnatal depression. Journal of Obstetrics and Gynaecology 23(4):341–346

Koltyn KF, Schultes SS 1997 Psychological effects of an aerobic exercise session and rest session following pregnancy. Journal of Sports Medicine and Physical Fitness 37:287–291

Lanir N, Aharon A, Brenner B 2003 Haemostatic mechanisms in human placenta. Best Practice & Research Clinical Haematology 16(2):183–195

Letsky E 1998 The haematological system. In: Chamberlain G, Broughton Pipkin F (eds) Clinical physiology in obstetrics, 3rd edn. Blackwell, Oxford

Lewis PR, Brown JB, Renfree MB, Short RV 1991 The resumption of ovulation and menstruation in a well-nourished population of women breastfeeding for an extended period of time. Fertility and Sterility 55:529–536

Macklon NS, Greer IA 1997 The deep venous system in the puerperium: an ultrasound study. British Journal of Obstetrics and Gynaecology 104:198–200

Magiakou MA, Mastorakos G, Rabin D, Dubbert B, Gold PW, Chrousos GP 1996 Hypothalamic corticotrophin-releasing hormone suppression during the postpartum period: implications for the increase in psychiatric manifestations at this time. Journal of Clinical Endocrinology and Metabolism 81(5):1912–1917

Miller AWF, Hanretty KP 1998 Obstetrics illustrated, 5th edn. Churchill Livingstone, New York, p 336

Ohlin A, Rossner S 1994 Trends in eating patterns, physical activity and socio-demographic factors in relation to postpartum body weight development. British Journal of Nutrition 71:457–470

Peschers UM, Schaer GN, DeLancey JO, Schuessler B 1997 Levator ani function before and after childbirth. British Journal of Obstetrics and Gynaecology 104:1004–1008

Quillin SL 1997 Infant and mother sleep patterns during the 4th postpartum week. Issues in Comparable Pediatric Nursing 20:115–123

Richter C, Huch A, Huch R 1995 Erythropoiesis in the postpartum period. Journal of Perinatal Medicine 23:51–59

Salamonsen LA 2003 Tissue injury and repair in the female human reproductive tract. Reproduction 125(3):301–311

Steiner M 1998 Perinatal mood disorders: position paper. Psychopharmacology Bulletin 34(3):301–306

Stern JM 1997 Offspring-induced nuturance: animal–human parallels. Developmental Psychobiology 31:19–37

Stone PJ, Franzblau C 1995 Increase in urinary desmoline and pyridoline during postpartum involution of the uterus in humans. Proceedings of the Society for Experimental Biology and Medicine 210:39–42

Swain AM, O'Hara MW, Starr KR, Gorman LL 1997 A prospective study of sleep, mood, and cognitive function in postpartum and nonpostpartum women. Obstetrics and Gynecology 90:381–386

Sweet B, Tiran D 1996 Mayes' midwifery, 12th edn. Baillière Tindall, London, pp 405, 406

Tekay A, Jouppila P 1993 A longitudinal Doppler ultrasonographic assessment of the alterations in peripheral vascular resistance of uterine arteries and ultrasonographic findings of the involuting uterus during the puerperium. American Journal of Obstetrics and Gynecology 168:190–198

Thranov I, Kringelbachh AM, Melchior E, Olsen O, Damsgaard MT 1990 Postpartum symptoms: episiotomy or tear at vaginal delivery. Acta Obstetrica et Gynecologica Scandinavica 69:11–15

Wang IY, Fraser IS 1994 Reproductive function and contraception in the postpartum period. Obstetrical and Gynecological Survey 49:56–63

The transition to neonatal life

Learning objectives

■ To identify the key steps in the transition to successful neonatal life.

■ To describe the vulnerability of the neonate, with particular reference to the potential risk of respiratory problems, jaundice and hypoglycaemia.

■ To outline the principles of thermoregulation in the newborn.

■ To compare the fetal and neonatal circulatory and respiratory systems, describing the transition stages.

■ To describe factors relating to the neonatal gastrointestinal, renal and nervous systems that make breast milk the ideal food.

Introduction

During fetal life, the placenta carries out the crucial physiological roles of gas exchange, nutrition, elimination of waste products and additional aspects of circulation. Within minutes of birth, the placental support ceases so the baby's own cardiovascular, respiratory, gastrointestinal, renal and metabolic systems must function independently. The transition from fetal to neonatal life needs to be smooth, swift and successful; the majority of infant deaths occur within the neonatal period (first 28 days) (Bernal et al 1993) and these are linked to inadequate progression to neonatal physiological functions.

The transition to extrauterine life depends on the degree of maturation in late gestation, the process of delivery itself and establishment of independent physiological processes for regulating homeostasis after placental separation. These physiological processes include establishing continuous respiration, changing from a parallel to a serial circulatory organization and ceasing the right-to-left shunting, establishing oral feeding and independent thermoregulation and glucose homeostasis (Gluckman et al 1999).

The process of birth is physiologically stressful with fluctuations in placental blood flow resulting in a degree of hypoxia and respiratory acidosis. Increased secretion of adrenal catecholamines, stimulation of the sympathetic nervous system and the subsequent mobilization of glycogen and lipid stores are fundamental in the activation of essential physiological mechanisms that result in an alert and active baby at birth. However, a prolonged or difficult delivery and marked hypoxia/anoxia and acidosis can result in an overstressed or seriously asphyxiated baby.

Both the fetus and the neonate can tolerate degrees of hypoxia and anoxia that would result in serious morbidity or mortality in an adult. The neonate retains the capability to divert a considerable proportion of its cardiac output to the brain thus protecting it. Although the brain is vulnerable to hypoxia, the compensatory mechanisms can increase tolerance to hypoxic states (Parer 1998). However, severe asphyxia can cause cerebral microhaemorrhages resulting in a spectrum of damage from impaired intellectual development to spasticity and irreversible brain damage.

Although there is usually a good correlation between gestational length and degree of maturity, infants affected by intrauterine growth retardation (IUGR) may have precocious organ development because undernutrition and the resulting fetal stress promote increased fetal cortisol secretion thus enhancing fetal organ maturation. In humans, fetal cortisol appears not to have a role in inducing labour as has been demonstrated in other species (see Ch. 13). The major problems of premature infants can be attributed to a shorter duration of glucocorticoid exposure (even though fetal stress results in actual levels being higher); this results in an increased risk of persistent fetal circulation, increased likelihood of lung immaturity and respiratory diseases syndrome and immaturity of thermoregulatory responses, the gastrointestinal system and enzymes involved in maintaining glucose homeostasis.

The glucocorticoid system is pivotal in the preparation for birth (Gluckman et al 1999). Fetal cortisol levels rise from about 35 weeks. Glucocorticoids influence surfactant production and maturation of the alveoli and other respiratory tissue thus promoting lung maturation. They also induce hepatic gluconeogenesis enzymes by promoting adrenaline synthesis (and potential effective response to stress), inducing hormone receptors and affecting thyroid hormone synthesis. Fetal corticotrophin-releasing factor (CRF) and antidiuretic hormone (ADH) and placental CRF orchestrate the increase in fetal cortisol production, which influence adrenocorticotrophin (ACTH) production by the maturing fetal pituitary gland; increased ACTH stimulates cortisol production.

At birth, there are also changes in the regulation of growth. Fetal growth is substrate-limited and actively constrained to optimize successful delivery (see Ch. 9). The prenatal rise in gluco-corticoids also induces growth hormone receptors and changes in expression of insulin-like growth factor I (IGF-I).

Chapter case study

The midwife officially recorded Zak as having an Apgar score of 9 at approximately 1 minute of age. Following the delivery James was surprised how alert Zak was, that he seemed to be aware of his surroundings and appeared to be actively looking around. What factors could have contributed to Zak's behaviour and what are the possible explanations for Zak being so alert following his delivery?

The cardiovascular system

Blood

Before birth

Fetal blood (Table 15.1) is structurally and functionally different to adult blood; it contains larger and more numerous erythrocytes (red blood cells) with a higher haemoglobin content which maximizes their uptake of oxygen (Palis & Segel 1998). Fetal haemoglobin with its two α-chains and two γ-chains has a higher affinity for oxygen in the slightly more acid fetal environment. Less-effective binding of 2,3-bisphosphoglycerate (or 2,3-diphosphoglycerate) means that the oxygen–haemoglobin dissociation curve of the fetus and neonate is shifted to the left (Fig. 15.1). Shifts of pH in the placenta further increase both dissociation of oxygen from maternal haemoglobin and its uptake by fetal haemoglobin. This means that, although fetal haemoglobin has an increased oxygen take-up, it is less efficient at releasing oxygen to the tissues.

At term, the ratio of fetal haemoglobin to adult haemoglobin (HbF:HbA) is 80:20; by 6 months production of the β-chain replaces the γ-chain so the ratio is 1:99 (Fig. 15.2). Preterm infants tend to have an even higher HbF level and a decreased 2,3-bisphosphoglycerate concentration therefore oxygen unloading at the tissue level is even less efficient. The raised levels of HbF in the neonate mean that haemoglobinopathies caused by altered synthesis of β-chains (such as β-thalassaemia) or altered structure of β-chains (such as sickle-cell anaemia) are not evident immediately at birth but manifest themselves when the infant is at least 2 months old. It is possible to detect fetal blood cells in the maternal circulation, an observation that is utilized in the management of Rhesus incompatibility (see Ch. 10) (Lamvu & Kuller 1997).

Table 15.1   *Fetal and adult blood*

	Fetal/neonatal	Adult
Blood volume	80–100 ml/kg 90–105 ml/kg (preterm)	75 ml/kg
Red blood cell number	6–7 × 10⁶/ml	female: 4.8 × 10⁶/ml male: 5.4 × 10⁶/ml
Haemoglobin content	20.7 g/dl	female: 14 g/dl male: 16 g/dl
Oxygen content of 100 ml saturated blood	21 ml (theory) 13 ml (practice)	16 ml (theory) 15.7 ml (practice)
Red blood cell lifespan	80–100 days 60–80 days (preterm)	120 days
Haemoglobin type	HbF: $\alpha_2\gamma_2$	HbA: $\alpha_2\beta_2$

Note: the theoretical value is the amount of oxygen the blood can be saturated with whereas, in practice, the blood is saturated to a lesser degree because the transfer of oxygen across the placenta is less efficient than the transfer of oxygen across the alveoli.

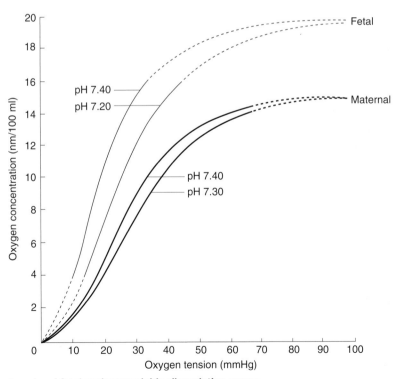

Fig. 15.1   *The maternal and fetal oxyhaemoglobin dissociation curves.*

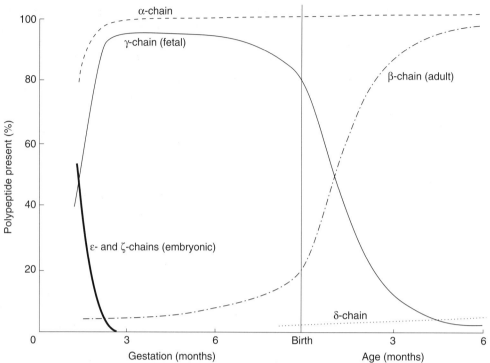

Fig. 15.2 *Changes in fetal:adult haemoglobin (HbF:HbA) ratios in fetal and infant blood. (Reproduced with permission from Begley et al 1978.)*

After birth

At birth, fetal blood has an increased population of nucleated erythrocytes (even more so if the baby has been subjected to increased stress, is immature or has Down's syndrome). For the first 3 months of life, the erythrocytes are more fragile, have an increased metabolism and a shorter half-life and erythropoietin production is suppressed (Box 15.1).

Haemostasis

Neonates, particularly those born prematurely, have an increased risk of haemostatic problems (Andrew 1997). The most common example (Kuehl 1997) is disseminated intravascular coagulation (DIC) due to accelerated inappropriate coagulation, which depletes the body's supply of platelets and clotting factors and paradoxically increases the risk of haemorrhage. Susceptibility is increased because, first, the immature neonatal reticuloendothelial system has a decreased capacity to remove intermediary products of coagulation so they can further stimulate coagulation and consumption of clotting factors, and, second, synthesis of clotting factors by the immature liver is ineffi-

Box 15.1

Physiological anaemia of infancy

Haemopoiesis (red blood cell production) is controlled by the hormone erythropoietin, which increases when oxygen delivery to the kidney is reduced; it stimulates red blood cell production by the bone marrow. The increased oxygen levels inhibit erythropoietin levels in the neonate postnatally (Strauss 1994). Levels remain low for 2–3 months (longer in preterm infants) and then increase, resulting in increased bone marrow activity and red blood cell production. As the neonate appears to tolerate the fall in haemoglobin concentration without ill-effects, it is deemed to be physiological. The haemodilution effects are increased by rapid growth being matched by total blood volume, which precedes any change in red blood cell number.

cient. Vitamin K levels in the neonate are about 50% of adult values, which affects the efficiency of the clotting cascade. Vitamin K levels are low because placental transport of the vitamin is poor and colonization of the gut by bacteria that synthesize vitamin K is not immediate. The consequent reduced level of all vitamin K-dependent clotting factors is associated with an increased bleeding tendency, which can predispose to haemorrhagic disease of the newborn (HDNB) (Box 15.2). Neonatal platelets exhibit decreased aggregation and adhesiveness because their production of thromboxane A_2 (TxA_2) is impaired. This appears to protect the term neonate against thrombosis but to increase the vulnerability to bleeding of the preterm or sick baby. Placental transfer of maternal drugs such as aspirin can affect coagulation in the neonate.

The circulation

Before birth

As the fetal oxygen source is the placenta rather than the lungs, blood in the fetal circulation flows in a circuit that perfuses the placenta and largely bypasses the lungs (Fig. 15.3). In order to do this, the fetal circulation has several additional structures: the umbilical vein, which carries blood rich in oxygen and nutrients

---

Box 15.2

Haemorrhagic disease of the newborn (HDNB)

- Bleeding from the gut, umbilicus, circumcision wounds and oozing from puncture sites
- Evident 2–3 days after birth
- Associated with antibiotics, which affect colonization of the gut with vitamin K-synthesizing bacteria
- Associated with anticonvulsant drugs (e.g. phenobarbitol, diphenylhydantoin), which concentrate in the fetal liver and antagonize the effect of vitamin K
- Associated with maternal warfarin treatment, which decreases levels of vitamin K-dependent clotting factors and prolongs prolonged clotting times
- Prophylactic vitamin K is routinely administered to all babies born in the UK (Hilgartner 1993) but studies have implicated intramuscular vitamin K administration in childhood cancer (Golding et al 1992)
- Term babies respond well to vitamin K therapy but synthesis of clotting factors is further limited in preterm babies by inadequate hepatic synthesis of precursor proteins

---

to the underside of the liver to the ductus venosus (a venosus is a shunt that connects a vein to a vein), which inserts into the inferior umbilical vein en route to the right side of the heart. The hypogastric arteries, which branch off the internal iliac arteries, are contiguous with the umbilical arteries of the umbilical cord, returning blood to the placenta. The lungs are bypassed by two structures: the foramen ovale, which allows blood to move directly from the right atrium to the left, and the ductus arteriosus, which connects the pulmonary arterial trunk to the descending aorta.

The oxygenated and nutrient-enriched blood is taken from the placenta in the umbilical vein that goes through the abdominal wall to the underside of the liver. This is the only unmixed blood and is about 80% saturated with oxygen; the blood goes through the ductus venosus to the inferior vena cava where it mixes with oxygen-depleted blood returning to the heart from the lower body (Fig. 15.4A). The inflows of blood from the inferior and superior venae cavae do not mix thoroughly because of their angle of entry and the shape of the right atrium. Because the entry of the inferior vena cava is aligned with the foramen ovale, most of the blood from the inferior vena cava travels from the right atrium through the foramen ovale into the left atrium and thence to the left ventricle and the ascending aorta.

Most blood entering the right atrium from the superior vena cava passes through the tricuspid valve into the right ventricle and to the pulmonary arterial trunk. The ductus arteriosus is inserted into the vessel at the bifurcation of the right and left pulmonary artery (taking blood to the right and left lung, respectively); it shunts blood from the pulmonary arterial route into the descending aorta. The pulmonary circulation is vasoconstricted and has a high vascular resistance. Only about 10% of the output of the right ventricle continues into the pulmonary circulation; the rest is diverted through the ductus arteriosus. From the descending aorta, the blood supplies the remaining organs and the lower body. The hypogastric arteries branch off the internal iliac arteries and return to the placenta via the umbilical arteries.

The upper body and head are fed from arteries which branch off from the aortic arch before the insertion of the ductus arteriosus and the subsequent mixing of slightly less-well-oxygenated blood. The early branching of the coronary and carotid arteries means the heart and brain receive slightly better oxygenated blood. The advantages conferred by the early branching of the subclavian arteries which supply the upper

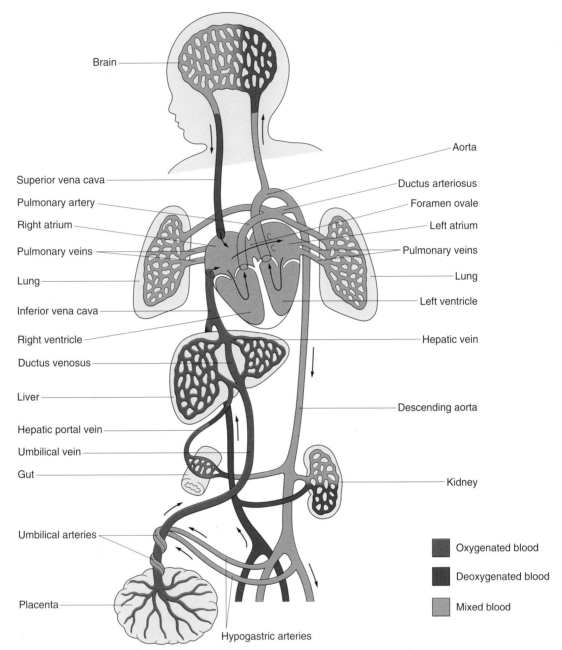

Brain

Aorta

Superior vena cava

Ductus arteriosus

Pulmonary artery

Foramen ovale

Right atrium

Left atrium

Pulmonary veins

Pulmonary veins

Lung

Lung

Inferior vena cava

Left ventricle

Right ventricle

Hepatic vein

Ductus venosus

Liver

Descending aorta

Hepatic portal vein

Umbilical vein

Gut

Kidney

Umbilical arteries

■ Oxygenated blood

■ Deoxygenated blood

■ Mixed blood

Placenta

Hypogastric arteries

Fig. 15.3   *The fetal circulation. (Reproduced with permission from Goodwin 1997.)*

limbs can be illustrated by the enhanced development of arms compared to the legs.

After birth

One of the most important transitional stages in the adaptation to extrauterine life is the establishment of the neonatal circulation. In fetal life, the source of oxygen is the placenta so most of the blood flow bypasses the fetal lungs. At birth, circulation perfuses the lungs and flow through the fetal vascular structures ceases. At birth, these changes that mark the transfer of the fetal into adult-type circulation (see Fig. 15.4B) are not rapid or immediate. They are initiated within 60 seconds of delivery but may not be fully completed for a few weeks. The two determining events that initiate the closure of the fetal shunts are

A

Head

Superior
vena cava
31%

Carotid
arteries
62%

Foramen ovale

RA   LA

Pulmonary
veins

RV   LV

Lungs

Pulmonary
arteries

Aorta

Ductus arteriosus

Inferior
vena cava
67%

25%   Body   52%

Ductus
venosus

80%   52%

Umbilical vein   Umbilical
arteries

Placenta

B

Head

Superior
vena cava

Carotid
arteries

Lungs

Pulmonary
veins

RA   LA

RV   LV

(ligamentum
arteriosum)

Inferior
vena cava

Pulmonary   Aorta
arteries

Body

Umbilical   tied   Umbilical
vein   arteries
(ligamentum
teres)   Placenta

Fig. 15.4 *Changes in circulation at birth: A fetal circulation showing oxygen saturation of blood; B neonatal circulation. (Reproduced with permission from Chamberlain et al 1991.)*

the arrest of the umbilical circulation, and therefore placental perfusion, and lung inflation and expansion, which results in increased pulmonary blood flow. The first breath results in lung expansion and vasodilatation of the pulmonary vessels in response to increased partial pressure of oxygen. The tortuosity of the capillaries is reduced and the pulmonary circulation changes from a high-resistance to a low-resistance pathway so 90% of the blood flows through the pulmonary vascular bed. There is a brief reversal of flow through the ductus arteriosus, which vasoconstricts in response to the change in oxygen level, mediated by prostaglandins, especially decreased prostaglandin PGE_2 (Thorburn 1992).

The smooth muscle of the umbilical artery walls is not innervated but is irritable. Vasoconstriction is stimulated by stretching and handling the cord, by cooling and in response to stress-related catecholamine release. The thicker walls of the umbilical arteries are able to generate high intraluminal pressure, which arrests the placental circulation, preventing flow from the infant to the placenta. This is augmented by the increased synthesis of prostaglandins and thromboxanes in response to the raised oxygen level due to breathing, which increases vessel irritability and vasoconstriction. The umbilical vein remains dilated; blood flow from the placenta to the infant can continue via gravity. Thus initial neonatal blood volume is affected by the timing of clamping of the umbilical cord and by the relative positions of the infant and placenta at the time of clamping. The usual practice is to clamp the umbilical cord earlier if the baby is subject to fluid overload (hydropic), or if the baby is polycythaemic (e.g. infants of diabetic mothers or growth-retarded), to limit the transfer of maternal analgesic agents or antibodies or to avoid possible baby-to-baby transfusions in the cases of multiple births (Kinmond et al 1993).

The flap of the foramen ovale (Fig. 15.5) is pushed closed because the decreased umbilical flow results in a decreased venous return from the inferior vena cava so the pressure in the right atrium falls. The increased pulmonary blood flow results in an increased return to the left atrium and consequent increase in pressure. Thus the pressure gradient across the foramen ovale is reversed.

The closure of the fetal structures may not be immediate or permanent and may never be completed. The closure of the foramen ovale is reversible at first; interruption of ventilation or a drop in alveolar oxygenation results in constriction of the pulmonary capillaries and consequent reversal of pressure across the atria and reversion to fetal circulation. The incomplete closure can result in intermittent and reversible cyanotic episodes. After a few days of functional closure, the tissue associated with the foramen ovale fuses and closure becomes permanent. In many adults, a patent foramen ovale can be demonstrated (a probe can be passed through) although the pressure gradient main-tains effective functional closure. Intermittent flow through the ductus arteriosus may initially occur during each cardiac cycle when aortic pressure is maximal following ventricular contraction. Bradykinin released from the newly inflated lungs mediates the constriction of the ductus arteriosus. Production of prostaglandins by the lungs, which had maintained the open ductus arteriosus in the fetus, is decreased as oxygenation increases. Fibrolysis and obliteration of the lumen of the ductus arteriosus are usually complete within 8 days; continued patency is very serious and can result in left ventricular failure. The ductus venosus constricts when umbilical flow is halted. The obliterated vessels remain as anatomical ligaments; the slow closure of the umbilical vein and its degeneration into ligamentum teres is utilized as a route for neonatal blood transfusions if required.

The nervous control of the cardiovascular system is well developed in the neonate with mature physiological control of blood pressure and cardiac output demonstrable. The systemic arterial blood pressure is relatively low in the first few weeks as vascular tone develops which increases vascular resistance. Pulmonary arterial blood pressure is initially high but falls to mature values as pulmonary resistance falls. The neonate's heart rate is fast, as in the fetus. As in the fetus, control of cardiac output is largely achieved by changing heart rate. At birth, the wall of the right ventricle is thicker than the left, which hypertrophies in response to the changed postnatal circulation.

 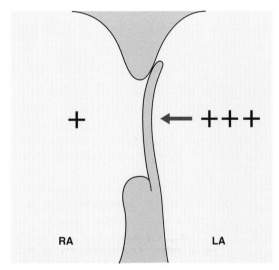

Fig. 15.5 *Initiation of neonatal circulation and closure of the foramen ovale between the right atrium (RA) and left atrium (LA).*

The respiratory system

The primitive air sacs are developed by the 20th week of gestation, and by 26 weeks respiratory bronchioles with a rich capillary supply are evident. Although the enzymes for synthesis of phospholipid/lipoprotein components of surfactant are present from week 18, the type II pneumocytes secrete surfactant only from week 26 with a surge in production after week 30. Surfactant, a detergent-like wetting agent, allows increased compliance, so the force required to inflate the alveoli is reduced thus increasing compliance. A lack of surfactant causes respiratory distress syndrome (RDS) (see below). The lecithin:sphingomyelin (L:S) ratio of the surfactant can be determined by amniocentesis indicating the maturity of the respiratory system (Fig. 15.6). By week 35, the L:S ratio in a healthily developing fetus is 2:1. This ratio is decreased in preeclampsia, prematurity, narcotic addiction, maternal diabetes and other problems in pregnancy. Administration of cortisol (dexamethasone) to the mother prior to delivery of a baby born from 24 to 34 weeks' gestation increases fetal surfactant production within 24 hours and can be used to decrease the risk of RDS (Hutchison 1994). Premature infants may require instillation of exogenous surfactant down endotracheal tubes to alleviate respiratory distress.

The lungs

Before birth

In fetal life, the lungs are filled by fluid secreted by the lungs, which exchanges with amniotic fluid. At birth, 10–25 ml/kg fluid will be expelled or resorbed. Fetal breathing movements (FBM) are observed on ultrasound from the first trimester. Initially, they are intermittent, rapid and irregular. As gestation progresses, FBM increase in strength and frequency, occurring up to 80% of the time in an organized episodic pattern (Nijhuis 2003). The lung fluid is 'breathed' out by the fetus into the amniotic fluid;. Patterns of FBM dominate during the daytime and are correlated with fetal behavioural states. Fetal wakefulness and arousal are associated with sustained vigorous respiratory patterns. Quiet sleep is associated with fewer FBM. Adrenergic and cholinergic compounds, prostaglandin synthesis inhibitors and raised maternal carbon dioxide levels stimulate FBM. They are inhibited by hypoglycaemia, cigarette smoking, alcohol consumption and accelerated labour. Despite the relatively low partial pressure of oxygen and high partial pressure of carbon dioxide, the fetus makes only shallow respiratory movements although severe hypoxia and acidosis may stimulate gasping. Mild hypoxia leads to quiet sleep and reduced energy expenditure and oxygen consumption, which may be protective. The movement of the diaphragm generates about 25 mmHg pressure for between 1 and 4 hours per day in a pattern that coincides with rapid eye movement (REM) sleep. FBM are important in lung development (Harding & Hooper 1996), promoting growth and allowing rehearsal of the respiratory actions. The fluid volume in the fetal airways correlates with the functional residual capacity in postnatal life (Strang 1991).

After birth

The most urgent need after delivery is the initiation of ventilation. Many factors interact to stimulate the first breath, including changes in temperature and state. The mild asphyxia and acidosis induced by clamping the cord sensitizes the medullary chemoreceptors that increase ventilatory drive. Tactile stimulation, such as

Fig. 15.6 *Lecithin:sphingomyelin (L:S) concentration in the amniotic fluid; the concentration rises very sharply after 30 weeks' gestation. (Reproduced with permission from Chamberlain et al 1991.)*

that which occurs during delivery, also promotes respiration. The fluid-filled lung with collapsed alveoli and undispersed surfactant proffers a high resistance to inflation and the first breath requires considerable effort. The diaphragm contracts strongly and the complaint flexible ribs and sternum of the newborn baby are pulled concave in the effort of the first breath. Once the lungs are inflated, the lung fluid is forced into the alveoli where it aids dispersal of surfactant and is rapidly resorbed into the pulmonary lymphatic vessels. Subsequent breaths require fewer changes in pressure and less mechanical work. The thoracic compression of a vaginal delivery aids fluid loss from the upper respiratory tract. Most babies gasp within 6 seconds and have patterns of normal breathing and gas exchange within 15 minutes. Initially the newborn infant has metabolic and respiratory acidosis due to decreased oxygen concentrations (resulting in increased lactic acid) and increased carbon dioxide levels respectively; this acid–base imbalance is corrected as ventilation improves. The risk of transient tachypnoea is increased in babies who are delivered by caesarean section or those who experience perinatal hypoxia.

The rate of ventilation of the newborn is high compared with an adult but is similar when relative size is taken into account. Ventilation is often irregular with the baby exhibiting periods of fetal-like shallow breathing. The reflexes associated with lung inflation also appear to be different. As well as the Hering–Breuer Reflex (where filling of the lungs increases expiratory centre activity), the newborn infant demonstrates Paradoxical Reflex of Head (where filling the lungs excites the inspiratory centre thus stimulating further inspiration) (Givan 2003). For the first few weeks, babies breathe via the nose and suck via the mouth. Control of ventilation by chemoreceptors is functional but qualitatively different in that hypoxia tends to increase depth of respiration (rather than respiratory rate) and that the response is temperature-dependent and is abolished in cold temperatures. The chemoreceptors seem to be more sensitive to raised carbon dioxide levels.

Babies have a relatively large oxygen consumption, which reflects their heat generation and that their more metabolically active tissues (e.g. liver and brain) are proportionately larger. The high airway resistance means that the energy cost of respiration is higher. Pulmonary vascular resistance drops 6–8 weeks after birth when the diameter of the small arterioles increases. The relatively high requirement for oxygen means that neonates are more susceptible to asphyxia than other age groups. Neonatal resuscitation aims to prevent mortality and morbidity. The aims of neonatal resuscitation are to promote and maintain adequate ventilation and oxygenation, to initiate and maintain adequate cardiac output and perfusion and to maintain body temperature and adequate blood glucose levels.

Respiratory distress syndrome

RDS is caused by a deficiency in surfactant, which results in alveolar collapse and increased airway resistance. Surfactant deficiency is usually inversely related to gestational age and lung maturity. Abnormal pH, stress and inadequate pulmonary perfusion also inhibit surfactant synthesis and recycling. RDS is worsened by asphyxia and is the most common cause of respiratory failure in the preterm infant. The reduced surface tension affects alveoli expansion. Small alveoli tend to collapse and normal alveoli are overdistended. Segments of the lung close and hypoxaemia and carbon dioxide retention progressively increase. The resulting metabolic and respiratory acidosis further limits the production of surfactant from the type II pneumocytes. Hypoxaemia causes vasoconstriction of the pulmonary arteries thus compromising pulmonary perfusion and increasing the likelihood of right-to-left shunting through the foramen ovale and ductus arteriosus. Local ischaemic damage affects the alveolar tissue and capillary endothelium. Changes in pulmonary pressure brought about by the infant attempting to maintain adequate air flow, together with the low plasma protein level common in preterm infants, tends to cause displacement of fluid into the alveoli. Fibrinogen in the exudate is converted into fibrin and lines the alveoli thickening the membrane. The thickened membrane and excess fluid increase the diffusion distance and impair gas transfer.

The infant responds to the respiratory difficulties by increasing respiratory rate and effort. The clinical signs appear early and increase in severity over 2 or 3 days. The infant may grunt and exhibit oedema and cyanosis. Cyanosis tends to be progressive and is due to high levels of deoxygenated haemoglobin in the capillaries. It is enhanced by right-to-left shunting, alveolar hypoventilation and impaired gas diffusion across the alveolar membranes. The baby grunts because expiration is against a partially closed glottis, which increases pressure and retards expiratory flow so increasing gas exchange. RDS risk is increased in prematurity, babies of diabetic mothers (because insulin is antagonistic to cortisol), antepartum haemorrhage and second-born twins. Male babies are twice as susceptible to RDS. Chronic hypertension, maternal heroin addiction, pre-eclampsia and growth retardation appear to protect against RDS.

Temperature regulation

Before birth

In utero, the fetus depends on its mother for temperature regulation. It loses heat via the placenta and via conduction (from skin to amniotic fluid to uterus). The fetus is a net heat producer although raised maternal temperature may compromise it (Edwards et al 1997). Brown fat is actively inhibited and fetal oxygen consumption is about 30% of postnatal levels (Gluckman et al 1999), so fetal temperature is maintained at about 0.5°C above maternal temperature. Research has focused on raised maternal temperature due to fever, exercise and external raised temperature (such as hot baths and saunas). The results are inconclusive. However, maternal fever has effects not only on temperature gradients but also on oxygen consumption and haemodynamics and may be associated with teratogenesis and preterm labour.

After birth

As environmental temperature is usually lower than maternal temperature, the baby will experience a temperature loss at birth. Heat transfer is affected by two gradients: the internal gradient involving transfer from the core to the surface of the baby and the external gradient involving heat transfer from the body surface to the environment. Transfer of heat through the internal gradient depends on insulation and blood flow. Neonates have less subcutaneous fat than adults do (about 16% body fat compared with 30%) and a higher surface area:mass ratio (about three times the relative surface area of an adult). Should the baby be born small, it will not only have an even larger surface area:mass ratio but the insulation provided by its subcutaneous fat will also be further compromised and skin permeability will be increased. Small-for-dates babies have proportionately bigger heads and higher metabolism and are disadvantaged in that their heat losses are higher. Changes in peripheral circulation affect heat loss via conduction.

Heat loss across the external gradient depends on the temperature difference between the body and the environment. Conduction, convection, evaporation and radiation transfer heat from the baby. Warming objects that will come into contact with the neonate, and increasing insulation by wrapping, limit heat loss by conduction. Evaporation offers the greatest route for heat loss immediately after delivery but drying the baby, especially the head, immediately after delivery is effective at reducing the loss. Skin keratinization is inadequate in immature infants so evaporative heat losses are higher. Evaporative insensible heat loss increases with respiratory problems, activity, the use of radiant heaters or phototherapy and low relative humidity. Convective losses are related to draughts and are affected by ambient temperature and humidity. Higher air temperatures, minimal air circulation, swaddling and baby hats reduce heat loss by convection. Radiation is the major form of heat loss from babies in incubators. It involves the transfer of radiant energy to surrounding objects not directly in contact with the baby. Consideration therefore has to be given to the temperature of objects in the local environment including the incubator, walls and windows. Skin-to-skin contact with the mother immediately following birth is a very efficient way of reducing heat loss from the neonate. The large skin area and the softness of the breasts enables a large amount of maternal skin to come into direct contact with the baby's skin surface.

The mechanisms of heat conservation and generation mediated by the peripheral nervous system are insufficient in the neonate (Okken 1991). Infants can produce heat from metabolic processes and by increasing activity. Postural changes are also important in conserving heat. Shivering is not so important in infants but heat generation by non-shivering thermogenesis (NST) is important. NST takes place in brown adipose tissue (BAT), a specialized type of adipose tissue that is well vascularized and has cells densely packed with mitochondria (Fig. 15.7). Adults have little brown adipose tissue, around the kidneys and great blood vessels, which generates minimal heat. However, 2–7% of the term infant's body weight is BAT, which has a major role in heat production in the neonate. BAT is formed from about 30 weeks' gestation until about 4 weeks' postbirth. Fat mass is significantly altered by maternal nutrition and gestational length; stores of BAT (and white fat) are lower in preterm infants. BAT comprises about 2% of birth weight and is predominantly located around the core

A

1
Developing cell
Rounded nucleus
Small fat vacuoles
One large fat vacuole

2
Mature cell
Nucleus compressed
Mitochondria are few,
small and rounded

3
Fat-depleted cell

B

1
Developing cell
Round nucleus
Numerous large mitochondria
Many fat vacuoles
Good innervation and vascularization

2
Mature cell
More cytoplasm
More fat

3
Fat-depleted cell
Few small fat vacuoles
Many mitochondria

4
Fat-storing cell
Vacuoles coalesce into a
single large vacuole

Fig. 15.7 *Structures and development of white and brown adipose tissue. (Reproduced with permission from Robinson 1994.)*

organs (Fig. 15.8). It generates heat by uncoupling electron transport from oxidative phosphorylation in the mitochondria so the energy released by electron transport will not be used to synthesize ATP but will be liberated as heat instead (Fig. 15.9). The unique uncoupling protein, which when maximally activated allows the production of at least 100 times as much heat from BAT compared to other tissue, is synthesized during the maturation of fetal fat (Symonds et al 2003). At birth, the activation of BAT is accompanied by mobilization of fat and a marked increase in lipolysis. Thermogenesis by BAT is inhibited in the fetus. The placenta produces both PGE_2 and prostacyclin (PGI_2) which inhibit BAT; it also suppresses formation of active T_3 (tri-iodothyronine) from T_4 (thyroxine) (see below).

Heat production per unit mass of the neonate is higher than that of an adult; thermogenesis begins when a critical temperature difference of 12°C between the environment and the skin is exceeded. The drop in temperature stimulates release of noradrenaline from sympathetic nerve endings that stimulate the brown adipose cells (Gunn et al 1991). At birth, catecholamines from the adrenal medulla and rise in T_3 production by the thyroid gland augment the effect of noradrenaline. Inhibition of BAT by the

Fig. 15.8 *Location of brown adipose tissue in the human infant.*

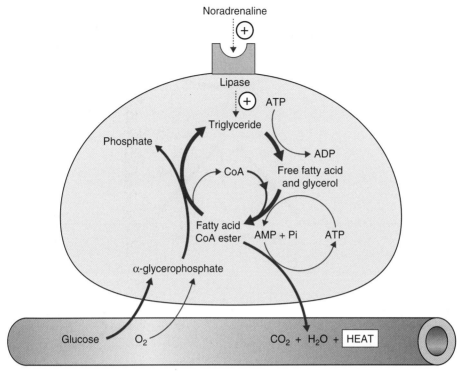

Fig. 15.9 *Metabolic pathways in brown adipose tissue: triglycerides break down to yield useful heat (about 160 kcal/mol are produced during each turn of the cycle). (Reproduced with permission from Begley et al 1978.)*

placenta ceases. Oxygen consumption and metabolic rate increase markedly in response to a drop in temperature. Heat generation involves lipolysis of BAT, which depends on the availability of oxygen, ATP and glucose. There is a strong interrelationship between ventilation, feeding and temperature regulation, which means that hypoglycaemia, hypoxia or acidosis can affect the ability of the neonate to produce heat (Fig. 15.10).

Mechanisms for losing heat are not well developed in the neonate (Power 1992). The neonate can lose some heat by sweating (which increases evaporation) but peripheral vasodilatation is the main source of heat loss. Although the density of neonatal sweat glands is high in some areas, they are less responsive and less efficient at sweat production. Phototherapy increases water loss. Sweating is more inefficient in preterm babies and those with central nervous system dysfunction. As the baby gets older and can rely on physical methods of generating heat, NST becomes less important. Brown adipose tissue gradually diminishes in the first year.

White adipose tissue provides both insulation and an energy reserve. Development of body fat in the fetus is under nutritional constraint whereas postnatal growth is controlled by genetic potential. Compared to other mammals, human infants are not only extremely fat at birth but they continue to increase in adiposity during early postnatal life. Although it has been suggested that the role of the fat is insulation required as compensation for human hairlessness, evidence to support this is weak. A more likely explanation is that the adipose tissue acts as an energy reserve both to support the demands of a large brain and to protect the infant from nutritional disruption at birth and weaning or during infection (Kuzawa 1998).

The neonatal liver

Bilirubin

The functions of the neonatal liver are similar to those of an adult but are relatively immature. The ability to synthesize plasma proteins and to metabolize foreign substances is inefficient. This, together with immature intestinal processes, means the neonate is at increased risk of developing hyperbilirubinaemia (Blackburn 1995). Before birth, bilirubin is cleared by the placenta and then handled by maternal metabolism. If bilirubin accumulates in the neonate, jaundice (or icterus) can occur. As the blood–brain barrier of the neonate is more permeable, free bilirubin can cross easily and in

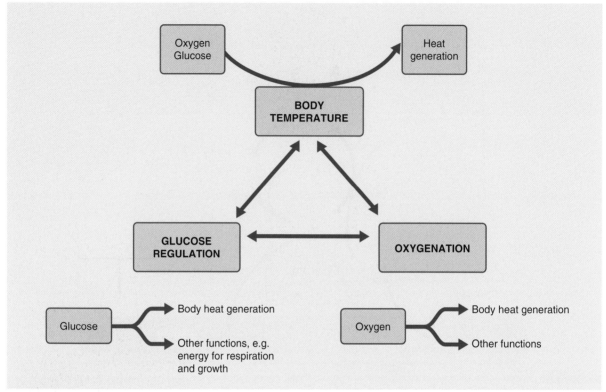

Interrelationship between temperature regulation, glucose concentration and respiration.

sufficient concentrations can cause kernicterus, resulting in a range of symptoms from convulsions and abnormal behaviour to cerebral palsy, deafness or death.

Bilirubin is a breakdown product of haemoglobin from red blood cells (Fig. 15.11). Iron from red blood cells is recycled. Haem, the pigment, is degraded by macrophages of the reticuloendothelial system to biliverdin and then to bilirubin. Unconjugated (indirect) bilirubin is insoluble and cannot be excreted. It is transported bound to plasma albumin to the liver to be metabolized into conjugated (direct) bilirubin, which is soluble. Conjugation involves binding of glucuronide sugars to bilirubin forming bilirubin diglucuronate. Conjugated bilirubin is excreted into bile and so into the intestines. It is a major component of bile and faeces. In the intestine, conjugated bilirubin is further metabolized by bacterial flora to produce urobilin and stercobilin (which give the characteristic colour of faeces). Some of the breakdown products of bacterial metabolism of bilirubin are deconjugated and absorbed across the gut wall to be recirculated. Small amounts of bilirubin are also excreted via the kidneys.

Decreased production of plasma proteins can result in raised unconjugated bilirubin levels. The pathways in the liver that deconjugate bilirubin to its water-soluble, and therefore excretable, metabolite may also be compromised. As meconium is rich in bilirubin, delayed passage of meconium increases the possibility that bilirubin will be deconjugated, absorbed and re-enter the circulating pool. Production of bilirubin in neonates is inversely correlated to gestational age and remains high for a few weeks (Lockitch 1994). This is partly due to high circulating levels of blood cells, which are then removed, and also to having more fragile red blood cells with a shorter lifespan (see Table 15.1). The risk of hyperbilirubinaemia is further increased by other conditions that stress this pathway such as excess blood cell breakdown (as in excessive trauma at birth or due to infection) or increased red blood cell breakdown (as in polycythaemia due to maternal diabetes).

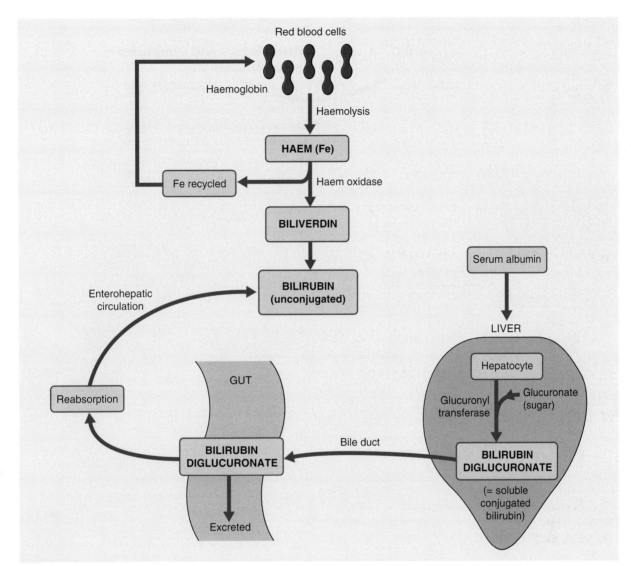

Fig. 15.11   *Breakdown of haemoglobin to form bilirubin.*

Fuel storage

Fetal metabolism is dominated by anabolic pathways, whereas the neonate has to catabolize fuel stores to provide nutrients between periodic neonatal feeds (Hay 1994). The last weeks of gestation are an important time for laying down lipids and glycogen. During fetal life, glycogen is stored in the skeletal muscle and, to a lesser extent, in the liver. Glycogen provides the substrate for energy metabolism during delivery and the first few hours of postnatal life (Nelson 1994). Fat stores serve as an alternative energy source; the neonate markedly increases fatty acid oxidation and uses ketone bodies for energy production. In the first few days of life, the respiratory quotient falls from 1.0 (as glucose sources are exhausted) to about 0.7 (a value similar to that seen in adult diabetics) as fat and protein are mobilized until adequate milk is consumed.

Glucose regulation

Thyroxine (T_4) is relatively inactive and is usually converted to active tri-iodothyronine (T_3). Fetal T_3 levels are low because fetal liver levels of outer-ring deiodinase are low and placental levels of inner-ring deiodinase are high, both of which drive preferential production of inactive reverse T_3. The resulting low level of the active thyroid hormone T_3 can support brain development but suppresses oxygen consumption by non-neural tissues and inhibits thermogenesis. In late gestation, the rise in glucocorticoids induces expression of outer-ring deiodinase in the fetal liver so production of fetal T_3 increases markedly. The rise in T_3 plays a role not only in hepatic enzyme activity but also in tissue maturation and lung and bone development. At birth, the T_3 levels increase further as the inner-ring deiodinase is reduced on placental separation, and evaporative cooling induces a rise in thyroid-stimulating hormone (TSH, thyrotrophin), which further stimulates hormone production by the thyroid gland. Adipose tissue significantly contributes to the conversion of T_4 to T_3 after delivery; smaller fat depots result in less thyroid hormone production, potentially further compromising thermogenesis in premature infants.

Blood glucose levels in the neonate tend to fall after delivery because the immature liver is better at promoting glycogen synthesis than glycogenolysis, and because the baby has increased activity and metabolism at birth. The large brain and large red blood cell number have a high requirement for glucose. The stress of delivery and cooling at birth stimulate the release of catecholamines, which stimulate glucagon release and suppress insulin release and are important in activating the metabolic pathways in the liver. The neonate is unable to regulate blood glucose efficiently (Smith 1995) and is usually hypoglycaemic (glucose levels are about 2 mmol/l) (Box 15.3). The enzymes involving glucose metabolism do not reach optimal levels in the liver for 2–3 weeks, so glycogenolysis and gluconeogenesis are relatively slow in correcting falls in blood glucose. If the delivery is protracted, the neonate may deplete its glycogen stores. Also the response to raised levels of glucose is slow; although adequate concentrations of insulin are present in the pancreas, the β-cells initially lack sensitivity to glucose, responding better to amino acids. Thus, neonatal blood glucose levels fluctuate. Values as low as 1.0 mmol/l have been recorded. In an adult, such a level of hypoglycaemia would cause convulsions, hypoglycaemic coma and probable neurological damage, whereas in the newborn they might cause an apnoeic attack. The central nervous system of the neonate exhibits a degree of plasticity and is partially protected as it can utilize fatty acids and ketones efficiently.

Box 15.3

Risk factors and symptoms of hypoglycaemia

Risk factors

- Hypothermia, evaporation, draughts, cold room
- Babies who do not feed or have a poor response to feeding in the early postnatal period
- Intrauterine growth retardation (IUGR)
- Prematurity
- Maternal diabetes
- Stress

Symptoms

- Lethargy: 'floppy baby' (normal muscle tone is reduced to conserve glucose usage of skeletal muscle)
- Drowsiness: difficult to rouse, indicating neurological function is impaired by lack of glucose
- Jitteriness: an adverse tremor in response to stimulation such as loud noise or touch, indicating neurological inhibition of reflexes is affected
- Coldness: may be a cause or consequence of hypoglycaemia

Note: many babies may be hypoglycaemic without clinical symptoms, indicating that they are maintaining normal neurological function by other metabolic pathways. The clinical symptoms indicate these pathways are failing and the infant is at risk. Hypoglycaemic screening of the neonate involves measuring the level of glucose in the infant's blood by analysis of a small amount obtained from a heel prick.

The gastrointestinal system at birth

The gut completes anatomical development by week 24 and the term neonate is able to digest and absorb milk from birth. Species-specific growth factors in milk are important in promoting postnatal development of the gut. The neonatal gut has immature digestive and absorptive capacities but there are a number of compensatory mechanisms, particularly for babies who are breastfed who receive both digestive enzymes and growth factors that stimulate gut development in the milk (Lonnerdal 2003).

Feeding reflexes

From birth, a normal infant can suck from the breast, convey milk to the back of the mouth and swallow it for a period of 5–10 minutes while breathing normally. There is an innate programme of reflexes and behaviour, which become evident within an hour or so following delivery, including the ability to move from the mother's abdomen to her breast, coordinated hand–mouth activity, rooting for the nipple, attaching to the breast and feeding vigorously before falling asleep. Touching the palate triggers the sucking reflex. The neonate exhibits rhythmic jaw action, which creates a negative pressure, and the peristaltic action of the tongue and jaw strips milk from the breast and moves it to the throat thus triggering the swallowing reflex. These breastfeeding reflexes are strong at birth in the normal neonate and are evident in preterm babies from about 32 weeks (about 1200 g). Extremely preterm babies and those that are sick or have a very low birth weight have markedly decreased or absent reflexes. Other babies who experience feeding problems include those with physical problems such as cleft lip or palate and those subjected to obstetric sedation, analgesia or extreme stress at birth.

The sucking and swallowing reflexes are aided by the particular morphological configuration of the neonate's mouth, which has a proportionately longer soft palate. The neonate also has an extrusion reflex in response to the presence of solid or semisolid material in the mouth. This reflex is lost at 4–6 months and is replaced by a pattern of rhythmic biting movements coinciding with the development of the first teeth at 7–9 months.

Hormone and enzyme production

Gastric secretion is developed but low; responses to gut regulatory hormones appear also to be low. The effect is that the gastric juice has a pH close to neutral (compared with a pH of 2 in an adult's stomach). The high gastric pH means that salivary amylase is not inactivated in the stomach so starch digestion can continue. Reflux of gastric contents is common, as the lower oesophageal sphincter is immature in both musculature and neurological control. Less-acidic gastric juice does not cause painful tissue damage to the oesophageal mucosa but also it is less effective at denaturing proteins including microorganisms. It has been suggested that a reflux of human milk is advantageous as very small amounts of milk may reach the upper part of the respiratory tract conferring an immunological benefit there. Breastfed babies have a lower incidence of respiratory problems. Decreased acid production in the stomach means that the activation of pepsinogen to pepsin is restricted, limiting protein digestion in the stomach. The decreased acidity and protein digestion may enhance the defence mechanism promoting the activity of immunoglobulins and antigen recognition in the gastrointestinal tract as these proteins survive the gentler gastric environment.

Pancreatic amylase levels are low in the newborn but breast milk contains mammary amylase, which can augment starch digestion. Colostrum is particularly rich in mammary amylase. Lactase activity is relatively late in developing, reaching adequate levels after 36 weeks' gestation. However, many preterm babies can digest lactose satisfactorily as unabsorbed lactose can be metabolized by colonic bacteria to short-chain fatty acids, which can then be absorbed thus salvaging the energy. The low pancreatic lipase levels are compensated for by lingual and gastric lipase produced by the neonate (stimulated by suckling) and by bile salt-stimulated lipase in human milk. Bile acid formation is low but human milk is rich in taurine, which is used for neonatal conjugation of bile salts.

Bowel movements

Passage of meconium, a mix of mucus, epithelial cells, fatty acids and bile pigments (which gives it the characteristic greenish-black colour), confirms that the lower bowel is patent. Passage of a changing stool (meconium and food residue), usually within 24 hours, indicates the whole gut is patent. At birth, the stomach capacity is 10–20 ml, which rapidly increases to 200 ml by 1 year.

The kidneys

Before birth

In utero, from 9 to 10 weeks' gestation, the fetus produces large volumes of dilute urine, which is an important source of amniotic fluid (Box 15.4). However, the regulatory and excretory functions of the kidneys are minimal before birth (Guillery 1997). The placenta

Clinical symptoms of Potter's syndrome

- Bilateral renal agenesis (absence of kidneys)
- Urine is not excreted into amniotic fluid
- Results in oligohydramnios (defined as less than 500 ml of amniotic fluid at term)
- Incidence: about 1 in 3000 livebirths
- Incompatible with postnatal life; most affected babies die within a few hours of birth
- Causes: pulmonary hypoplasia because of restricted space for thoracic expansion and an imbalance of fluid for filling the lungs; musculoskeletal abnormalities because fetal movement is constrained; abnormal facies because face is moulded by compression; cord compression in labour and fetal distress (Scott & Goodburn 1995)

corrects any osmotic imbalance. Mature kidney function is not developed until about 1 month; until then the urine is fetal-like. The neonatal kidneys, weighing about 12.5 g each, have a low glomerular filtration rate (GFR) and relatively low surface area. The ability to reabsorb or excrete sodium (Na^+) is poor so the urine produced is of low specific gravity and hypotonic, reaching 1.5 times plasma concentration (700–800 mOsm) compared to adult values of 3–5 times plasma concentration (1200–1400 mOsm).

After birth

At birth, the normal obligatory water loss means the baby loses 5–10% of its birth weight in the first 4 days as a result of the loss of water and Na^+. Neonatal renal function can efficiently prevent dehydration and eliminate the lower level of metabolic waste products of the breastfed infant. Changing fluid intake (or increasing the solute load) can result in osmotic imbalance, acidosis or dehydration. The risks are lower if the baby is feeding on demand; however, the very immature renal function of preterm babies requires careful calculation of fluid and electrolyte balance as Na^+-rich urine may be produced despite low plasma Na^+ levels. This can be crucial if there is high extrarenal water loss, for instance in the presence of fever or high ambient temperature.

The ability to excrete protons or hydrogen ions (H^+) is also limited, thus increasing the neonate's susceptibility to acidosis. Elimination of drugs such as antibiotics cleared by the renal system is decreased so the half-life of the drug in the circulation is increased necessitating a requirement for decreased frequency of dose. The neonate should urinate within 24 hours of delivery. Initially, 15–30 ml/kg of urine is produced per day increasing to 100–200 ml/kg by day 7 as the fluid intake increases. Mature renal function is not achieved until 12 months to 2 years.

The nervous system

Before birth

The fetus responds to noises, intense light, noxious stimulation of the skin and decreased temperature by changing autonomic responses such as heart rate and by moving. Fetal movements can be felt from about week 14; the 'exercise' is thought to aid muscle growth and limb development. By term, the nervous system is prepared to process and receive information. Human cortical function is relatively immature compared with that of some other mammalian species. Complete myelination of the long motor pathways occurs after birth, therefore fine movements of the fingers, for instance, are not evident until several months after birth.

After birth

After birth, the nervous system undergoes accelerated development in response to increased sensory input. Reflexes may be slightly depressed for the first 24 hours, particularly if there has been transplacental transfer of narcotic analgesia, after which several reflexes can be elicited. In cases of severe asphyxia, low Apgar scores (see p. 395) or neurological damage, reflexes are depressed and may take longer to appear. The grasping reflex and the Moro embrace are used to assess the reflex ability of the newborn. Babies also demonstrate a strong palmar grasp and a rhythmic stepping movement. Many reflexes common to the neonate disappear unless there is pathological interference, in which case they may be exhibited in the adult. The baby exhibits general awareness to its surroundings and reacts to sound and light.

Babies are born with active sensory pathways. Studies have demonstrated that neonates can recognize the smell of their mother's milk. They can differentiate between tastes and appear to have a preference for sweet tastes. Although babies can see at birth, there are big postnatal developments in visual capability, particularly in the first 6 months. The neonate has limited visual acuity but appears to focus at a distance of 20 cm. From birth, babies can discriminate between contrast and contours and can follow movement. The neonate is able to hear and discriminate between sounds particularly those of low- to middle-range frequency. Studies have demonstrated a neonate's ability to recognize the characteristics of their mother's voice and to demonstrate a preference for rhythmic sing-song intonation. Neonates are reassured by the rhythmic sounds of breathing, heartbeat and gut peristalsis, which they hear, for instance, while being held. Newborn infants can be trained to activate a tape-recorder by sucking non-nutritively on a modified nipple; they demonstrate that they recognize not only their mother's voice but also particular passages of a book that they were read in utero (Lipsitt & Rovee-Collier 2001). The development of motor function is described by the 'Jacksonian principle', a hierarchical model whereby the last reflexes to develop are the first to be lost when the organism degenerates and dies. This pattern occurs because the first reflexes to develop are well-rehearsed and require less oxygen to be initiated than more recent reflexes. The order of sensory development (tactile, vestibular, thermal, chemical, auditory and visual) is also reversed during injury, disease or ageing.

Sleep and behavioural states

The fetus exhibits slow-wave and REM sleep between patterns of wakefulness. The neonate sleeps about 16 hours per day, 40% in REM sleep, compared with a total of 12 hours asleep at 2 years of age (20% in REM sleep). Sleep patterns are not diurnal and do not follow a light–dark cycle. Six sleep–wake states are recognized: quiet (deep) sleep, active (light) sleep, drowsy state, awake (quiet) alert, active alert and crying (Wolff 1966). The proportion of time in each state varies with postconceptual age. Quiet deep sleep is restful and the baby is in an anabolic state when growth hormone secretion is high, mitotic rate is high, oxygen consumption is low and there is little movement. In active sleep, the eyes are closed but the baby moves its face and extremities. Respiration and heart rate are irregular. The baby exhibits 'paradoxical' REM sleep, in which the brain activity is similar to awake states. This state is associated with learning and synapse development. The drowsy state is transitional between being awake and asleep. The eyes are open and the baby is alert but has little movement. The baby appears to focus on visual stimuli and appears to be processing sensory information. In the active alert state, respiration rate is increased and is irregular. There are skin colour changes, much activity and the baby has increased sensitivity to stimuli. Crying is the method of communication usually in response to unpleasant stimuli. Characteristically, neonates close their eyes, grimace and make sounds. However, preterm infants may not be capable of making a noise.

At one time, it was believed that the immature degree of myelination and lack of experience meant that neonates were unable to perceive pain. In fact, not only does the anatomical and functional requirements for pain perception develop early and the fetus, preterm and term infant demonstrate similar physiological responses to the adult, but there is also evidence that pain perception is more intense and that early experience of pain has long-term developmental and behavioural consequences (Taddio & Katz 2004). Catecholamine and cortisol release increases, heart rate and respiration rates change, metabolic rate and oxygen consumption increase and blood glucose levels rise. The rate of transmission may be slower but a probable shorter distance between the pain receptor and brain compensates for this. Assessment of pain can be difficult as pain may be expressed differently; facial expressions may be used but some babies tend to withdraw and increase passivity and sleep patterns in response to pain.

The skin and immune system

The skin of a neonate appears relatively transparent and soft and velvety. It is important in temperature regulation, as a barrier and as a sensory organ. Part of the appearance is due to the lack of large skin folds and localized oedema. Melanin production and pigmentation are low in the newborn so the skin is vulnerable to damage by ultraviolet rays. However, residual levels of maternal and placental hormones can produce transient pigmentation of certain skin areas. During delivery, the skin is subject to changes in blood flow and mechanical stress from the pressure of contractions and from maternal structures which can result in abrasions and ischaemia. Obstetric interventions, for example fetal monitoring, scalp sampling and use of amnio-hooks, forceps and vacuum extraction, also compromise the integrity of the skin.

Immediately after birth, most fair-skinned babies have characteristic pink coloration with blue but warm extremities.

Vernix caseosa is a superficial fatty substance that coats the fetal skin from the middle of gestation and subsequently decreases as gestation progresses. Lanugo is the first generation of downy body hair that is fine and unpigmented; it appears from the 12th week and is mostly shed before birth. Vernix caseosa tends to accumulate at the sites of dense lanugo growth and is evident on the preterm baby on the face, ears and shoulders and in folds. At term, traces of vernix are present on the brow, ears and in the skin creases. Vernix caseosa is composed of sebaceous gland secretion and skin cells and is rich in triacylglycerides, cholesterol and fats. Its role is to protect the fetus from the amniotic fluid and to prevent loss of water and electrolytes. It provides insulation for the skin and helps to reduce friction at delivery; it may also have antibacterial properties.

The barrier properties of the stratum corneum of the skin increase with increased gestational age, especially after 24 weeks (Rutter 1996). The epidermis of a preterm baby might be only five layers thick compared with about 15 layers in a term infant. A thinner epidermal layer results in increased transepidermal water loss, decreased ability to cope with friction, thermal instability because of the increased blood supply to the surface and increased permeability to microorganisms and chemicals (such as topically applied substances and reagents on clothes). Premature babies have translucent shiny red skin that becomes pinker through to the white thick skin of term infants. Drying out of the skin is a normal maturation process. Substances that interfere with the keratinization process, such as emollients, can delay the development of the skin becoming effective as a barrier. The transepidermal water loss can be limited by use of a thermal blanket, altering the air flow and maintaining an insulating layer of saturated air in contact with the skin.

The neonate is a compromised host, vulnerable to nocosomial (cross) infection. Host defence mechanisms are immature, partly because of lack of previous exposure to common organisms and partly because the neonate has limited cellular responses (see Ch. 10). Breaks in the delicate mucosa and skin from delivery and invasive obstetric procedures provide opportunities for the entry of pathogenic bacteria. In relation to artificial feeding, neonates are at increased risk of developing gastrointestinal infections, which may be associated with later development of allergies. Preterm infants, especially those of less than 34 weeks' gestation, are very vulnerable as they have less maternal IgG transfer. At birth, the neonate leaves the sterile fetal environment for one loaded with microorganisms (Jarvis 1996). Ingestion and inhalation provide routes for bacterial colonization after birth, initially with organisms derived from the maternal genital tract. The neonate's skin, umbilical cord and genitalia are colonized first, followed by the face, respiratory system and gut. Skin flora is increased in infants with little vernix caseosa and is limited by antiseptic agents and alkaline soaps. Initially gut colonization is with organisms that the infant comes into contact with at and immediately after delivery. The profile of organisms is affected by the diet; breastfed babies have optimal conditions for the growth of the protective lactobacilli and bifidobacterium. Different patterns are seen in babies of very low birth weight and those who require feeding or ventilatory assistance. Meconium in vivo is usually sterile but when excreted provides rich culture conditions for microorganisms. The use of antibiotics changes the pattern of bacterial colonization of the neonate and can encourage the growth of resistant bacteria.

Case study 15.1 gives an example of neonatal infection.

Case study 15.1

During a routine visit, the midwife examines Tracy, a 3-day-old baby, who was delivered in hospital and discharged the day before. Her umbilicus appears moist and sticky so the midwife takes a swab for culture and sensitivity. Two days later it is revealed that Tracy's umbilicus has been colonized with methicillin-resistant *Staphylococcus aureus* (MRSA). The infant appears well, has been exclusively breastfed and has regained her birth weight.

- What treatment, if any, would Tracy require and what reasons could be applied to argue against the use of antibiotic therapy?
- Do you think it is necessary to try to identify the source of the infection?
- What should the midwife do to ensure that further cross-infections do not occur?
- What factors may put other individuals at risk?

Examination of the newborn

After delivery, the baby is always examined by a midwife who, in accordance with professional legislative requirements, must refer any deviation from the normal to a medical practitioner. There is a statutory requirement to document findings.

The Apgar score

The baby's condition, including mental and physical development and level of awareness, is assessed using the Apgar score (Table 15.2).

Although the interpretative value of the Apgar score has been questioned, it is a means of assessing a baby for the absence or presence and degree of birth asphyxia. It is quick and simple and no other test has been routinely adopted. The Apgar test scores the baby's heart rate, respiratory effort, colour, muscle tone and reflex responses at 1 and 5 minutes following birth. It is repeated at 5-minute intervals when active resuscitation measures are undertaken. The 1-minute score may be low as the baby has been subjected to physical stress including a drop in temperature. Dark-skinned babies are assessed out of a total score of 8 omitting evaluation of skin colour.

Measurement of heart rate can be done by palpating the heart via the anterior chest wall or listening to the heart with a stethoscope. A heart rate of 110–150 beats per minute is considered normal. A baby who is crying is obviously breathing in order to produce sound. Breathing can be seen easily, even on quiet babies. The respiratory rate of a healthy newborn baby is about 40–60 breaths per minute and should not be punctuated by grunting. A high-pitched or irritable cry may indicate brain damage or cerebral irritation due to oedema or haemorrhage.

The colour of the mucous membranes inside the mouth and the eyelids is assessed. If the blood flow is good, as in a healthy baby, these areas will be pink. If the tissues are being deprived of oxygen, they appear purplish or navy blue if the deprivation is severe. Healthy babies often appear bluish at the extremities but this may be due to cold rather than poor circulation. The face may appear congested if the cord was around the neck or if pressure from the delivery was prolonged. Pale babies may be anaemic, and polycythaemic babies (with an excess of red blood cells) tend to look very red.

The rooting reflex, turning of the head towards a touch on the cheek, is noted. Alternative reflexes include the baby curling the toes if the sole of the foot is stroked or responding with a grabbing movement if the palm of the hand is stroked (palmar grasp reflex). Abnormal responses such as the toes curling upwards are often associated with abnormalities. The Moro reflex is looked for by startling the baby. If the head is allowed to drop back a few centimetres, the baby responds by flinging the arms outwards, usually accompanied by crying.

Muscle tone is more difficult to assess. All newborn babies have poorly developed musculature and seem fairly floppy, but babies who are especially floppy because they have immature coordination do not resist limb movement. Healthy babies have flexed limbs and respond to handling; the normal procedure is to lay the baby on the midwife's hand resting on its stomach and to observe position of the limbs.

A baby that needs urgent resuscitation is pale and floppy, has a sluggish pulse and makes no respiratory effort. This is apparent and needs immediate response

Table 15.2 *Apgar score*

	0	1	2
Heart rate	Absent	Slow (<100 beats per minute)	Fast (>100 beats per minute)
Respiratory effort	Absent	Irregular, slow	Regular, cry
Muscle tone	Limp	Some flexion in limbs	Well-flexed limbs
Reflex irritability	Nil	Grimace	Cough, cry
Colour	White, blue	Body pink, extremities blue	Completely pink

without having to calculate the Apgar score first. The Apgar score indicates the baby's capability to survive without intervention. If the Apgar score is above 7, little intervention is required, but a baby with an Apgar score of 5–7 will often need suction and oxygen via a face mask. A score of 3–5 usually requires administration of oxygen via an 'Ambu' bag or equipment that allows facial oxygen to be delivered under cycles of positive pressure to inflate the lungs. A lower score requires immediate active treatment usually requiring ventilation via an endotracheal tube.

Case study 15.2 is an example of a baby possibly in need of resuscitation.

Body measurements and inspection

Once these tests are completed, further examination of the newborn can take place. An initial development check is followed by a paediatric check 24 hours later. The baby's weight, length and head circumference are measured and recorded. Babies with birth weights above the 90th centile or below the 10th centile have an increased risk of becoming hypoglycaemic. Examination of the genitalia allows assignation of the sex of the baby. In male infants, the scrotum is felt for the presence of both testes and the position of the urethral exit on the penis is checked. In female babies, the vaginal and urethral orifices are inspected. Presence of meconium demonstrates patency of the anus; this may become evident on rectal temperature measurement although rectal temperature recording should be avoided unless the baby is very cold and the core temperature needs assessing due to the increased risk of developing necrotizing enterocolitis.

Moulding of the head and oedema of the scalp are common at birth because of the pressure imposed by

the birth canal (see Ch. 13). The normal term infant is well endowed with subcutaneous fat and usually has vernix caseosa in the skin folds. Postmature babies may have dry and peeling skin. The fontanelles and suture lines are observed. Bulging fontanelles may indicate an increased pressure and sunken fontanelles that the baby is dehydrated. An abnormal-shaped head indicates abnormal moulding (see Ch. 13). Eyes and ears are checked for abnormalities; the eyes should be clear and free from discharge. Low-set, absent or deformed ears may be associated with chromosomal abnormalities. The baby's mouth is inspected for the presence of teeth, which can be removed, or other extraneous material. Both the soft and hard palate are checked; the baby should demonstrate a sucking reflex. Minor skin blemishes are common. Hypertrophic sebaceous glands or milia present as white spots on about 40% babies. Both these spots and 'stork marks'—minor capillary haemangiomas—usually on the nose or eyelids, disappear within a few months of delivery.

The overall morphology of the baby should be symmetrical. The insertion of the umbilicus should be central, and is checked for swellings. The nipples, of either male or female babies, may be swollen and producing milk in response to circulating maternal hormones. Respiratory movement of the chest of a healthy baby is symmetrical and the abdomen is rounded. The limbs are checked for equal length and free movement; short limbs can indicate achondroplasia. The digits are counted; extra digits and webbing between the digits are relatively common. The feet and ankles are examined for talipes and other abnormalities.

Visible signs of congenital dislocation of the hips (CDH) are asymmetry of the pelvis, asymmetrical creases in the groin and apparent differences in leg length. Midwives may be discouraged from undertaking manipulative tests of the hips as there is a danger of malpositioning the head of the femur into the acetabular cup, which can trap the femoral blood flow resulting in necrosis of the head of the femur. Midwifery units usually have local policies and protocols for the screening of hips for congenital dislocation.

The neck is observed for shortness, webbing or folds of skin on the back of the neck; these characteristics are associated with chromosomal abnormalities, such as Turner's syndrome. The spine is checked for swellings or defects and for pilonidal dimples or hairy patches, which may indicate occult spina bifida. Before the baby is discharged from the postnatal ward, there should be confirmation that the baby is feeding normally; excretion of urine and meconium

---

Case study 15.2

Paul is only 10 seconds old. He appears blue, not moving and limp and does not respond to touch. The midwife summons help and a paediatrician is called. The paediatrician arrives 4 minutes later to find a healthy, well-perfused infant, crying while being held by his mother.

- Was the midwife justified in being cautious by summoning a paediatrician early?
- How many midwives in practice wait a full minute before their initial assessment of the newborn?

normally occurs within 24 and 48 hours of delivery, respectively. Early screening is important both to reassure the parents and to detect any abnormality or problem requiring further investigation.

Key points

- Many changes must occur at birth for successful transition to neonatal life, including initiation of breathing, conversion from fetal to neonatal circulation and physiological homeostatic control of thermoregulation and metabolism.

- The transition to neonatal circulation requires closure of the fetal shunts and vasodilatation of the pulmonary circulation; oxygen is a major stimulant.

- Successful breathing requires adequate maturation of the lungs, particularly the presence of adequate surfactant and neuromuscular control, and clearance of lung fluid.

- The relatively large surface area of neonates means they are vulnerable to excessive heat loss; body temperature is maintained by non-shivering thermogenesis. Efforts to reduce heat loss at birth are essential.

- Normal newborn infants are able to maintain adequate blood glucose levels; this can be compromised by a stressful labour, a shortened third trimester and abnormal maternal metabolism.

- Human milk and early physiological conditions compensate for the immature development of the neonatal gut.

Application to practice

An understanding of the transition to neonatal life is important for the following reasons. Many infants require some degree of intervention to enable establishment of respiration after birth. An infant who does not appear to adapt fully at birth (i.e. is cyanotic) may have an underlying cardiac defect.

The midwife should use her assessment of adaptation as part of the neonatal check and not check solely for visible abnormalities.

Many parents are distressed at the appearance of a baby that has just been born and need reassurance that the transition is not always completely spontaneous and that this is quite normal.

Annotated further reading

Baston H, Durward H 2000 Examination of the newborn: a practical guide. Routledge
A practical step-by-step guide to examining the newborn infant which covers normal developments, parental concerns, labour and delivery, clinical examination and identification of abnormalities as well as professional and legal implications.

Blackburn ST, Loper DL 2002 Maternal, fetal, and neonatal physiology: a clinical perspective. 2nd edn. Saunders, Philadelphia
An in-depth and well-illustrated description of physiological adaptation to pregnancy and development of the fetus and neonate that draws from physiological research studies. The chapters are clearly organized by physiological systems and link physiological concepts to clinical applications, including the assessment and management of low- and high-risk pregnancies.

di Renzo GC, Simeoni U 2004 An atlas of the newborn: the transition to extrauterine life. Taylor and Francis
This book provides a guide to recognizing and assessing the visual signs and symptoms of the neonate and differentiating those that are normal from those that indicate an underlying condition or disease.

Henderson C, Jones K (eds) 1997 Essential midwifery. Mosby, London
A research-based midwifery textbook covering biological, social and psychological aspects of midwifery care applied to conception, pregnancy, infancy and development of the family. It has a holistic approach, integrates theory and practice well and includes factors influencing midwifery such as politics.

Kelnar CJH 2004 Sick newborn baby. Saunders
A revised and updated guide to care of the sick neonate, covering a comprehensive range of topics with a baby-centred and holistic perspective.

Lowe NK, Reiss R 1996 Parturition and fetal adaptation. Journal of Gynaecology and Neonatal Nursing 25: 339–349
This article focuses on how the process of labour facilitates the fetus in the transition to extrauterine existence.

Polin RA, Fox WW, Abman SH (eds) 2003 Fetal and neonatal physiology. Saunders, Philadelphia
This in-depth reference book provides a comprehensive description of normal and abnormal physiology of the fetus and neonate, stressing developmental aspects and the clinical significance of abnormal physiology including pathophysiology and management of many of neonatal diseases.

Rennie JM, Roberton NRC (eds) 1998 Textbook of neonatology, 3rd edn. Churchill Livingstone, New York
This is a comprehensive reference book covering care of the normal neonate and the pathophysiology, diagnosis management and prognosis for disorders in the newborn; includes consideration of cost of care and legal issues.

Silver RA, Soll RF 1996 Physiological adaptation at birth. In: Hillier SG, Kitchener HC, Neilson JP (eds) Scientific essentials of reproductive medicine. Saunders, Philadelphia
This chapter, from a textbook focusing on molecular and cellular fundamentals of reproductive biology, provides a comprehensive guide to the physiological basis of neonatal transition to extrauterine life.

Sinclair JC, Bracken MB (eds) 1992 Effective care of the newborn infant. OUP, Oxford
This book provides an invaluable review of the research evidence on the effects of the various care practices carried out during pregnancy, childbirth and the early days after birth.

....

References

Andrew M 1997 The relevance of developmental hemostasis to hemorrhagic disorders of newborns. Seminars in Perinatology 21:70–85

Begley DJ, Firth JA, Hoult JRS 1978 Human reproduction and developmental biology. Macmillan, New York, pp 160, 199

Bernal AL, Watson SP, Phaneuf S, Europe-Finner GN 1993 Biochemistry and physiology of preterm labour and delivery. Baillière's Clinics in Obstetrics and Gynaecology 7:523–552

Blackburn S 1995 Hyperbilirubinaemia and neonatal jaundice. Neonatal Network 14:15–25

Chamberlain G, Dewhurst J, Harvey D 1991 Illustrated textbook of obstetrics. Gower Medical (Mosby), London, pp 14, 15, 16

Edwards MJ, Walsh DA, Li Z 1997 Hyperthermia, teratogenesis and the heat shock response in mammalian embryos in culture. International Journal of Developmental Biology 41:345–358

Givan DC 2003 Physiology of breathing and related pathological processes in infants. Seminars in Pediatric Neurology 10(4): 271–280

Gluckman PD, Sizonenko SV, Bassett NS 1999 The transition from fetus to neonate: an endocrine perspective. Acta Paediatrica Supplement 88:7–11

Golding J, Greenwood R, Birmingham K, Mott M 1992 Childhood cancer, intramuscular vitamin K and pethidine given during labour. British Medical Journal 305:341–346

Goodwin B 1997 Health and development: conceptions to birth. Open University, Milton Keynes, p 259

Guillery EN 1997 Fetal and neonatal nephrology. Current Opinion in Pediatrics 9:148–153

Gunn TR, Ball KT, Power GG, Gluckman P 1991 Factors influencing the initiation of nonshivering thermogenesis. American Journal of Obstetrics and Gynecology 164(1 Pt 1):210–217

Harding R, Hooper SB 1996 Regulation of lung expansion and lung growth before birth. Journal of Applied Physiology 81:209–224

Hay W Jr 1994 Placental supply of energy and protein substrates to the fetus. Acta Paediatrica Supplement 405:13–19

Hilgartner M 1993 Vitamin K and the newborn. New England Journal of Medicine 329:957

Hutchison AA 1994 Respiratory disorders of the neonate. Current Opinion in Pediatrics 6:142–153

Jarvis WR 1996 The epidemiology of colonisation. Infection Control and Hospital Epidemiology 17:47–52

Kinmond S, Aitchison TC, Holland BM, Jones JG, Turner TL, Wardrop CA 1993 Umbilical cord clamping and preterm infants: a randomised trial. British Medical Journal 306:172–175

Kuehl J 1997 Neonatal disseminated intravascular coagulation. Journal of Perinatal and Neonatal Nursing 11:69–77

Kuzawa CW 1998 Adipose tissue in human infancy and childhood: an evolutionary perspective. American Journal of Physical Anthropology Supplement 27:177–209

Lamvu G, Kuller JA 1997 Prenatal diagnosis using fetal cells from the maternal circulation. Obstetrical & Gynecological Survey 52:433–437

Lipsitt LP, Rovee-Collier C 2001 Prenatal and infant development. In: Smelser NJ, Baltes PB (eds) International encyclopedia of the social and behavioral sciences. Elsevier, London, pp 11994–11997

Lockitch G 1994 Beyond the umbilical cord: interpreting laboratory tests in the neonate. Clinical Biochemistry 27:1–6

Lonnerdal B 2003 Nutritional and physiologic significance of human milk proteins. American Journal of Clinical Nutrition 77(6):1537S–1543S

Nelson N 1994 Physiology of transition. In: Avery GB, Fletcher MA, MacDonald MG (eds) Neonatology, pathophysiology and management of the newborn, 4th edn. Lippincott, Philadelphia, pp 223–247

Nijhuis JG 2003 Fetal behavior. Neurobiology of Aging 24(Suppl 1):S41–S46

Okken A 1991 Postnatal adaptation in thermoregulation. Journal of Perinatal Medicine 19(Suppl 1):67–73

Palis J, Segel GB 1998 Developmental biology of erythropoiesis. Blood Reviews 12(2):106–114

Parer JT 1998 Effects of fetal asphyxia on brain cell structure and function: limits of tolerance. Comparative Biochemistry and Physiology A: Molecular and Integrative Physiology 119:711–716

Power GG 1992 Fetal thermoregulation: animal and human. In: Polin RA, Fox WW (eds) Fetal and neonatal physiology. Saunders, Philadelphia, p 447

Robinson D (ed) 1994 Temperature and exercise. S324 Animal physiology Book 2. Open University, Milton Keynes, p 96

Rutter N 1996 The immature skin. European Journal of Pediatrics 155(Suppl 2):s18–20

Scott RJ, Goodburn SF 1995 Potter's syndrome in the second trimester: prenatal screening and pathological findings in 60 cases of oligohydramnios sequence. Prenatal Diagnosis 15:519–525

Smith SL 1995 Hypoglycaemia in the neonate. In: Alexander J, Levy V, Roch S (eds) Aspects of midwifery practice: a research-based approach. Macmillan, Basingstoke, pp 154–176

Strang LB 1991 Fetal lung liquid: secretion and reabsorption. Physiological Reviews 71:991–1016

Strauss RG 1994 Erythropoietin and neonatal anemia. New England Journal of Medicine 330:1227–1228

Strickberger MW 1968 Genetics. Macmillan, New York

Symonds ME, Mostyn A, Pearce S, Budge H, Stephenson T 2003 Endocrine and nutritional regulation of fetal adipose tissue development. Journal of Endocrinology 179:293–299

Taddio A, Katz J 2004 Pain, opioid tolerance and sensitisation to nociception in the neonate. Best Practice & Research Clinical Anaesthesiology 18(2):291–302

Thorburn GD 1992 The placenta, PGE_2 and parturition. Early Human Development 29:63–73

Wolff PH 1966 The causes, controls and organization of behaviour in the neonate. Psychological Issues 5(Monogram 1):1

16 Lactation and infant nutrition

Learning objectives

- To describe the anatomical structure of the breast.
- To outline the hormonal control of lactation.
- To describe how the physiology of lactation can be applied clinically.
- To describe the mechanisms of milk secretion.
- To discuss maternal adaptations during lactation: the effects on fertility, maternal behaviour and nutritional requirements.
- To explain why breastfeeding provides optimal nutrition of the neonate.
- To describe the non-nutritional advantages of breast milk.

Introduction

Infant feeding is the result of multifaceted interactions between infant nutritional demand and maternal physiology. The physiological basis of lactation is important in understanding and facilitating successful breastfeeding. Despite increased awareness of the health benefits of human milk, many women discontinue breastfeeding because they perceive that they have insufficient milk supply. Most breastfeeding problems have identifiable physiological, rather than pathological, causes and are best addressed by considering the interactions between the mother and baby. Successful breastfeeding has nutritional, emotional, developmental and economic benefits. It can be argued that the nutrient requirement of the infant is one of the best understood areas of nutrition. Human milk, however, does not just provide the optimal balance of nutrients in a form appropriate to the developmental needs of the infant, it also compensates for the immature digestive capability and vulnerable immune status of the neonate. Breast milk is the most appropriate food for growth, development and protection of the neonate.

Chapter case study

Almost immediately following his birth, Zara placed Zak in her arms and he instinctively latched onto the breast and started feeding before the cord was cut. Zak fed on the breast for over 45 minutes before detaching himself. What are the advantages of offering the baby the breast as soon as possible after delivery for both mother and baby? What factors could have a negative influence on the early establishment of breastfeeding and how can the midwife optimize breastfeeding?

Anatomy of the breast

The tissue of the breast extends from about the second to the sixth rib (depending on posture). The extension of the tail of the tissue into the axilla (Fig. 16.1) can result in discomfort in the early puerperium when it may become swollen. The mammary gland is made up of a branching network of ducts ending in lobular–alveolar clusters which are the sites of milk secretion. The breast also has a variable amount of adipose tissue and connective tissue. The breast is divided into sections or lobes by fibrous septae, which run from behind the nipple towards the pectoralis

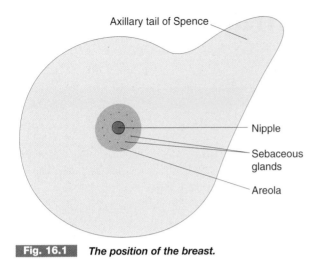

Axillary tail of Spence

Nipple

Sebaceous glands

Areola

Fig. 16.1 *The position of the breast.*

muscle. These septae are important in localizing infections, which are often visually evident as a wedge of red inflamed skin on the surface of the breast. Each of the 8–12 lobes, separated by connective tissue, contains glandular tissue composed of clusters of alveoli and small ducts (Fig. 16.2). The alveolar secretory cells are grouped in grape-like lobules around an extensive branching system of small ducts, which lead to the nipple. Fat is interspersed throughout the lobules. Ultrasound studies of babies feeding at the breast show that there are no discernible lactiferous sinuses in the human breast and that the ducts, even close to the nipple, can branch and be very small and compressible (Ramsay et al, 2005)

The nipple is surrounded by the areola, a pigmented area of varying size, which darkens during pregnancy and has a rich vascular supply and sensory nerve inputs. Surrounding the nipple are Montgomery's tubercles which are sebaceous glands that hypertrophy and become prominent during pregnancy, providing lubrication and protection. Heavy use of soap can increase the risk of nipple damage, particularly drying and cracking. The sensitivity of the nipple and surrounding area increases markedly immediately after delivery. Suckling results in an influx of afferent nerve impulses to the hypothalamus controlling lactation and maternal behaviour.

Each lobe consists of 20–40 lobules, each containing 10–100 alveoli, the glandular physiological units. Alveolar cells are cuboidal in the resting non-pregnant breast and change remarkably to develop full secretory features during lactation. The alveolar cells secrete milk into the lumen of the small ducts. These

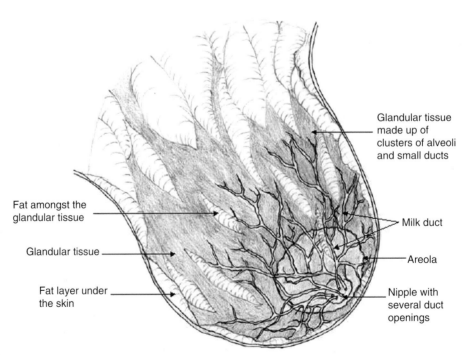

Glandular tissue made up of clusters of alveoli and small ducts

Fat amongst the glandular tissue

Glandular tissue

Fat layer under the skin

Milk duct

Areola

Nipple with several duct openings

Fig. 16.2 *Anatomy of the human breast. (Reproduced with permission from Ramsey et al 2005.)*

secretory cells are surrounded by oxytocin-sensitive myoepithelial (contractile) cells, which are important in milk ejection. The ducts are also lined by contractile cells that open the ducts widely during the milk ejection reflex to assist flow.

Breast growth and development

Mammary growth and development can be divided into four phases: resting, development (pregnancy), milk-secreting (lactation) and involution. At birth, the structure is simply the nipple and a few rudimentary ducts, with few or no alveoli, reflecting their evolutionary origin of modified apocrine sweat glands. Until puberty, the only degree of development may be a little branching of the ducts. There is a decreased incidence of breast cancer in populations with a high consumption of phytoestrogens (oestrogen-like compounds derived from plants). It is suggested that the phytoestrogens stimulate development of the mammary cells in childhood and puberty before pregnancy; these well-differentiated cells may be more resistant to tumour formation (Adlercreutz 1995).

The human is unusual, even compared with other primates, having extensive breast development at puberty, rather than at pregnancy, resulting in an erotic significance. During puberty, the proliferation of the milk ducts, which elongate, sprout and branch, is primarily dependent on secretion of oestrogen with further contributions from growth hormone (GH) and adrenal hormones. The modest alveolar development at this stage is stimulated by progesterone, providing the tissue has been primed by oestrogen. Prolactin may also play a role although the interaction between the adrenal and pituitary glands and the ovaries is not fully understood. The hormonal fluctuations of the menstrual cycle give repeated exposure of the tissue to oestrogen and progesterone, which allow additional but limited growth. Many non-pregnant women experience cyclical changes, especially premenstrually, in breast volume, which is associated with water retention. Occasionally, some secretory activity may occur within the alveoli and a mammary secretion may be expressed premenstrually.

Once an adult woman has developed breasts, minimal stimulation is required to begin milk secretion (Box 16.1). Growth in breast size is most marked in early pregnancy (Hytten 1995). The hormones required for breast development during pregnancy are

Relactation

Relactation, or induced lactation, is the process whereby lactation is initiated at a time not associated with delivery. For instance, an adoptive mother who has not borne a child may wish to breastfeed her adopted baby or a mother may want to resume feeding her own child. Relactation is easier if the woman has previously lactated or been pregnant and if the infant is young. Hormonal support such as oxytocin nasal sprays may be used. The woman is advised to eat well and rest, and to stimulate the nipple and breast often, either by hand or with a breast pump. Supplementary formula milk is given to the baby by spoon or dropper; bottle teats and dummies are avoided. Use of a 'Lact-Aid' supplementer is often found helpful. This device allows the baby to feed on formula milk from a tube attached to the mother's nipple. As the baby feeds, it stimulates the nipple and increases endogenous prolactin secretion. The formula milk is in a bag maintained at body temperature because it is in contact with the mother's body. As breast milk production increases, the amount of formula milk can be reduced.

less than those required for other species. In humans, neither human placental lactogen (hPL) nor GH is essential.

In early pregnancy, breast size and areolar pigmentation increase. The tubercles of Montgomery enlarge and the nipples become more erect. Blood flow to the breast doubles so blood vessels become more prominent and the skin may appear to have a translucent marbled appearance. There is a sharp increase in ductal and glandular elements so the breasts tend to feel slightly lumpy in early pregnancy. This initial hyperplasia is followed by alveolar cell hypertrophy and initiation of secretory activity in later pregnancy.

Oestrogen plays the dominant role in development of the ducts and progesterone in the development in glandular tissue, although insulin and other growth factors, such as epidermal growth factor (EGF) and transforming growth factor (TGFα), have a role in regulation. Changes in pregnancy depend on the lactogenic hormones prolactin and hPL, with placental oestrogen and progesterone playing important modulatory roles. Under these hormonal influences, prominent lobules, resembling bunches of grapes, form in the breast so the alveolar lumen becomes dilated by mid-pregnancy and the secretory cells fully differentiated (Box 16.2). The areola becomes pigmented and a secondary patchily pigmented areola may develop. The nipple enlarges and becomes more mobile and protractile, as the connective tissue anchorages soften and become more stretchable with the oestrogen-driven increase in hydration (see Ch. 11). By the 4th month of pregnancy, the epithelial cells accumulate substantial amounts of secretory material and the mammary glands are fully developed. Prolactin levels progressively increase throughout the pregnancy and are maximal at term. Although it is possible to expel a breast secretion in pregnancy, this is not true colostrum. Full colostrum and milk production is inhibited by high progesterone levels so copious milk production is not established until after parturition. Placental hPL may also contribute to blocking of prolactin responses in pregnancy. Even if very small amounts of the placenta are retained after delivery, lactation is inhibited (see Chs 13 and 14).

Physiology of lactation

Mammary differentiation and milk secretion are coordinated by the endocrine system and involve three categories of hormones: reproductive hormones which change during reproductive development and affect mammary gland development and coordinate milk delivery; metabolic hormones which regulate metabolic responses to nutrient intake or stress; and mammary hormones produced by the lactating mammary gland (Neville et al 2002). Lactation can be considered as two phases: lactogenesis, the initiation of lactation; and galactopoiesis, the maintenance of milk secretion. Lactogenesis itself has two stages; stage 1 is the enzymatic and cellular differentiation of the alveolar cells, which results in colostrum formation, and uptake of immunoglobulins prior to parturition but very little milk synthesis and secretion. Lactogenesis stage 2 is the onset of copious secretion of all milk components about 2–4 days after parturition following the progesterone withdrawal at parturition and concurrent stimulation by prolactin and cortisol. Lactogenesis is normally robust but may be delayed with stressful deliveries and in poorly controlled diabetes (Neville & Morton 2001) and in obese women, probably because adipose tissue abrogates the decrease in progesterone concentration (Rasmussen et al 2001). Once lactation is commenced, it is maintained by the removal of milk which is orchestrated by prolactin, which stimulates production of milk, and oxytocin, which is involved in milk ejection (Table 16.1, Fig. 16.4).

Prolactin

Suckling results in the firing of afferent impulses via the anterolateral columns of the spinal cord to the brain stem and hypothalamus. The hypothalamus subsequently decreases release of dopamine (formerly described as prolactin inhibitory factor) into the portal circulation to the pituitary gland. It was postulated that a dopamine-stimulating factor existed but, although several hormones positively modulate prolactin secretion, control is largely by the lifting of the tonic inhibition from dopamine. The abrogation of the dopamine inhibition stimulates the release of prolactin from the cells of the anterior pituitary. Secretion of prolactin is modified by oestrogen and thyroid-stimulating hormone (TSH). Studies in rats have demonstrated that vasoactive intestinal peptide (VIP), released from the pituitary gland, is an extremely potent prolactin-releasing factor and affects mammary blood flow. The number of signals affecting prolactin release indicates a complex neuroendocrine axis (Ben-Jonathan et al 1991). β-Endorphin and melanocyte-stimulating hormone (MSH), which are co-released from the intermediate lobe of the pituitary gland, also seem to have a role. β-Endorphin blocks dopamine inhibition of prolactin and MSH stimulates the release

---

Box 16.2

Changes to the breasts in pregnancy

- Increased vascularization—may cause tingling
- Dilatation of superficial veins—fair skin appears 'marbled'
- Hypertrophy—full development of lobules
- Dilatation of alveoli and ducts—may feel nodular
- Thickening of nipple skin
- Pigmentation of nipple and areolar—persists after pregnancy
- Secondary areola may appear in dark-skinned women
- Montgomery's tubercles become prominent
- Small quantity of clear colostrum can be expressed in latter half of pregnancy

Table 16.1 *Prolactin and oxytocin*

	Prolactin	Oxytocin
Source	Anterior pituitary gland	Posterior pituitary gland (but synthesized in hypothalamus)
Primary control	Lifting of dopamine inhibition	Neural pathway
Modulating factors	Positively stimulated by oestrogen, TSH, VIP	Neurotransmitters
Peak response	30 minutes	30 seconds
Stimulus	Suckling	Suckling, sound, sight and thought of baby
Target cell	Alveolar cell	Myoepithelial cell
Effect	Milk synthesis	Milk ejection

of prolactin by lowering the threshold of the lactotrophs (Porter et al 1994).

Levels of prolactin begin to rise within 10 minutes of suckling, peak about 30 minutes after initial stimulation and then progressively fall back to basal levels within a further 3 hours. This delay in prolactin secretion following suckling led to the concept that the rise in prolactin was the 'order for the next meal'. Areolar stimulation is essential for prolactin release; negative pressure alone is not adequate and denervation of the nipple prevents prolactin release in response to nipple stimulation.

Prolactin levels fall abruptly about 2 hours before delivery then dramatically rebound. These fluctuations in prolactin level probably relate to changing oestrogen concentrations. The level of prolactin seems to be important in establishing lactation but levels are much diminished after 6 weeks at a rate dependent on suckling frequency and duration (Johnston & Amico 1986). The peak prolactin levels in response to suckling also fall progressively.

Prolactin has a pulsatile release. A diurnal rhythm of prolactin secretion is apparent, with higher circulating levels during sleep. The exact quantitative relationship between prolactin levels and milk production is not clear. In the early puerperium bromocriptine, a dopamine D_2 receptor agonist, causes a fall in prolactin levels and abolishes milk secretion. Dopamine-receptor blockers (such as metoclopramide, haloperidol, domperidone and sulpiride) increase prolactin levels and milk production. Dopamine binds to receptors on the pituitary and is internalized resulting in the increased breakdown of prolactin within the secretory

granules. However, women who have had pituitary surgery and have prolactin levels just above non-pregnant level can breastfeed. The evidence seems to suggest that a threshold prolactin level is required but then there is no correlation between prolactin level and milk production (Howie et al 1980).

Prolactin binds to receptors on the secretory alveolar cells, acting at several sites to increase synthesis of several components of the milk including casein, lactalbumin and fatty acids. During pregnancy, secretory alveolar cells proliferate and acquire the characteristics of highly active secretory cells including numerous mitochondria, an extensive endoplasmic reticulum, well-developed Golgi apparatus and many secretory vesicles.

Biosynthesis of milk

The secretory cells of the alveoli (Fig. 16.3) synthesize or extract the components of milk, which are secreted into the alveolar lumen. The cells are joined near their apical surface by adherins and tight junctions. The apical plasma membrane has a smooth surface with few microvilli, in contrast to the tightly folded basal membrane, which facilitates uptake of substrates such as amino acids, glucose, acetate and fats from the extracellular space. Proteins, fats and lactose are synthesized in the cell and packaged into vesicles. The vesicles move to the apex of the cell where exocytosis takes place.

The composition of the maternal diet can influence the components of breast milk, especially those passing from blood to milk with little modification by the

Fig. 16.3 *The alveolar secretory cells of the breast. (Reproduced with permission from Pond 1992.)*

alveolar cell, such as lipids. The alveolar cells have a unique mechanism for lipid secretion whereby microlipid droplets coalesce forming progressively larger lipid droplets that are eventually enclosed by a specialized milk fat droplet membrane prior to secretion (McManaman & Neville 2003). Aqueous solutes including the proteins, oligosaccharides, lactose, citrate, phosphate and calcium are secreted into the milk by exocytosis after being packaged into secretory vesicles by the Golgi apparatus. Macromolecular substances derived from maternal serum, such as serum proteins (IgA, albumin and transferrin), endocrine hormones (insulin, prolactin and oestrogen), cytokines and lipoprotein lipase are transported by a transcytosis pathway. Various membrane transport pathways transfer small molecules and ions such as glucose, amino acids and water. Large blood cells and serum

follow a paracellular route, squeezing between the alveolar cells.

Oxytocin

Oxytocin levels control the milk ejection reflex, which is responsible for the transfer of the milk from the breast to the baby. Oxytocin stimulates the myoepithelial cells so the alveolar sacs are compressed, increasing the pressure, and the ducts shorten and widen. Although secretion of oxytocin is under a similar neuroendocrine reflex to prolactin, it is physiologically independent. Oxytocin synthesis in the hypothalamus, and its release from the posterior lobe of the pituitary gland, is increased in response to handling the baby, hearing cries or thinking about feeding as well as by tactile stimulation at the nipple. Oxytocin is released in short-lived bursts of less than a minute immediately in response to stimuli. Frequently, the largest response is to the baby crying before feeding so maximum release of oxytocin may occur before suckling starts. Between feeds, isolated pulses of oxytocin are released (McNeilly 2001) possibly in response to other babies' cries or fleeting images of the baby. Unlike prolactin secretion, the milk ejection reflex can be conditioned, as demonstrated by dairy farmers who clang their buckets to stimulate oxytocin and a good milk yield. Similarly, a baby's cry can often trigger oxytocin secretion, which is why the practice of babies 'rooming-in' with their mothers (sleeping close to their mother's bed) is often associated with successful breastfeeding.

The milk ejection reflex is very sensitive to inhibition by physical and psychological stresses such as pain and discomfort, anxiety, emotional swings, tiredness, embarrassment, worry and alcohol. The limbic system, which coordinates the body's responses to emotions, is involved in oxytocin release. The likely mechanism is catecholamine inhibition of oxytocin release and adrenergic vasoconstriction of mammary blood vessels limiting access of the oxytocin to the myoepithelial cells. Women experiencing problems in establishing milk flow are often helped by covering their breasts with warm flannels which appears to aid blood flow and oxytocin access.

Surprisingly, denervation of mammary glands in experimental animals appears to have little effect on milk production (Williams et al 1993). This suggests that the afferent nerve pathway may not be so important as the interactions of neurotransmitters. Transmitters that have been implicated in the control of the milk ejection reflex include noradrenaline, β-endorphin, serotonin and dopamine. As with control of prolactin secretion, the number of factors influencing oxytocin secretion suggests that the pathway is much more complicated than originally thought. Stimulation of the female reproductive tract, especially the vagina and cervix, increases oxytocin release so milk may be ejected from the breasts during coitus.

Oxytocin binds to specific receptors on the myoepithelial cells around the milk-secreting cells and to longitudinal cells in the duct walls. Contraction of the myoepithelial cells results in milk being expelled into the ducts, which shorten as the longitudinal cells contract. Oxytocin-induced contraction generates pressure waves within the breasts and is responsible for prickly sensations associated with breastfeeding. When the milk ejection reflex is well established, milk may be spontaneously ejected from both breasts.

Oxytocin pulses increase in amplitude during labour and are involved in the positive-feedback amplification in labour (see Ch. 1). Oxytocin is associated with changes in maternal behaviour and increased alertness at delivery. The pulses of oxytocin induced by feeding have an effect on the uterus, stimulating uterine contractions and involution. Multiparous women tend to feel these contractions or 'after-pains' with increased intensity. Women who do not want to breastfeed may find the physiological changes in the breasts at delivery uncomfortable; various techniques are recommended to inhibit lactation (Box 16.3).

Suckling and milk transfer

In feeding from the breast, the baby takes the whole nipple into its mouth and places its tongue under the adjacent areola. When the baby's tongue moves down, ducts in the nipple fill with milk which is expelled when the tongue moves upwards.

Babies exhibit two distinct patterns of suckling (Turgeon-O'Brien et al 1996). Nutritive suckling is a continuous stream of strong slow sucks, which efficiently allows milk transfer. This occurs predominantly in the early part of the feed. Non-nutritive suckling increasingly replaces nutritive suckling during the progression of the feed. It is characterized by alternation of rapid shallow bursts of suckling and rests. It is thought that patterns of thumb sucking may reflect these two conducts. Breastfed babies have two distinct rhythms of thumb sucking and tend to put more of the root of the thumb into their mouths. Although non-nutritive suckling is associated with a decreased transfer of milk, it is still very effective in stimulating

---

Box 16.3

Methods for suppression of lactation

- Bromocriptine (dopamine agonist) (use with great caution)
- Treatment with sex steroids to antagonize prolactin effects
- Breast-binding
- Application of ice-packs

prolactin release and so may be important in successful lactation.

The amount of milk produced is extremely variable; that mothers can feed multiple babies and produce additional milk for banking or storage suggests that the mammary synthetic capacity exceeds the normal requirement of single infants. A demand-fed baby consumes irregular quantities of milk at irregular times. The suggestion that the baby determines milk yield by local control is supported by the strong correlation between degree of breast emptying and rate of milk synthesis. Some women feed exclusively from one breast (and not at all from the other). The autocrine factor capable of overriding the central hormone control, feedback inhibitor of lactation (FIL), was first identified in goats (Wilde et al 1995). This protein inhibitory factor has also been found in the whey fraction of human milk. It is secreted from the alveolar cells and accumulates in milk. The factor inhibits secretion of lactose, probably by blocking the action of prolactin, and therefore provides the mechanism to adjust supply to demand. When milk is not removed from the breast, the concentration of the factor increases and blocks the action of prolactin thus reducing the rate of milk synthesis. It helps to explain why maternal dietary intake has relatively little influence on the amount of milk produced. Women in traditional societies have a much greater frequency of breastfeeding so their production of FIL is probably not enough to have an autocrine effect on lactation; milk synthesis is most likely to be influenced solely by metabolic and endocrine mechanisms (Hartmann et al 1998).

Involution

After cessation of lactation, involution takes about 3 months. Milk accumulates in the alveoli and small lactiferous ducts, which causes distension and mechanical atrophy of the epithelial cells and rupture of the alveolar walls, creating large spaces. Milk secretion is therefore suppressed by local mechanical factors rather than by diminishing prolactin levels. Phagocytosis of the cells and glandular debris results in fewer and smaller lobular–acinar structures. The alveolar lumens decrease in size and may disappear. The alveolar lining changes from a single secretory layer to a non-secretory double layer. If breastfeeding is stopped suddenly, the process is more intense and

painful. The breasts remain larger after lactation as the deposits of fat and connective tissue are increased. Involution after lactation is different to the structural atrophy and loss of adipose tissue occurring in postmenopausal mammary cells deprived of oestrogen.

Problems associated with lactation

Milk insufficiency

Most problems have an identifiable physiological basis; breast milk insufficiency is frequently overdiagnosed and is usually simply resolved (Woolridge 1996). The majority of women with apparently insufficient milk supply have unsubstantiated worries and require confidence, improved technique (especially positioning), encouragement or advice. This can be supported by physiological strategies such as electric breast pumps and pharmacological (anti-dopamine) agents. Iatrogenic low milk supply may be attributed to excessive down-regulation of supply probably during the calibration period. It is possible that baby milk manufacturers inadvertently exploit the importance of the calibration period by offering free milk samples early in lactation. If the initial calibrated volume cannot be increased, the mother will then be unable to increase her milk supply later and will be forced to provide alternative inferior sources of milk, which are expensive and can be harmful if water supplies are contaminated, as happens in a number of developing countries.

Behavioural problems that are acquired by the baby as coping strategies to avoid aversive events may also induce a low milk supply. These problems include discomfort during positioning at the breast and problems with breathing. Self-limitation of intake and lack of persistence may account for the condition described as 'contented underfed babies' (Woolridge 1996). Pathophysiological failure is rare and probably affects less than 2% of women with apparent milk insufficiency. Rare causes include mammary hypoplasia, or absence of normal breast development at puberty or in pregnancy. Retained placental products affect lactation reversibly but Sheehan's syndrome, necrosis of the anterior pituitary due to acute hypovolaemic shock, as in antepartum haemorrhage (e.g. due to placental abruption) or postpartum haemorrhage, is more serious.

Drugs

Many drugs are secreted into breast milk, but the data on the effects of specific drugs on the breastfed infant is often not available. Of particular concern are those drugs with central nervous system (CNS) activity as the postnatal development of the infant's nervous system is vulnerable. The benefits of maternal treatment and the advantages of breastfeeding have to be balanced against the risk of exposure of the neonate to the medication. Passive diffusion of the unbound, unionized form of the drug into the breast milk is the major mechanism of transfer. Therefore, it is affected by maternal compartmentalization and molecular properties and the composition of the breast milk (McManaman & Neville 2003). Assessment of adverse drug reactions in infants is difficult. Drugs that are minimally excreted into the breast milk, are metabolized quickly by the neonate and are not associated with adverse effects are obviously the preferred choice.

Socially used drugs such as alcohol (Mennella & Beauchamp 1991), nicotine and illicit drugs (heroin and cocaine) (Golding 1997) also cross into the milk. How much these affect the baby is not clear. Women who smoke are less likely to want to breastfeed, or initiate breastfeeding, and more likely to breastfeed for a shorter duration (Amir & Donath 2003). Drug metabolism and elimination by the neonate is often limited so exposure to apparently low doses of the drug in milk can have a cumulative effect, particularly in premature babies and those who have prolonged exposure. Drugs tend not to accumulate in the milk but have a bidirectional transfer. Therefore, the amount of drug received by the infant will be reduced if the mother takes the drug immediately after a feed so the baby does not feed when the drug is at peak concentration in the maternal plasma and milk. Production of breast milk is also a method of excretion and contains drugs, viruses, food additives, chemical contamination (such as lead), pesticides and radioactivity. Chemical residues of pollutants are detected in most human milk throughout the world. Heavy metals are of concern because of the susceptibility of the infant's nervous system. Mammals do not have a mechanism to excrete pesticide residues such as polychlorinated biphenyls and 1,1,1-trichloro-2,2-bis(p-chlorophenyl)ethane (DDT). However, the residues do cross the blood–breast barrier so lactation is the only way to reduce the body load. The burden is then transferred to the breastfed infant (Rogan et al 1987). Usually breastfeeding is not contraindicated.

Viruses

Maternal viruses may enter the milk. Vertical transmission and subsequent infection of the infant via breastmilk has been confirmed for human immunodeficiency virus (HIV), tuberculosis (TB), cytomegalovirus (CMV) and hepatitis B. It is probably inadvisable for mothers with TB to breastfeed as the infection tends to be reactivated by maternal tiredness and stress (Box 16.4). However, advice for HIV-positive mothers is unclear. The immunological properties of breast milk are probably important in protecting against illnesses that accelerate the development of AIDS (acquired immune deficiency syndrome), particularly in areas of the world where it is endemic (Van de Perre 1995). The likelihood of HIV transmission is affected by maternal viral load, the volume of the milk consumed, the duration of breastfeeding, inflammation of the breast (e.g. caused by cracked nipples), the presence of oral thrush and the introduction of formula milk (Warner & Sapsford 2004). (Note that several medications used in HIV prophylaxis can transfer to the breastmilk and have potentially serious side-effects, including anaemia, seizures, hepatitis and feeding difficulties.)

Case study 16.1 is an example of concerns about breastfeeding.

Inhibition of fertility

Breast milk is also important to the infant because suppression of fertility is an advantage. An adequate birth interval is important for both maternal and child health. Lactational amenorrhoea may last from 2 months to 4 years. It is particularly important in developing countries where breastfeeding prevents more pregnancies than all the other methods of contraception put together. The variability in duration of suppressed fertility seems to be related to a number of

---

Box 16.4

Contraindications to breastfeeding
- Maternal illness
- Maternal drug consumption
- Congenital abnormalities, e.g. cleft palate
- HIV-positive—controversial
- TB infection (depending on strain and treatment)

Case study 16.1

Elma expressed concerns about breastfeeding throughout her pregnancy. She complained that the midwives running the antenatal classes were biased towards breastfeeding and that bottle-feeding was just as good. Elma described her own family as an example; she is the oldest of five children all of whom were bottle-fed by her mother and were well and healthy. Two days after delivery, Elma experienced breast discomfort and tentatively asked a midwife whether it was too late to try breastfeeding.

- How would you as the midwife explain and encourage Elma to breastfeed throughout the antenatal period?
- What factors would increase her chances of being successful in breastfeeding?
- What support would she require from the midwives?
- Would breastfeeding or anything else help to relieve the breast discomfort?

factors; the most important seems to be frequency of suckling. At the end of pregnancy, levels of gonadotrophins are very low because high levels of oestrogen continue to impose negative feedback. At delivery, the placental hormones begin to disappear, at different rates depending on their half-life. hPL disappears from the plasma within hours. Oestrogen and progesterone levels fall to prepregnant levels within a week of the placental loss (Hytten 1995). Levels of human chorionic gonadotrophin (hCG) are negligible about 3 weeks after delivery. There is a gradual recovery in the ovarian–pituitary axis over the first 4 months after delivery; this recovery is delayed by regular suckling.

In non-lactating women, body temperature measurements and the first menstrual bleeding suggest that the earliest ovulation may occur at 4 weeks after delivery but is usually delayed until 8–10 weeks (McNeilly 2001); most women have resumed normal menstrual patterns by 15 weeks. The first menstrual cycle is often anovulatory or associated with an inadequate luteal phase. Most women ovulate by the third cycle. 50% of non-lactating women who do not use contraception conceive within 6–7 months.

Menstruation and ovulation return more slowly in a lactating woman. Ovarian activity usually returns before the end of lactational amenorrhoea. Therefore, menstruation is a poor indicator of fertility; conception can occur without menstruation. Neither ovulation nor menstruation normally occurs within 6 weeks, but about half of all contraceptive-unprotected breastfeeding mothers conceive within 9 months of lactation, 1–10% during lactational amenorrhoea. Between 30% and 70% of first cycles are ovulatory; the longer the period of lactational amenorrhoea, the more likely the woman is to ovulate prior to the first menstruation.

The precise mechanisms involved in lactational amenorrhoea are not clear. High prolactin levels abolish the pulsatile luteinizing hormone (LH) secretion and decrease the pituitary response to gonadotrophin-releasing hormone. The mid-cycle positive feedback in response to oestrogen is absent. The sensitivity to negative feedback is enhanced and that to positive feedback is decreased. So, even if enough LH and follicle-stimulating hormone (FSH) are present to stimulate follicular development, the inhibitory effect of oestrogen results in an inadequate luteal phase. Prolactin is inhibitory at the level of the ovary, blocking the effects of LH and FSH. It also has a direct effect on the brain, possibly affecting libido.

As prolactin secretion has a pulsatile rhythm with larger amounts being released at night, the frequency of stimulation by suckling and the night-time feeds are particularly important in maintaining prolactin levels high enough to suppress fertility (McNeilly 2001). The duration and number of feeds are important because the prolactin levels are augmented before they return completely to the basal secretory level. Prolonged amenorrhoea is associated with maternal malnutrition (Rogers 1997). Poor nutrition is associated with suppression of fertility in non-lactating women. The extra nutrient requirement for milk production can increase the degree of maternal malnutrition. Also, although women receiving less than optimal nutrition can breastfeed their babies adequately, they secrete milk more slowly so the infants feed more often and for longer which raises their circulating prolactin levels.

Maternal behaviour

Maternal commitment to reproduction is more than pregnancy; it involves the establishment of lactation and appropriate maternal behaviour (Grattan 2002). The demands of the parents and offspring during lactation may conflict. It is suggested that parents will tend to maximize the survival of their young but not to the extent that would limit investment in other off-spring, including those as yet unborn (Peaker 1989). This theory means that, although mothers will try to recoup the investment of pregnancy by favouring the offspring's survival, should this cost compromise their future reproductive ability there are definite advantages in discontinuing this investment in favour of a more favourable future offspring. There may be genetic components affecting the time-course of lactation or the upper limit of milk production. The rate of milk secretion and duration of lactation vary with nutritional state. Some mammals respond to decreased food supply in ways that favour the succeeding pregnancies, such as killing some or all of the litter. Species with long gestation and long-term commitment to the offspring, such as humans, tend to favour the well-being of live offspring.

Behavioural changes include preparatory behaviour such as nest building and increased aggression. Care and protection are associated with lactation. These behavioural patterns are associated with the progressive independence of the young. In humans, this behaviour is more difficult to observe than in other species.

The nutritional status of the mother may affect feeding and interaction with her infant (Britton 1993). The effect of maternal malnutrition can affect infant development, depending on its duration and the timing. Infants malnourished in utero may have decreased capacity to respond to appropriate cues and therefore an increased likelihood of social and further nutritional deprivation. Malnourished infants have poorer muscle tone, increased lethargy, irritability and frequency of illness, decreased attention and responsiveness and altered sleep–wake states. Malnourished mothers experience more fatigue, which can affect their own sensitivity to cues from the baby, such as responses to stress and attention–behavioural patterns.

Nutrition of the lactating mother

Human growth rate is much slower than that of other animals. Neurological development is relatively late and the duration of human lactation is longer. During lactation, daily nutrient input and reserves laid down in pregnancy are juggled. Milk output is largely independent of the mother's ethnic origin and nutritional status. A balanced diet in lactation appears to favour the health of the mother. However, it should be noted that substrates required for milk synthesis are not flexible. Mammary glands are not able to synthesize essential amino acids or long-chain polyunsaturated fatty acids (LC-PUFAs); they also require non-essential amino acids for protein synthesis and glucose or glucose precursors for lactose and oligosaccharide synthesis. These have to be provided from the maternal diet or from maternal body reserves. Indeed, it has been suggested that the maternal brain may act as a reservoir of PUFAs for both fetal and neonatal brain requirements (Dewar & Psych 2004) and that increased transfer of nutrients to the developing brain during pregnancy and lactation might contribute to postnatal depression.

Energy requirements for milk production

The energy output of milk is a significant proportion of the total energy output of the lactating woman; it is suggested that peak lactation requires an increase of energy intake of about 25%. In dairy animals, the level of food intake strongly correlates with milk yield. In a number of species, lactation results in a significant increase in size and complexity (such as villus size) of the maternal intestine (Hammond 1997), but it is obviously not possible to study any such adaptive changes in lactating women. It may not be valid to apply knowledge of nutrition and physiology of dairy animals, which are completely milked twice a day, to mammals who suckle their young according to natural patterns of behaviour. Anthropological studies on human hunter–gatherer communities suggest that babies feed every half hour at 2 weeks and every 4 hours at 4 months. The characteristics of mammalian milk relate directly to the interaction between the mother and child. Marsupials and animals that bear their young during hibernation and are always present produce milk that is dilute and has a low fat content. In contrast, in animals where the mother nurses her young at widely spaced intervals, for instance a hunting lioness, the milk is very concentrated and high in fat. Human milk has most resemblance to the former; it is dilute with a low fat content suggesting that humans have evolved as a species where the young have unlimited access to milk and there is high attentiveness shown by a constantly present mother (Prentice & Prentice 1995). The stress of human lactation is relatively low compared with species with faster growing or multiple young, but this is countered by the high cost of maintaining a dependent infant for a prolonged period. The high level of maternal investment in pregnancy and slow reproductive cycle mean that humans are committed to sustain a conception.

There is a discrepancy between the theoretical calculated energy requirement for milk production and the actual intake of lactating women, even taking into account the fat reserves laid down in pregnancy. Current recommendations are that an exclusively breastfeeding woman requires an additional 2700 kJ (650 kcal) per day and an increase of 20 g of protein per day (Dewey 1997). However, it is thought that about 600 kJ (150 kcal) per day will be provided by the maternal fat stores for the first 6 months so the net increment needed is 2100 kJ (500 kcal) per day. In practice, these requirements are much higher than the observed intakes in successfully lactating women even when offered unlimited access to food. Lactational performance is particularly resilient in humans as demonstrated by the efficiency of lactation in undernourished and impoverished communities. In animals, a decrease in non-shivering thermogenesis (inhibition of brown-fat heat generation) (NST) and therefore the provision of extra energy for milk production is suggested to account for this difference. The mechanism in humans is not thought to be mediated by changes in NST but the lactating woman has increased sensitivity to insulin (Illingworth et al 1986). This energy-sparing effect and efficient energy utilization of lactating women has a particularly big implication in developing countries.

Increased incidence of obesity in Western societies is of concern with about a third of women having a body mass index (BMI) greater than 25 kg/m². Pregnancy is a risk factor for the development of obesity and it is suggested that postpartum weight loss may not be inevitable (Ohlin & Rossner 1996). Possibly the changes in energy metabolism associated with pregnancy and lactation may remain after weaning. If so, lactation could contribute to the problem. Different species of mammal lay down body fat during pregnancy to different degrees. In lactation, mammals rely on the deposited fat to different extents. Whales and seals, for instance, rely entirely on body fat and protein reserves to sustain lactation whereas dairy cows and laboratory rats are very dependent on increased intake to provide energy for milk yield. Pregnant women deposit fat and have a changed hormonal environment. The reported studies tend to conflict and do not show significant differences in weight loss with different patterns of infant feeding. However, interpretation of the studies is confused by confounding factors such as different duration and extent of feeding and the increased tendency of women who are not breastfeeding to reduce their weight deliberately. There is also a large variation in the energy content of the milk produced (see below). Lactating women produce adequate-to-abundant quantities of milk of sufficient quality to promote growth of healthy infants, even when maternal nutrition is not adequate. Whereas the health of the breastfeeding infant is apparently protected should maternal nutrition be compromised, it is probably at the cost of depletion of maternal nutrient stores and potential effects on subsequent pregnancies. Deliberate weight loss in well-nourished healthy breastfeeding woman has no effect on the yield or composition of breast milk. However, it is recommended that weight loss should not be more than 1–2 kg per month (Institute of Medicine 2002). Although reduction in energy intake does not affect milk synthesis, lower intakes of food mean that micronutrient intake might be compromised. As energy intake falls, the likelihood of a number of nutrients failing to reach the recommended intake progressively increases. In order of vulnerability, the nutrients most likely to be affected are calcium, zinc, magnesium, thiamin, vitamin B_6, vitamin E, riboflavin, folate, phosphorus and iron (Lawrence 1999).

Minerals

Both pregnancy and lactation present a tremendous challenge to maternal calcium status (Prentice 2000). The fetal skeleton requires 5 mmol of calcium per day. The lactational drain of calcium is greater; average daily production of 800 ml of milk contains 6.25 mmol of calcium. It is estimated that about 10% of total maternal calcium stores (about 105 g) is transferred to the fetus/neonate, predominantly duration lactation (Wysolmerski 2002). One or more of the following can meet demand for calcium: increased dietary calcium, increased absorption, decreased excretion, or increased bone demineralization (net loss of bone). In the third trimester, absorption of calcium increases together with a modest increase in bone resorption. Calcium demands of lactation are met by an increase in the rate of bone resorption and a decrease in renal calcium excretion which is speculated to have evolved from the adaptations in bone and mineral metabolism that supply calcium for egg production in lower vertebrates (Wysolmerski 2002). The oestrogen level during lactation is relatively low so the bone mass is not protected to the same extent.

Lactation is the period of most rapid bone loss in a woman's life; there is a net drain of calcium from the body, with a selective decrease in trabecular bone. This reduction is independent of parathyroid hormone and vitamin D levels. So lactation may appear to increase future risk of osteoporosis, but risk factors shown to be associated with fractures do not necessarily include breastfeeding (Sowers 1996). During weaning, an imbalance between bone resorption and bone formation results in a rapid and complete recovery of bone mass. The implications for birth spacing and prolonged breastfeeding are not clear. Modern practices of delaying childbearing resulting in decreased time for recovery before menopause are probably countered by the cumulative effect of having fewer children. Prolonged lactational amenorrhoea may help to restore maternal iron status

Concentrations of major minerals including calcium, sodium, potassium, phosphorus and magnesium are not affected by the diet. Milk iron, zinc and copper concentrations are independent of maternal mineral status suggesting active transport mechanisms for these nutrients in the mammary gland (Domellöf et al 2004). When milk production falls during weaning, milk iron levels decrease and milk zinc levels increase. Maternal intakes of iodine and selenium do affect levels in milk.

Water and fluids

The volume of milk produced is robust; only very severe dehydration and extreme malnutrition affect the volume of milk produced. There is no evidence that increasing fluid intake increases the volume of milk produced or that reducing fluid intake prevents engorgement. When fluids are restricted, urine output decreases and the woman is at risk of dehydration. Breastfeeding women should be advised to drink when they are thirsty and to be aware that they will need more fluid than normal.

Infant nutrition and the composition of human milk

Human milk optimally fulfils the nutritional requirements of the human neonate. It has a unique composition that is particularly suitable for the rapid growth and development of the infant born with immature digestive, renal and hepatic systems. Unique features of human milk are able to compensate for the under-developed neonatal capabilities. Human milk contains not only the macronutrients, vitamins and minerals but also non-nutrient growth factors, hormones and protective factors.

There are at least 100 components of human milk, including substances yet to be identified and their roles elucidated. In the Koran, breast milk is described as 'white blood'. This is a particularly apt description because the early milk has more white blood cells than blood itself. Milk is a solution in which other substances are dissolved, emulsified or colloidally dispersed. The value of breast milk is undisputed; rarely should breastfeeding be discouraged.

Both the volume and composition of human milk is extremely variable. Some of this variability is genetic (any genetic mutation leading to inadequate mammary development in humans would no longer be eliminated as alternatives to human milk are available). Postponing childbearing until long after sexual maturity has an effect on breast development as advancing age causes some atrophy of the mammary tissue (Hytten 1995). However, there is little relationship between the size of the breast and milk output.

The unique characteristic of humans is the large complex brain, which undergoes much development in the first 2 years of life. Human milk provides levels of lactose, cysteine, cholesterol and thromboplastin, which are required for CNS tissue synthesis. However, as breast milk provides a model of optimum nutrition, analysis of its composition has allowed good substitutes to be produced as formula feeds. Infant formula milk will never completely mimic human milk, however, as the quality of the nutrients is not reproducible and the immunological aspects of the milk make it superior.

Although breast milk may be considered perfect nutrition, its composition is variable. It varies from woman to woman, from one period of lactation to another, and hourly through the day. Its composition is related to the timing of the feed, how much is produced and parameters relating to the last feed (Emmett & Rogers 1997); it has also been suggested that maternal age, parity, health and social class affect the composition of the milk. Mothers of premature infants produce milk that has a higher concentration of some nutrients, but this probably reflects the small volumes produced for small infants. Except for vitamin and fat content, the composition is largely independent of maternal nutrition unless the mother experiences severe malnutrition. Supplementation may improve maternal health rather than affect milk composition and volume.

There are many difficulties encountered in the estimation of the volume of milk produced. Weighing either the mother or baby before and after the feed is fraught with problems. Although double-labelled water measurements have allowed more accurate estimations (Lucas et al 1987), the variability within a feed and from feed to feed make it very difficult to ascertain precisely the nutrient consumption of a healthy growing baby. These estimates of about 60 kcal per 100 ml are lower than UK food composition tables (69 kcal per 100 ml). The volume of daily milk intake by healthy infants has a wide range. Factors that influence frequency, intensity or duration of feeds will affect volume consumed. Breastfed infants appear to self-regulate their energy intake and consume more milk if it has a lower energy level. This is thought to be related to the lower incidence of obesity in individuals who were breastfed as infants (Dewey 2003). Breastfeeding allows infants to learn self-regulation of energy intake whereas bottle-fed infants may be encouraged to finish the bottle which suppresses their autoregulatory mechanism. Breast milk may also contain appetite inhibitors and stimulators. It is suggested that different modes of infant feeding have different metabolic programming effects. Formula-fed infants tend to receive more protein which results in an increased insulin response. Insulin stimulates adipose tissue deposition (increased number and fat content of adipocytes) which is associated with weight gain and obesity. Alternatively breastfeeding may affect leptin metabolism; the higher level of fatness in formula-fed infants may programme reduced sensitivity to leptin in later life. However, it should be noted that there is confounding by parental attributes and the family environment. Parents who choose to breastfeed tend to have a healthier lifestyle with more optimal dietary habits and higher levels of physical activity; they also exert less parental control over child-feeding practices (Dewey 2003).

The low levels of gastric secretion and other immature digestive characteristics of the neonatal gut confer a number of immunological advantages which were described in Chapter 15 (p. 391).

Colostrum

In the first 3 days postdelivery, the mother produces about 2–10 ml of colostrum per day. More colostrum is produced sooner if the woman has had previous pregnancies, particularly if she has lactated before. In some cultures, colostrum is thought to be old milk or 'pus' and is discarded rather than fed to infants.

Colostrum is transparent and is yellow from the high β-carotene content. Mature milk in contrast looks less viscous and slightly blue. Colostrum has more protein and vitamins A and K and less carbohydrate and fat than mature milk. It is easily digested and well absorbed. It has a lower energy content of 58 kcal per 100 ml compared with 70 kcal per 100 ml in mature milk. Levels of sodium, potassium, chloride and zinc are high in colostrum but reflect the low volume produced rather than the infant's requirements for a bolus dose of certain nutrients. The composition is extremely variable, which reflects its unstable secretory pattern.

Colostrum facilitates the colonization of the gut with *Lactobacillus bifidus* (Wharton et al 1994). Meconium also contains growth factors for *Lactobacillus bifidus*. Colostrum seems to have a laxative effect, stimulating the passage of meconium. The high protein content is largely due to the abundant antibodies, which protect against gastrointestinal tract infection. IgA forms 50% of the protein content of colostrum, falling to 10% by 6 months.

During the first 30 hours or so, the secretion (colostrum) has a high protein:lactose ratio. In the following days, as the baby suckles more and stimulates milk production, the resulting increase in prolactin secretion stimulates production of the major whey protein α-lactalbumin, which is a specific component of the enzyme lactose synthetase and so regulates lactose production. The effect of increasing lactose production is that water is drawn into the secretion to maintain osmotic equilibrium so the volume increases thus diluting the protein content. The absolute amounts of protein secreted into the milk are maintained or increased even though the concentration falls.

The composition of the milk becomes relatively stable from about day 5 but is variable in volume. The amount of breast milk produced is related to the weight and requirement of the infant; there is a steady increase in volume in the first few weeks. Milk production appears to get under way regardless of the size and requirements of the baby, although hPL levels may play a role in the increased production of milk in mothers of twins. The early weeks of lactation can be considered to be a time of calibration between maternal production and the infant's demand. The volume of milk produced is usually increased to match demand. Down-regulation may be irreversible. It is suggested that mothers of small or preterm babies should express as much milk as they can (i.e. peak yield rather than only enough for the baby's transiently limited requirement).

Milk secretion in women who do not suckle their baby may persist scantily for 3 or 4 weeks while prolactin levels are still high. The effect of suckling is to stimulate the release of prolactin and oxytocin, which are essential for the maintenance of lactation (Fig. 16.4). Provided breastfeeding is regular, lactation can last for several years. Most studies suggest that the average daily volume of milk produced is about 800 ml. Measurement of the milk produced is notoriously difficult but it is clear that there is much variation depending on demand: mothers of twins produce about twice as much milk.

Protein

Protein is the limiting nutrient for growth and development. It also provides nitrogen and amino acids required for membrane and transport proteins, hormones, enzymes, growth factors, neurotransmitters and immunoglobulins. Human neonates have a slow growth rate compared with other species which is reflected in the low protein concentrations (0.7–0.9 g protein per 100 ml compared with 3.5 g per 100 ml in cow's milk). (Note that early estimates of protein neglected the high concentration of non-protein nitrogen thus significantly overestimating protein level; see below.) Excess protein intake can present an excessive solute load to the immature kidneys, which results in acid–base imbalance and metabolic acidosis. Chronic

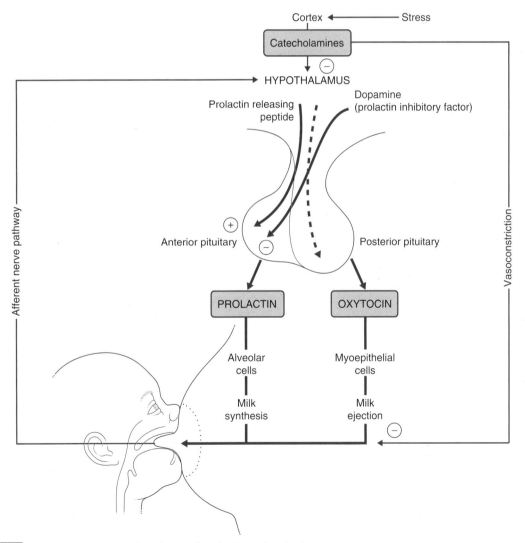

Fig. 16.4 *Suckling stimulates the release of prolactin and oxytocin.*

protein undernutrition or prolonged lactation may result in changes in the protein composition of milk. Protein supplementation of the mother's diet tends to increase milk volume rather than affecting protein concentration but has an important role in supplementing maternal health.

When milk proteins are exposed to the relatively acidic environment of the neonatal stomach they separate into casein (proteins that precipitate, forming curds) and whey (those proteins that remain soluble). This means that there is a continuous flow of nutrients, initially as soluble lactose and whey proteins, and later from digested curd. Whey proteins include serum albumin, α-lactalbumin, lactoferrin, secretory IgA and some enzymes and protein hormones transported from the maternal circulation. Whey proteins are easy to digest by a human neonatal gut, which has particularly low levels of trypsin and pepsin. The whey-dominant content of milk reduces the risk of lactobezoars (obstructive milk curd balls) forming in the stomach. Human α-lactalbumin is easier to digest than bovine β-lactalbumin.

The ratio of whey to casein in human milk is 60:40 (1.5). The β-casein in human milk forms curds that are soft and flocculent with a low curd tension, which are easily digested. Bioactive peptides formed from partial hydrolysis of human milk casein may be important in stimulating the neonatal immune system (Ebrahim 1990). In contrast, cow's milk has a whey:casein ratio of 20:80 (0.25). Bovine casein is predominantly α-casein, which forms a tough rubbery precipitate unless heat-treated, which is more difficult for human infants to digest and decreases the bioavailability of calcium and other cations. Human β-casein tends to form smaller micelles incorporating minerals that are easier for the neonate to digest. κ-Casein in cow's milk has a marked effect on the development of the bovine gastrointestinal physiology, stimulating the secretion of chymosin, which is the dominant protease of the fourth stomach. Casein associates with calcium, phosphate and magnesium in the micelles.

The immune response to cow's milk

A high proportion of dietary casein of bovine origin is associated with an increased incidence of intestinal allergy and inflammation and is implicated as one of the possible triggers of necrotizing enterocolitis. As the neonatal gut is permeable, large proteins can be absorbed intact across the gut. Some of these proteins stimulate maturation of the gut and immune system. However, others may present an immunological challenge that produces a response which can cause problems later in life. It has been controversially hypothesized that proteins in cow's milk formula are associated with an increased incidence of diabetes (Karjalainen et al 1992). The hypothesis suggests that a large bovine protein crosses the infant's gut and stimulates the immune system (Monte et al 1994). Because of similarities between this protein and proteins of the endocrine pancreas, the immune system may direct an autoimmune response against the cells of the pancreas destroying the insulin-producing β-cells. For whatever reason, the incidence of insulin-dependent diabetes mellitus is lower in children who have been breastfed.

Essential amino acids

Proteins are formed of chains of 20 amino acids. Some of the amino acids cannot be made in the body; these are essential or indispensable amino acids (see Table 12.1, p. 284). Non-essential amino acids can be synthesized from glucose and ammonia via the Krebs cycle or from free amino acids by transamination. Some amino acids are conditionally essential for the neonate because the neonate has limited synthetic capability. The amounts and proportions of essential amino acids determine the quality of a protein. A protein that is rich in all essential amino acids has a high biological value or net protein utilization which means all the amino acids supplied are converted into proteins. A food with a deficiency of an amino acid has a low biological value. Human milk has a very high biological value because it is fully utilized by the neonate as its amino acids are exactly in proportion to requirement. Few other foods have such a high value. By the end of the second week of life, 90% of the ingested nitrogen-containing substances in milk are absorbed, suggesting that milk contains the optimal pattern of amino acids.

The amino acid content of human milk, especially whey proteins, is ideal for the growth requirements of the human infant. Neonatal metabolism of certain amino acids (e.g. phenylalanine, tyrosine and methionine) is initially limited because the enzymes involved in their metabolism are expressed late in development. If these amino acids reach high concentrations, they can cause damaging effects. Human milk is relatively low in tyrosine, phenylalanine and methionine but high in amino acids that the infant cannot synthesize in adequate amounts. The inability to synthesis adequate quantities of histidine, cysteine and taurine means that these become conditionally essential for infants and need to be provided in the diet. The enzyme that converts methionine to cysteine, cystathionase, is low or undetectable in the neonate. Cysteine is required for growth and development. Infants, especially preterm infants, fed unmodified cow's milk may develop hyperphenylalaninaemia and hypertyrosinaemia, which can increase the net acid load and adversely affect development of the CNS.

Taurine is the second most abundant free amino acid in human milk. Infants use taurine for bile acid conjugation (in contrast to adult conjugation by glycine) so this amino acid is important in the digestion and metabolism of cholesterol and fats. There are also high levels of taurine in fetal brain tissue where it may act as a neurotransmitter or neuromodulator, and be involved in myelinization of nerves and the optimal maintenance of retinal integrity (Chesney et al 1998). The absolute requirement for taurine is unknown but it is added to formula milk at the levels found in human milk.

Aspartame is a sweetener composed of aspartic acid and phenylalanine. If maternal consumption of foods containing aspartame is increased, there is an increase in plasma levels of phenylalanine but levels in milk only increase marginally suggesting that the mammary gland regulates the transfer of amino acids into the milk.

Non-protein nitrogen

More than 25% of the nitrogen found in human milk comes from sources other than protein. This is the non-protein nitrogen (NPN) fraction (Box 16.5). Methods for protein determination usually rely on measuring the total nitrogen in a foodstuff and calculating the average amount of protein that would contain that much nitrogen. Therefore, the protein content of human milk was overestimated before it was clear how large the proportion of NPN was. Each mammalian species has a characteristic amount and profile of NPN, which is of nutritional significance. The NPN of human milk includes a variety of compounds such as peptides and free amino acids (such as those that are conditionally essential), nucleotides, traces of inorganic compounds, urea, creatinine, N-acetyl sugars and glycosylated amines. Some of the NPN compounds are of developmental importance

---

Box 16.5

Non-protein nitrogen (NPN)

The protein content of human milk was initially overestimated because it was based on the assumption that the nitrogen fractions within the milk would all be components of protein. In fact, about 25% of the nitrogen-containing components in the milk are not within proteins. This is high compared with other species; for instance, cow's milk contains only 5% of the total nitrogen as NPN.

NPN includes:

Amino sugars	which promote the growth of *Lactobacillus bifidus* and are also incorporated into neural tissue and gut epithelial membrane
Taurine	a free amino acid that is a component of bile salts and therefore contributes to fat digestion
Peptides	these have roles as growth factors and hormones
Cysteine	a free amino acid that is conditionally essential in the infant because the conversion of methionine to cysteine is limited
Binding factors	these facilitate absorption of other nutrients
Urea Creatine Creatinine Uric acid	the role of these factors is not clear

---

but the biological significance of others is uncertain. Urea is high in early milk, reflecting high plasma levels due to uterine involution (see Ch. 14).

Fat

Fat is the main source of energy in the milk. The nutritional status of the mother can affect the fat concentration of the milk and therefore the energy content, fatty acid composition and immunological properties. Of all the macronutrients in milk, fat is the most variable component; it is influenced by the maternal diet, parity, the season of the year and amount of milk removed at the last and current feed, the length of the time between feeds and the fat content of the last feed (Mitoulas et al 2002). The sampling method used to measure fat is important as hindmilk has 3–5 times the fat content of foremilk. Averaging foremilk and hindmilk is unlikely to produce a good estimate of the overall composition. The fat content of milk is lowest in the early morning (about 6 a.m.) and then rises to a peak mid-morning (about 10 a.m.) before falling during the day (Hytten 1995). There is also a progressive decline in the average fat content with increasing maternal age but with much individual variability. The diurnal rhythm of milk composition is related to GH secretion. The fatty acid pattern is variable, reflecting maternal energy intake and dietary fat consumption. It is possible to discriminate between the milk of vegetarian and non-vegetarian mothers (Sanders, Ellis & Dickerson 1978). If maternal energy and fat intake fall, the fat composition of the milk resembles maternal adipose fat composition as fat stores are mobilized. If the maternal diet is high in energy but low in fat, milk triglycerides are higher in medium-length fatty acids (lauric acid, C_{12}, and myristic acid, C_{14}) indicating synthesis of fatty acids from carbohydrates is increased (Lawrence, 1999). Women of high parity (greater than 10) may have decreased capacity for milk synthesis and therefore produce milk of lower fat (and energy) level.

As fat concentration affects the energy content of the milk, these variations in fat content make it particularly difficult to arrive at the average energy content of human milk. Previous overestimation of energy levels in breast milk resulted in formula milk providing too high an energy level which may have led to overfeeding and potential obesity problems of previous generations.

Ninety per cent of fat is present as triacylglycerides. The remaining 10% is made up of free fatty acids, phospholipids, cholesterol, diglycerides and monoglycerides, glycolipids and sterol esters. Fat provides the vehicle for fat-soluble vitamins and essential fatty acids required for brain development. Phospholipids are critical components of cell membranes and are a component of surfactant. The fatty acid composition of human milk is very different to that of cow's milk. Human milk has more essential fatty acids (linoleic and α-linolenic acids), has a higher proportion of unsaturated fatty acids and is rich in long-chain fatty acids. Cow's milk has more short-chain fatty acids (C_4–C_8) and a higher content of saturated fatty acids. The products of lipase digestion are predominantly 2-monoglycerides and free fatty acids, which can be absorbed. Most of the triacylglycerides in human milk have palmitic acid (16:0) or oleic acid (18:0) at position 2 of the molecule. Bovine triacylglycerides usually have palmitic acid at position 1 or 3 so digestion of cow's milk fat can release free palmitic acid, which is precipitated by calcium as soap. This can result in the loss of absorption of both fat and calcium.

Human milk and vegetable oil fats are better absorbed than is the saturated fat of cow's milk. Long-chain fatty acids require bile salt micelle formation and lipase activity. Short- and medium-chain fatty acids can be absorbed intact.

Human milk has a high content of cholesterol, which is required for myelin synthesis (important for the CNS development). The cholesterol content of breast milk is not affected by maternal diet. There may be a connection between cholesterol exposure early in life and the development of enzymes for cholesterol degradation and amounts of endogenous cholesterol synthesized (Bayley et al 1998), which results in lower cholesterol levels in individuals who were breastfed as infants.

As lactation progresses, triacylglyceride levels increase and cholesterol levels fall but phospholipid content remains stable. Usually, 20% of the milk in a feed remains in the breast; this contains about half of the fat. This effect may be due to absorption of fat globules on the surface of the alveolar cells in the secretory and ductal surfaces of the breast. It has been observed that babies suck in longer bursts and decrease the rest intervals when they are feeding on hindmilk (Woolridge & Fisher 1988).

Essential fatty acids

Essential fatty acids (see Ch. 12) (Table 16.2) are required for cell proliferation, retinal development and myelinization of the CNS. The LC-PUFAs docosahexaenoic acid (DHA) and arachidonic acid (AA) are essential constituents of cell membranes, particularly of the nervous system, occurring at notably

Table 16.2 *Long-chain polyunsaturated fatty acids*

	Omega-6 (*n-6*) family	Omega-3 (*n-3*) family
Predominant source	Vegetable oils	Marine oils
Essential fatty acid	Linoleic	α-Linolenic
Converted to	Arachidonic acid	Docosahexaenoic acid

high concentrations in the brain and retina. The neonate has a limited ability to desaturate and elongate fatty acid chains thus limiting the conversion of linoleic acid into AA and α-linolenic acid into DHA, so these PUFAs may be conditionally essential in the neonatal diet. Infants acquire PUFAs prenatally via the placenta and postnatally in milk. Human milk is particularly rich in DHA which is suggested to be associated with the raised IQ levels and better visual perception of breastfed infants (Lucas et al 1992). Maternal PUFA status, and therefore milk levels, vary with fish and omega-3 fatty acid intake but there is no evidence that supplementation of healthy women consuming good diets is beneficial.

LC-PUFAs are important for synaptogenesis in the visual system which is assessed by measuring visual acuity and speed of processing in infants. Breastfed infants appear to have a slight neurodevelopment advantage which is attributed to the high PUFA level of human milk. However, it should be noted that there are a number of selection biases, as women who choose to breastfeed tend to have higher IQ, educational level and socioeconomic status. Patterns of parent–child interactions may also be different.

The variation in milk fat probably reflects the variation in maternal diet (Sanders et al 1978). A low-fat maternal diet may maximize de novo synthesis of fatty acids for milk triacylglycerols but should contain adequate quantities of LC-PUFAs. As a species, humans have a uniquely large brain, which is composed of about 60% lipid. The essential dietary requirement for LC-PUFAs required for the development of the human cerebral cortex has some interesting evolutionary aspects. It has been proposed that the freshwater lakes of the Rift Valley in East Africa provided the optimal environment to promote development of *Homo sapiens* (Broadhurst, Cunnane & Crawford 1998). Freshwater fish and shellfish are particularly rich in LC-PUFAs and have an AA:DHA ratio similar to that of the human brain.

The importance of the long-chain fatty acid ratios may explain some of the observed benefits of breast milk such as the decreased incidence of multiple sclerosis (Pisacane et al 1994). Animal fats, including human milk, tend to be rich in omega-6 fatty acids (Crawford 1993). Formula milks are supplemented with fat derived from vegetable sources so tend to be far richer in linoleic acid than the omega-3 family of long-chain polyunsaturated fats. Several manufacturers of milk intended for preterm babies now supplement their formula milk with AA and DHA because

premature babies have a very limited capability in elongating and desaturating fatty acids.

Lipases

Human milk contains lipases, which are supplemented by unique production of neonatal lipases; these together compensate for limited pancreatic lipase activity. Lipoprotein lipase (serum-stimulated lipase) may appear in milk because of leakage from mammary tissue. Refrigerated and frozen milk undergo lipolysis. The enzyme responsible for this appears to have activity similar to that of pancreatic lipase; it is present in the fat fraction of the milk and is inhibited by bile salts. The most important lipase is the bile salt-stimulated lipase, which occurs in milk of humans and other primates. This enzyme, which is stable and active in the gut, has a significant effect on hydrolysis of milk triacylglycerides and is activated by concentrations of bile salts even lower than those required for micelle formation.

Lipase activity occurs in the saliva (and there may be additional gastric lipase activity). This lingual lipase is stimulated by the presence of milk in the mouth and by suckling, even non-nutritive suckling. Human milk fat digestion is 85–90% efficient compared with less than 70% efficiency of the fat digestion in cow's milk-derived formulas. Human milk fat globules are enclosed in maternal alveolar cell membranes, which aid in maintaining optimal surface area for emulsification and absorption and also protect the fat from lipolysis and oxidation. These factors mean that human milk stores well.

Carnitine

Human milk contains carnitine, which has an important role in facilitating the entry of long-chain fatty acids into mitochondria where they are oxidized. Carnitine is synthesized from the essential amino acids lysine and methionine, but neonates may have limited synthetic capacity. Carnitine also is involved in the initiation of ketogenesis and in the regulation of heat generation from brown adipose tissue. As infants use fat as a major source of energy and have limited ability to synthesize carnitine, they have an increased need for carnitine.

Carbohydrate

Lactose, which is unique to mammalian milk (and probably therefore important in the development of the mammalian order), is the principal carbohydrate of milk, present at about 7 g per 100 ml. The lactose concentration of mature human milk is thought to be related to the size of the adult brain. Levels of lactose are stable as lactose drives the volume of milk produced. There is no evidence that maternal nutrition affects lactose concentration. As well as lactose, there are also trace amounts (about 10%) of 130 other sugars, the most prevalent of which are glucose, galactose, glucosamine and other oligosaccharides (see below). Some of the non-lactose sugars may contribute to favourable gut colonization. Nitrogen-containing oligosaccharides, including the complex sugar L-fucose, promote the growth of *Lactobacillus bifidus* resulting in increased gut acidity, which suppresses the growth of pathogenic bacteria and may facilitate calcium absorption.

Lactose is a disaccharide that is digested by the enzyme lactase into its component monosaccharides, glucose and galactose. Lactase activity develops rapidly in late gestation and is adequate from 36 weeks; its activity cannot be prematurely induced by exposure. Most mammals and many humans do not produce lactase after infancy. The ability to produce lactase throughout life seems to be related to continual exposure to lactose in communities that have a strong economic dependence on dairy farming.

Lactose is relatively insoluble and is slowly digested and absorbed in the small intestine. It promotes the growth of microorganisms that produce organic acids and synthesize many B vitamins. The acidic environment is inhospitable to many pathogenic bacteria. Lactose forms soluble salts so the absorption of calcium, phosphorus, magnesium and other metals is increased in the presence of lactose.

Clinical application: nutritional problems of preterm infants

Human milk is nutritionally inadequate for preterm infants, leading to poor growth rates and osteopenia. However, it does have clear advantages. It has valuable immunological properties, protecting against necrotizing enterocolitis. It is associated with improved cognition and it stimulates gut maturity. The ideal food for a preterm infant able to tolerate lactose is the baby's own mother's milk fortified with additional calories, protein and minerals. Babies requiring parenteral feeding benefit from receiving some milk in the gut. One of the problems of tube feeding is the loss of energy, as the fat tends to stick to the tubes. If the mother has a good supply of milk, fractionating the milk and feeding the baby the fat-rich hindmilk can increase the energy content. Skin-to-skin contact has also been found to be important for premature babies and it helps to stimulate the mother's lactational capabilities. It also increases the maternal IgA in the milk, which is specific to the nocosomial flora of the hospital environs.

In preterm babies, with low lactase activity, a large proportion of lactose reaches the large intestine in an undigested form. Here it is metabolized by colonic bacteria to produce organic acids, hydrogen and carbon dioxide. The organic acids are absorbed across the intestinal mucosa and a proportion of the energy is recovered. This means that preterm babies are able to utilize a large proportion of the energy contributed from lactose. The extent of colonic salvage can be determined by measuring the amount of hydrogen in the baby's breath and can be severely compromised by antibiotics or surgery disrupting the colonic flora. It is suggested that over-accumulation of organic acids in the lower gut may be a factor in the initiation of necrotizing enterocolitis (Lucas & Cole 1990) (Box 16.6).

Although the evolution of mammalian species has obviously depended on the unique properties of lactose, intolerance to lactose may occur. Although galactose is directly involved in the synthesis of glycoproteins and glycolipids of the CNS, it is not essential in the diet. Galactose can be synthesized from glucose in the liver so glucose can substitute for lactose in a lactose-free diet. Alternatively, lactase can be added directly to bottles or milk or milk can be fermented prior to ingestion.

Box 16.6

Necrotizing enterocolitis

- Seen predominantly in premature infants
- Associated with infection, hypertonic feeds, hypovolaemia and perinatal asphyxia
- Most prominent in jejunum, ileum and colon
- Clinical signs usually appear at 3–10 days old
- Symptoms may include abdominal distension, blood in stools, vomiting, lethargy, respiratory distress and poor thermoregulation
- Human milk fed enterally is protective, possibly by stimulating gut maturity and integrity, providing substrates for enzymes and increasing perfusion

Table 16.3 compares the composition of human colostrum, mature human milk and cow's milk.

Starch

Starch digestion in young babies is possible. Infant saliva contains some amylase activity but levels rapidly increase from 3 to 6 months. Pancreatic amylase activity is minimal in the first 3 months and remains low until about 6 months. Mammary amylase in human milk has a high activity in colostrum, which is retained for about 6 weeks. Intestinal mucosa has both disaccharidases and glucoamylase, which hydrolyses oligosaccharides and disaccharides. Glucoamylase is a brush-border enzyme that can hydrolyse glucose polymers in formula milk. Formula feeds derived from cow's milk often contain maltodextrin, a polymer of maltose and glucose. This has the advantages of being easily digested and increasing the viscosity and mineral

Table 16.3	Comparison of human colostrum, human milk and cow's milk			
	Colostrum	**Mature human milk (100 ml)**	**Cow's milk (100 ml)**	**Comments**
Energy Water		70 (kcal)	66 (kcal)	Colostrum is produced in small but easier to digest amounts—produced during first 3 days of life; neonate may feed frequently as metabolic process adapts from the constant feed environment of the uterus to an extrauterine fast/feed cycle
Protein	Immunoglobulins account for increased protein content	1.3 g (mostly whey); lactalbumin; immunoglobulins; lactoferrin; lysozyme; enzymes; hormones	3.5 g (high casein content)	Colostrum rich in passive immunity factors to provide initial protection to infant; cow's milk harder to digest owing to increased casein, also contains lactoglobulin not found in breast milk (may be responsible for cow's milk allergy); protein ratios differ owing to the calf having a faster growth trajectory than the human infant
Lactose	Less lactose	7.0 g provides 37% of energy requirement	4.9 g	Breast milk tastes sweeter than cow's milk
Fat	Less fat	4.2 g (98% triglycerides) provides approx. 50% of energy requirements	3.7 g	All mammalian milks are rich in fats owing to the high-yielding energy from fat metabolism
Sodium Potassium Chloride Calcium Phosphorus		15 mg 60 mg 43 mg 35 mg 15 mg	22 mg 35 mg 29 mg 117 mg 92 mg	Higher concentrations of organic ions in cow's milk; the neonatal kidney may be unable to regulate higher ion concentrations owing to immaturity
Magnesium		2.8 mg		
Vit A	Increased level	60 μm	less	
Vit D		0.01 μm		
Vit E	Increased level	0.35 μm		
Vit K	Increased level	0.21 μm	6 μm	

Continued

Table 16.3   *Comparison of human colostrum, human milk and cow's milk—Cont'd*

Colostrum	Mature human milk (100 ml)	Cow's milk (100 ml)	Comments
Thiamin	16 μm	44	
Riboflavin	30 μm	175 μm	
Nicotinic acid	230 μm		
B_{12}	0.01 μm	0.4 μm	
B_6	6 μm		
Folates	5.2 μm	5.5 μm	
Pantothenic acid	260 μm		
Biotin	3.8 μm		
Vit C	3.8 mg	1.1 mg	
Iron	76 μm	5 mg	Breast milk has low levels of iron; however, it is absorbed approx. 20 times more efficiently than iron supplements
Copper	76 μm		
Zinc	295 μm		
Iodine	7 μm		

content of the formula. Babies are born with relatively high levels of glucoamylase activity, which further increases after birth. Glucoamylase is less susceptible to being affected by intestinal mucosal damage and is distributed along the length of the small intestine, which increases the efficiency of hydrolysis and uptake of its products.

There is evidence that the ability to digest starch can be induced if starch is present in the diet. Adaptation is not quick and may take days to weeks. Undigested starch causes gastrointestinal disturbances, such as diarrhoea, interfering with the absorption of other nutrients, so affected infants may exhibit symptoms of failure to thrive. Hypoxia and ischaemia result in decreased intestinal perfusion, which alters the structure of the epithelial cells affecting uptake of monosaccharides.

Oligosaccharides

Milk contains about 130 different oligosaccharides. Human milk seems to have a particular diverse profile of oligosaccharides, which vary genetically and with the duration of lactation and the time of day. The role of oligosaccharides in milk is protective. They are not absorbed and appear to act as substrates for beneficial bacteria and to bind pathogens competitively thus mopping them up (McVeagh & Miller 1997). Oligosaccharides thus promote a particular bacterial flora in the gut of breastfed babies, which results in a characteristic pH and may protect against urinary infections. The oligosaccharide sialic acid occurs in high concentrations in breast milk. It is found in high concentrations in the brain and is associated with brain development and increased learning behaviour in animals (Tram et al 1997).

Vitamins

A plentiful supply of breast milk from a well-nourished woman contains all the vitamins required by a term neonate, with the possible exceptions of vitamins

D and K. Dietary taboos practised during lactation in some cultures may affect the vitamin content of breast milk. As fat is the most variable constituent of the milk, the level of fat-soluble vitamins is relatively unstable. There is a seasonal variation in the vitamin A content of cow's milk. Water-soluble vitamins in breast milk fluctuate with maternal intake as they move readily from maternal serum to milk. Human milk has a high level of vitamin C; there may be a seasonal variation in vitamin C content and both infant and maternal requirements for vitamin C increase with stress (including lactation). B vitamin levels in milk are acutely affected by maternal diet. Vitamin B_{12}, which is found in animal protein, is likely to be deficient in the milk from strict vegetarian or vegan women who should take vitamin B_{12} supplements during pregnancy and lactation. Transfer of folate from maternal plasma into milk occurs against a steep concentration gradient so the nursing infant is well protected against maternal folate deficiency. However, maternal folate reserves may be depleted during lactation which would have important consequences for the mother and her own folate status, especially if the interpregnancy interval is short.

Vitamin D

Breastfed babies rarely develop rickets although the level of vitamin D in breast milk is low. The vitamin D content of foods is measured by assessing the vitamin D content of the fat fraction. However, breast milk may contain an aqueous vitamin D sulphate, which is not included in the fat fraction, so the vitamin D content of breast milk may be underestimated. Neonates have stores of all fat-soluble vitamins, including vitamin D, and they are able to synthesize vitamin D on exposure to sunlight from an early age. Vitamin D-deficient milk is associated with low exposure to sun, long winters, Northern climes, use of sun screen, dark skins and cultural practices such as covering the skin. Increased levels of pollution may also affect vitamin D synthesis in the skin. Certain ethnic groups, such as Rastafarians in the UK, have an increased risk of vitamin D deficiency.

Vitamin E

Vitamin E, mostly in the form of α-tocopherol, is an antioxidant. Deficiency compromises the integrity of the red blood cell membrane and can lead to microhaemorrhages if severe. In formula feeds, the α-tocopherol:polyunsaturated fat ratio is held constant (1 IU vitamin E per gram of linoleic acid).

Vitamin K

Vitamin K deficiency is associated with haemorrhagic disease of the newborn (see Ch. 15) and is usually due to low stores of vitamin K rather than low levels in the milk. There is a critical need for vitamin K during birth and in the first days of life when the risk of bleeding, particularly intracranially, is high. Vitamin K is not efficiently transferred across the placenta. The major source of vitamin K in postnatal life is from the by-products of bacterial metabolism, but the baby is born with a sterile gut, and gut colonization capable of producing vitamin K is not adequate until the baby is at least 6 weeks old as lactobacilli do not synthesis menaquinones. Concentrations of vitamin K are higher in colostrum and early milk, particularly the hindmilk as the vitamin is fat-soluble. Breast milk stimulates colonization of the gut by vitamin K-producing bacteria. A prophylactic dose of vitamin K is routinely given at birth to protect against haemorrhagic disease of the newborn.

Vitamin A

Vitamin A requirement is increased if stores are inadequate or there are problems with fat absorption. A deficiency of vitamin A in infancy is associated with bronchopulmonary dysplasia. This may result from a low intake or increased requirement for the vitamin in healing the damaged lung epithelium. Breastfeeding women are advised to select plenty of vegetables and fruit rich in provitamin A.

Minerals

The mineral content of milk is slightly affected by maternal diet but milk provides all the major minerals and trace elements required by the normal term infant. Usually the mother's dietary deficiency or excess intake of mineral does not affect the composition of her milk very much as maternal homeostasis protects the infant against fluctuations of most minerals in the maternal diet. Parenteral feeding of infants, rather than frank deficiencies, has elicited most information about mineral requirements. Deficiencies are usually associated with short gestation or severe placental insufficiency.

The concentration of most minerals remains generally low but the bioavailability is high. Human milk has a number of binding proteins, notably for iron, calcium and zinc. The absorption of iron from human milk is particularly efficient, aided by the lactoferrin and transferrin content of milk and its low pH. The binding of iron is bacteriostatic.

The sodium content of human milk is inversely related to the volume of milk produced so it is higher initially and at weaning. Cow's milk has four times the sodium content of human milk. Hypernatraemia, caused for instance by hot weather, mild infection or over-concentrated formula reconstitution, can result in dehydration.

Calcium absorption is affected by vitamin D, calcium and phosphorus concentrations, fatty acids and lactose. It is particularly enhanced by the acid environment and low phosphorus content of human milk. The calcium:phosphorus ratio of human milk is 2:4 (compared with 1:3 in cow's milk). If phosphorus levels are high, there is increased phosphorus absorption at the expense of calcium absorption as they compete for the same mechanism of transfer across the gut wall. The resulting fall in plasma calcium concentration can cause hypocalcaemia with symptoms of jitteriness, tetany and convulsions.

Milk-borne trophic factors

As well as nutritive and immunological factors, human milk contains a group of biologically active factors that affect nutritional status and somatic growth. These factors can be classified into four groups: hormones and peptide growth factors, nucleotides and nucleosides, polyamines and digestive enzymes. The hormone group includes insulin, GH, insulin-like growth factors (IGF-I and IGF-II), somatostatin, EGF, prolactin, erythropoietin and GH-releasing factor. Some of these hormones and growth factors are absorbed across the permeable neonatal gut into the body where they affect metabolism and promote growth and differentiation of organs and tissues. Other hormones, such as somatostatin, appear not to be absorbed but resist proteolysis, having an effect directly on the wall of the gut. They may protect gastrointestinal cells and therefore reduce the risk of necrotizing enterocolitis.

Both human and bovine colostrum are rich in nucleotides, which are precursors of nucleic acids. Nucleotides appear to have a role in enhancing growth and differentiation. They are particularly involved in liver cell function, lipid metabolism and lipoprotein synthesis. They also affect the development of the gut-associated lymphoid tissue (GALT). Unlike cow's milk, mature human milk maintains high levels of nucleotides. Up to a fifth of the breastfed neonate's requirement for nucleotides is derived from milk. Dietary nucleotides may facilitate iron absorption and promote development of the immune response.

The polyamines spermine and spermidine are present in all cells but human milk has about 10 times as much polyamine content as cow's milk. Levels of polyamines are particularly high in the first days of lactation. They may have mitogenic, metabolic and immunological effects promoting gut development of the newborn. Enzymes include amylase, lipase and proteases which aid digestion.

Case study 16.2 is an example of concerns about newborn nutrition.

Special considerations

Breast milk can vary in taste and colour and can affect the infant's digestive system. Some components of the mother's diet such as artichokes, asparagus, peppers, legumes, brassica (vegetables from the cabbage family) and alliums (vegetables from the onion family) may occasionally result in a reaction from the infant though the evidence that maternal diet is the cause of infant colic is inconsistent. The taste and flavour of breastmilk can be altered by components of maternal

---

Case study 16.2

Isla is 11 days old and has just regained her birth weight. She has been breastfed since birth and appears to be very healthy and alert. Julia, her mother, contacts the midwife because she is concerned about Isla who is sleeping 12 hours at night and feeds only four times a day. Julia's elder sister also gave birth recently and her 21-day-old baby feeds every 2 hours, day and night, and has been progressively gaining weight. Julia's sister reported that her midwife told her that this is how a newborn baby normally behaves and advises Julia to stop breastfeeding because her baby is not growing properly.

- How can the midwife reassure Julia that Isla is well, feeding normally and gaining adequate nutrition?
- What concerns, if any, would you have for Julia's niece or how would you reassure Julia that all was normal?
- Why do some babies have different patterns of feeding and weight gain?

diet such as garlic (Mennella et al 2001). When the breastfeeding mother consumes garlic, the infant consumes more milk. These early flavour and odour experiences may programme later food preferences including those at weaning. Rarely, breastmilk colour has been reported to be affected by excessive maternal consumption of food colouring (usually in soft and sports drinks) and drug therapy (Lawrence 1999).

It has been suggested that susceptible infants might be exposed to environmental allergens and dietary antigens via their mother's breast milk. In some cases, where there is a history of allergy, mothers may be advised to avoid potential allergens whilst breastfeeding such as nuts, eggs, cow's milk, berries and tropical foods. However, responses vary widely and foods should not be eliminated without medical supervision.

Caffeine passes into breast milk as does alcohol. With all substances including caffeine, nicotine, alcohol and drugs, the levels are reduced in the milk if maternal consumption is timed immediately after a feed with the longest possible time before the next feed.

Breastfeeding women are encouraged to exercise, time providing. Exercise increases blood lactic acid levels and there may be some transfer of lactic acid into breast milk. Human milk is sweet and lactic acid has a sour bitter taste which may result in infants displaying puckering facial expressions and even rejecting milk if they are offered it close to exercise. However, not all infants are sensitive to the taste of lactic acid and discarding the first few millilitres of milk by manual expression often remedies the situation (Lawrence 1999). Physical activity and energy intake must be balanced.

Immunological properties of human milk

Neonates are particularly susceptible to infection (see Ch. 15). Milk has an important non-nutritive protective role. Human milk discourages bacterial growth whereas cow's milk promotes bacterial growth in the upper small bowel, which is optimal for ruminants (Jackson & Golden 1978). Breastfed infants have fewer infections (Box 16.7), but some of this effect may be due to a decreased exposure to other foods bearing microorganisms (Golding et al 1997). The protective properties of milk are also important in protecting the breasts themselves from infection. Many cultures use breast milk topically, for instance to

---

Box 16.7

Advantages of breastfeeding

- Optimal infant nutrition
- Convenience, cost and lack of contamination
- Reduced risk of mortality from necrotizing enterocolitis and sudden infant death syndrome
- Reduced infection: gastrointestinal, respiratory, urinary tract, ear, meningitis, intractable diarrhoea
- Reduced atopic disease and allergy: eczema, asthma
- Increased intelligence
- Reduced overweight and obesity in childhood and adulthood
- Reduced risk of autoimmune disease
- Enhanced immunity
- Reduced risk of maternal cancer: breast, ovarian
- Increased maternal oxytocin levels: promote expulsion of placenta, minimize postpartum blood loss, facilitate rapid uterine involution (see Ch. 14)

---

treat eye infections. Immunological properties of human milk are increased with better maternal nutrition (Chang 1990).

Immunoglobulins

The immunoglobulins (antibodies) in milk are distinct from those found in maternal serum. The major immunoglobulin is secretory IgA which is produced from plasma cells in the breast; milk also contains minor amounts of monomeric IgA, IgG and IgM. Secretory IgA is at very high concentrations in the colostrum but declines to lower levels by day 14 as milk volume increases. The mother will produce specific immunoglobulins to every pathogen she encounters. The transfer of IgA into the milk is a form of passive immunity (see Ch. 10), augmenting the placental transfer of IgG to the fetus. The baby's own immune system is further stimulated by factors in the milk. Breastfed babies have superior responses to vaccination programmes and have higher IgA in their saliva, nasal secretions and urine (Prentice 1987, Prentice et al 1987).

IgA is stable at low pH and resistant to proteolytic enzymes so it survives in the gastrointestinal tract. IgA has an important role in the defence against infection, slowing bacterial and viral invasion of the mucosa. It adheres to the gastric mucosa and prevents adhesion of microorganisms. IgA promotes closure of the gut and so decreases its permeability to allergens such as cow's milk β-lactoglobulin and serum bovine albumin.

Binding proteins

Lactoferrin is an iron-binding protein that facilitates the absorption of iron from milk. In binding iron, it reduces the amount of free iron available for microorganisms in the gut, thus inhibiting the growth of certain pathogenic bacteria. It is suggested that lactoferrin in breast milk helps to reduce the incidence of gastrointestinal tract infections. Excess free iron is associated with increased bacterial pathogens in the gut. These bacteria have a high iron requirement and can cause gut damage and microhaemorrhages, which themselves can lead to iron-deficiency anaemia.

Other protective properties

Breast milk contains high levels of lysozyme, which is protective against Gram-positive bacteria and viruses. Breast milk contains prebiotic substances, called bifidogenic factors, which together with lactose stimulate the growth of lactobacilli thus promoting an acidic and protective environment. Fibronectin, which is present in high concentrations in human milk, is a non-specific opsonin (see Ch. 10) that increases phagocytosis of bacteria. Milk also contains other protective factors (Table 16.4).

Milk is not sterile but contains about 4×10^9 cells per litre including lymphocytes from maternal Peyer's patches and scavenger macrophages and neutrophils. Levels of cells are particularly high in the colostrum. Proteins and mucins of the milk lipid globule membrane itself may also confer immunological advantages (Keenan 2001). Other factors in human milk with anti-infective or immunological properties include anti-proteases, which inhibit the breakdown of anti-infective immunoglobulins and enzymes, free fatty acids which have antiviral properties and cytokines which stimulate an inflammatory response from the immune cells.

Formula feeding

Human milk substitutes existed before the modern age of infant formulas. There were two approaches, either using a surrogate mother or wet nurse, or feeding milk from another mammal. In Western countries, where dairy farming is established, cow's milk is modified and processed into the formula feeds, which are the basis of bottle feeding. Human children in other cultures are reared on buffalo, goat, horse, camel and yak milk. Mammalian milks may be quantitatively similar but the quality is variable, being species-specific.

Cow's milk is supplemented with carbohydrate, either lactose or maltodextrin, which dilutes the higher mineral and protein content. Cow's milk fat (which has a high commercial value as butter and cream) is substituted with vegetable oil-fat blends. This increases the absorption efficiency; unabsorbed fat decreases the energy content, lowers calcium absorption and produces steatorrhoea.

For whey-dominant formulas, demineralized whey (which is expensive) is blended with skimmed milk to increase the whey:casein ratio and decrease the electrolyte content. The profit margin of whey-dominant formulas is lower than that of casein-dominant formulas. Casein-dominant formulas are marketed for the 'hungrier baby' and, although the energy content is constant, are considered to be a progressive step in feeding. Mothers often demonstrate a strong brand loyalty when choosing formula milk.

Soy-based formulas were originally designed for infants intolerant of cow's milk protein. The early problems of loose malodorous stools, nappy rash and stained clothing associated with soy milk have been remedied by the use of isolated soy protein rather than soy flour.

Trace minerals and vitamins are added in line with legal limits. Taurine is added to formula milk and, more recently, nucleotides have been added; they probably act as growth factors and may have immune effects. Packaging of formula feed is important. Anaerobic storage and copper supplementation help to reduce fatty acid oxidation. Scoop and granule size are carefully designed to optimize precision in reconstitution.

Breastfed infants grow at a slightly slower rate and have a different body composition than formula-fed infants. They consume less milk (about 85% of that consumed by formula-fed infants) and have lower energy expenditure. Breastfed infants have a lower risk for later obesity and possibly insulin resistance, obesity and type II diabetes mellitus. Gastric emptying is faster and there is less gastro-oesophageal reflux and loss of intake in breastfed infants. They also have less infectious disease (see below) and a lower rate of necrotizing colitis.

Table 16.4 *Protective factors in milk*

Factor	Function
Cells B lymphocytes T lymphocytes Macrophages Neutrophils	Produce antibodies against specific microbes Kill infected cells Produce lysozyme and activate parts of the immune system Phagocytose bacteria
Lacto bifidus factor	Promotes an acidic environment favourable for the growth of *Lactobacillus bifidus* and inhibits the growth of pathogenic microorganisms
Immunoglobulins (antibodies IgA, IgG, IgM, IgD and IgE)	Active against specific organisms, i.e. poliomyelitis, salmonella
Immunoglobulin A (IgA)	Lines the gut to discourage adhesion of pathogenic microorganisms and limits allergen entry
Lactoferrin	Decreases iron available by binding to iron for bacterial growth Acts as a bacteriostatic agent
Lysozymes Lactoperioxidase Complement	Act in a non-specific way by damaging the cell walls of microorganisms
Lipids	Inhibit growth of staphylococcus and viruses by disrupting cell membranes
Fibronectin	Promotes macrophage activity and aids repair to damaged gut tissue
γ-Interferon	Promotes activity of immune cells
Mucins	Adhere to microorganisms inhibiting attachment to the gut wall
Oligosaccharides	Inhibit attachment of microorganisms to mucosal surfaces
Bile salt-stimulated lipase	Acts as an antiprotozoal
Bile salt-stimulated lipase Lipoprotein lipase, α-amylase	Promote fat and protein digestion
α_1-Antitrypsin α_1-Antichymotrypsin	Prevent breakdown of protective factors
Epidermal growth factor	Promotes maturation of the gut wall
Binding proteins B_{12}-binding protein Lactoferrin Transferrin Folate-binding protein Somatomedin C	Increase absorption of nutrients and limit availability of nutrients utilized by bacteria

Weaning

Weaning can be defined as the progressive transition from milk to a normal family diet. Before 4 months, it is considered unnecessary, being associated with increased incidence of diarrhoea and interference with the maintenance of breastfeeding (the nutritional value of the complement is usually lower than that of breast milk). An increase in dietary cereals and vegetables tends to affect the absorption of iron, which can be delicately balanced in younger infants. By 6 months, many babies will require complementary feeding and will have sufficiently developed to cope with it. Deciduous teeth erupt at about 6 months. Incisors, which cut food, are the first teeth to appear, followed by molars at about 12 months, which allow grinding of food.

Determination of the appropriate time to introduce foods other than milk is not just by age but should also take into consideration the food available, conditions to prepare it, the growth velocity and the neuromuscular development of the infant. It is not clear which pattern of growth is optimal. Growth charts are based on weight and height data from clinical surveillance. Ethnicity and both environmental and genetic factors affect growth. Practically, the high weight velocity, which is seen in the first 3 months of life, is not related to overfeeding. The deceleration of growth after 3 months is not in itself an indicator to wean. Early weaning is associated with an increased number of respiratory symptoms (Forsyth et al 1993).

By 6 months, normal physiological development can support the introduction of alternative foods. The baby is able to hold its head erect and can control the movement of its hands to mouth. The tongue extrusion reflex is waning and can be overcome. Indeed, it is suggested that there is a critical window for introducing solid food and if it is not done within this window the baby tends to develop a preference for liquid feeds and may become a child with feeding problems. The kidneys are mature enough to cope with a solute load.

Although the health benefits of breastfeeding are not disputed, opinions and recommendations are divided on the optimal duration of exclusive breastfeeding. In March 2001, the World Health Organization convened an expert consultation committee to systematically review the evidence and make recommendations about the optimal duration of exclusive breastfeeding. The committee called for exclusive breastfeeding of infants until 6 months old and continued breastfeeding with appropriate complementary feeding until 2 years old. Despite this, many authorities argue that there is a lack of clear evidence to either support or refute recommendations for the age of introduction of complementary foods to the breastfed or formula-fed infant to be between 4 and 6 months. Although exclusive breastfeeding for the first 6 months of life can support growth and development in some infants, subgroups have been identified within certain populations who may require complementary feeding prior to this age, particularly larger, and often male, infants (Lanigan et al 2001). To be confident that exclusive breastfeeding does not increase the risk of undernutrition (growth faltering) in healthy term infants, it may be necessary to make recommendations per infant weight rather than infant size.

Weaning is an important biological and social learning process as well as offering foods of higher nutrient and energy density than milk. Exposing different tastes to children has already begun in milk feeding. Compounds ingested by the mother are transported into the milk (Mennella 1995). This may present an important learning experience not received by bottle-fed babies.

Key points

- The physiological unit of the mammary gland is the alveolus. Prolactin, from the anterior pituitary, stimulates milk production from the alveolar cells. Oxytocin, from the posterior pituitary, stimulates contraction of the myoepithelial cells lining the alveoli and the ducts, resulting in milk ejection or 'let-down'.

- Prolactin secretion slowly reaches a peak following stimulation at the nipple. Secretion is pulsatile and circadian and is controlled by the abrogation of tonic inhibition from dopamine produced by the hypothalamus. Prolactin inhibits ovulation thus suppressing fertility.

- Oxytocin release is stimulated by nipple stimulation and by thinking about or hearing the baby. Secretion of oxytocin immediately follows stimulation and can be inhibited by stress.

- The effects of prolactin are locally controlled by the production of FIL (feedback inhibitor of lactation) in the milk. Increased concentrations of FIL suppress the response to prolactin thus inhibiting milk production. This is important in mammary gland involution when breastfeeding is curtailed.

- Lactating women appear to have increased efficiency of energy utilization. The nutritional composition of the milk is not affected greatly by maternal diet unless the mother is extremely undernourished; however, concerns have been expressed about effects on maternal calcium balance and the tendency to develop obesity. Breastfeeding is associated with a reduced risk of maternal breast and ovarian cancer.

- Human milk provides optimal nutrition for the human neonate, which has immature renal, hepatic and gastrointestinal functions and a rapidly developing nervous system. Breastfed babies have a lower incidence of infection.

- Colostrum is the early secretion from the breast; it provides important anti-infective properties and promotes favourable colonization of the gut.

- Protein requirements are relatively low as the human neonate has a relatively slow growth rate. Human milk has a high concentration of whey proteins and non-protein nitrogen components, which include growth factors. The amino acid composition of human milk protein compensates for the neonate's limited ability to convert essential amino acids to non-essential amino acids; the net protein utilization of human milk is high.

- Fat is the main energy source in milk and the most variable constituent. The proportion of fat is higher in hindmilk. The fatty acid composition of human milk allows optimum absorption. Human milk fat is rich in polyunsaturated fatty acids required for development of the brain and nervous system.

- Lactose is the major carbohydrate of milk; it provides energy, aids absorption of other nutrients and promotes an environment favourable to beneficial microorganisms.

- Human milk has important immunological properties and is associated with a lower incidence of infections and a persistently more responsive immune system in breastfed babies.

Application to practice

It is consistently shown that breastfeeding is influential in the reduction of many disease states and thus should be encouraged. The midwife is uniquely placed to influence the overall health of the nation.

Knowledge of lactation and its benefits are important if the midwife is to promote breastfeeding in practice.

. . . .

Annotated further reading

Black RF, Jarman L, Simpson JB 1998 The science of breastfeeding. Jones & Bartlett, Toronto
Module 3 of the Lactation Specialist Self-Study series which is based on the competencies published by the International Lactation Consultant Association. This volume covers anatomy and physiology in relation to lactation and infant feeding, nutritive and non-nutritive components of human milk, maternal nutritional requirements and practical considerations.

Fomon S 2001 Infant feeding in the 20th century: formula and beikost. Journal of Nutrition 131(2):409S–420S
A history of changing infant feeding practices in the 20th century, including the effects of sanitation, dairying practices and milk handling on home- and commercially prepared formulas.

Howard BA, Gusterson BA 2000 Human breast development. Journal of Mammary Gland Biology and Neoplasia 5:119–137
A comprehensive well-illustrated review of physiological states of the human breast including prenatal, prepubertal and pubertal development, adult resting state, pregnancy, lactation and postinvolution.

Lawrence RA 1999 Breastfeeding: a guide for the medical profession, 5th edn. Mosby, St Louis
An excellent textbook of evidence-based clinical information covering all aspects of breastfeeding, anatomical, physiological, biochemical, nutritional, immunological and psychological aspects of human lactation, as well as the problems of clinical management of breastfeeding including drugs in human breast milk, breastfeeding and infectious disease, induced lactation and relactation, feeding infants with problems and milk expression and storage.

Lonnerdal B 2003 Nutritional and physiologic significance of human milk proteins. American Journal of Clinical Nutrition 77(6):1537S–1543S
A review of the proteins that contribute to the unique qualities of human milk, including those that assist in the digestion and utilization of nutrients and those with antimicrobial, prebiotic and immunomodulatory properties

Palmer G 1993 The politics of breastfeeding. Pandora, London
Discusses social, historical and economic factors affecting a woman's decision to breastfeed and the implications of the type of infant feeding method on health, the environment and the global economy.

Prentice A 2000 Calcium in pregnancy and lactation. Annual Reviews of Nutrition 20:249–272
An in-depth review of the calcium requirements in pregnancy and lactation and how these are met by physiological adaptation, including altered bone metabolism.

Riordan J, Auerbach KG 1999 Breast feeding and human lactation, 3rd edn. Jones & Bartlett, London
A comprehensive text on breastfeeding aimed at midwives, breastfeeding consultants, antenatal teachers, dietitians and nutritionists. Covers cultural aspects, anatomy and physiology, breastfeeding education and practical considerations such as breast pumps, donor milk and breastfeeding the ill child.

Rogers IS 1997 Relactation. Early Human Development 49:S75–S81
This article discusses the possibility of re-establishing lactation in certain situations and includes information on promoting lactation in women who have never been pregnant.

Shennan DB, Peaker M 2000 Transport of milk constituents by the mammary gland. Physiological Reviews 80(3):925–951
A thorough review of the cellular mechanisms that transport milk constituents into, out of and across the mammary secretory cell.

Weaver LT, Prentice A 2003 Nutrition in infancy. In: Morgan JB, Dickerson JWT (eds) Nutrition in early life. Wiley, Chichester, pp 205–232
A comprehensive review of the mammary gland and lactation, the composition of human milk in relation to infant nutrition requirements and alternatives to human milk.

References

Adlercreutz H 1995 Phytoestrogens – epidemiology and a possible role in cancer protection. Environmental Health Perspectives 103:103–112

Amir LH, Donath SM 2003 Does maternal smoking have a negative physiological effect on breastfeeding? The epidemiological evidence. Breastfeeding Review 11(2):19–29

Bayley TM, Alasmi M, Thorkelson T et al 1998 Influence of formula versus breast milk on cholesterol synthesis rates in four-month-old infants. Pediatric Research 44:60–67

Ben-Jonathan N, Laudon M, Garris PA 1991 Novel aspects of posterior pituitary function: regulation of prolactin secretion. Frontiers in Neuroendocrinology 12:231–277

Britton H 1993 Mother–infant interaction: relationship to early infant nutrition and feeding. In: Suskind R M, Lewinter-Suskind L (eds) Textbook of pediatric nutrition. Raven Press, New York, pp 43–48

Broadhurst CL, Cunnane SC, Crawford MA 1998 Rift Valley lake fish and shellfish provided brain-specific nutrition for early *Homo*. British Journal of Nutrition 79:3–21

Chang S-J 1990 Antimicrobial proteins of maternal and cord sera and human milk in relation to maternal nutritional status. American Journal of Clinical Nutrition 51:183–187

Chesney RW, Helms RA, Christensen M, Budreau AM, Han X, Sturman JA 1998 The role of taurine in infant nutrition. Advances in Experimental Medicine and Biology 442:463–476

Crawford MA 1993 The role of essential fatty acids in neural development: implications for perinatal nutrition. American Journal of Clinical Nutrition 57(Suppl): S703–S710

Dewar CS, Psych MR 2004 Enhanced nutrition of offspring as a crucial factor for the evolution of intelligence on land. Medical Hypotheses 62(5):802–807

Dewey KG 1997 Energy and protein requirements during lactation. Annual Review of Nutrition 17:19–36

Dewey KG 2003 Is breastfeeding protective against child obesity? Journal of Human Lactation 19(1):9–18

Domellöf M, Lönnerdal B, Dewey KG, Cohen RJ, Hernell O 2004 Iron, zinc and copper concentrations in breast milk are independent of maternal mineral status. American Journal of Clinical Nutrition 79:111–115

Ebrahim GJ 1990 The scientific contribution of breast feeding research. Maternal Child Health March:92–93

Emmett PM, Rogers IS 1997 Properties of human milk and their relationship with maternal nutrition. Early Human Development 49:S7–S28

Forsyth JS, Ogston SA, Clark A, Florey C du V, Howie PW 1993 Relationship between early introduction of solid food to infants and their weight and illnesses during the first two years of life. British Medical Journal 306:1572–1576

Golding J 1997 Unnatural constituents of breast milk: medication, lifestyle, pollutants, viruses. Early Human Development 49:S29–S43

Golding J, Emmett PM, Rogers IS 1997 Does breast feeding have any impact on non-infectious, non-allergic disorders? Early Human Development 49:S131–S142

Grattan DR 2002 Behavioural significance of prolactin signalling in the central nervous system during pregnancy and lactation. Reproduction 123(4):497–506

Hammond KA 1997 Adaptation of the maternal intestine during lactation. Journal of Mammary Gland Biology and Neoplasia. 2:243–252

Hartmann PE, Sherriff JL, Kent J 1995 Maternal nutrition and the regulation of milk synthesis. Proceedings of the Nutrition Society 54:379–389

Hartmann PE, Sherriff JL, Mitoulas LR 1998 Homeostatic mechanisms that regulate lactation during energetic stress. Journal of Nutrition 128:394S–399S

Howie PW, McNeilly AS, McArdle T, Smart L, Houston M 1980 The relationship between suckling-induced prolactin response and lactogenesis. Journal of Clinical Endocrinology and Metabolism 50:670–673

Hytten F 1995 The clinical physiology of the puerperium. Farrand Press

Illingworth PJ, Jung RT, Howie PW, Leslie P, Isles TE 1986 Diminution in energy expenditure during lactation. British Medical Journal 292:437–442

Institute of Medicine 2002 Dietary reference values for energy, carbohydrates, fiber, fat, protein and amino acids (macronutrients). IOM Standing Committee on the Scientific Evaluation of Dietary Reference Intakes, Food and Nutrition. National Academy of Sciences, Washington DC

Jackson AA, Golden MHN 1978 The human rumen. Lancet 1978:764–767

Johnston JM, Amico JA 1986 A prospective longitudinal study of the release of oxytocin and prolactin in response to infant suckling in long term lactation. Journal of Clinical Endocrinology and Metabolism 62:653–657

Karjalainen J, Martin JM, Knip M et al 1992 A bovine albumin peptide as a possible trigger of insulin-dependent diabetes mellitus. New England Journal of Medicine 327:302–307

Keenan TW 2001 Milk lipid globules and their surrounding membrane: a brief history and perspectives for future research. Journal of Mammary Gland Biology and Neoplasia 6(3):365–371

Koppe JG 1995 Nutrition and breast-feeding. European Journal of Obstetrics, Gynecology and Reproductive Biology 61:73–78

Lanigan JA, Bishop J, Kimber AC, Morgan J 2001 Systematic review concerning the age of introduction of complementary foods to the healthy full-term infant. European Journal of Clinical Nutrition 55(5):309–320

Lawrence RA 1999 Diet and dietary supplements for the mother and infant. In: Breastfeeding: a guide for the medical profession, 5th edn. Mosby, St Louis, pp 297–333

Lonnerdal B 1985 Dietary factors affecting trace element bioavailability from human milk, cow's milk and infant formulae. Progress in Food and Nutrition Science 9:36–62

Lucas A, Cole TJ 1990 Breast milk and neonatal necrotising enterocolitis. Lancet 336:1519–1523

Lucas A, Ewing G, Roberts SB, Coward WA 1987 How much energy does the breast fed infant consume and expend? British Medical Journal 295:75–77

Lucas A, Morley R, Cole TJ, Lister G, Leeson-Payne C 1992 Breast milk and subsequent intelligence quotient in children born preterm. Lancet 339:261–264

McManaman JL, Neville MC 2003 Mammary physiology and milk secretion. Advanced Drug Reviews 55:629–641

McNeilly AS, Robinson ICAF, Houston MJ, Howie PW 1983 Release of oxytocin and prolactin in response to suckling. British Medical Journal 286:257–259

McNeilly AS 2001 Lactational control of reproduction. Reproduction, Fertility and Development 13(7–8):583–590

McVeagh P, Miller JB 1997 Human milk oligosaccharides: only the breast. Journal of Paediatrics and Child Health 33:281–286

Mennella JA 1995 Mother's milk: a medium for early flavor experiences. Journal of Human Lactation 11:39–45

Mennella JA, Beauchamp GK 1991 The transfer of alcohol to human milk: effects on flavor and the infant's behavior. New England Journal of Medicine 325:981–985

Mennella JA, Jagnow CP, Beauchamp GK 2001 Prenatal and postnatal flavor learning by human infants. Pediatrics 107(6): E88

Mitoulas LR, Kent JC, Cox DB, Owens RA, Sherriff JL, Hartmann PE 2002 Variation in fat, lactose and protein in human milk over 24 h and throughout the first year of lactation. British Journal of Nutrition 88:29–37

Monte CS, Johnston CS, Roll LE 1994 Bovine serum albumin detected in infant formula is a possible trigger for insulin dependence diabetes mellitus. Journal of the American Dietetic Association 94:314–316

Neville MC, Morton J 2001 Physiology and endocrine changes underlying human lactogenesis II. Journal of Nutrition 131:3005S–3008S

Neville MC, McFadden TB, Forsyth I 2002 Hormonal regulation of mammary differentiation and milk secretion. Journal of Mammary Gland Biology and Neoplasia 7:49–66

Ohlin A, Rossner S 1996 Factors related to body weight changes during and after pregnancy: the Stockholm pregnancy and weight development study. Obesity Research 4:271–276

Peaker M 1989 Evolutionary strategies in lactation: nutritional implications. Proceedings of the Nutrition Society 48:53–57

Pisacane A, Impagliazzo N, Russo M et al 1994 Breast feeding and multiple sclerosis. British Medical Journal 308:1411–1412

Pond C (ed) 1992 Reproductive physiology. Open University, Milton Keynes, pp 197, 200

Porter TE, Grandy D, Bunzow J, Wiles CD, Civelli O, Frawley LS 1994 Evidence that stimulatory dopamine receptors may be involved in the regulation of prolactin secretion. Endocrinology 134:1263–1268

Prentice A 1987 Breast feeding increases concentration of IgA in infants' urine. Archives of Disease in Childhood 62:792–795

Prentice A 2000 Calcium in pregnancy and lactation Annual Review of Nutrition 20:249–272

Prentice AM, Prentice A 1995 Evolutionary and environmental influences on human lactation. Proceedings of the Nutrition Society 54:391–400

Prentice A, Ewing G, Roberts SB et al 1987 The nutritional role of breast-milk IgA and lactoferrin. Acta Paediatrica Scandinavica 76:592–598

Ramsay DT, Kent JC, Hartmann RL, Hartmann PE 2005 Anatomy of the lactating human breast redefined with ultrasound imaging. Journal of Anatomy 206:525–534

Rasmussen KM, Hilson JA, Kjolhede CL 2001 Obesity may impair lactogenesis II. Journal of Nutrition 131(11):3009S–3011S

Rogan WJ, Gladen BC, McKinney JD et al 1987 Polychlorinated biphenyls (PCBs) and dichlorodiphenyl dichloroethane (DDE) in human milk: effects on growth, morbidity and duration of lactation. American Journal of Public Health 77:1294–1297

Rogers IS 1997 Lactation and fertility. Early Human Development 49(Suppl):S185–S190

Sanders TAB, Ellis FR, Dickerson JWT 1978 Studies of vegans: the fatty acid composition of plasma choline-phosphoglycerides, erythrocytes, adipose tissue, breastmilk and some indicators of susceptibility to ischemic heart disease in vegans and omnivore controls. American Journal of Clinical Nutrition 31:805–813

Sowers M 1996 Pregnancy and lactation as risk factors for subsequent bone loss and osteoporosis. Journal of Bone and Mineral Research 11:1052–1060

Tram TH, Miller JCB, McNeil Y, McVeagh P 1997 Sialic acid content of infant saliva: comparison of breast fed with formula fed infants. Archives of Disease in Childhood 77:315–318

Turgeon-O'Brien H, Lachapelle D, Gagnon PF, Larocque I, Mahen-Robert LF 1996 Nutritive and non-nutritive suckling habits. Journal of Dentistry for Children 63:321–327

Van de Perre P 1995 Postnatal transmission of human immunodeficiency virus type 1: the breast-feeding dilemma. American Journal of Obstetrics and Gynecology 173:483–487

Warner BB, Sapsford A 2004 Misappropriated human milk: fantasy, fear and fact regarding infectious risk. Newborn and Infant Nursing Reviews 4(1):56–61

Wharton BA, Balmer SE, Scott PH 1994 Faecal flora in the newborn: effect of lactoferrin and related nutrients. Advances in Experimental Medicine and Biology 357:91–98

Wilde CJ, Prentice A, Peaker M 1995 Breast-feeding: matching supply with demand in human lactation. Proceedings of the Nutrition Society 54:401–406

Williams GL, McVey WR, Hunter JF 1993 Mammary somatosensory pathways are not required for suckling-mediated inhibition of luteinizing hormone secretion and delay of ovulation in cows. Biology of Reproduction 49:1328–1337

Woolridge MW 1996 Breastfeeding: physiology into practice. In: Davies DP (ed) Nutrition in child health. RCOP, London, pp 13–31

Woolridge MW, Fisher C 1988 Colic, 'overfeeding', and symptoms of lactose malabsorption in the breast-fed baby: a possible artefact of feed management? Lancet ii:382–384

Wysolmerski JJ 2002 The evolutionary origins of maternal calcium and bone metabolism during lactation. Journal of Mammary Gland Biology and Neoplasia. 7:267

Glossary

Aerobic metabolism   The production of ATP requiring oxygen.

Aetiology   The cause of.

Afferent   Conducting or leading towards a target or centre.

Agonist   A substance that interacts with a receptor molecule that initiates the same response as the hormone/transmitter usually binding to that site.

Aliphatic   An organic compound that contains carbon atoms arranged in a chain rather than a ring formation.

Alkalosis   An increase above that within the normal pH range of the body.

Allograph   Implanted tissue that is of different genetic origin to the donor.

Alopecia   The loss of body and scalp hair.

Amoeboid   Appearing and behaving like the large single-celled organism called an amoeba.

Amplitude   The difference between the highest and lowest measurement within a regular cycle.

Anabolic metabolism   The synthesis of biological compounds involving the expenditure of energy.

Anaerobic metabolism   The production of ATP in the absence of oxygen.

Anastomose   The joining up of two tubes, vessels, etc., ensuring that the lumen remains patent between them.

Androsperm   A sperm carrying a Y chromosome.

Aneuploidy   Presence of an abnormal number of chromosomes.

Angiogenesis   The formation of new blood vessels.

Anisogamy   The existence of different forms of gametes related to sexual dimorphism.

Antagonist   A substance that blocks receptor sites and then inhibits any further responses.

Anteflexed   Curved inwards.

Anteverted   Folded over.

Antibody (immunoglobulin)   A 'Y'-shaped molecule that combines with an antigen (foreign protein) as part of the immune response, synthesized by white blood cells.

Antigen   A molecule that initiates the immune response found within foreign tissue.

Antral   A cavity within the body.

Apoptosis   The genetic programming resulting in the death of a cell.

Aquatic   Pertaining to an underwater environment.

Arborize   To grow in a branch-like formation.

Asynclitism   To be tilted laterally on either side of the anterior/posterior mid-plane.

Asphysia   The death of a cell through a lack of oxygen.

Atresia   The abnormal narrowing or closure of the lumen in a tube or vessel.

Atretic   Having the characteristics of or pertaining to atresia; without an opening.

Atrophy   Decreased functioning due to hypoplasia with increasing age.

Attenuated   Modified to have less of an effect than normal.

Bactericidal   Containing substances that can kill bacteria.

Bacteriostatic   Containing substances that inhibit the reproduction of bacteria.

Basal metabolic rate   The amount of energy expenditure required for the maintenance of essential body function only.

Behaviour   The study of how organisms interact within the environment.

Biosynthesis   The manufacture of body tissues and substances.

Breech   Pertaining to the fetal rump.

Carotenoid   Naturally occurring fat-soluble pigment that colours plants red, yellow, orange or brown.

Catabolic metabolism   The breakdown of compounds requiring the expenditure of energy.

Cephalic   Pertaining to the fetal head.

Chemoattractant   A substance that acts as an attractant.

Chemostasis   The maintenance of a chemical balance.

Chorioamnionitis   Infection of the chorion and amnion during pregnancy.

Circadian   About one day.

Clonal expansion   The ability of white blood cells to duplicate rapidly as part of the immune response.

Cloning   Reproduction of an organism identical to an organism from which non-gamete genetic material is obtained.

Co-dominant   Expression of both of two differing alleles in the phenotype when present in the genotype.

Coitus   The act of sexual intercourse.

Colloid   A protein suspended in a liquid.

Contraception Prevention of pregnancy by intervention.

Cortex The outer tissue layer or part of a structure.

Cranial Pertaining to the skull.

Cyanosis The bluish appearance of body tissues in situations of hypoxia.

Cyclical Repeated on a regular basis.

Cytoplasm The intercellular tissue contained within the cell membrane.

Decidualization The formation of the decidua of pregnancy.

Deletion The loss of part of a chromosome.

Dermatome Area of skin supplied by a single spinal nerve; derived from segmental development during embryonic stage.

Desquamation The loss of the outer layers of a continuously growing squamous tissue.

Detumescence The resolution of the inflammatory response.

Diapedesis The passage of blood cells through the blood vessel wall into the surrounding tissue.

Diastolic The period of relaxation of the ventricles of the heart.

Dichrotic A notch observed on the downstroke of the arterial pressure waveform that indicates the closure of the aortic valve.

Differentiation The division of cells resulting in the daughter cells becoming different owing to the activation of particular genes.

Dimorphism The existence of an organism in distinct forms such as male and female.

Diploid The normal number of paired chromosomes.

Discoid Disc-like.

Dorsal Pertaining to the back.

Dysgenesis Abnormal formation.

Dyspnoea Difficulty in breathing.

Ectopic pregnancy Implantation occurs outside the uterine cavity, usually in a uterine tube.

Efferent Carrying away from a centre (e.g. a blood vessel or nerve).

Endocytosis The process by which substances are transported into the cell within envelopes formed out of the outer cell membrane.

Endogenous Pertaining to the internal physiological environment.

Entrained Reset by an external factor.

Enzyme A protein that is able to speed up a chemical reaction without being structurally altered by the process itself.

Epitopes A cluster of antigens that evoke an immune response.

Ergometrine A drug derived from alkaloids of ergot that causes a sustained, strong contraction of the myometrium.

Erythropoietin A hormone produced chiefly by the kidneys (in the adult) and by the liver (in the fetus) that initiates red blood cell production.

Eugenics The science aimed at producing the perfect individual.

Euploidic Contains the normal number of chromosomes.

Evolution The study of genetic variation and change within generations of populations.

Exogenous Pertaining to the external environment.

Extended Tilted away from.

Flexed Tilted towards.

Follicle Tissue structure that is fluid-filled.

Free radical An oxygen molecule containing an unpaired electron.

Gametogenesis The formation of gametes.

Gastrulation The formation of the inner layers of the embryo by cell migration in a process of invagination.

Gene manipulation The science of artificially adding or removing genes to effect a change within an individual.

Gene pool The total number of genes within a population.

Genome The total number of genes within a single organism.

Gluconeogenesis The synthesis of glucose from non-carbohydrate sources.

Glycolytic The breakdown of glucose.

Graft rejection The rejection of donor tissue by the recipient's immune system.

Grey matter of brain Unmyelinated axons, nuclei and dendrites in the brain.

Gynosperm A sperm carrying an X chromosome.

Haemoptysis The presence of blood in sputum.

Half-life The time taken for the reduction by half of the quantity present.

Haploid Half of the normal chromosomal number (containing only one chromosome from the normal paired chromosomes).

Hermaphrodism The presence of male and female sex organs within the same individual.

Heterozygous Alleles at a particular locus of paired chromosomes each coding for a different phenotype.

Hirsutism The presence of excess body hair.

Homeothermic A warm-blooded animal (sometimes referred to as endothermic).

Homozygous   Alleles at a particular locus of paired chromosomes both coding for the same phenotype.

Hydrolytic   Dissolving in water.

Hyperaemia   An excessive quantity of blood.

Hyper/hypoglycaemia   Abnormally high/low level of glucose within the blood.

Hyperprolactinaemia   Abnormally raised levels of the hormone prolactin.

Hyperventilation   Overbreathing resulting in alkalosis.

Imprinting   A behaviour pattern initiated by specific stimulation of a neural pathway that cannot be further influenced once it has occurred.

Incompatible   Not tolerated and so initiating the immune response.

Inherent   Having a genetic basis, hereditary, innate.

Innate   Present from birth, congenital, e.g. a behaviour pattern that is not learnt but instinctive.

Invaginate   To fold inwards to form a pouch.

Inversion   The translocation of a portion of a chromosome comprising an upside-down switch.

Ischaemia   The death of tissues due to a reduction or loss of the blood supply.

Keratinized   Containing the protein keratin.

Ketotic   Detectable amounts of ketone bodies present indicating that metabolism of fats is occurring.

Lipolysis   The release of fatty acids from the breakdown of adipose tissue.

Lipophilic   Having an affinity for fat.

Luteolysis   The degradation of the corpus luteum.

Macromolecules   Large organic compounds.

Macrosomic   Larger than normal body size.

Maturation   The achievement of full function following a period of growth and/or development.

Medulla   The central tissue layer or part of a structure.

Menarche   The commencement of the menstrual cycles.

Menopause   The cessation of the menstrual cycles.

Menses   The period of shedding of the endometrium during the menstrual cycle.

Mentum   Pertaining to the fetal chin.

Methylation   The addition of a methyl group ($-CH_3$) to a compound.

Micturition   The voiding of urine.

Mitogen   A substance that initiates the process of mitosis.

Morphogenesis   The formation of body structure.

Morphology   The development of form and size.

Necrotic   The bacterial decomposition of dead tissue.

Neuronal   Pertaining to the nervous system.

Neurotransmitter   A chemical that crosses a synaptic gap to initiate an action potential in the receiving neuron.

Neurulation   The embryonic formation of the neural tube from the neural plate.

Nidation   The process of implantation of the blastocyst into the uterine endometrium.

Nocturia   The need to void urine frequently at night.

Nomenclature   Terminology describing systematic naming.

Occiput   A bone at the posterior lower part of the skull.

Oedema   Excess fluid in the extracellular compartments.

Opsonization   The process by which bacteria and other cells are made susceptible to phagocytosis.

Oxidative   The combination of oxygen with other molecules.

Pathogen   A foreign organism that causes harm.

Penile   Pertaining to the penis.

Perfusion   The blood flow.

Peristaltic   Coordinated contraction of smooth muscle around the lumen of a tube or vessel that facilitates the unidirectional movement of the contents within the lumen.

Phagocytic   The ingestion of foreign material by phagocytes.

Phosphorylation   The addition of an organic phosphate group to a molecule (often activating an enzyme).

Photoperiod   The period of natural daylight exposure.

Placebo   An inert/harmless substance that has no pharmacological effect, used in double-blind trials in comparison with drugs to assess their clinical effectiveness.

Placentation   The formation of the fetal and maternal components of the placenta.

Placentome   A lobe of the placenta.

Poikilothermic   A cold-blooded animal (sometimes referred to as exothermic).

Polycythaemic   An abnormally high number of red blood cells.

Polysperm   Fertilization by more than one sperm.

Postprandial   The period following the consumption of a meal.

Preantral   Before the antral phase.

Precursor   A substance that is altered into another substance.

Primordial   Existing from the beginning.

Proliferative The ability to increase quickly in numbers.

Prophylaxis Treatment aimed at prevention rather than cure.

Pseudopodia A temporary protrusion in the cell membrane.

Psychogenic The development of the mind.

Pulsatile Released episodically rather than continuously.

Pyrexia An abnormally high body temperature.

Rate-limiting A process that proceeds in relation to the amount of precursor available.

Receptor A molecule that combines with a chemical signal that initiates a response within the cell.

Reticulocyte An immature red blood cell.

Sacrum The bony vestigial remains of the prehensile tail that forms the posterior part of the pelvis.

Senescence Old age.

Septum (pl. septa) A structure that divides the body or body area/organ.

Sinciput Pertaining to the fetal forehead.

Sinusoids An irregularly shaped blood vessel.

Specific gravity The relative density of a fluid in relation to pure water.

Sphincter A ring of muscle that can occlude a tube or vessel when contracted.

Steroidogenesis The production of steroid hormones.

Stroma The structural framework of a cell or organ.

Syncytium A mass of cells in which the cellular membranes have broken down forming a continuous mass.

Syntocinon A synthetic analogue of naturally occurring oxytocin used in obstetrics as a pharmacological method of augmenting uterine contractions via a controlled intravenous infusion.

Tactile Pertaining to touch.

Teratogen A chemical that interferes with the formation of the embryo.

Thermostasis The maintenance of a constant body temperature.

Totipotent A cell that has the capability of dividing to form a complete new individual.

Transcription The process of synthesizing mRNA from a DNA template.

Translation The process of forming an amino acid chain from a coded sequence of mRNA bases.

Transudation Blood plasma that collects within the interstitial space.

Unicellular Made up of one cell.

Uterotonins Substances that encourage the myometrium to contract.

Vascularization The growth of blood vessels into tissue.

Vascularized Perfused with blood vessels.

Vasoactive Has an effect on vascular smooth muscle.

Vasoconstriction Contraction of smooth muscle within the blood vessels.

Vasodilation Relaxation of the smooth muscle within blood vessels.

Ventral Pertaining to the front.

Vestigial A physical characteristic (structure) in evolutionary decline, i.e. remaining present but no longer necessary for survival.

Villus (pl. villi) A finger-like projection from a membrane surface.

Volatile Evaporates at ambient temperatures.

White matter of brain Bundles of myelinated axons within the brain.

Zygote A totipotent cell formed from the fusion of two gametes.

Index

Numbers in *italic* refer to figures.